W.

Medicolegal Reporting in Orthopaedic Trauma

Third edition

Commissioning Editor: *Deborah Russell*
Project Development Manager: *Paul Fam*
Project Manager: *Scott Millar*
Designer: *Andy Chapman*
Illustrations Manager: *Mick Ruddy*

Medicolegal Reporting in Orthopaedic Trauma

Third edition

Edited by

Michael A Foy BM, FRCS
Consultant Orthopaedic Surgeon
Princess Margaret Hospital
Swindon
Wiltshire
United Kingdom

Phillip S Fagg MB, BS, FRCS
Consultant Orthopaedic Surgeon
Doncaster and Bassetlaw Hospital
Doncaster
South Yorkshire
United Kingdom

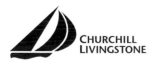

CHURCHILL LIVINGSTONE

Edinburgh • London • New York • Oxford • Philadelphia • St Louis • Sydney • Toronto 2002

Churchill Livingstone
An imprint of Elsevier Science Limited
© Harcourt Publishers Limited 2002
© Elsevier Science Limited 2003

First published 1990
Second edition 1996
Third edition 2002
Reprinted 2003

ISBN 0 443 06374 5

British Library Cataloguing in Publication Data
A catalogue record for this book is available from the British Library

Library of Congress Cataloging in Publication Data
A catalog record for this book is available from the Library of Congress

Note
Medical knowledge is constantly changing. As new information
becomes available, changes in treatment, procedures, equipment and
the use of drugs become necessary. The authors and the publishers
have taken care to ensure that the information given in this text is
accurate and up to date. However, readers are strongly advised to
confirm that the information, especially with regard to drug usage,
complies with the latest legislation and standards of practice.

your source for books,
journals and multimedia
in the health sciences
www.elsevierhealth.com

The
publisher's
policy is to use
**paper manufactured
from sustainable forests**

Printed in China

Contents

Contributors

Roger M Atkins
Consultant Orthopaedic Surgeon
Department of Orthopaedic
    Surgery
Bristol Royal Infirmary
Bristol
United Kingdom

Orla MB Austin
Specialist Registrar in Plastic
    Surgery
Dept of Plastic and Reconstructive
    Surgery
St James University Hospital
Leeds Teaching Hospitals
NHS Trust
Leeds
United Kingdom

Gordon Bannister
Consultant Orthopaedic Surgeon
Southmead Hospital
Bristol
United Kingdom

Rolfe Birch
Consultant Orthopaedic
    Surgeon
Peripheral Nerve Injury Unit
Royal National Orthopaedic
    Hospital
Stanmore
Middlesex
United Kingdom

Roger N Bloor
Senior Clinical Lecturer
University of Keele
Mental Health Directorate
Bucknall Hospital
Bucknall
Stoke-on-Trent
United Kingdom

Christopher J Briggs
Partner
Hempsons
Portland Tower
Manchester
United Kingdom

Andrew S Cole
Consultant Trauma and
    Orthopaedic Surgeon
Southampton University
    Hospitals
Southampton
United Kingdom

Jack Collin
Consultant Vascular Surgeon
Nuffield Department of Surgery
John Radcliffe Hospital
Oxford
United Kingdom

Tim RC Davis
Special Professor in Trauma and
    Orthopaedic Surgery and
    Consultant Hand Surgeon
University Hospital
Queens Medical Centre
Nottingham
United Kingdom

David K Evans
Emeritus Consultant Orthopaedic
    Surgeon
Derbyshire
United Kingdom

Phillip S Fagg
Consultant Orthopaedic Surgeon
Doncaster and Bassetlaw
Hospital
NHS Trust
Doncaster
United Kingdom

Jeremy CT Fairbank
Consultant Orthopaedic
    Surgeon
Nuffield Orthopaedic Centre
Oxford
United Kingdom

Michael A Foy
Consultant Orthopaedic Surgeon
Princess Margaret Hospital
Swindon
Wiltshire
United Kingdom

Grey EB Giddins
Consultant Orthopaedic and
    Hand Surgeon
Royal United Hospital and
Royal National Hospital for
    Rheumatic Diseases
Bath
United Kingdom

John Hutchinson
Consultant Spinal Surgeon
Frenchay Hospital
Bristol
United Kingdom

John P Ivory
Consultant Orthopaedic
    Surgeon
Princess Margaret Hospital
Swindon
Wiltshire
United Kingdom

Bryan Jennett
Professor Emeritus of
Neurosurgery
Institute of Neurological Sciences
Glasgow
Scotland

Contributors

Simon PJ Kay
Consultant Plastic, Reconstructive
and Hand Surgeon
Dept of Plastic and Reconstructive
Surgery
St James University Hospital
Leeds Teaching Hospitals
NHS Trust
Leeds
United Kingdom

M Bertie Leigh
Senior Partner
Hempsons
London
United Kingdom

Jeff Livingstone
Frenchay Hospital
Bristol
United Kingdom

Peter Lunn
Derby
United Kingdom

Colin McEwen
McEwen Solicitors
Swindon
Wiltshire
United Kingdom

Mike Rigby
Orthopaedic Registrar
The Royal United Hospital
Bath
United Kingdom

Guy Selmon
Orthopaedic Registrar
Guy's Hospital
London
United Kingdom

J Campbell Semple
Hand Surgeon
Harley Street
London
United Kingdom

John R Silver
Honorary Consultant in Spinal
Injuries
National Spinal Injuries Centre
Wendover
Buckinghamshire
United Kingdom

Gordon J Turnbull
Consultant Psychiatrist and
Honorary Senior Lecturer
Traumatic Stress Unit
The Priory Ticehurst House
Ticehurst
East Sussex
United Kingdom

Cynthia Watts
McEwens Solicitors
Swindon
Wiltshire
United Kingdom

G Philip Wilde
Consultant Trauma and
Orthopaedic Surgeon
Oxford Radcliffe NHS Trust
Oxford
United Kingdom

David J Wilson
Consultant Radiologist
Nuffield Orthopaedic Centre
NHS Trust
Oxford and John Radcliffe
Hospital
Oxford
United Kingdom

Preface

It is now over ten years since the first edition of this book was published. We believe that it filled a void that existed within the orthopaedic literature on the important subject of personal injury litigation, and the fact that we have been invited to prepare a third edition would suggest that we have come some way towards filling that void.

We are of course aware that a book of this nature cannot answer all the questions that the courts will wish answered. There is plenty of scope for learned orthopaedic discussion on causation and prognosis, but we hope that this book allows such debate to be carried out from an evidence-based starting point.

As always, we are grateful to our contributors and their families who have given up valuable time to provide their chapters.

Last and not least we are grateful to the staff of Harcourt Health Sciences for their help and advice along with their encouragement to meet deadlines!

PS Fagg
MA Foy
2001

Acknowledgements

The editors would like to thank Eileen Austin and Kate Ireland for invaluable secretarial help and James Simpkin for his tireless work as a research assistant. We would like to thank our contributors for the precious family time that was given up in the preparation of their chapters. As always, we would like to acknowledge the support of our wives, Judith and Denise, and apologise for the family time that was lost whilst the book was being prepared. Finally, we would like to thank the staff at Harcourt Health Sciences for their support during this project.

Section 1

Medicolegal practice

Chapter 1

The orthopaedic surgeon's viewpoint

Gordon Bannister

▇ Introduction

Medico-legal reporting is a very focused application of the clinician's normal work. The same history, examination and investigations are the basis but the emphasis is different. The clinician's principal role when consulting is to give patients an accurate diagnosis and discuss the relative risks and benefits of any interventions undertaken on their behalf. Inability to work resulting from the presenting illness is dealt with by a sickness certificate, or very occasionally referral to a social worker. The automatic assumption is that the patient is giving a truthful history and is solely interested in getting better.

The medico-legal consultation is different. There are fewer fractures and more back and neck injuries than in clinical trauma practice. The history from the Claimant may be unreliable. Physical signs are more likely to be influenced by psychological overlay and therapeutic interventions are often less effective. If a treatable condition can be identified, this should be regarded as a bonus rather than an expectation. The outcome of medico-legal consultation is usually financial compensation and the emphasis is on areas of disability that the law compensates.

English law recognises three forms of loss for which compensation may be awarded:

1. Losses of a non-monetary type, such as pain and suffering, interference with life-style or inability to obtain a job as enjoyable as anticipated (loss of congenial employment). Awards in this area are modest.
2. Monetary losses, such as
   (a) future loss of earnings
   (b) impairment of job prospects
   (c) need for future medical treatment or care
   Awards in this area have to be estimated and are potentially large.
   These are collectively known as **General Damages** (Table 1.1).
3. Losses that can be precisely calculated such as previous loss of earnings, damage to property and expenses incurred because of injury. These are known as **Special Damages**.

The greater the potential compensation, the more keenly a case will be contested.

The areas of contention in medico-legal reporting are whether the accident caused the presenting symptoms (Causation), whether the symptoms are as severe as the Claimant professes, whether the Claimant gives a reliable account of them (Reliability) and whether symptoms and signs are compatible with a recognised medical condition with a known prognosis (Medical expertise). The medico-legal report, therefore, concentrates on these areas and is important because Courts generally decide compensation once and for all at one hearing. They do not have the advantage of case review that is the norm in medical practice.

The medico-legal process

The Court dictates certain requirements of format which should be observed (Table 1.2).

The medico-legal process begins with an independent report and may progress to examination of covert video surveillance, supplementary correspondence on issues lawyers need clarifying, review of other medical experts' reports, conference with legal advisors and other experts, preparation of combined reports with other medical witnesses and, finally, giving evidence in Court. Most cases should not go through the entire process, only a single figure percentage finishing up in Court.

The medico-legal report

The basis for the medico-legal report is a history that details areas likely to attract compensation and addresses potential sources of contention.

A medico-legal (Appendix I) questionnaire that can be completed before attending is useful because it allows the Claimant time to consider the severity and effect of the symptoms experienced. The Claimant's background, occupational history, family support and domestic commitments should be recorded, along with home telephone number, so that matters arising can be checked. The family practitioner, physiotherapy and alternative practitioner records and relevant X-rays should be available, along with any statement of claim on which the Claimant will rely. The medical records are best obtained by the Claimant's solicitors who are initiating the action. These

Table 1.1 General damages in english Courts (from Judicial Studies Board Guidelines. Assessment of general damages in personal injury cases. Blackstone 5th ed.; Butterworths Personal Injury Litigation Services. Eds Ian Goldrein, Maragaret De Haaf. Butterworths)

Injury	Compensation (£)
Uncomplicated fractures of hand, wrist, scaphoid, forearm and humerus	3250–9500
Fractured tibia, ruptured knee ligaments, vertebral fractures	10 000
Whiplash depending on residual symptoms	2000–15 000
Os calcis fractures	20 000
Fractured femur or hip requiring hip replacement	20 000–26 000
Above-knee amputation one leg	47 500–70 000
Amputation arm at shoulder	70 000
Neurological effects of back injury, e.g. incontinence	50 000–85 000
Paraplegia	90 000–110 000

Table 1.2 Form and content of experts' reports

1.1 An expert's report should be addressed to the Court and not to the party from whom the expert has received his instructions.

1.2 An expert's report must:

  (1) give details of the expert's qualification,

  (2) give details of any literature or other material which the expert has relied on in making the report,

  (3) say who carried out any test or experiment which the expert has used for the report and whether or not the test or experiment has been carried out under the expert's supervision,

  (4) give the qualifications of the person who carried out any such test or experiment, and

  (5) where there is a range of opinion on the matters dealt with in the report

    (i) summarise the range of opinion, and

    (ii) give reasons for his own opinion,

  (6) contain a summary of the conclusions reached,

  (7) contain a statement that the expert understands his duty to the Court and has complied with that duty (rule 35.10(2)), and

  (8) contain a statement setting out the substance of all material instructions (whether written or oral). The statement should summarise the facts and instructions given to the expert which are material to the opinions expressed in the report or upon which those opinions are based (rule 35.10(3)).

1.3 An expert's report must be verified by a statement of truth as well as containing the statements required in paragraph 1.2(7) and (8) above.

1.4 The form of the statement of truth is as follows:

'I believe that the facts I have stated in this report are true and that the opinions I have expressed are correct'.

can be photocopied, filed in chronological order and used by all parties in the Courts. It is particularly important that all the family practitioner records are made available to assess the medical history of the Claimant before the incident under investigation.

At the onset it is sensible to advise the Claimant that the clinician's duty is to provide an independent medical report to the Court and that conclusions will not be influenced by the aims of the instructing party or by suggestions of opposing teams of lawyers.

Accident history

The history should record the date and mechanical nature of the accident. In industrial accidents, it is important to establish whether the trauma was of a type to which the Claimant was subjected to on a daily basis or whether it was unusually violent. In road traffic accidents, the Claimant will wish to emphasise the negligent driving of the other party and it is wisest for the clinician to pre-empt this by explaining that his expertise is medical and any opinion he may express on road traffic safety would have to be ignored by the Court. The onset of symptoms, attendance at Accident and Emergency Departments, family practitioners, physiotherapists or alternative practitioners should be recorded. Description of onset of symptoms some months after the accident makes causation questionable, severity of symptoms is useful for future comparison and a pain analogue score of 0 (no pain) to 10 (the worst pain imaginable) allows progress to be assessed and gives some indication of the Claimant's pain threshold. A claim of discomfort of 8–9 out of 10 for symptoms that do not merit analgesia suggests enhanced pain appreciation or exaggeration. Progress of symptoms, should be noted. Most skeletal trauma improves, then stabilises. Resolution of symptoms, followed by relapse months or years later, is recorded in the literature but is atypical. The time symptoms stabilise should be noted, along with any physical, alternative or psychological intervention that may have assisted and continues to be helpful.

Medical history (Tables 1.3 and 1.4)

Symptoms associated with the accident may have predated it, albeit in less severe form. The clinician should record the pain severity and functional restriction of these and the difference caused by the accident detailed.

Subsequent symptoms

The development of any subsequent disease that may affect function and the severity should also be recorded. This includes subsequent accidents or disorders of other parts of the locomotor system not injured at the time of the index event (e.g. backache) or other systems that may affect function (cardiovascular, respiratory or malignant diseases).

Present state

Next the clinician should record symptoms in order of intrusion, their severity, the factors that aggravate or improve them and the use of medication. Patients describing chronic severe pain often take no medication, stating that they do not like taking tablets and emphasising their stoicism. In clinical practice, patients with severe hip or back pain usually discontinue medication only because of recognised side effects.

Table 1.3 Inconsistent symptoms

1. Delay of onset of symptoms by weeks or months
2. Continuing deterioration after plateau
3. Resolution and later relapse
4. Reluctance to take analgesia
5. Unrealistic aspirations based on past performance
6. Poor sickness record and high job turnover in favoured occupation
7. Increased pain after medical examination
8. Disparity of activities on video surveillance

Table 1.4 Consistent symptoms

1. Unusual physical injury
2. Continuous history from time of accident
3. Documentation by doctors or therapists
4. Symptomatic improvement
5. Realistic pain assessment
6. Working despite discomfort

Functional state

There are usually a number of activities of which the Claimant is incapable. These should be recorded in detail, along with the reasons making the tasks impossible. It is particularly useful to identify difficulties in walking, shopping, driving, car maintenance, gardening and recreational activities, as these are activities generally covered in covert video surveillance.

Likewise, activities that of necessity are performed but cause pain should be noted. The Claimant who limps into the consulting room with a stick, reports inability to walk more than 50 yards without pain, yet is seen briskly progressing to his car after the interview, is giving an inconsistent account.

Psychological symptoms

Psychological sequelae are present in approximately 20% of trauma victims in clinical practice (Mayou et al 1993) and are under-perceived in fracture clinics because of training and constraints of time. In medico-legal practice, they appear more frequently and with greater severity. The orthopaedic surgeon is not a psychiatrist but can identify non-organic disease and should point this out, emphasising the limits of his expertise in making a precise diagnosis. The common presenting disorders are somatoform, post-traumatic stress disorder and reactive depression. These express as widespread pain, flashbacks and nightmares, emotional lability, and disturbance of concentration, memory, sleep pattern and libido. Driving anxiety is frequently reported.

Employment

The Claimant's work capacity, work record before and after the accident, educational achievements, present and past employment and potential for re-training must all be assessed by the clinician. It is the duty of Claimants to try to make the best of the changed circumstances brought about by the injury (mitigate their losses). The clinician's report should establish any restriction in work practice, its effect on earning capacity or likely promotion and the reasons given for this. Past performance in competitive examinations is a useful guide to future potential. The Claimant who has poor grades at GCSE, is attempting two applied subjects a 'A' Level, yet feels that a lucrative career in the professions has been denied him, is probably being unrealistic. Most candidates at 'A' Level achieve results 1–2 grades lower than their GCSE performance. Advice is, however, best obtained from the educational institution concerned. Claimants may report a particular dedication and high job satisfaction in a field of employment now denied them. Time regularly lost for minor ailments and frequent changes of occupation bear scant testimony to this.

If the Claimant is unlikely to work again, it is important to establish when he would normally have retired because this affects loss of future earnings. Orthopaedic surgeons are not occupational health physicians and indeed the normal retirement age for most occupations is not known. Police officers are a group that have traditionally taken early retirement on grounds of ill health and many building site workers move to more supervisory roles in the latter years of their career, as their locomotor system ceases to cope with heavy labouring demands. Restriction in domestic activities such as home renovation, gardening and housework necessitating help should be noted, as well as disturbance in recreational and personal activities.

Finally, in Claimants whose disability prevents even the most basic self-care, requiring wheelchairs, appliances and attendants, it is worth the clinician recording a typical day in their life to establish if there is potential at least to improve its quality, if not to return Claimants to gainful employment. Occupational therapists are often engaged to report on the needs of such Claimants and in practice inspect their living accommodation and detail functional history without examining their physical ability to carry out tasks. Clinicians called as experts are asked to comment on the recommendations of such a report and the above history helps to give a more balanced assessment of the claims made.

Examination (Table 1.5)

A pain map is useful in identifying sites of maximum pain and the organic nature of its distribution. Copious indications of a variety of pain types indicate distress (Fig. 1.1). Presence, or absence, of discomfort on a pain map completed early in protracted legal proceedings may be helpful in establishing the time of onset of symptoms as the claim progresses and time confounds the memory of the Claimant.

The examination needs to be as objective and reproducible as possible to be comparable with other reports. Walking disability, capacity to dress and undress, sites of tenderness, range of motion measured by goniometer, power of grip by dynamometer and neurological findings should all be noted, as indicated by the presenting condition. Potential muscle wasting should be measured at a defined site. Inspection reveals the state of the hands and attention to personal appearance. The claims of inability to carry out manual work are inconsistent with dirt-ingrained fingers with thickened skin.

Table 1.5 Inconsistent signs

1. Non-anatomical heavily marked pain map
2. Thickened and dirt-ingrained hands
3. Grooming in inaccessible locations
4. Immaculate appearance in depression
5. Overreaction to examination
6. Distracted movement
7. Global weakness and non-anatomical sensory deficit
8. Variation of physical signs in contemporaneous examinations

Please fill out the pain drawings.
This will tell us where your pain is NOW and something about it.
Using the appropriate symbols, mark the areas on your body
where you feel the pain.

Pins & Needles ooo Burning ✕✕✕ Aching +++ Stabbing /// Other •••

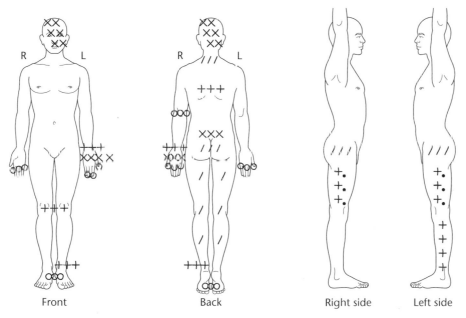

Front   Back   Right side   Left side

Fig. 1.1 Pain map of young lady with widespread pain, inability to self-care and a marked somatoform disorder following a low violence soft tissue injury.

The inability to flex the neck and back, or raise the upper limb, makes hair care, painting toenails or removal of body hair from inaccessible locations physically impossible. A description of extreme depression, restricted mobility and poverty is generally inconsistent with an immaculate personal appearance requiring hairdressers and beauty therapists.

Over-reaction by movement at a speed more likely to cause pain than the local pressure eliciting such a response is inconsistent with the presentation of pure organic disease, as is global weakness and regional sensory deficit. Non-organic signs may result from psychological distress or conscious exaggeration. The ageing orthopaedic surgeon who has long tolerated the musculoskeletal aches and pains that the litigant claims are ruining his life may find the litany of complaints, inconsistencies of evidence and absence of hard physical signs sufficiently irritating that he dismisses the claim as conscious malingering in search of a meal ticket for life. While understandable, this may be a medical oversight of psychological disease. In such circumstances, a validated objective test for psychological disease is useful and Goldberg's General Health Questionnaire is a widely used screen for this (Appendix 2). Finally, if there is a validated scoring system for the disability reported, it gives greater objectivity and comparative information for future and other reports.

Medical evidence

The hospital, family practitioner, occupational health, physiotherapy and alternative practitioner records give valuable evidence about pre-existing disease, the presentation of symptoms, the history and physical signs recorded at the time of the accident and their progress. However, such records will often be incomplete: Casualty Officers and family practitioners are constrained by time and orthopaedic expertise. They record and attend to the principal complaints and ensure that potentially life or limb threatening conditions are averted. Time constraints similarly apply to fracture clinic appointments. The omission to mention specifically an area of discomfort that proves ultimately to be the most troublesome to the patient is common. It is unsafe to assume that symptoms did not exist just because they are not recorded in the circumstances described above. Physiotherapists and chiropractors have specific skeletal training, often use pain maps and allocate 30 minutes to their initial consultation. Their training emphasises the global nature of musculoskeletal disorder and more reliance can be placed on omission of symptoms from their initial consultation. In fracture clinics the injury will be documented in hospital records until the surgeon feels he has nothing further to offer the patient, in the family practitioner notes until complaints cease or are overtaken by other ones and in the chiropractor's until both parties feel that further expense is not justified. Physiotherapists emphasise self-help and discharge with optimistic appraisals; chiropractors and osteopaths tend to advise regular maintenance therapy. Remission of symptoms, followed by relapse many months later, may suggest separate pathology and the degree of recovery usually depends on the recollection of the Claimant. It is, therefore, important that the clinician document entries in chronological order, indicating the nature of other conditions causing the Plaintiff to present in the interim and noting the reason for provision and duration of sick notes. Following the incident in question, there are often many entries in the family practitioner records for minor complaints for many months before the skeletal injury that forms the basis of the claim is noted. This is inconsistent with the normal presentation of trauma. The works occupational health record can indicate a change in attendance and the reason given for absence, just as family practitioner records document the change in rate of consultation. The medical history before the accident helps to establish the presence of symptoms but rarely their severity. An episode of backache years before the accident in a manual worker is less persuasive than increasing GP attendances and time off work before the index event. Time off work may be obtained from the occupational health and family practitioner records and if there has been a previous accident, the personal injury report before settlement is an invaluable account.

Prognosis and opinion

Having accumulated the evidence, the task now facing the clinician is to make a diagnosis, indicate whether any intervention can improve matters, and if not the future level of discomfort, disability and care requirements.

Precise diagnoses cannot be given for the vast majority of cases of back and neck pain, although the natural history is sufficiently well known to allow an accurate prognosis. In general, the longer symptoms persist the less likely they are to remit, and the longer the Claimant has been off work the less likely he is to return. If the Claimant cannot return to his original work, an estimation of potential for work is essential. Civil law requires a probability of more than 50%. Causation diagnoses and prognosis are a synthesis of consistent and inconsistent symptoms and signs. The relevant ones should be listed and a reasoned conclusion drawn. The burden of proof is on the Claimant. If the third party records are incomplete and place substantial reliance on the Claimant's uncorroborated account, its reliability must be assessed. If there are sufficient inconsistencies to doubt the account given, they should be recorded and the strength of the Claimant's case detailed. There should be little disagreement among experts about the consistency of symptoms with the medical literature (the medical literature relating to fractures is contained in this volume). Most debate among experts will relate to causation, the Claimant's reliability and the prognosis of neck, back and repetitive strain syndromes.

The instructing solicitors may ask for an estimate of aggravation or acceleration. If disease processes were completely understood and progression regular, such estimates would be possible. In fact, neither is the case and these assessments are almost entirely speculative. When reliance is placed on radiological changes in previously asymptomatic patients, they are little improved and any such assessment must be appropriately qualified. It is much wiser for the expert clinician to make this clear from the start than to have to admit it in cross-examination as a preliminary as to how much the rest of his opinion is poorly informed guesswork.

Supplementary correspondence

The expert's report, once prepared, will be read by the instructing solicitors and their clients, and if it contains any typographical errors or factual inaccuracies, these should be corrected immediately. Any change of evidence by the Claimant should be discussed by phone and justified before any changes to the report are made. If any changes are made, the report should be re-dated to the final draft. Alterations or selective omissions at the instructing solicitor's request were never good practice and under the 1998 Civil Procedure Rules (CPR) thoroughly discouraged (Table 1.2). Questions clarifying an expert's report may be put by either party, and a copy of those questions should be sent to the opposing party's solicitors. The solicitor posing the question is responsible for the fee.

Other experts' reports

A practice encouraged by 1998s CPR is a direction that experts communicate to produce a schedule of areas of agreement and disagreement at the direction of the Court.

If the report is presented by an expert's instructing solicitor for comment without such a direction, the latter may be anticipated and the exercise addressed accordingly. Ideally, the instructing solicitors should detail the points that need to be addressed but all too often the medical experts are left to their own devices. It is usually wisest for one expert to take on a comparison of the reports under the headings, history, examination and opinions. There will be disabilities recorded by one expert but not the other and there may be differences in physical findings. There may also be discrepancies in detail of history and completeness of examination. If the Claimant is a responsible person in law, states that one expert conducted an interview and examination in a matter of minutes without his being asked to undress and the details of the report are scanty, it is sensible to concentrate on common points, attributing the findings of the more detailed report to the expert who prepared it.

Differences of opinion will usually depend on the importance placed on the various consistencies and inconsistencies and depend on the Claimant's credibility. If the opposing expert's interpretation of the natural history of the presenting condition is at odds with the published literature, this should be pointed out with appropriate references. The formulation of such a response as areas of agreement and disagreement will pre-empt a precipitous request for a combined report from the Court.

Video evidence

In cases that attract high levels of compensation, the credibility of the Claimant will be tested by covert video surveillance by private detectives. These are usually retired police officers who sometimes provide enthusiastic commentaries of variable medical accuracy that should not influence the expert's opinion. Rather, the expert should read the Claimant's statement and all the medical records, note the restrictions described and the ranges of movement documented, arm himself with a video recorder with freeze-frame facility and assess the activity, discomfort and ranges of movement. Observer error using a goniometer is 10° and differences of 30° can be regarded as inconsistent. Video surveillance is often inconclusive but identifies gross changes and is valuable when conscious exaggeration is suspected.

Agreed reports

The aim of agreed reports is to focus the Court's attention on genuine areas of disagreement to save time at Trial. The Claimant's expert is usually instructed to make contact and a preliminary phone call to arrange discussions should be made as soon as possible after the Court direction. If one expert has evaluated the other's report, the letter should be faxed and can be used as a basis for the final document. The reasons for disagreement should be stated clearly, as these will form the basis of evidence should the case proceed to Court.

Conference with counsel

Conferences can be useful but the travel involved is time consuming and expensive. Phone conferences can be set up at a fraction of the cost and are equally effective. Under the CPR the Court will usually order that evidence be exchanged well in advance of the Court hearing. Conferences were previously used as an opportunity for experts to state their candid views rather than those in exchanged reports. However, this practice was never appropriate and is now even less so. Conferences are acceptable for clarification in complex cases but most of the time correspondence should be sufficient.

Court attendance

If an expert prepares medico-legal reports, he must accept that he will occasionally be called to Court. Court appearances are highly unsatisfactory. The Courts prefer medical evidence from experts in active clinical practice but issue a witness summons (formerly subpoena) for a window of time, often over a week, preventing the very practice on which clinicians' expertise depends. There is a shortage of Judges and the Court administration is designed to maximise the use of their time. Because many cases settle just before the hearing, more cases are booked than can be heard. Thus teams of lawyers and medical experts are found sitting outside courtrooms waiting their turn and often being dismissed half way through the day. The problem for experts is that there is also a shortage of orthopaedic surgeons, the time spent sitting outside a Court is time lost from patient care and this practice is an expensive waste of everybody's resource. It usually takes the medical expert 1–2 weeks to reinstate work, yet a huge number of cases still settle within days of hearings or on the steps of the Court. If the Judge has read the papers, is familiar with personal injury practice and proactive with the more loquacious barristers, it should be possible to hear medical evidence in a single agreed session, saving the orthopaedic surgeon's time and the Court's money.

The instructing solicitor is likely to compel the expert's attendance by service of a witness summons to avoid bearing costs if his absence holds up the case. Before Court, the expert should re-read his reports and correspondence so that he is thoroughly familiar with the arguments and, having arrived, wait to be called. He will have in front of him a paginated bundle of documents including his own reports and correspondence. He will be asked to swear on the Bible or comparable religious document. Then the barrister appointed by his instructing solicitor will ask him to tell the Court his name, qualifications and experience. His report will normally be served as his evidence in chief but he may then be asked to clarify one or two points of evidence before cross-examination commences. The barrister for the opposing side will attempt to persuade the expert to modify the views expressed in his report and correspondence. His qualifications, experience and reasoning will all be questioned in an attempt to find inconsistencies, question his credibility and devalue his views. It is important the clinician remains cool, refers to entries in his evidence to ensure they are being quoted in context, considers the questions and addresses his answers to the Judge. The Judge will make notes if the evidence is useful and should be given time to complete them. If necessary, the expert should repeat his answer to make the task easier. On conclusion of cross-examination, the barrister who opened will re-examine to clarify matters further and the expert will then be permitted to stand down. His barrister may ask him to remain to advise on any technical points raised by the opponent's expert. The clinician may not at this juncture produce fresh evidence in the form of published work but he may point out inconsistencies in the opposing expert's argument to the legal advisors instructing him. Normally, the Judge will give permission for medical experts to leave when their evidence is complete. This then concludes the clinician's involvement in the case.

Terms and conditions

A letter of instruction from solicitors normally concludes by agreeing to pay the clinician's 'reasonable fee'. What the instructing solicitor regards as reasonable may not concur with the expert's view and no assurance will be given as to when the fee will be settled. Personal injury lawyers face cash flow problems, have an ethic of paying their barristers long after cases are settled and prefer to do the same with their experts. Personal injury cases are funded by the private resources of the Claimant, trade unions, insurance companies or increasingly contingency. Under no circumstances should an expert undertake a report for which payment is contingent on the outcome of litigation. The British Orthopaedic Association and Law Society (Law Society 1985) recommend a contract and this should be signed by both parties before work commences (Appendix 3). A clause may be added stipulating the time within which the account is to be settled, or experts may decline to release the report until the fee is received. Cases vary in complexity and the fee scale should reflect this. Solicitors charge per unit of time and this is a method experts may choose. With the advent of 1998's CPR, experts spend more time on supplementary correspondence and preparing combined reports. Fee scales based on time are the fairest reflection of this. Occasionally a contract will be returned signed with the addendum 'subject to the assessment of costs'. The legal costs are usually borne by the losing side, subject to assessment by a cost Judge, who may reduce them. This process may take many months. The expert's contract is with the instructing solicitor, who is liable for fees regardless of assessment. The expert may prefer to decline instructions modified in this manner. The scale of fees is determined by local practice and the expert's skill and experience. The newly appointed consultant who overcharges will find he is not instructed again and is wise to take advice from both consultant colleagues and solicitors to ensure the fairest arrangement for all parties. Should disputes arise, the matter is best discussed with the instructing solicitor or a senior partner of the firm. Unlike barristers, medical experts can sue solicitors for unpaid fees and it is useful for a clinician to have a solicitor of his own for the most intransigent accounts. The solicitor will be much more familiar with the law of contract and will be able to advise the expert if there has been a breach of professional practice when firms fail to honour contracts, having made use of the expert's time. If a solicitor refuses to honour a signed contract after all other avenues have been pursued, the matter can be taken to a Small Claims Court. Small Claims Courts are likely to enforce a signed contract and deal with claims of up to £5000. The expert can arrange to be represented by his own solicitor but will not have the costs of this awarded.

Acknowledgement

The views expressed in this chapter are the author's own based on 20 years of medico-legal practice. The author is extremely grateful to District Judge Mike Daniel, who kindly read the chapter and gave advice on points of law.

■ References

Civil Court Service 1999 Section 3 P 1084–1086 Jordan Publishing Ltd

Mayou R, Bryant B, Duthie R 1993 Psychiatric consequences of road traffic accidents. British Medical Journal 307: 647–651

The Law Society 1995 Code of practice for medico-legal reports in personal injury cases

Medico-legal questionnaire

Background

Name: Date of Birth: Home Telephone No:

What is your job?

How long have you been working in this field?

What other jobs have you done?

How many days' sickness did you usually take before your accident?

Are you right or left handed?

Are you married?

How many dependent children do you have?

What sort of a house do you occupy?

Accident

Date of accident:

Where did it hurt immediately afterwards?

Did any other parts of your body hurt later?
If so when?

	Parts of body	Time pain started
1)		
2)		
3)		

Have you ever had pain in these parts of the body before the accident?

	Parts of body	Time pain started
1)		
2)		
3)		

Did you attend hospital?

If So which hospital?

Did you see your own doctor?

What treatment were you given?

Did your pain improve subsequently?

Are you: improving staying the same getting worse?

If your symptoms are not changing when did they reach their present state?

Present state

Where do you get pain? severity out of 10

0 = No Pain. 10 = Worst Pain Imaginable

Site

1)

2)

3)

4)

What medication do you take?

And how often?

Of which activities are you absolutely incapable?

1)	4)
2)	5)
3)	6)

Which activities cause you particular discomfort?

1)	4)
2)	5)
3)	6)

How has the injury affected your relationships or mental health?

Effect of injury on employment and recreation

Work

How long were you off work after the accident?

If you have returned to work in what ways are you restricted?

1)	2)

Does the injury affect your earning capacity?

Are you restricted in domestic activities?
If so which?

1)	3)	5)
2)	4)	6)

What are your favourite recreations?

Recreation	Frequency before accident	Frequency now
1)		
2)		
3)		
4)		
5)		
6)		

Appendix 2

The general health questionnaire GHQ 28

David Goldberg

Please read this carefully.

We should like to know if you have had any medical complaints and how your health has been in general, *over the past few weeks*. Please answer ALL the questions on the following pages simply by underlining the answer which you think most nearly applies to you. Remember that we want to know about present and recent complaints, not those that you had in the past.

Score 0 for the two left columns and 1 for the two right. Maximum possible score is 28. The upper limit of normal is 5.

It is important that you try to answer ALL the questions.

Thank you very much for your co-operation.

Have you recently

A1 – been feeling perfectly well and in good health?	Better than usual	Same as usual	Worse than usual	Much worse than usual
A2 – been feeling in need of a good tonic?	Not at all	No more than usual	Rather more than usual	Much more than usual
A3 – been feeling run down and out of sorts?	Not at all	No more than usual	Rather more than usual	Much more than usual
A4 – felt that you are ill?	Not at all	No more than usual	Rather more than usual	Much more than usual
A5 – been getting any pains in your head?	Not at all	No more than usual	Rather more than usual	Much more than usual
A6 – been getting a feeling of tightness or pressure in your head?	Not at all	No more than usual	Rather more than usual	Much more than usual
A7 – been having hot or cold spells?	Not at all	No more than usual	Rather more than usual	Much more than usual
B1 – lost much sleep over worry?	Not at all	No more than usual	Rather more than usual	Much more than usual
B2 – had difficulty in staying asleep once you are off?	Not at all	No more than usual	Rather more than usual	Much more than usual
B3 – felt constantly under strain?	Not at all	No more than usual	Rather more than usual	Much more than usual
B4 – been getting edgy and bad-tempered?	Not at all	No more than usual	Rather more than usual	Much more than usual
B5 – been getting scared or panicky for no good reason?	Not at all	No more than usual	Rather more than usual	Much more than usual
B6 – found everything getting on top of you?	Not at all	No more than usual	Rather more than usual	Much more than usual
B7 – been feeling nervous and strung-up all the time?	Not at all	No more than usual	Rather more than usual	Much more than usual

Have you recently

C1 – been managing to keep yourself busy and occupied?	More so than usual	Same as usual	Rather less than usual	Much less than usual
C2 – been taking longer over the things you do?	Quicker than usual	Same as usual	Longer than usual	Much longer than usual
C3 – felt on the whole you were doing things well?	Better than usual	About the same	Less well than usual	Much less well
C4 – been satisfied with the way you've carried out your task?	More satisfied	About same as usual	Less satisfied than usual	Much less satisfied
C5 – felt that you are playing a useful part in things?	More so than usual	Same as usual	Less useful than usual	Much less useful
C6 – felt capable of making decisions about things?	More so than usual	Same as usual	Less so than usual	Much less capable
C7 – been able to enjoy your normal day-to-day activities?	More so than usual	Same as usual	Less so than usual	Much less than usual
D1 – been thinking of yourself as a worthless person?	Not at all	No more than usual	Rather more than usual	Much more than usual
D2 – felt that life is entirely hopeless?	Not at all	No more than usual	Rather more than usual	Much more than usual
D3 – felt that life isn't worth living?	Not at all	No more than usual	Rather more than usual	Much more than usual
D4 – thought of the possibility that you might make away with yourself?	Definitely not	I don't think so	Has crossed my mind	Definitely have
D5 – found at times you couldn't do anything because your nerves were too bad?	Not at all	No more than usual	Rather more than usual	Much more than usual
D6 – found yourself wishing you were dead and away from it all?	Not at all	No more than usual	Rather more than usual	Much more than usual
D7 – found that the idea of taking your own life kept coming into your mind?	Definitely not	I don't think so	Has crossed my mind	Definitely has

A [   ] B [   ] C [   ] D [   ] TOTAL [   ]

Scoring the GHQ 28, award 0 for the first two responses on the left (not at all and no more than usual) and 1 for the two on the right. More than 5 is abnormal

Published by the NFER-NELSOL Publishing Compnay Ltd.,
Darville House, 2 Oxford Road East, Windsor, Berks. SL4 1DF.

First published 1978

Medico-legal contract

Terms and Conditions of Mr [ ] FRCS in Relation to Medico-legal practice

1. Instructing solicitors shall treat all information supplied by Mr [ ] as confidential and shall not disclose indirectly or directly or otherwise use this information except for the purpose of the specified litigation without the prior consent of Mr [ ].

2.1 Mr [ ]'s charges for preparing a report will be based on the complexity and length of the report but are likely to be in the range of £ [ ] to £ [ ].

2.2 Mr [ ]'s hourly rate of £ [ ] will apply to all work other than preparation of the report.

2.3 If required to attend a conference in chambers, Mr [ ]'s charge will be £ [ ] per half day.

2.4 If required to appear in Court, Mr [ ]'s charge will be £ [ ] per day.

2.5 Mr [ ] shall be fully reimbursed for all travelling time at £ [ ] per hour first class train travel, car mileage at £0.80 per mile together with overnight stay and subsistence if necessary.

2.6 The amount due to Mr [ ] shall not be subject to taxation by the Court. Instructing solicitors shall:

(a) ensure that Mr [ ]'s charges are no higher than reasonably necessary for the purpose of the litigation, bearing in mind his professional expertise; and

(b) where necessary, obtain prior approval from the Legal Aid Board of Mr [ ]'s charges.

3.1 Instructing solicitors shall pay all sums due within 4 weeks of the date of invoice. Late payment will be subject to interest of [ ]% per annum. In the event of late payment, further reports and co-operation will be withheld until payment is received.

3.2 Mr [ ] reserves the right to require advance payment for work undertaken prior to supplying that work to instructing solicitors.

4. In the event of cancellation of a Court appearance or settlement, instructing solicitors shall pay the full fee unless the settlement is made [ ] days in advance. A cancellation charge of half a day's Court fee per day is liable unless the case is cancelled or otherwise settled [ ] days in advance, in which case Mr [ ] shall waive the charges set out in clause 2.4 above.

5. Instructing solicitors shall be responsible for giving adequate instructions and shall check also that all matters are covered in the reports. Instructing solicitors shall be responsible for any claim made against Mr [ ] resulting from their failure to do so.

6. The liability of Mr [ ] to instructing solicitors and/or their clients for negligence howsoever arising in respect of any loss or damage caused by an act or default of Mr [ ] shall be limited to the amount received by Mr [ ] for his services.

Chapter 2

The legal viewpoint

Christopher Briggs and Bertie Leigh

■ Introduction

Since the last edition of this volume there has been a vast change in the practice of civil litigation in this country. This has been occasioned by the far-reaching review undertaken by Lord Woolf, resulting in the demise of the old rules of practice and the creation of a new code: the Civil Procedure Rules (CPR).

The intention of the changes is to create a system whereby parties may enjoy access to justice in a quicker and more cost-effective manner. To this end, parties are encouraged to employ a greater 'cards on the table' approach and in doing so are forced to address the real issues of a case at an earlier stage. The Courts themselves actively manage cases, seeking strict adherence to set timetables for the progress of the litigation and there are punitive penalties which may be imposed upon parties who fail to do so.

The role of the expert witness, always important, is now pivotal, particularly at the early stages of a case. The CPR specifically impose a duty on the expert to help the court—a duty which overrides any duty owed to the party instructing the expert, and this is emphasised by the requirement that any report be addressed to the Court itself.

In the past at the back of every lawyer's mind while instructing an expert to prepare a report in the course of litigation is the knowledge that the report will have to be disclosed to the other side if it is to be used at trial. The lawyer is anxious, therefore, to ensure that the report will present the client's case in its best light and there is a temptation to play down any potential weaknesses. As a result there used to be a trend for lawyers to become increasingly involved in the preparation of reports until the so-called 'expert' report assumed the colour of a special pleading rather than an impartial opinion. The apogee of this practice was in the mid-1970s when the House of Lords dealt with the case of *Whitehouse* v. *Jordan* [1981] 1 ALL ER 267. There a joint report was prepared on the Claimant's behalf by two eminent obstetricians after a long conference between the doctors and counsel, and, although it appeared otherwise, the final report was actually settled by counsel. The result was disastrous. The joint report did not stand up against the defendants' reports and, after rigorous cross-examination, the experts

were forced to recant from crucial parts of their report. On the subject of medical reports Lord Wilberforce said:

While some degree of consultation between experts and legal advisers is entirely proper, it is necessary that expert evidence presented to the Court should be and should be seen to be, the independent product of the expert, uninfluenced as to form or content by the exigencies of litigation.

(*Whitehouse* v. *Jordan* [1981] 1 ALL ER 267)

The duties and responsibilities of expert witnesses were usefully set out in the more recent case of *Ikarian Reefer* [1993] 2 Lloyds Rep 68.81 from which there was a plethora of expert evidence much of which offered little or no assistance. The court endorsed Lord Wilberforce's comments in *Whitehouse* v. *Jordan* and added that if an expert had insufficient expertise or lacked information in a certain area then the expert must say so.

It is clear that a lawyer must not exert undue influence over an expert in the preparation of reports and must endeavour to limit his role to what is considered a proper level of consultation. The lawyer's involvement has been further diminished with the introduction of the CPR, which came into effect on 26 April 1999 and which have put the relationship between the expert, the Court and parties on a fixed basis for the first time. The overriding duty of all experts is to the Court and the expert's report must now be addressed to the Court rather than to the lawyer who has instructed the expert. Part 35 of the CPR (see Appendix 3) sets out the expert's duties as follows:

■ Expert evidence shall be restricted to that which is reasonably required to resolve the proceedings.
■ It is the duty of an expert to help the Court on the matters within his expertise.
■ This duty overrides any obligation to the person from whom he has received instructions or by whom he is paid.

Having seen the lawyers' role in the preparation of reports curtailed, it should not be forgotten that an expert's report is an important document which will play a crucial role in the course of litigation. There are two types of medical report: those dealing with liability and those describing the Claimant's present condition and prognosis. The first category is used predominantly to establish liability in medical negligence cases, and as such is outside the scope of this volume. This chapter is concerned with reports as to condition and prognosis which are common to all types of Personal Injury litigation.

Reports for service with proceedings

An expert may be approached at any time by any party to an action to produce a report upon condition and prognosis. The CPR provide for a pre-action protocol to be followed which includes a detailed Letter of Claim being served by a Claimant which *inter alia* must describe the patient's injuries and present condition and prognosis, and so a medical report will have to be obtained at this stage by the Claimant. Additionally, the protocol provides for the Claimant making an offer to settle at this stage supported by a medical report, unless there is no significant continuing injury. If proceedings are issued, the Rules provide:

Where the Claimant is relying on the evidence of a medical practitioner the Claimant must attach to or serve with his Particulars of Claim a report from a medical practitioner about the personal injuries which he alleges in his claim.

The Rules are in their infancy and it is unknown how the Courts will define such a medical report. The previous Rules referred to 'a report substantiating all the personal injuries alleged in the Statement of Claim which the [Claimant] proposes to adduce in evidence as part of his case at trial'. Two schools of thought formed as to the precise meaning of this definition. The first took the view that all this report needed to do was to confirm the existence of the medical conditions listed in the pleading. The second took the view that not only should the existence of the medical conditions pleaded be confirmed, but also it was necessary for the expert to attribute those medical conditions to the accident or other event of which complaint is made. The question was considered in the Ativan and Valium group litigation by the Honourable Mr Justice Ian Kennedy, who said:

The purpose of [the Rule] is to ensure that a [Claimant] has proper medical evidence before beginning an action for personal injuries. A defendant can at once decide whether or not he needs to obtain medical evidence of his own, so contributing to the early settlement or speedy trial of the claim.

It is tempting to say that all that is required is a confirmation of the presence of the several conditions listed in the pleadings, but that in my view overlooks two cardinal factors. Firstly the purpose of the Rule is not well served unless a defendant knows whether there is medical support for the attribution of present conditions to the event in question. Secondly the requirement is for injuries to be substantiated: by definition a condition is not an injury unless its presence is attributable to the accident. Often there are medical conditions present in a [Claimant] other than those which result from the event in

question. It is not in my view correct to argue that one must look to the defence to see whether there is an issue as to attribution.

He went on to say:

What is required is a report which substantiates all the injuries with the sufficient particularity that one is not left in any doubt what is and what is not attributed to the accident or other event.

It is clear, therefore, that any report prepared by an expert for the purpose of assisting a Claimant to commence proceedings must address the question of whether or not the medical conditions complained of are attributable to the accident alleged. These matters may, in fact, be fairly obvious from the circumstances of the case, such as injuries resulting from a road accident. Particular care must be given, however, when considering pre-existing conditions, and conditions alleged to have been caused, for instance, by the administration of drugs.

Condition and prognosis reports: general

The purpose of a report as to condition and prognosis is usually to assist the Court to quantify the Claimant's claim in the event that the defendant is found to have been negligent. In most cases a victim of personal injury will be able to obtain compensation for two types of damages—pecuniary and non-pecuniary. Broadly speaking, pecuniary damages are those which can be translated into monetary terms, while non-pecuniary damage covers immeasurable elements such as pain and suffering. In legal terms a pecuniary loss is called 'special damage' and non-pecuniary loss is 'general damage'.

The underlying principle in awarding special damages is *restitutio integrum*. In the words of Lord Blackburn in 1880, the Court should award 'that sum of money which will put the party who has been injured, or who has suffered, in the same position as he would have been in if he had not sustained the wrong for which he is now getting his compensation or reparation' (*Livingstone* v. *Reywards Coal Co.* [1880] 5 App Cas 25). It is not possible to calculate non-pecuniary damages on the same basis since the value of the loss of a leg cannot be quantified, so the better view would be to consider this as 'fair' compensation for the injury that the Claimant has suffered as a result of the defendant's negligence.

Examples of damages which may be awarded are as follows.

Medical and other expenses

A successful Claimant may be able to recover, as part of his special damages, any medical or other expenses which have been reasonably incurred as a result of the injury.

Any prospective expenses will be awarded as part of the general damages. The expenses will have been 'reasonably incurred' if they were not too excessive and were reasonably necessary to improve the quality of the Claimant's life. He should thus be able to recover the cost of any special equipment needed as a result of the injuries, the cost of adapting his house and of any special attendances which might be required at home. Thus reports should describe the needs of the patient in each of these respects and the reasonableness of solutions proposed (see particularly Chapter 20).

In the case of medical expenses the Claimant is entitled to seek private treatment and, to the extent that he wishes to do so, he is able to recover such sums as he would have to bear if he received private care (Law Reform (Personal Injuries) Act 1948 s. 2(4)). If his care requires him to stay in a special hospital or institution, the cost will be recoverable. Similarly, the expert should describe the likely future course of the Claimant's condition and any operations which might be necessary.

Third party expenses

If a third party incurs financial loss as a result of the Claimant's injury, such sums are recoverable from the defendant. Thus, if a third party has to give up work in order to care for the Claimant he should be able to recover damages in respect of reasonable loss of earnings. Similarly, if the third party has incurred expense in providing the Claimant with the medical or nursing care or equipment, the sums are recoverable as special damages. In addition, a third party may be entitled to recover such expenses as were incurred in visiting the Claimant in hospital. The medical expert's role is not to list the equipment or the visits, but to describe the needs of the patient so that a Judge can assess whether the sums claimed are reasonable. The expert may help to tell the Court whether the expenditure claimed is reasonable: doctors are wise to err on the side of explicitness in expressing medical opinions for the laity.

Loss of earnings

The Claimant will be awarded damages in respect of any loss of earnings incurred, together with compensation for the loss of any benefits—such as a company car—if this results from the accident. Such damages will be calculated from the date of the cause of action to the date of trial and will form part of the Claimant's special damages. Thus if the Claimant claims for the loss of employment, the expert should assess the extent to which the injury is responsible and is a handicap in the labour market.

Prospective loss of earnings will be calculated separately. The Claimant may be prevented from working in the future for a number of reasons totally unconnected with the accident. In addition, his future earning power will not be obvious as it will depend on a number of factors, such as future employment prospects and redundancy. For these reasons future loss of earnings is not calculated on a straight mathematical basis. Instead, a reasonable figure for the Claimant's net annual loss (the multiplicand) is multiplied by a figure (the multiplier) to reflect the number of years during which the loss is expected to last, discounted to allow for the interest the money will earn. The multiplier will reflect the age, sex and life expectancy of the Claimant. A report should always say if and by how much a Claimant's life expectancy has been diminished.

Loss of earnings capacity

The Claimant is entitled to receive compensation if he is placed at a disadvantage in the labour market as a result of the defendant's negligence. This is so even if the Claimant is at present in employment: probable difficulties in finding another job in the event of losing this one have a bearing on damages.

Pain and suffering

Damages are recoverable in respect of pain and suffering, both actual and prospective, which are directly attributable to the Claimant's injuries. Damages recoverable under these headings include the pain and suffering attendant on any operation which is necessary as a result of the defendant's negligence. The Court will be helped by the clinician's description and assessment of the pain and discomfort involved, and the experiences that the claimant has already suffered.

Loss of amenity

A Claimant will be entitled to compensation under this heading in respect of loss of enjoyment of life consequent to the injury. The Court tries to assess the damages according to the severity of the injury, and thus the Claimant who has lost a finger will receive a smaller amount of compensation under this heading than a Claimant who has lost an arm. The amount of an individual award is necessarily conventional, if not arbitrary. The law assesses such awards on the basis of precedents, so that the amount of an award is derived from the Judge's understanding of what has been awarded in previous cases involving similar injuries. It is relatively easy, therefore, for a lawyer to predict the probable level of damages in any particular case. This figure may then be adjusted according to the Claimant's pre-accident circumstances. If, for example, the Claimant was an enthusiastic sportsman and as a result of the injury is no longer able to participate in the sport, his damages under this heading will be increased to reflect the diminution in his enjoyment of life. Similarly, if a Claimant is disfigured by the accident and as a result his professional prospects or social life are impaired, he will be entitled to recover increased damages. All of these things should be described in appropriate cases, because the medical expert has a vital role to play in describing to a Judge what the effect of a given injury has been to a specific individual.

Presentation of medico-legal reports
Background information

A medical report may be commissioned by either party to an action at any time during the course of litigation or by a potential litigant exploring his case before deciding to issue proceedings. The expert will usually be approached by a solicitor who will give a brief explanation of the case, and ask the expert whether he would be prepared to give an opinion.

In many cases the expert consulted by the patient's solicitor will have actually treated the patient and will therefore have access to the notes and documents. In other cases the instructing solicitor will arrange for a full set of papers to be sent to the clinician. These should usually include a copy of the Claimant's medical records and X-rays together with a detailed account of the circumstances giving rise to the injury. If proceedings have already begun the solicitor will inform the expert of how much progress has been made, sending copies of the relevant pleadings.

The instructions forwarded to the expert by the patient's solicitor are no longer privileged against disclosure, although the Court will only order that the other party or parties be given sight of any written instructions or be allowed to ask the expert questions in court about his instructions, whether written or oral, if there are reasonable grounds to believe that the summary of his instructions is inaccurate or incomplete.

This rule follows the decision in *Clough* v. *Tameside and Glossop Health Authority*. In this case the defendant commissioned an expert's report from a consultant psychiatrist and as part of his instructions the expert was given a copy of a report obtained from another clinician. The defendant disclosed the expert's report which recited the receipt by him of the particular medical report and the Claimant thereupon applied for disclosure of the medical report referred to. The Judge decided that service of the expert's report did waive privilege over the medical report referred to therein. Having referred to the expert's

duties as described in the *Ikarian Reefer* case, Mrs Justice Bracewell said:

An expert must state the facts or assumptions on which the opinion was based and should not omit to consider material facts which detract from any concluded opinion. An essential element of the process is for a party to know and to be able to test in evidence the information supplied to the experts in order to ascertain if the opinion is based on a sound factual basis or on disputed matters or hypothetical facts yet to be determined by the Courts.

It is only by proper and full disclosure to all parties than an expert opinion can be tested in Court: in order to ascertain whether all appropriate information was supplied and how the expert dealt with it... fairness dictates that a party should not be forced to meet a case pleaded or an expert opinion on the basis of documents he cannot see.

(*Clough* v. *Tameside and Glossop Health Authority* [1998] 2 ALL ER 971)

Following service of the expert's report all other parties are now entitled under Part 35 of the CPR to put one list of written questions to the expert, but only in order to clarify the report. In practice, it is courteous and preferable for these questions to be sent to the lawyer who instructed the expert but the rules do entitle a party to send the questions to the expert direct and simply forward a copy to the lawyer. The questions must be put to the expert within 28 days of service of his report so an expert is entitled to check with the party instructing him the date when the report was served before answering. In any event, the expert does not have to respond to any correspondence sent direct by another party's solicitor without first contacting the party who has instructed him. The Claimant is not entitled to ask the expert oral questions. The questions must be answered in writing by the expert and will form part of the original report. There is no set timetable for response but it is likely that answers will need to be prepared within 28 days of receipt. If any of the questions put are not answered by the expert then the Court may order that the party instructing the expert cannot rely upon the report at trial.

Interestingly, Part 35 of the Rules also entitles an expert to write to the Court direct to request directions to assist in carrying out his function as an expert, and an expert may do this without giving notice to any party. Therefore any clarification required or concern held as a result of an expert's instructions can be addressed in this way.

The venue: High Court or County Court

All cases of a value up to £50 000 must be commenced in the County Court, and all those of a value up to £25 000 must be tried there unless the Court otherwise directs. The Court will exercise its discretion to have an action tried in the High Court notwithstanding its value having regard to such matters as the financial substance of the claim, whether questions of general public interest are raised, and whether the transfer will result in a more speedy trial. It has been suggested that, *inter alia*, cases involving professional negligence, fatal accidents or claims against the police might be considered important and therefore suitable for transfer to the High Court. However, even so, they must be commenced in the County Court and subsequently transferred. It is suggested, therefore, that an expert is more likely to receive instructions in a case which is proceeding in the County Court rather than in the High Court, but this makes little difference to the expert in the preparation of his report.

The Claim Form

Legal proceedings in both the High Court and County Court are now begun when the Claim Form is served on the defendant. The Claim Form is a formal document which notifies the defendant that the Claimant intends to pursue a claim against him. The Claim Form must be issued at the Court within 3 years of the date of the cause of action, or within 3 years of the Claimant realising that his injuries were caused by the defendant's negligence. If there is a medical reason why the Claimant would not have known of his cause of action, then this may usefully be described in the report. If the Claimant is a minor at the relevant date, the 3-year period does not begin until he is 18. Once issued, the Claim Form must be served on the defendant within 4 months unless the Court authorises an extension of time for service.

Particulars of Claim

The Claim Form may contain Particulars of Claim or these may be served separately. Particulars of Claim are now also referred to as a 'Statement of Case'. This sets out the details of the Claimant's claim against the defendant, and lists the alleged acts of negligence which caused the Claimant's damage. It will also itemise the Claimant's injuries and claim damages together with interest.

The expert should still take his own history of the injury, and should note any discrepancy with the Statement of Case.

The defence

The defence contains the defendant's response to the allegations made against him, any of which he can either admit, deny or not admit. If the defendant does not admit a fact he is neither admitting nor denying it but merely inviting the Claimant to prove the point. If he denies an allegation he gives notice that the alleged fact is in issue. Under the old Rules a defence could be a simple blanket denial of the allegations; however, under CPR, it is clear that a defendant when denying an allegation must state his reasons for doing so, and if he intends to put forward

a different version of events from that given by the Claimant he must state this version.

Request for further information

Either party to a claim can ask for further information or clarification of any matter which is in dispute in the proceedings or request additional information in relation to any such matter. Where the expert would be assisted by more information he should say so, since those instructing him may be able to obtain it.

The format of the report

Following the decision of the House of Lords in *Whitehouse* v. *Jordan* [1981] 1 ALL ER 267 the form and content of an expert's report must be left to his own discretion. The following format is thus intended to act as a general guide only (see also Appendix 1). However, an expert's report must contain certain information as described by Part 35 of the Rules and the practice direction (see Appendix 3) and these requirements are italicised.

The heading

First and foremost, the report should be addressed to the Court. The heading of the report should begin with its title, making clear that it is a report on condition and prognosis, giving the date of the examination and where it took place. *The report must contain a statement setting out the substance of all material instructions, summarising the facts and instructions given to the expert which are material to the opinions expressed in the report or upon which those opinions are based.* Therefore, the information and documents available to the expert should be specified and any restrictions or adverse circumstances spelled out.

Particulars of the patient

This part of the report should state the name, age and pre-accident occupation of the Claimant. If any injury to the upper limbs has been sustained, it is important to state the handedness of the patient. The report should also include a brief account of the Claimant's relevant medical history prior to the accident.

General

Where there is a range of opinion on the matters dealt with in the report, an expert must summarise the range of opinion and give reason for his own opinion.

The history of the present injury

1. The date of the accident.
2. A note of how the accident occurred. This record should be kept as brief as possible. It should merely set the scene rather than providing a definitive account of what occurred. It is not the medical expert's role to give

an opinion on the non-medical circumstances giving rise to the injury.

3. A comment on the management of the Claimant's case to date. This should include a description of the type of treatment which the Claimant has received, together with the number of attendances and operations undergone. If the treatment has been unpleasant or uncomfortable, the expert should mention this and explain why.

The present condition

This should explain the expert's findings on examination:

1. The patient's appearance and demeanour
2. The type of examination undertaken and its results
3. Whether any investigations were carried out, and, if so, the results
4. Interpretation of X-rays.

If the injury is disfiguring the expert may illustrate the report with photographs.

If an expert has used any test or experiment for the report he must say who carried this out, give the qualifications of the person, and state whether or not the test or experiment was carried out under the expert's supervision.

The present complaint

The expert will ask the Claimant whether he experiences any residual pain as a result of the injury. If he does, the clinician should state whether the pain is continuous or whether it is brought on in certain circumstances. He should also describe the type of pain and its severity, as well as any analgesia necessary. The Claimant may complain of a restriction of mobility or difficulty in adjusting to his post-accident lifestyle. He may have problems adapting to special aids. If the Claimant mentions marital or social problems arising from the injury, these should be included in the report. The expert should also bear in mind the possibility of psychological trauma and its likely significance in the present case. The whole should add up to an accurate assessment of the cause of the Claimant's injury and present disabilities.

The prognosis

1. Whether any further treatment is required and, if so, its nature, extent, likely duration and gravity.
2. Whether the Claimant will need to take any more time off work and, if so, how much and whether it is likely to interfere with earning capacity.
3. The risks or complications associated with the particular injury or course of treatment.
4. Whether the Claimant is able to go back to his pre-accident work and, if not, what other type of work he would be suited for.

5. Whether the Claimant is still able to enjoy his pre-accident hobbies and pastimes.
6. The Claimant's cosmetic appearance and whether it is likely to improve or deteriorate.
7. The Claimant's psychological state and its likely prognosis.
8. Whether there are any other problems arising from the injury and the likely duration of these problems.
9. If the Claimant's injuries are so serious that his life-expectancy is reduced, a report should include an estimate of how long the Claimant is likely to live. This is usually an unanswerable question which the expert should approach by imagining 100 patients in the position of the Claimant; what is required is the date when, doing the best he can, he thinks it most likely that the 50th patient would die.
10. Whether the Claimant has any special needs, i.e. special care and attendance, housing, transport and special equipment.
11. Whether the Claimant will be likely to benefit from paramedical help, such as physiotherapy, speech therapy, occupational therapy or social workers.
12. Whether, in the clinician's opinion, the Claimant should qualify for benefits such as mobility or attendance allowance.

Use of published works and statistics

It is not intended that a medical expert should conduct a thorough search of the medical literature to find any printed material to support his opinion. *But an expert must give details of any literature or other material which he has relied upon in making his report. It is good practice therefore to provide copies of the literature with the report.*

The conclusion

The report must contain a summary of the conclusions reached.

The report must give details of the expert's qualifications and specialist knowledge.

The report must contain a statement that the expert understands his duty to the Court and has complied with that duty.

The report must then be verified by a Statement of Truth, the form of which is as follows:

'I believe that the facts I have stated in this report are true and that the opinions I have expressed are correct' and then signed by its author.

Proceedings for Contempt of Court may be brought against a person who makes or causes to be made a false statement in a document verified by a Statement of Truth without an honest belief in its truth.

Any medical report should be written in clear and unambiguous terms. The expert should explain his findings as fully as possible, bearing in mind that the report will be read by lay people.

The joint expert

The CPR provide for the Court to direct that where two or more parties wish to submit expert evidence on a particular issue, that the evidence on this issue is given by one expert only. Joint instructions of experts as to condition and prognosis is likely to become the norm. Where the Court gives a direction for a single joint expert to be used each instructing party may give instructions to the expert and must at the same time send a copy of the instructions to the other instructing party.

Giving evidence in court

The majority of Personal Injury actions will be settled before the matter comes to Court. An action can be settled at any stage in the proceedings and it is not uncommon for the settlement to take place 'at the door of the court'. However, the aim of the new Rules is to encourage settlement at a very early stage. In reality, however, a settlement is not always possible and the parties must try to prove their cases in Court.

Every doctor asked to prepare a report should assume that he will be required to give evidence. He should thus ensure that he is able to rearrange his commitments, sometimes at short notice, in order to give this evidence. In most cases a clinician may be given a long period of notice of the trial date. In the High Court in London, at the time of writing, the present waiting time for a 3-day hearing is approximately 1 year. This time is considerably shorter in the case of trials outside London. As both parties expect to call expert evidence, it is the normal practice in Personal Injury cases to request a fixture. This means that the trial is fixed to take place on a certain date or dates, as opposed to floating in a list and being slotted in when a vacancy arises, often at very short notice. An expert should expect, as a matter of courtesy, to be asked by his instructing solicitors for a list of dates upon which it would not be convenient for him to attend Court before the trial date is fixed.

At some stage in the proceedings the expert's report will have been disclosed to the other side. If the report can be agreed the other side will not need to produce their own expert evidence, and it may not be necessary for the original expert to give oral evidence as his report could be read in open Court.

If the reports are not agreed the expert will be shown the report of his counterpart and asked to comment. If it seems that the parties are not too far apart it may still be possible to agree one report. If not, the expert must be equipped to deal with any opposing findings in his opponent's report.

An expert may now be asked to attend a meeting between the experts of all parties. The CPR now expressly provide for this and the Court has power to order such a meeting to take place for the purpose of identifying those parts of the evidence which are an issue, and the preparation of a joint statement indicating those parts of the evidence of the witnesses on which all are agreed, and those on which they are not. An expert should, therefore, be prepared to attend such a meeting if requested by his instructing solicitor.

As the date of trial draws nearer, the expert is likely to be asked to attend a conference with the counsel who will be arguing the case in Court. This will give counsel the opportunity to question the expert in detail on his report and discover whether there are any areas of vulnerability. The expert must also be prepared to educate counsel if necessary about the medical aspects of the case by explaining the report in lay terms. In civil cases there is normally no reason why the expert should not sit through the entire case and hear all the evidence, including that of his opponent. This is particularly important when acting for a defendant, as it will give the clinician time to consider the weight of his opponent's evidence, but it is also helpful for a claimant's expert, as he will be on hand to advise counsel about the medical points raised.

When called to give evidence the expert may take into the witness box a copy of his report and all the papers on which he relies. He will be asked to swear an oath in a form suitable for his religion or, if he so chooses, simply to affirm that the evidence he gives will be the truth.

The expert will then be examined in chief by the Barrister instructed by the solicitors who instructed him. This means that the Barrister will guide the expert through his report and raise any supplemental points which have come out during the course of the trial. The expert should think carefully about the evidence that he is to give and should try to stick as closely as possible to his original report. It is usually counterproductive if an expert surprises his counsel by coming up with a new idea in the box.

When the evidence in chief has been completed the counsel will sit down and the Barrister for the other party will rise to his feet. He will then conduct a cross-examination, challenging those points of the evidence which do not fit in with his client's case and putting forward an alternative view. This examination is rarely acrimonious but counsel will be trying very hard to get the expert to tone down his evidence. An expert must be aware of this and avoid falling into any carefully laid traps. He should take time to consider his replies and think very carefully before conceding any issue. The line of attack should not take the expert too much by surprise, as he will have seen the report of his opponent beforehand and this will form the basis of the cross-examination.

When the cross-examination is completed the expert may be re-examined by his own Barrister. This gives the Barrister the opportunity to cover points raised in cross-examination and not dealt with in the examination in chief. It also gives counsel the chance to set the record straight on any issue which has become clouded.

When the re-examination is ended the expert may step down from the witness box. The Judge will usually order that each witness is free to leave the Court as soon as his evidence is completed.

The question of an expert's fee should not be overlooked. The expert is entitled to charge for time spent reconsidering the papers and preparing any supplemental reports which may be necessary. He is also entitled to charge for time and expenses incurred in attending the trial. These are matters which should be discussed with and recovered from his instructing solicitors. This is particularly important as the Court has the power to restrict experts' fees.

A witness can be compelled to attend Court in order to give evidence by means of a witness summons. This is an order of the Court requiring the witness to attend on a specified day and remain in the Court until such time as the case is completed. Failure to comply with this order is Contempt of Court, punishable by a fine and/or imprisonment. In most cases an expert will be happy to attend Court voluntarily, but on occasion he may require a witness summons before his employers will allow him the time off. In these cases a witness summons will be issued and served on the doctor.

Specimen format for a medico-legal report

Note that this is not the only format for a medico-legal report. It is introduced more as an *aide-mémoire* for those who may be unfamiliar with the information required by the legal profession.

Title page

Name, address, telephone number of reporting surgeon. Medical report on:

Name	Mr John Smith
Address	23 South Street, Westford
Date of birth	8 December 1952
Date of report	20 October 1994
Status	Married
Date of injury	20 October 1993
Occupation at time of injury	Lorry driver
Present occupation	Unemployed
Time lost from work as a result of injury	Six months
Report prepared for the assistance of the Court	Eastford County Court
Your ref.	XY2/P3 dated 10 July 1994
Our ref.	ABC/DJF
Documents available	1. Southern General Hospital notes
	2. Medical report from Mr AB Lee

Suggested further headings

History of injury

Brief details of the patient's recollection of the incident. If a Road Traffic accident, was the patient wearing a seat belt or crash helmet?

Treatment to date

This will give an account of the management of the problem up to the present time from:

1. The patient's account
2. The hospital notes.

This section will include a precise account of the injuries recorded at the time of admission to or attendance at hospital.

Present condition

This will detail the patient's current symptoms and signs and discuss X-rays:

1. Symptoms:

   - pain
   - stiffness
   - sleep loss
   - marital or social problems
   - functional impairment
2. Signs:

   - deformity
   - loss of joint movement
   - description of scars
   - shortening
   - wasting, weakness (Consider use of clinical photographs)
3. X-rays, if appropriate.

Effect of accident on occupation

Effect of accident on social activities

How have the patient's social and sporting activities been affected by the accident/injury? What is he unable to do now that he could do before the accident/injury?

Literature

Opinion and prognosis

An opinion as to whether the injuries sustained are compatible with the mechanism described is essential.

The prognosis is particularly important and should consider:

1. Is further treatment required? (If *yes*, describe its nature, duration and gravity.)
2. Is further time off from work expected?
3. What is the likelihood of complications developing?
4. If there is a cosmetic abnormality; is it likely to improve or to deteriorate?
5. Is there any reduction in the patient's life-expectancy?
6. Describe the psychological state of the patient.
7. Does the patient have any special needs? If so, are they on-going?

Conclusions

A summary of the conclusions reached must be given.

I understand my duty to the Court in preparing this report and I have complied with that duty.

I believe that the facts I have stated in this report are true in that the opinions I have expressed are correct.

Signature

The report's author must record his qualifications and position so that the origin and standing of the provider of the report are clear to whoever is reading it.

Appendix

2

Part 35   Experts and assessors

Contents of this part

Duty to restrict expert evidence

35.1   Expert evidence shall be restricted to that which is reasonably required to resolve the proceedings.

Interpretation

35.2   A reference to an 'expert' in this Part is a reference to an expert who has been instructed to give or prepare evidence for the purpose of Court proceedings.

Experts—overridng duty to the Court

35.3   (1)   It is the duty of an expert to help the Court on the matters within his expertise.

(2)   This duty overrides any obligation to the person from whom he has received instructions or by whom he is paid.

Court's power tp restrict expert evidence

35.4   (1)   No party may call an expert or put in evidence an expert's report without the Court's permission.

(2)   When a party applies for permission under this Rule he must identify:

(a) the field in which he wishes to rely on expert evidence; and

(b)   where practicable the expert in that field on whose evidence he wishes to rely.

(3)   If permission is granted under this Rule it shall be in relation only to the expert named or the field identified under paragraph (2).

(4)   The Court may limit the amount of the expert's fees and expenses that the party who wishes to rely on the expert may recover from any other party.

General requirement for expert evidence to be given in a written report

35.5   (1)   Expert evidence is to be given in a written report unless the Court directs otherwise.

(2)   If a Claim is on the fast track, the Court will not direct an expert to attend a hearing unless it is necessary to do so in the interests of justice.

Written questions to experts

35.6   (1)   A party may put to.

(a)   an expert instructed by another party; or

(b)   a single joint expert appointed under rule 35.7.

Written questions about his report.

(2)   Written questions under paragraph (1):

(a)   may be put once only;

(b)   must be put within 28 days of service of the expert's report; and

(c)   must be for the purpose only of clarification of the report; unless in any case

(i)   the Court gives permission; or

(ii)   the other party agrees.

(3)   An expert's answers to questions put in accordance with paragraph (1) shall be treated as part of the expert's report.

(4)   Where

(a)   a party has put a written question to an expert instructed by another party in accordance with this rule, and

(b)   the expert does not answer that question,

the Court may make one or both of the following orders in relation to the party who instructed the expert:

(i) that the party may not rely on the evidence of that expert; or

(ii) that the party may not recover the fees and expenses of that expert from any other party.

Court's power to direct that evidence is to be given by a single joint expert

35.7 (1) Where two or more parties wish to submit expert evidence on a particular issue, the Court may direct that the evidence on that issue is to be given by one expert only.

(2) The parties wishing to submit the expert evidence are called 'the instructing parties'.

(3) Where the instructing parties cannot agree who should be the expert, the Court may:

(a) select the expert from a list prepared or identified by the instructing parties; or

(b) direct that the expert be selected in such other manner as the Court may direct.

Instructions to a single joint expert

35.8 (1) Where the Court gives a direction under Rule 35.7 for a single joint expert to be used, each instructing party may give instructions to the expert.

(2) When an instructing party gives instructions to the expert he must, at the same time, send a copy of the instructions to the other instructing parties.

(3) The Court may give directions about:

(a) the payment of the expert's fees and expenses; and

(b) any inspection, examination or experiments which the expert wishes to carry out.

(4) The Court may, before an expert is instructed:

(a) limit the amount that can be paid by way of fees and expenses to the expert; and

(b) direct that the instructing parties pay that amount into Court.

(5) Unless the Court otherwise directs, the instructing parties are jointly and severally liable(GL) for the payment of the expert's fees and expenses.

Power of court to direct a party to provide information

35.9 Where a party has access to information which is not reasonably available to the other party, the Court may direct the party who has access to the information to:

(a) prepare and file a document recording the information; and

(b) serve a copy of that document on the other party.

Contents of report

35.10 (1) An expert's report must comply with the requirements set out in the relevant practice direction.

(2) At the end of an expert's report there must be a statement that:

(a) the expert understands his duty to the Court; and

(b) he has complied with that duty.

(3) The expert's report must state the substance of all material instructions, whether written or oral, on the basis of which the report was written.

(4) The instructions referred to in paragraph (3) shall not be privileged(GL) against disclosure but the Court will not, in relation to those instructions:

(a) order disclosure of any specific document; or

(b) permit any questioning in Court, other than by the party who instructed the expert.

unless it is satisfied that there are reasonable grounds to consider the statement of instructions given under paragraph (3) to be inaccurate or incomplete.

Use by one party of expert's report disclosed by another

35.11 Where a party has disclosed an expert's report, any party may use that expert's report as evidence at the trial.

Discussions between experts

35.12 (1) The Court may, at any stage, direct a discussion between experts for the purpose of requiring the experts to:

(a) identify the issues in the proceedings; and

(b) where possible, reach agreement on an issue.

(2) The Court may specify the issues which the experts must discuss.

(3) The Court may direct that following a discussion between the experts they must prepare a statement for the Court showing:

(a) those issues on which they agree; and

(b) those issues on which they disagree and a summary of their reasons for disagreeing.

(4) The content of the discussion between the experts shall not be referred to at the trial unless the parties agree.

(5) Where experts reach agreement on an issue during their discussions, the agreement shall not bind the parties unless the parties expressly agree to be bound by the agreement.

Consequence of failure to disclose expert's report

35.13   A party who fails to disclose an expert's report may not use the report at the trial or call the expert to give evidence orally unless the Court gives permission.

Expert's right to ask Court for directions

35.14   (1) An expert may file a written request for directions to assist him in carrying out his function as an expert.

(2) An expert may request directions under paragraph (1) without giving notice to any party.

(3) The Court, when it gives directions, may also direct that a party be served with:

(a) a copy of the directions; and

(b) a copy of the request for directions.

Assessors

35.15   (1) This rule applies where the Court appoints one or more persons (an 'assessor') under section 70 of the Supreme Court Act 1981 [41] or section 63 of the County Courts Act 1984 [12].

(2) The assessor shall assist the Court in dealing with a matter in which the assessor has skill and experience.

(3) An assessor shall take such part in the proceedings as the Court may direct and in particular the Court may:

(a) direct the assessor or prepare a report for the Court on any matter at issue in the proceedings; and

(b) direct the assessor to attend the whole or any part of the trial to advise the Court on any such matter.

(4) If the assessor prepares a report for the Court before the trial has begun:

(a) the Court will send a copy to each of the parties; and

(b) the parties may use it at trial.

(5) The remuneration to be paid to the assessor for his services shall be determined by the Court and shall form part of the costs of the proceedings.

(6) The Court may order any party to deposit in the Court office a specified sum in respect of the assessor's fees and, where it does so, the assessor will not be asked to act until the sum has been deposited.

(7) Paragraphs (5) and (6) do not apply where the remuneration of the assessor is to be paid out of money provided by Parliament.

---

(41) 1981 c. 54.
(42) 1984 c. 28c Section 63 was amended by S.I. 1998/2940.

Practice direction—experts and assessors

This practice direction supplements CPR Part 35

Note *Part 35 is intended to limit the use of oral expert evidence to that which is reasonably required. In addition, where possible, matters requiring expert evidence should be dealt with by a single expert. Permission of the Court is always required either to call an expert or to put an expert's report in evidence.*

Form and content of expert's reports

1.1 An expert's report should be addressed to the Court and not to the party from whom the expert has received his instructions.

1.2 An expert's report must:
(1) give details of the expert's qualifications,
(2) give details of any literature or other material which the expert has relied on in making the report,
(3) say who carried out any test or experiment which the expert has used for the report and whether or not the test or experiment has been carried out under the expert's supervision,
(4) give the qualifications of the person who carried out any such test or experiment, and
(5) where there is a range of opinion on the matters dealt with in the report,
   (i) summarise the range of opinion, and
   (ii) give reasons for his own opinion,
(6) contain a summary of the conclusions reached,
(7) contain a statement that the expert understands his duty to the Court and has complied with that duty (rule 35. 10(2)), and
(8) contain a statement setting out the substance of all material instructions (whether written or oral). The statement should summarise the facts and instructions given to the expert which are material to the opinions expressed in the report or upon which those opinions are based (rule 35. 10(3)).

1.3 An expert's report must be verified by a statement of truth as well as containing the statements required in paragraph 1.2 (7) and (8) above.

1.4 The form of the statement of truth is as follows:

'I believe that the facts I have stated in this report are true and that the opinions I have expressed are correct.'

1.5 Attention is drawn to rule 32.14 which sets out the consequences of verifying a document containing a false statement without an honest belief in its truth.

(For information about statements of truth see Part 22 and the practice direction which supplements it.)

1.6 In addition, an expert's report should comply with the requirements of any approved expert's protocol.

Information

2. Where the Court makes an order under rule 35.9 (i.e. where one party has access to information not reasonably available to the other party), the document to be prepared recording the information should set out sufficient details of any facts, tests or experiments which constitute the information to enable an assessment and understanding of the significance of the information to be made and obtained.

Instructions

3. The instructions referred to in paragraph 1.2(8) will not be protected by privilege (see rule 35.10(4)). But cross examination of the expert on the contents of his instructions will not be allowed unless the Court permits it (or unless the party who gave the instructions consents to it). Before it gives permission the Court must be satisfied that there are reasonable grounds to consider that the statement in the report of the substance of the instructions is inaccurate or incomplete. If the Court is so satisfied, it will allow the cross-examination where it appears to be in the interests of justice to do so.

Questions to experts

4.1 Questions asked for the purpose of clarifying the expert's report (see rule 35.6) should be put, in writing, to the expert not later than 28 days after receipt of the expert's report (see paragraphs 1.2 to 1.5 above as to verification).

4.2 Where a party sends a written question or questions direct to an expert and the other party is represented by solicitors, a copy of the questions should, at the same time, be sent to those solicitors.

Single expert

5. Where the Court has directed that the evidence on a particular issue is to be given by one expert only (rule 35.7) but there are a number of disciplines relevant to that issue, a leading expert in the dominant discipline should be identified as the single expert. He should prepare the general part of the report and be responsible for annexing or incorporating the contents of any reports from experts in other disciplines.

Assessors

6.1 An assessor may be appointed to assist the Court under rule 35.15. Not less than 21 days before making any such appointment, the Court will notify each party in writing of the name of the proposed assessor, of the matter in respect of which the assistance of the assessor will be sought and of the qualifications of the assessor to give that assistance.

6.2 Where any person has been proposed for appointment as an assessor, objection to him, either personally or in respect of his qualification, may be taken by any party.

6.3 Any such objection must be made in writing and filed with the Court within 7 days of receipt of the notification referred to in paragraph 6.1 and will be taken into account by the Court in deciding whether or not to make the appointment (s, 63(5) County Courts Act 1984).

6.4 Copies of any report prepared by the assessor will be sent to each of the parties but the assessor will not give oral evidence or be open to cross-examination or questioning.

Chapter 3

Recent developments in the law and their effect on medico-legal practices

Colin McEwen, Cynthia Watts

Developments in the Law

The implementation of the Civil Procedure Rules (CPR) on 26th April 1999 heralded the most radical shake up of the civil justice system in recent times. Coupled with changes in the funding of civil litigation, (public funding through Legal Aid (now Community Legal Funding) has all but disappeared and been replaced by Conditional Fees), the impact has been profound for all participants in the conduct of civil cases and specifically personal injury and clinical negligence claims. These changes were directly prompted by the recommendations of Lord Woolf's review of the whole system of civil justice published in his 1996 report Access to Justice.

This chapter describes some of the more significant effects of this new procedural code for conducting civil litigation and summarises some of the important legal principles relevant to medico-legal practice. The CPR are frequently updated. It is therefore recommended that the latest version of the CPR is checked before relying on any specific statement in this chapter.

The old regime

Traditionally, it has been for the solicitors handling the case on behalf of the injured person to determine the pace of the claim both in gathering evidence and in pursuing the claim through the Courts. This is no longer so.

The new approach

April 1999 brought fundamental changes, which even included changes of terminology. We now have Claimants instead of Plaintiffs, Court proceedings are commenced by issuing a Claim Form rather than a High Court Writ or a County Court Summons and Pleadings have been replaced by Statements of Case.

To remedy the defects he identified in the old system, Lord Woolf wanted to develop a new system that offered appropriate procedures at reasonable cost. His solution was to take the control of litigation out of the parties' hands and place it in the hands of the Court. The aim: to force litigants and their legal teams to focus on the issues

and to adopt a new culture of co-operation to resolve claims as quickly and cheaply as possible.

Consequently we now have a new set of rules – the CPR, drafted in much simpler language and hopefully more comprehensible to litigants in person as well as lawyers. However, the ongoing pace of change has not lost momentum and frequent updates continue to both amend and extend the scope of the CPR.

The Principal Changes
The Overriding Objective

All cases must be dealt with justly in accordance with five basic principles.
At all stages the Court will try to:

a) ensure that the parties are on an equal footing;
b) save expense;
c) deal with the case in a way which is proportionate to the amount of money involved, the importance of the case, the complexity of the issues and the parties' financial positions;
d) ensure the case is dealt with expeditiously and fairly
e) allot to it an appropriate share of the Court's resources while taking into account the need to allot resources to other cases.

Any party failing to conduct litigation in accordance with the overriding objective will risk severe costs sanctions. The overriding objective is stated simply, but its effect is not so certain.

Pre-action Protocols

It is intended that the CPR will incorporate a series of pre-action protocols designed to enable the parties to resolve disputes before resorting to litigation. In the present context the relevant protocols are the Personal Injury and the Clinical Disputes pre-action protocols. Further protocols are in the process of development e.g. the Road Traffic Accident protocol. The Personal Injury pre-action protocols apply directly to fast track litigation (see below) although the clear expectation is that the spirit of the protocols will be followed in all cases irrespective of their tracking or the existence of a relevant pre-action protocol. There must be good justification for not adopting the relevant protocol. The Court will not be concerned with minor infringements, but will look at the effect of non-compliance on the other party when deciding whether to impose cost sanctions.

The protocols promote an early 'all cards on the table' approach to litigation. Under the Personal Injury Pre-action Protocol, Defendants will normally have 3 months and 21 days in which to investigate and respond to a detailed Letter of Claim (based on standard letter templates annexed to the protocol), although an initial acknowledgement is required within 21 days. An admission of liability will bind the Defendant for all claims up to a value of £15 000.

Choosing Experts

The protocols envisage the use of jointly selected experts accessible to both parties. Early expert evidence will usually be desirable. The names of at least one, and preferably two or more, alternative experts in the appropriate specialty should be proposed to the Defendant who has 14 days to accept, reject or suggest alternatives. If a Defendant does not respond or objects to all the experts proposed, the parties can go ahead and instruct their own respective experts and if proceedings are subsequently issued, the Court will decide whether either party acted unreasonably. A Defendant who does not object will not be entitled to rely upon their own evidence unless the Claimant agrees or the Court directs or the first party's report has been amended and the first party refuses to disclose the original report.

If the Claimant intends to instruct a medical agency to arrange the medical report the Claimant's solicitor ought to obtain the Defendant's consent.

A party who instructs an expert outside a protocol and prior to obtaining permission from the Court risks not being allowed to call that particular expert and/or to recover the expert's fees.

Where a jointly selected expert is instructed either party may put written questions to the expert on the report, relevant to the issues via the first party's solicitors. The expert's answers should be sent separately and directly to each party. A jointly selected expert's fee for reporting will usually be paid by the instructing first party, whereas the expert's costs of responding to questions will usually fall to the party asking the questions.

If a medical report is being obtained from a jointly selected medical expert but has not yet been received, and liability is admitted, proceedings should not be issued until the Defendant has had 21 days after receipt to consider the report and make, if desired, an offer in settlement.

The Court as Case Manager

Generally speaking, the Court can now make any order it considers appropriate at any stage. It must be proactive and so can exercise many of its powers on its own initiative. Sanctions are to be applied strictly. The trial date is sacrosanct so an extension of time or relief from sanctions will not be given if it would result in a failure to meet the trial or some other important date. Consequently, solicitors will need to agree strict time scales for examinations and production of reports with experts from the outset if they are to avoid falling foul of Court timetables.

Tracking

After a Defence is served and both parties have submitted Allocation Questionnaires to the Court cases are allocated to one of three categories known as tracks, principally on the basis of the value of the claim. Other factors to be weighed in the balance include the nature of the remedy being sought; the likely complexity of the facts, law or evidence; the number of parties; the value of any counterclaim, the required oral evidence, the importance of the claim to non-parties and the views and circumstances of the parties involved.

Small Claims Track

Claims where the personal injury element (if any) will not exceed £1000 and the total value of the claim will not exceed £5000 will automatically be allocated to this track. Each party will bear its own legal costs. Consequently, a Claimant will not be able to retain the services of a solicitor and expect the Defendant to pay his or her legal costs. Therefore, solicitors will normally commence Court proceedings only in respect of claims where the Personal Injury element exceeds £1000, which is one reason why particular care should be taken by experts when preparing reports on relatively minor claims. The use of expert evidence will be minimal because of the costs rule.

Parties can mutually consent to a higher value claim being allocated to the small claims track and avoid the risk of being responsible for their opponents' costs. The Court must be satisfied that this is appropriate for the claim. However, the small claims procedure lends itself particularly to disputes between individuals living within the same area, and District Judges have been given increased powers to assist litigants in presenting their cases.

Fast Track

For personal injury claims valued at above £1000 up to a maximum £15 000. As soon as a case is allocated to this track the Court will set a timetable with a trial date or window not more than 30 weeks ahead. The parties will have to keep the case moving and work towards this date.

Trials will usually be limited to 1 day, with oral, lay and expert witness evidence being discouraged and the trial costs are fixed. Experts are limited to one per field and to two expert fields. It is expected that a single jointly instructed expert will be the norm. Experts are not required to attend unless the Court decides that it is necessary in the interests of justice bearing in mind the need to balance the cost of attendance against the value and complexity of the claim.

Multi-Track

For claims valued at more than £15 000. Only the larger Personal Injury and Clinical Negligence claims will fall within this track. The spirit of the pre-action protocols should still be followed, although they are not directly applicable. Clinical Negligence claims are likely to be placed in a specialist list. The timetable for the case will frequently be set at a 'case management conference' during which it is expected that the parties will reduce the areas of dispute as far as possible. Party instructed experts will probably be more common than in the fast track, although single joint experts will be preferred wherever possible.

It is possible for Claimants to limit their claims to £15 000 to keep within the fast track. A complicated claim worth less than £15 000 can be allocated to the multi track, but a simple claim worth more than £15 000 cannot be allocated to the fast track.

The Court may transfer a case between tracks on its own motion at any time.

Experts (CPR 35)

Consultants involved in medico-legal work should be familiar with CPR 35 and the Practice Direction which supplements it (see appendix to Chapter 2). Experts will need to become equally au fait with the draft Code of Guidance for Experts, which will ultimately be converted into a Practice Direction; breaches of it are expected to attract consequences more severe than would flow from a breach of protocol. It is likely to have wider significance than the existing protocols and relate to the use and actions of experts both *before* and *after* the issue of proceedings. The code seeks to promote best practice in the use of experts.

One of Lord Woolf's main concerns was the delay and unnecessary costs generated by the uncontrolled use of experts who had become increasingly partisan to the extent that in some cases there was doubt as to how much reliance a judge could place upon their evidence. The solution was to require an expert who reports to the Court to owe his primary and overriding duty to the Court rather than to the party instructing him or by whom he is being paid.

CPR 35 applies only to experts who have been instructed to report for the purpose of Court proceedings. An expert who is instructed to *advise* a prospective litigant on whether he has a claim is outside the remit of the CPR and in this advisory capacity owes a duty to the client. If the matter proceeds to litigation then the expert's overriding duty is to the Court. In practice the dividing line between these dual functions is not always clear. In certain circumstances the duty to the Court may arise before proceedings are issued, e.g. if a doctor is asked to prepare a condition and prognosis report to be served when a Personal Injury claim is subsequently issued.

CPR 35.1 empowers and imposes a duty on the Court to 'restrict expert evidence to that which is reasonably required to resolve the proceedings' and a party may not call an expert without the permission of the Court (CPR 35.4 (1)). Prior to obtaining the Court's permission there is no 'expert', although the respective parties may have been using 'advisors'. The Court may also limit the amount of the expert's fees that the party who wishes to rely on the expert evidence may recover from the other party, applying the 'overriding objective' principle. Where expert evidence is necessary the expert's overriding duty is 'to help the Court on the matters within his expertise' (CPR 35.3). This requirement has, in effect, statutory force.

The Court will consider three aspects:

a) whether expert evidence is necessary;
b) whether it can be given by a single joint expert; and
c) whether the cost is proportionate to the value of the claim.

Solicitors are likely to engage in more pre-instruction discussions with potential experts on whether a Court would consider their evidence is 'reasonably required' in a particular case. It may become necessary in the future for potential experts to explain the reasonable requirement for their input to the Court in writing or orally (Tinham 2000). In practice the CPR seeks to restrict the number of experts involved in a case and then imposes a clear duty on those who are used.

CPR 35.10 (1) requires the expert's report to comply with the specific requirements set out in the Practice Direction. Most importantly, at the end of his report the expert must include a statement that:

a) he understands his duty to the Court; and
b) he has complied with that duty (CPR 35.10(2)).

The expert's report must state the substance of all material instructions whether written or oral, on the basis of which the report is written (CPR 35.10(3)). This new transparency has caused solicitors to consider carefully the instructions they give and the documentation they provide to an expert as they may not wish to risk having to disclose privileged material to their opponent. Generally, it is better for solicitors to be completely frank with experts from the outset so that the expert is fully informed and is able to reach the correct view within his field of expertise as economically as possible. In effect, experts are now required to explain exactly what they have applied their expertise to. This should help to identify and resolve the expert issues early on (Phipps 2000). The Practice Direction, which must be read alongside CPR 35, prescribes the form and content of experts' reports. Experts are encouraged to restrict their report to cover only what is reasonably required to resolve the proceedings justly.

Experts may also have to answer questions clarifying their report from either party. The instructing party pays the experts' fees for responding to the questions. The responses will be treated as forming part of the report and should repeat the formal requirements that he understands his duty to the Court and has complied with that duty. A failure by the expert to co-operate will result in sanctions such as a party not being permitted to rely upon the expert's evidence or recover his fees and expenses from the other party. There is no direct sanction against the defaulting expert. We will have to see if solicitors or their clients can obtain redress from experts who let them down by such failures.

The Court has power to order that evidence on a particular issue be given by a single expert jointly instructed by the parties (CPR 35.7) and make specific orders in relation to the payment of his fees e.g. to be shared between the parties or paid into Court. This may lead to difficulty for the unfunded Claimant, but not for the insurance companies. In practice, funding arrangements are being developed to enable Claimants to borrow the costs of disbursements until the conclusion of their claims.

In a case where a single joint expert report has been obtained, which is unsatisfactory, in certain circumstances the Court may allow a party to instruct a further expert, e.g. in a case of substantial value (*Daniels v. Walker* [2000] 1 WLR 1382).

In cases where there are opposing experts the Court will frequently order a discussion (preferably by telephone) between experts to identify the issues and, where possible, reach agreement (CPR 35.12). This may also involve the preparation of a statement for the Court showing the areas of agreement and disagreement and the reasons for disagreement. The content of the discussion between the experts is not to be referred to at the Trial unless the parties agree. Similarly, any agreement reached

on an issue during expert discussions will not bind the parties unless they have specifically agreed to be bound by the agreement. It is difficult to see how this will work in practice after the experts' joint statement has already been submitted to the Court. Experts should ensure that they receive clear instructions of the issues to be discussed and how the meeting is to be conducted before taking part in these discussions (which are likely to become the norm). *Tactically, an expert should try to prepare the first draft of any statement of agreed and disputed issues for approval by his opponent.*

Experts now have a right (CPR 35.14) to make a written request to the Court (without notifying either party) for directions in circumstances where they encounter or foresee a particular difficulty in fulfilling their function and duty to the Court. The Court is likely to notify the parties of the directions made. A Court may be persuaded to order sequential (as opposed to simultaneous) disclosure of experts' reports if it would result in a saving of costs.

The Court also has power under CPR 35.15 to appoint an expert as an assessor to assist it to deal with a matter, but it is unlikely that this power will be relevant in a Personal Injury context.

Where there has been non-compliance with the CPR, Court orders, practice directions or pre-action protocols, the ultimate sanction is that the Court can disallow the use of expert evidence. The case of *Stevens v. Gullis* [2000 1 All ER 527] demonstrates the Court's willingness to deal severely with non-compliant experts by debarring a party from calling his expert evidence. In that case a Defendant's expert whose report did not comply with the CPR and who had failed to comply with various directions made by the Court was debarred from giving evidence with the consequence that judgement was entered for the Claimant. The Master of the Rolls commented that the expert witness in that case had 'demonstrated by his conduct that he had no concept of the requirements placed upon an expert under the CPR'. The Court is taking a similarly strict line on experts' availability to attend trial; it is only concerned with true unavailability e.g. because the expert is attending a trial elsewhere, rather than inconvenience. It is not sufficient for an expert to provide the Court with a list of unavailable dates without reasons. In some instances the Court has not accepted the reasons for an expert's unavailability to attend trial and has ordered the instruction of a fresh expert.

Consequently, potential and existing experts need to consider seriously whether they can truly give the commitment and energy now required by the more interactive civil litigation process before entering the arena of medico-legal practice.

Offers to Settle and Payments into Court (CPR 36)

Previously, only Defendants had the advantage of the very effective tactic of paying a sum into Court to settle the claim. Failure to recover more than that sum had significant costs consequences for the Claimant. A well-pitched and timed offer could often force a Claimant to settle at an undervalue or at the lower end of an acceptable band for settlement.

Although the CPR have not only maintained this mechanism for Defendants (Part 36 Payment) they have now introduced a reciprocal mechanism for Claimants in the form of a Part 36 Offer to Settle. The Court has the power to make adverse costs and interest orders against a party who fails to obtain a more beneficial result than has previously been offered provided the offer was made in accordance with the CPR. The benefit of a Part 36 Offer is that it puts the opposing party at risk as to costs if they reject the offer and do not achieve a better outcome. Such offers may well accompany a Claimant's Letter of Claim under the relevant pre-action protocol. Medical and other experts may be requested to provide further input on disputed issues at short notice (to comply with the strict time limits) to assist a party in deciding whether to accept or reject such an offer. The Part 36 Offer and counter-offer structure is proving to be of fundamental importance in the post-CPR approach to civil litigation. Experts should have it in mind at all stages and especially when discussing the case with the other side's expert.

Other Points to Consider in Relation to Medico-Legal Practice

Pre-issue Medical Report

It is still the requirement that any Personal Injury claim submitted to the Court must have a brief description of the injury and medical condition of the Claimant supported by a medical report which complies with the requirements of the CPR. This report need not be as detailed or final as the report which will be used at trial, indeed in many cases it may be a GP or preliminary Consultant's report which will have to be supplemented in due course by a more detailed document. However, sufficient detail should be made available so that Defendants can assess the nature and size of any claim.

Striking out

With the onset of judicial case management solicitors and indeed experts are under increased pressure to deliver within the strict timetables set.

Under CPR 24, 'summary judgement' may be given to either party if the opposing party has no real prospect of succeeding with their claim. Such orders may be granted by the Court on its own initiative or on the application of a party.

There are in addition a host of other sanctions (not to mention the various costs sanctions) e.g. striking out all or part of a Statement of Case if it discloses no reasonable ground for bringing or defending a claim and striking out for failure to pay Court fees by their due date. The sanctions at the disposal of the Court are potentially draconian and it will take some time before the implications of the new regime are fully worked through.

Split trials

Judicial case management favours 'split Trials' where liability is dealt with separately and in advance of establishing the value ('quantum') of the claim if the medical position remains uncertain when other matters are ready for Trial. In most cases quantum can subsequently be negotiated or the costs of dealing with complex quantum can be avoided if liability is not established, e.g. in Clinical Negligence cerebral palsy claims. If liability is established the Defendant will have lost the opportunity to negotiate a discount on quantum on the basis of litigation risk.

Alternative Dispute Resolution (ADR)

Personal Injury lawyers have been required to consider alternative means of resolving disputes since 1995. The ADR Practice Direction and the Woolf reforms are likely to encourage more of these types of settlement.

The Court encourages the use of ADR and in general a less adversarial approach. The Allocation Questionnaires filed as soon as a Defence is filed specifically require the parties to tell the Court whether they have considered ADR. In Personal Injury and Clinical Negligence claims mediation is the most likely form of ADR in this country.

Mediation

This is the process whereby the parties to a dispute appoint a neutral person to mediate between them to assist them to reach a solution that they can both accept. The procedure is 'facilitative' if the mediator is not expected to advise the parties of his own views on the merits of the dispute. It is 'evaluative' if the mediator is expected to express his view.

Mediations may take several forms but there are certain common features:

a) The mediator is a trained but entirely independent person.
b) Neither party is bound by anything said in the mediation, except if agreement is reached at the end of the day, written down and signed by both parties.
c) To be effective a mediator requires that each party brings its full decision-making team e.g. experts, spouse etc. in order that a conclusion can be reached on the day.
d) The matter must have reached such a stage that settlement is possible and mediation appropriate. Often this will be after initial negotiations have failed.

It is a term of the mediation that the mediator cannot be called as a witness in any subsequent proceedings in the event that no settlement is achieved.

Mediation can be used for disputes involving any number of parties, and is appropriate in a wide variety of matters including personal injury. Because any settlement reached is tailored to the particular needs of the parties it is likely to be especially attractive where there is a continuing relationship between them, e.g. employer/employee situations. The parties also have the opportunity to incorporate issues that would not be legally enforceable e.g. an apology.

Written medico-legal reports are crucial in any Personal Injury mediation. However, personal attendance of the medical or care advisor may also be appropriate in more serious cases, particularly those involving long-term care.

Community Legal Service

Public funding of civil claims was severely curtailed from 1st April 2000. The Community Legal Service (CLS) replaced the Legal Aid scheme and the Legal Services Commission took over from the Legal Aid Board. The rules on obtaining assistance were made more stringent in an effort to restrict eligibility. A costs benefits matrix is applied to new applications which takes into account the chances of success and the likely benefit as well as an estimate of costs to be incurred. Clinical negligence claims may receive CLS funding to cover the cost at least of obtaining initial expert medical reports to determine whether there is a reasonable claim worth pursuing.

Conditional fee arrangements 'no win, no fee'

Conditional Fee Agreements (CFAs) have become an increasingly common method of funding Personal Injury litigation given the very limited circumstances in which public funding is now available. These permit a Claimant's solicitor to agree with a client that he or she will not be charged unless the case is won and to increase the fees which would normally be charged by up to 100% (the success fee) depending on the estimated prospects of success in a particular case. Both solicitors and barristers alike are prepared in appropriate cases to pursue claims for Claimants on this basis. From 1st April 2000 a successful Claimant is permitted to recover the success fee as part of his costs from the Defendant provided the first agreement entered into was signed after that date. Similarly, indemnity insurance premiums are recoverable in respect of policies issued after that date to insure against the risk of having to meet any proportion of the Defendant's costs.

Claimants who have the benefit of appropriate Legal Expenses Insurance (LEI) taken out before the accident will not require a CFA.

Should experts also be subject to payment by results?

The debate rumbles on as to whether experts should put their money where their opinion is. It has been argued that many experts are already offering free screening services for prospective litigants and therefore a no win, no fee service is the next logical step. The concern is that if an expert were to have a financial interest in the claim being won, this might undermine his independence. The counter-argument is that if an expert believes in his case he can maintain his primary duty to the Court. The Draft Code of Guidance for Experts under the CPR clearly prohibits payment to experts being conditional on the outcome of the case (McConnell 1999). Experts have, therefore, escaped the new conditional fee environment for the moment at least. However, in practice, a number of experts (including medical practitioners) have made such agreements. There is nothing to prevent experts who are acting in an 'advisory' (shadow expert) role from entering into alternative funding arrangements with solicitors for 'pre-expert appointment' work such as advising on whether expert evidence is reasonably required, identifying expert issues, assisting with case plans, statements of case, calculation of quantum and consideration of Part 36 Offers.

In certain situations a solicitor may still require 'advisory' expert input after the appointment of a single joint expert (e.g. if he is not satisfied with the joint expert) to assess the joint report, draft questions, assist with cross-examination, and consider Part 36 Offers, but if an 'advisor' is to become an 'expert' fresh instructions should be issued to clarify the new appointment. This may be at the stage when Court proceedings are issued or where a party is allowed to obtain a further opinion because he/she is unhappy with the opinion of a single joint expert.

Advisors' costs are usually recoverable if specifically approved by the Court or if they relate to advice provided prior to the appointment of an expert. It may legitimately be argued that the costs of advisory work which requires specialist skills that the lawyer may not have (e.g. analysing medical records) and which can be provided more cheaply by an appropriate advisor should be recoverable as part of the solicitor's disbursements if this work is contracted out and not duplicated by the solicitor. Such advisory work could also be undertaken on a CFA basis (Makin 2000).

Road Traffic Cases

With the increasing activity in the market and the inability (or reluctance) of accident victims to pay for various services up front and then seek indemnity, it is increasingly common for various services to be provided on credit, subject to the accident victim agreeing to include the cost in his claim against the other party's insurer.

The effectiveness of credit replacement car hire has itself been the subject of voluminous satellite litigation.

The Compensation Recovery Unit (CRU) of the Department of Social Security is also active on behalf of National Health Service Trusts in recovering treatment costs under the Road Traffic (NHS Charges) Act 1999 from Defendant insurers. The maximum amounts payable are £354 for an outpatient and £10 000 for an inpatient.

Credit medical reports

Increasingly Road Traffic and Personal Injury claims are being handled by either specialist solicitors' firms or solicitors' firms with specialist departments. Claims are frequently referred to them by motoring organisations, legal expense insurers and the like. Extensive use is made of computerised case management systems. The standard letters and responses under the pre-action protocols assist with this.

This undoubtedly leads to greater efficiency and an improved ability to monitor cases against the rigorous time limits imposed under the pre-action protocols and the CPR discussed above. However, solicitors are likely to build up substantial disbursement accounts in paying medical and other experts as the solicitor is not paid until the matter is concluded.

Coupled with the difficulties experienced in receiving timely reports, this has led to the development of arrangements whereby solicitors offer consultants a volume of referrals in exchange for agreement by the consultant to provide reports within specified times and to accept payment deferred to the conclusion of the case.

Credit medical treatment and rehabilitation

A number of solicitors are already entering into arrangements with physiotherapists and others for private treatment to be given to accident victims on a credit basis. If this is of interest to experts then an approach to one of their local specialist firms might be worthwhile. Additionally, national networks are developing to facilitate such referrals. The emphasis in the future will be on rehabilitation of the accident victim from the outset through to long-term care regimes where necessary.

For insurers this is a means of 'managing claim costs via playing a socially responsible, but economically viable, role in the compensation of the claimant' (Burtonshaw 2000). For Claimants' solicitors it represents a more complete and extended service over and above maximising damages. In serious cases this will require the appointment of a 'case manager' outside the litigation process probably a medical generalist (not an expert witness) who will assess the individual's needs and facilitate the rehabilitation process. Currently, such arrangements are in the embryonic stages, but they represent a welcome change in philosophy which many Claimants' solicitors have been pioneering for some time. A Code of Best Practice on Rehabilitation, Early Intervention and Medical Treatment in Personal Injury Claims has been agreed by a number of interested groups. Hence, there is clearly a place for timely medical intervention of various sorts depending on the nature and severity of the injury.

Charging for reports

It appears that consultants (and the agencies referring work to them) currently charge fees on the basis of 'what the market will bear', and get away with it. However, this is likely to come under increasing scrutiny in the future under the principle of 'proportionality'.

Costs (CPR 43–48)

In the CPR culture the Court is particularly proactive on the issue of costs, which are assessed at interlocutory hearings and at the end of a trial. Accurate assessments of past costs and the estimated costs of proceeding are requested from the parties at the Allocation and Listing Questionnaires stages respectively.

Costs have always been in the discretion of the Court. However, the CPR now require the Court to take into consideration matters such as the conduct of the parties (including compliance with the pre-action protocols) and the question of 'proportionality' (the amount of costs incurred in relation to the value of the claim). Excessively adversarial behaviour will no longer be tolerated and is likely to result in costs penalties, possibly against the solicitor personally. Whether a costs order can be made against an expert who has behaved unreasonably or failed to comply with an order of the Court is currently undecided. The Court will not allow costs that have been unreasonably incurred or are unreasonable in amount. The general rule remains that the loser pays the winner's costs but the Court may make a different order. In short, the Court has complete discretion as to whether costs are payable and by whom, the amount and when they are to be paid. It is important to note that a winning party who exaggerated his claim (or whose expert has been over optimistic) may be penalised in costs. Additionally, if no order for costs is made none will be recoverable!

Detailed assessment (which replaces taxation) will follow an order by the Court that the losing party pays the winner's costs (or some variation on this).

The solicitors for both parties will try to agree the costs to be paid. The calculation is based on how many hours have been spent on the matter, with untimed telephone calls and ordinary letters out being allowed at 6 minutes each. An hourly rate is applied based on the rate allowed in the local Court. This will vary according to the qualification and experience/grade of the fee earner concerned. VAT and 'disbursements' are then added.

A costs schedule for possible agreement might look as follows:

Time spent	7 h 30 min at £125 per hour	937.50
Letters out	50 at £12.50	625.00
Telephone Calls	20 at £12.50	250.00
Total		1812.50
VAT		317.19
Medical Reports		
Mr Bloggs (Orthopaedic)		400.00
Dr Smith (GP)		150.00
Court Fees		400.00
TOTAL		£2,762.50
VAT		317.19
GRAND TOTAL		£3,079.69

If agreement on these fees cannot be negotiated then the payee solicitor will send his papers to a costs draftsman who will prepare a detailed bill of costs, frequently many pages long, itemising all the work done by way of a general narrative and in the specific. If the parties still fail to agree costs the payee solicitor must commence the detailed assessment of costs procedure and both parties must comply with the prescribed timetable. This course of action is likely to remain as uneconomic and as much loathed as the previous taxation procedure, with solicitors thus aiming to resolve costs wherever possible, before resorting to the procedure. The extension of fixed costs remains under consideration.

The CPR's strong reliance on costs sanctions coupled with the apparent downward pressure on costs being exerted by the Lord Chancellor highlights the following issues:

a) If a medico-legal expert is paid when the report is submitted, his fee may subsequently be challenged on detailed assessment. The Court may request the solicitor to obtain from the expert a justification of his fees, possibly by way of a summary of his overheads in preparing the report plus his 'profit' element. Solicitors charging rates, on the other hand, are set by the local Court on an informal annual basis. There seems to be nothing similar for the medical profession, and the BMA and Law Society have agreed that experts' fees should not be subject to any reasonableness test.

b) However, if the expert's fee is reduced on detailed assessment, is it right that the expert accepts the reduction and repays the solicitor, or should the solicitor have to bear the financial burden of the shortfall? The current position seems to overlook the central role that experts now play.

c) The use of a jointly selected or single joint expert, or alternatively the requirement that experts meet to minimise their areas of disagreement, will mean that the attendance of experts at Court will become a rarity in all but the most difficult cases. However, it is still sensible for experts to reach agreement with their instructing solicitors well in advance of trial as to what will happen if the case is settled after the expert is booked to attend a trial. This is best done by the expert clearly detailing this in his terms of business at the time of accepting the original instructions for the report. In particular this will give the instructing solicitors the opportunity of warning their opponents of the potential costs of reaching a settlement late in the day.

What is a reasonable charge may well depend on the nature of the expert's practice. It may be that 50% of the attendance fee if the settlement is notified within 30 days of the hearing and 100% if it is notified within 7 days is reasonable. However, the expert should appreciate that recovery of this fee by his instructing solicitor will be subject to the Court's approval.

It is almost certain that experts' fees will be reduced in the new CPR regime. Specifically, CPR 35.4(4) empowers the Court to limit the amount a party may recover from any other party in respect of an expert's fees. So, in fast track cases the number of experts and their fees will be closely scrutinised and the principle of 'proportionality' is likely to be rigorously adopted.

From the Judges

Most Personal Injury claims have their legal basis in the tort of negligence, the essence of which is that:

a) The Defendant owed the Claimant a duty of care.
b) The Defendant acted in breach of that duty of care.
c) The Claimant sustained injuries and/or losses as a consequence of that breach.

Particular controversy and debate has arisen in relation to psychiatric injuries following accidents. Judges seem to have been concerned to stem a flood of claims from claimants ever more distant from the original incident.

However, it has now been confirmed that if a person is involved in an accident and suffers a *recognised psychiatric injury* as a result, then a claim can be mounted for those non-physical injuries whether or not there has also been a physical injury. This is to be contrasted with the situation of someone who may witness the accident and may have no claim even if his symptoms are identical.

- *Question.* Can compensation be claimed for shock and stress if no actual physical injury has also been suffered by a road traffic accident victim?
- *Answer.* The Courts are clear that an injured party cannot claim damages for suffering stress as the result of an accident. There must be a 'recognisable psychiatric injury'. However, such a claim for non-physical injuries can succeed in the absence of any physical injury.

- *Question.* Can a claim for 'nervous shock' be sustained?
- *Answer.* In practice, the general view is that this must amount to post-traumatic stress syndrome, i.e. a diagnosable state lasting for more than a month after the incident. However, the view is now becoming more prevalent that a claim can be mounted based either on 'phobic travel anxiety' or 'acute stress disorder', i.e.

diagnosable stress but lasting for less than a month. Solicitors seeing victims immediately after an accident should therefore make an enquiry of them not only as to their physical but also their mental condition and this should also be researched in some depth when later reports are prepared.

- *Question.* Can a claim be made by a person not directly involved in the incident?
- *Answer.* If a person is physically present at the scene of an accident or its immediate aftermath and sees their spouse, parent, child or close friend being harmed or endangered, and suffers significant long-term symptoms from this experience, a claim may be possible. However, the litigation following the Hillsborough disaster made it clear that the Courts are anxious to restrict the circumstances in which this kind of claim is brought. In particular it is now doubtful whether seeing any such scene on the television, knowing that your loved ones were in the crowd and then discovering they had been killed, is sufficient. It is probably necessary to either see or hear the incident or its immediate aftermath.

The balance of probabilities

It is well known that the standard of proof in civil cases is the 'balance of probabilities'. What was not so well known or understood was how this test was applied in practice.

In one case it was alleged that an anaesthetist had been negligent during an operation and that this had caused serious damage to a child. The case was defended. The Court was asked to consider, as a preliminary matter, how the case would be approached. In particular, would the Court award damages in proportion to the percentage chance that the child's condition had been caused by the doctor's alleged negligence, i.e. if there was a 40% probability that the doctor was to blame then would the child receive 40% of the full value of his condition? The answer was no. If it were the case that, on the balance of probabilities (i.e. a greater than 50% likelihood), the condition had been caused by the doctor's alleged negligence then the Defendant would have to pay full compensation for the child's injuries. On the other hand if such likelihood could not be made out then the child would receive nothing.

Medico-legal experts are pressed by solicitors to give an opinion on whether it is *probable* that 'such and such' has been caused by the accident or may occur in the future. This case explains why.

It may be helpful to give one or two examples of phrases which are *unhelpful* in establishing the legal test of the 'balance of probability' and so are to be avoided in good medico-legal reporting:

Had the accident not happened the pre-existing condition *might* have remained symptomless for some time.'

As this patient has not returned to my surgery since his initial visit I think we can assume that his whiplash injury was mild in extent and cleared up after a few days.

Rather more helpful are:

Of course it is not possible to be certain in such matters but I believe that the pre-existing condition would *probably* have remained symptomless for a further 2 or 3 years had it not been for the accident.

My best assessment is that *60%* of the continuing symptoms are attributable to the accident and the remainder to the pre-existing condition.

Whilst the accident undoubtedly caused an initial injury the continuing symptoms are *more likely than not* entirely due to the low standard of medical care which this patient subsequently received.

Criticising other medical practitioners

Whether or not one criticises a fellow professional has been a bone of contention for many years. Clearly one should do this only if one is relatively certain that such criticism is justified. But if one is certain, does one have a duty to the patient who has been injured, or is this outweighed by a number of factors and in particular the following?

a) It is ungentlemanly to criticise a fellow member of the profession.
b) In America such criticism is so 'normal' and the costs of the resulting litigation so great that the very availability of professional services is being put at risk.
c) Professional insurance for the medical profession is rising as a result of professional negligence claims, now averaging at about 1 or 2% of fee income. The cost of clinical negligence claims to the NHS is similarly rising.
d) 'Everybody knows' that the members of all professions look after their own.

Whether any such reasons make it right or not, to comment on shoddy workmanship which has damaged someone is of course a matter for the individual consultant. Insofar as lawyers have any right to comment the following ethical framework offers a comparison:

a) A duty to the Court
b) A duty to our client
c) A duty to our pocket

There is no duty to fellow solicitors.

Structured settlements

In more serious cases it is now relatively common for the Claimant to receive part of his compensation from the Defendant in periodic instalments during the remainder of his life, designed to meet specific needs at certain times in the future e.g. care costs. Such payments are usually index-linked and can be for a guaranteed minimum period or deferred for a period. They are self-funded by some Defendants e.g. the NHS or alternatively an annuity is purchased. The Courts sanction and indeed frequently encourage such voluntary arrangements, which can be tailored to suit the individual Claimant. The Courts will not impose such an arrangement on the parties but the practice has grown up for a trial Judge to indicate his likely decision and then adjourn to allow the parties to investigate whether a structure would be acceptable and if so on what terms.

In the past large lump sums have, in some cases, been spent unwisely by Claimants and their families, resulting in the Claimant becoming dependent on state benefit. A structured settlement avoids this problem. The periodic payments are treated as repayment of capital and are therefore tax-free.

The principal disadvantage of these types of arrangements is that they are inflexible once set up.

Conditional Settlement

Circumstances occasionally arise where there is the *possibility* of a catastrophic future event, but no way of predicting whether or not it *will* happen, for instance a substantial risk that epilepsy will develop in later life. In such cases the Court will contemplate making a 'Conditional' award which permits the Claimant to come back for a further payment if and when that catastrophic event occurs.

The Courts have made it clear that they will make such an award only in exceptional cases. Thus where, for instance, there is damage to a hip with probable substantial deterioration in the future then that probability, together with the costs of operations etc. will be factored into a single final award made on judgment.

It is thus essential that future prospects and their financial implications, together with the probability of their occurrence, are fully explored in the medical and other evidence available to the Court at trial.

■ Summary

Information technology, strict costs controls and effective training will feature prominently in the resolution of disputes in the new Woolf era. The implementation of the Human Rights Act 1998, which embodies the unqualified right to a fair trial, will also impact on the powers of the Court and in particular, its prerogative to restrict the right of an individual to call an expert witness of his choice or to limit the right to an oral hearing.

Conclusion

The rules governing the instruction and conduct of medico-legal experts are in a state of rapid change. Do not be embarrassed to ask your instructing solicitor if you are unclear on any point. Equally, do not be surprised if he or she cannot give a definitive answer!

References

Burtonshaw A 2000 The rehabilitation process as facilitated by case management – a view from the insurance industry. Association of Personal Injury Lawyers Newsletter Vol 10 Issue 1 February 2000

Makin C 2000 Will we ever see conditional fees for experts? Solicitors Journal Vol 144 No 1 14th January 2000 10–11

McConnell B 1999 No Win, No Fee, No Way. New Law Journal 26 November 1999 1760

Phipps C 2000 Being Frank with Experts. Solicitors Journal Vol 144 No 4 4 February 2000:90–91

Tinham A 2000 Expert Evidence: Use of the Single Joint Expert, Dual Experts, and Expert Advisors. The Personal and Medical Injuries Law Letter Vol 16 No 2 February 2000:7–9

The orthopaedic surgeon in court

David K. Evans

Introduction

Most orthopaedic surgeons do not like appearing in Court. There is a natural reluctance to be cross-examined on one's opinions, especially if there are deficiencies exposed, and more especially since one is on the stage as an 'expert' witness. There is some consolation in knowing that few actions are contested on questions of fact, and most well-informed orthopaedic surgeons will agree on the facts. The problems in Court arise when the case is fought on matters of opinion. There is a natural reluctance to disagree with one's colleagues openly in public, although there is no reticence in disagreeing with them in a closed orthopaedic meeting, or in private. It is helpful to remember that the Court wants to know one's opinion based on one's experience, and that one is there to help the Judge arrive at a conclusion. In many cases there is no question of black or white or right and wrong, but the question is decided on 'the balance of probabilities'.

In essence, the Court will want to know the orthopaedic surgeon's opinion on:

1 whether it is more likely than not that the accident as described produced the injuries;
2. whether recovery was as expected from such injuries;
3. the degree of disability remaining for everyday activities, for work activity, and for the patient's leisure pursuits;
4. the possibility of disability worsening in the future and the effect such worsening will have on working ability;
5. the possibility of a future surgical intervention; and
6. whether the patient will become physically dependent on mechanical aids, and in most serious cases whether he will require re-housing.

The new court procedure rules

Since April 1999 the changes in Civil Procedure Rules (CPR) suggest that only one jointly agreed orthopaedic expert will be instructed in a case if the value of the case is less than £15 000 and it has been routed onto the fast track.

Under CPR the duty of the expert is to the Court. Any other obligations are overridden, including those to the party issuing instructions and funding the report. Either party in the action is able to ask written questions of the expert (in effect a written cross-examination), and this correspondence is open between the parties and the Court. The fast track timetable is fixed, and it is expected that only rarely in such cases will the expert be required to attend Court to give oral evidence. Fewer medical reports will thus be required, and possibly fewer Court appearance will be necessary. It has to be said, however, that most low value cases were usually settled out of Court in any event, although CPR should despatch these cases expeditiously. The rules should certainly result in abolishing cases settled at the door of the Court (often following an irritating delay of several hours while the Barristers negotiated). Claims of more than £15 000 will be subject to Court Management. If they are of considerable value and of some complexity it is likely that two experts will still be required, especially if the facts of the case allow differences of interpretation. This may well apply in medical negligence cases. Nevertheless, there is likely to be much more correspondence between experts and representatives from both sides. Conferences between experts too will become commoner so that areas of agreement and disagreement can be narrowed, and a compromise solution perhaps agreed. If the case still goes to Trial, the Trial time is likely to be considerably reduced as a result of the preliminary ground work.

It is important to recognise if the case does proceed to a Hearing the examination and cross-examination may be restricted to the area of disagreement between the experts. It is essential, therefore, that any agreed joint report between the experts should detail at some length the evidence leading to the difference in views.

Planning ahead for a Court case

In the author's experience, solicitors will go out of their way not to inconvenience the doctor. In most cases a date suitable for all parties is arranged. Sometimes, however, the Court itself will fix a date, and only the surgeon's absence out of the country will be taken as a valid excuse to change it. It is usual practice for the surgeon to be subpoenaed to attend. This may seem unnecessary if the surgeon has agreed to attend Court on a particular day, but it safeguards the surgeon's solicitor from being overruled by a second solicitor with a case on the same day who does serve the surgeon with a subpoena, thus negating any verbal contract.

If the orthopaedic surgeon has no NHS commitments there is usually no difficulty in arranging to attend Court although he may have to cancel a day's medico-legal consulting. Difficulties do arise when the expert witness is in active NHS practice. Understandably, the NHS Trust Administrators are not anxious to lose the services of a consultant for a day. It is the author's belief that medico-legal reporting is a private activity, and, although allowed to take place in hospital buildings, should be done at the end of the working day, at lunch time, or at the weekends. Similarly, attendance at Court is a private activity. If a consultant is warned to attend Court, then he should apply for a day's annual leave. If the case is settled, the request for leave can always be withdrawn. The loss of holiday for the average orthopaedic surgeon will not be very great. In this author's practice Court bookings prior to 1999 averaged about 7.5% of the total number of reports done in any year. Of that 7.5%, less than one in five actually reached a hearing in Court, the rest being settled.

It is doubtful whether the average orthopaedic surgeon in NHS practice would be attending Court more than three or four times a year and this number may well reduce with the new rules. Nevertheless, the four out of five cases which are settled are still a great nuisance, since settlement is often reached only a few days before the hearing. Ideally, a thorough work-up of the case involving solicitors, barristers and witnesses should be possible even before a hearing date is fixed. The increasingly common practice of arranging a conference between these parties is to be applauded. In a complicated case the issues can be clarified and counsel can be briefed at length on the points of medical dispute. In cases of medical negligence, particularly, such a conference is often crucial. Frequently a reluctant doctor can be persuaded that he is in the wrong, and thus avoids an embarrassing Court appearance. Similarly, the reasons why the case should be defended can be gone into in detail over two or three hours rather than in half an hour at the door of the Court.

Should the orthopaedic surgeon be compensated for the late cancellation of a Court fixture? This obviously depends on what loss has been sustained. If the surgeon has already been granted annual leave for a day to attend Court and his appointments and operating lists have been cancelled, then it is surely fair that he be given compensation for the loss of a day of yearly entitlement. If he has had to cancel a session of private consultations, he may well lose those patients, and again should be compen-

sated. If, however, the expert witness is not in active NHS practice, then usually there is no financial loss as a rule. If booked for a two day case, which is concluded at the end of day one, however, there is little he can do to arrange consultations for the following day.

Whatever the circumstances of the expert, if a case is cancelled within 48 hours of the fixture, then he will usually have spent some time in preparing the case and going through the documents and often the literature. A fee for half a day, under such circumstances, would be reasonable.

The amount of fees for Court attendances are a continual source of worry. Many, if not most, lawyers charge fees on an hourly basis, and one would think it reasonable for medical experts to charge for attendance at Court on such a basis also. An hourly rate equal to that which one would expect to earn in a private consulting session would be appropriate.

Preparing for a Court appearance

As with every other public appearance, thorough preparation is important. Preparation to attend Court begins with the initial medical report. The agreement to write a report implies an undertaking to attend Court if necessary, and the basis of the orthopaedic surgeon's evidence in Court is the medical report or reports. It should go without saying that his opinion should be quite unbiased. Indeed the new rules emphasise that his prime duty is to the Court and not to his instructing solicitors. The surgeon's opinion should reflect his views honestly and it follows that it would be the same opinion whichever side was instructing him. Do not hesitate to state honest views, even if they should seem adverse and disappointing to the instructing solicitor, for such views will save the solicitor and his client a great deal of time and money. If medical negligence is alleged, and it is the expert's view that negligence has occurred, then he should say so. The acceptance of liability by the Defendants and the settlement of the action often saves a great deal of money by avoiding a lengthy Court hearing. On the other hand if there is no justification for claiming negligence then not only will the patient be saved the expense and trouble in pursuing a hopeless case, but if the surgeon's arguments are clear and understandable they may reassure the patient and set his mind at rest.

Preparation of the Barrister by the medical expert is an essential part of preparation for Court. Although the Barrister has probably appeared in Court fighting many similar cases, he is still grateful for guidance on the relevant anatomy, the meaning of physical signs, and the interpretation of imaging investigations. The surgeon should be sure the Barrister understands his views.

Before going to Court the expert must prepare his evidence. He must read and re-read his reports and those of the opposition. If it is a considerable time since he examined the patient he might suggest to the solicitor that he see the patient again and to bring his evidence up-to-date. He should put himself in the position of the opposing barrister, and examine his report for areas where cross-examination is likely. This is the time to back up his opinions with facts from the literature. It is often useful to take original articles or reprints to Court, and let the Barrister know what the facts are. It is best to let him bring these facts out in evidence if he so wishes.

It is important to review the evidence of the opponent. Areas where there is a difference of opinion should be identified. The expert's Barrister will almost certainly have noticed them, but he will want to know why there is a difference. The expert should confirm that his medical opponent is qualified to give an expert opinion on the case in question. Surprisingly, it is still possible for an opponent to be a specialist in a field which is not orthopaedics. This author has recently been involved in a case which went to trial and in which the opponent was a consultant neurologist. The ensuing argument was about a man with back pain who had no radiating pain and no neurological symptoms or signs! It is not unfair to point out to one's Barrister that such a consultant probably has little experience of the treatment and follow-up of such cases.

It is essential also to become completely familiar with the medical records. Both those from the hospital and the general practitioner should be carefully gone through. Memorise timing and detail of the important events. The surgeon should aim at being more conversant with the medical details of the case than his Barrister (although he will find that this is often difficult!).

Giving evidence

If the evidence cannot be agreed, then the case must be fought in Court. If the case turns on the medical evidence, then this evidence is taken early in the case immediately after the Plaintiff has been in the witness box. If the expert has been instructed by the Plaintiff's solicitors then he will be asked to give his evidence before his opponent. This gives the opponent the advantage of considering the strength of the expert's case, and the emphasis the expert's Barrister places on certain parts of the report. The expert for the Defence will then enter the witness box. The orthopaedic surgeon should remain in Court to hear his opponent's evidence, and to advise his counsel should there be a disagreement or a weakness which should be challenged.

The expert's evidence should be given clearly and audibly, so that the Judge and lawyers are in no doubt of his words. He should speak slowly, and address his remarks to the Judge. He should note whether the Judge is recording his evidence in long hand, or whether it is taped. If he is writing, the expert should slow his delivery to the Judge's speed of writing.

The expert's Barrister will concentrate on the report and may clarify and expand on it to reinforce his case. The surgeon should answer questions clearly and digress only to explain medical facts which have not been clearly stated. Reasons should be given for the views expressed. The opposing Barrister, when cross-examining, will question the expert's views and put forward views that are helpful to his own client's case. He will attempt to make the expert modify his opinion and suggest he is not as emphatic as appears in his written report. Such an approach may irritate, but the surgeon should not get upset. Consider replies, remain courteous, and if views are firmly held, as they should be at this stage, the surgeon should continue to press them and give reasons why the views proposed by the opposing Barrister are likely to be incorrect. Although cross-examination may be persistent and relentless, the expert will find that, as a rule, he will be treated courteously. Even though his pride may be a little hurt that he seems to be disbelieved, he should not lose his temper. The expert can influence the Judge only by remaining confident and unruffled, and that can be achieved only by a thorough preparation of the case, so that the expert has all the facts clearly in mind. He should never forget that he is there to help the Court reach a just verdict, and he is giving an honest and unbiased opinion.

Summary

- The amount of litigation involving orthopaedic surgeons as expert witnesses has increased but, nevertheless, 98% of accident cases do not reach Court.
- Simple fracture cases are usually straightforward, but those involving soft tissue and spinal injuries can be more contentious.
- The surgeon's opinion will be elicited on: whether the accident as described produced the injuries; whether recovery was as would be expected; the degree of disability remaining and whether the condition is likely to deteriorate; any further surgical intervention; and the effects on working capacity and life expectancy.

- The duty of an expert is to the Court and not to the instructing solicitors.
- The initial medical report, which is the basis of preparation for a Court appearance, should be unbiased and based on the Plaintiff's history, physical signs and symptoms and the surgeon's experience of similar cases.
- An exchange of medical reports between opposing sides can lead to agreement being reached by correspondence and may obviate the need for a Court appearance, as can a preliminary conference among solicitors, Barristers and expert witnesses.

- The Barrister will welcome guidance as to the correct interpretation of medical evidence from both sides in the case.
- Attendance at Court can present problems for surgeons with NHS commitments and may necessitate application for leave. Subsequent late cancellation of the Court fixture can raise the question of compensation. A personal view of fees for Court attendances is offered.
- When giving evidence in Court the expert should not forget that he is there to help the Judge. He should not allow himself to be bullied by the Barrister. He should not lose his temper.

Section 2

Results following upper limb fractures

The shoulder

Phillip S. Fagg

Sternoclavicular joint

Introduction

Sternoclavicular joint injuries are not common. Rowe & Marble (1958) found 10 injuries to the sternoclavicular joint in their analysis of 1603 shoulder-girdle injuries (0.6%). Only one of these cases was of a retrosternal dislocation of the sternoclavicular joint (0.06%).

Injuries of the sternoclavicular joint may be classified as follows:

- grade I—minor sprains and contusions
- grade II—subluxations, usually anterior
- grade III—complete dislocations, anterior or retrosternal
- grade IV—recurrent dislocation

Results of treatment

Grade I and II injuries

A grade I injury or sprain of the sternoclavicular joint results from a mild medially directed force applied to the lateral aspect of the involved shoulder or from the shoulder being suddenly forced forward. The ligaments remain intact. Treatment is symptomatic with a forearm sling and no long-term sequelae are expected. The patient would be expected to use the arm for everyday activities after 5–7 days (Rockwood 1991).

In the grade II injury or subluxation of the sternoclavicular joint there is rupture of the sternoclavicular ligaments and the intra-articular disc, but the continuity of the costoclavicular ligaments is maintained. There is little in the literature on the prognosis for these injuries, but generally it is good following conservative treatment. This was confirmed by Ferrandez et al (1988), who reported the results in six patients treated for 3 weeks in a sling. All six had excellent results in terms of pain, mobility and resumption of work, although 'slight deformity', of no clinical or cosmetic significance, was sometimes detectable. But while the results are generally good, Pierce (1979) described four examples of internal derangement of the intra-articular disc as a result of indirect trauma unassociated with frank dislocation. These patients complained of persistent tenderness, swelling and a clicking sensation over the joint. Surgery was required in each case, and in one patient who underwent surgery 8 years after the initial injury some degenerative changes were present in the joint. All these patients became asymptomatic with a full range of motion after surgery.

Grade III injuries: anterior dislocation

Anterior dislocations of the sternoclavicular joint are approximately 10 times more common than posterior dislocations. Not all of these dislocations are due to ligamentous and meniscal damage alone. Omer (1967) found an intra-articular subchondral clavicular fracture in all four of his patients who underwent clavicular osteotomy for the surgical reduction of their dislocation. All four had a stable reduction without recurrent dislocation, although one patient developed arthritic symptoms 2 years after the injury. Denham & Dingley (1967) described epiphyseal separation of the medial end of the clavicle in three patients: reduction was stable in all three. They pointed out that the medial epiphysis of the clavicle was only a few millimetres thick, did not ossify until age 18 and may not unite with the metaphysis until the age of 22–25 years.

The treatment of acute anterior dislocation of the sternoclavicular joint is by closed or open procedures. De Jong & Kaulesar Sukul (1990) reported that non-operative management was the treatment of choice in anterior sternoclavicular dislocations. Of the 10 patients followed up for a mean period of over 5 years and assessed by the scoring method of Eskola et al (1989), seven patients had a good result, two had a fair result and one patient had a poor result. Limitations of shoulder function were minimal and mostly due to other associated injuries. Eskola (1986), however, reported that five of his eight patients treated by closed reduction redislocated, and in three of these five patients the joint was painful. The range of motion of the shoulder joint was normal in all patients. He made a plea for primary open reduction in acute sternoclavicular dislocation as the treatment of choice. Rockwood et al (1997), however, have emphasised that they do not recommend open reduction of the sternoclavicular joint for anterior dislocation. They believe that open reduction of an unstable anterior dislocation is justified only for patients who continue to have severe pain and marked functional impairment.

Many surgical procedures have been advocated for what is in effect a relatively rare condition. These include the use of fascial loops, subclavius tenodesis, clavicular osteotomy or use of the sternomastoid muscle to reinforce the anterior capsule. There are insufficient cases reported fully to appraise the benefits of each particular procedure, but the four reported by Eskola (1986), in which either the ligaments and capsule were sutured or a tendon graft performed with Kirschner wires for fixation, all had a good result. Ferrandez et al (1988) reported seven cases of anterior dislocation treated by open reduction and Kirschner wire fixation. No patient had pain but one did have a slight loss of shoulder motion (10° limitation of rotation and 30° loss of abduction). Four of their patients had a 'slight deformity' on the affected site, and six resumed work. In two patients mediastinal migration of Kirschner wires occurred, but was of no clinical significance.

Complications from transfixing pins running from the clavicle to the sternum to reinforce some of the above procedures have often been reported. Brown (1961) noted a 30% complication rate in 10 cases of transfixing wires, including wire breakage and penetration of the pulmonary artery. However, despite these grave complications he felt that in view of the stable reduction achieved, the method was justified! Clark et al (1974) reported a case of fatal perforation of the aorta and reviewed three previous cases of perforation of the major vessels and trachea. The use of Kirschner wires, Steinmans pins, or any other type of metallic pins to stabilise the sternoclavicular joint has been condemned by Rockwood (1991).

While the functional results following reduction are generally good, recurrent dislocation is not uncommon, having been reported to occur in 22% of patients treated by closed reduction (Nettles & Linscheid 1968).

Recurrent anterior dislocation may cause little functional disability, but may lead to cosmetic problems, especially in young women. Of patients with recurrent anterior dislocation 60–79% had no pain, limitation of movement or functional disability (Nettles & Linscheid 1968, Savastano & Stutz 1978). Troublesome disability seems to be more common in men performing heavy labour or vigorous athletic activity.

Eskola et al (1989) described 12 patients in whom pain and instability necessitated operative repair. Five of these patients had a tendon graft to the first rib and the manubrium, and in three the medial end of the clavicle was attached to the first rib with a fascia lata graft. In four patients subperiosteal resection of the medial 2.5 cm of the clavicle was performed without stabilisation. Of the eight patients with tendon or fascia lata grafts, four had a good result and four a fair result using Eskola's points system.

The four patients who underwent subperiosteal resection all had poor results.

Fifteen cases of subperiosteal resection of the medial end of the clavicle to treat a painful sternoclavicular joint were reported by Rockwood et al (1997). Eight patients had a primary arthroplasty with preservation of the costoclavicular ligament. At an average follow-up of 7.7 years all had an excellent result. The other seven patients had a revision of a failed arthroplasty in which the costoclavicular ligament had to be reconstructed. Only three patients had an excellent result in this group.

Occasionally, habitual dislocation is seen, especially in young adolescent girls, occurring spontaneously or as the result of only minor trauma.

Grade III injuries: retrosternal dislocation

Retrosternal dislocation of the sternoclavicular joint are approximately 10 times less common than anterior dislocations. The diagnosis is often not immediately apparent, although the symptoms are frequently severe. The delay in diagnosis was reported by Noda et al (1997) based on 30 case reports. In only 48% of patients was the correct diagnosis made on first attendance. Thirty per cent were diagnosed within 1 week, 11% from the second to the fourth week, and 11% beyond 1 month. Serious complications are often quoted, but reported cases are not common. Death is rare but has resulted from laceration of the trachea or haemothorax (Kennedy 1949). Injury to the mammary vessels, subclavian vessels, brachial plexus and rupture of the thoracic duct may also occur (Peacock et al 1970, Buckerfield & Castle 1984, Noda et al 1997).

Not all cases of chronic retrosternal dislocation are necessarily symptomatic. Savasatano & Stutz (1978) reported one patient who redislocated almost immediately after closed reduction and who was asymptomatic 23 years later, and another who was asymptomatic 21 months post injury. However, almost all authorities believe that reduction of the dislocation is essential because of damage to the underlying major vessels from prolonged dislocation.

Obstruction of the subclavian vessels has been reported to occur up to 10 years after retrosternal dislocation (Howard & Shafer 1965, Mehta et al 1973).

Open and closed techniques of reduction of retrosternal dislocations have been reported. Buckerfield & Castle (1984) achieved a 100% success rate with the closed reduction of seven cases; Rockwood (1991) commented that open reduction is not usually required for acute posterior dislocation.

Unlike anterior dislocations, retrosternal dislocations are generally stable once reduced. If reduction by closed methods fails or redislocation occurs then open reduction is required. The presence of a thoracic surgeon is recommended by some authors in the event of vascular complications (Rockwood et al 1997).

Once reduced, most cases appear to have normal function. Some thickening of the medial end of the clavicle can occur. This thickening is variably reported. Though Ferry et al (1957) noted it in one-third of their six patients and Mehta et al (1973) in two of their four patients, it is probably overlooked in some reports. Heinig (1968) estimated that approximately half of his patients with stable reductions and full function were mildly symptomatic, with some crepitation on abduction and external rotation of the involved shoulder, and with mild discomfort on excessive use of the involved extremity.

Sternoclavicular injuries in children

Sternoclavicular injuries are occasionally reported in children. As stated previously, the medial epiphysis of the clavicle is only a few millimetres thick, does not ossify until the age of 18, and may not unite with the metaphysis until the age of 22–25 years. Thus some of the sternoclavicular dislocations reported may be unrecognised injuries to the epiphyseal plate.

Five cases of retrosternal dislocation in children were reported by Yang et al (1996). Reduction was usually obtained by retraction of the shoulders, but for persistent dislocations a towel clip was used to lift the medial end of the clavicle into its reduced position. Nettles and Linscheid (1968) reported two cases of anterior dislocation and one of retrosternal dislocation in newborn babies after difficult labours, but they made no specific comment as to their treatment or outcome. Normal return of function is the rule.

Traumatic floating clavicle

Panclavicular dislocation of the clavicle has occasionally been reported. Operative treatment is described as technically difficult and conservative treatment may provide satisfactory function.

Six cases were detailed by Sanders et al (1990): all six patients had an anterior dislocation of the sternoclavicular joint and posterior dislocation of the acromioclavicular joint. In all six, the anterior displacement of the sternoclavicular joint was mainly of cosmetic importance, with no functional disability. However, four of the six patients required reconstruction of the acromioclavicular joint for persistent aching.

Summary

- Sternoclavicular joint injuries account for 0.6% of all shoulder girdle injuries.
- Grade I sprains and grade II subluxations generally have a good prognosis, although occasionally indirect injury to the sternoclavicular joint will result in internal derangement of the intra-articular disc.
- Epiphyseal injuries may occur at the sternoclavicular joint at up to 25 years of age and may mimic true dislocations.
- Anterior dislocation of the sternoclavicular joint may occur spontaneously or after minimal trauma in adolescent girls with habitual dislocation.
- Because of the serious complication rate, which includes penetration of mediastinal structures, Kirschner wires and other transfixing pins should not be used to stabilise the sternoclavicular joint.
- There is a 22% recurrent dislocation rate following operative or closed reduction of anterior sternoclavicular dislocation. This produces a cosmetic deformity and may be painful, although in 60–79% of patients there are minimal symptoms. Heavy labourers and keen sportsmen are most likely to be troubled by symptoms.
- Retrosternal dislocations occasionally cause immediate damage to adjacent major vessels, occasionally with fatal results. Late complications may occasionally occur from unreduced dislocations many years after the initial injury.
- In over 50% of patients the diagnosis of retrosternal dislocation is not made at initial presentation.
- Thickening of the medial end of the clavicle may occur following open or closed reduction, and approximately 50% of patients with stable reductions may have mild symptoms despite full function.
- Dislocation of the sternoclavicular joint in children is uncommon but may occur in infants following difficult labour, although normal function is invariably reported after treatment.

Acromioclavicular joint
Introduction

Acromioclavicular injuries are classified into six types (Rockwood 1991). Type I include strains and contusions of the acromioclavicular joint with no gross deformity. Type II injuries are due to rupture of the capsule and acromioclavicular ligament with an intact coracoclavicular ligament, while type III injuries are due to rupture of the acromioclavicular and coracoclavicular ligaments. In the type IV injury the clavicle is displaced posteriorly into or through the trapezius muscle, while the type V injury is an exaggeration of the type III injury with major vertical separation of the clavicle from the acromion. Inferior dislocation into either a subacromial or subcoracoid position typifies a type VI injury.

The incidence of complete acromioclavicular dislocations is estimated at three or four per 100 000 population per annum (Larsen et al 1986). Rowe & Marble (1958) found 52 acromioclavicular injuries in 1603 shoulder-girdle injuries (3.25%).

The incidence of injury in the common types taken from four papers is shown in Table 5.1. The figure of 25% for type I injuries is probably artificially low, as many of these patients may not report to a doctor or hospital with their injury.

Results of treatment

Type I and II injuries

There are a few reports documenting the results of type I and II injuries. Of 24 patients with a type I injury treated with immobilisation, Park et al (1980) reported a disability period of 6 weeks. Using a standard rating system in which the total for perfect recovery was 100, the mean rating was 94 at an average follow-up of 6.3 years. However, two of these 24 patients required subsequent resection of the distal clavicle for painful degenerative arthritis of the acromioclavicular joint. The symptoms, physical findings and radiographic changes in two larger series of type I injuries are compared in Table 5.2. Thirty-eight percent of these patients had some persistent symptoms at follow-up, of which 9% were major symptoms. Nuisance symptoms were pain, clicking and feelings of instability that did not affect the function of the individual. Major symptoms were pain and instability that affected mainly athletic activities. Positive physical findings were visual deformity, swelling, decreased mobility, pain with stress or palpation and crepitation on movement. The difference in the incidence of positive radiographic changes in these two papers was due to even minor changes, being reported by Cox (1981).

The disability period for 25 type II injuries treated by immobilisation, reported by Park et al (1980), was 6 weeks. Using their standard rating system the mean rating was slightly lower, at 90 out of a maximum of 100 at an average of 6.3 years' follow-up.

The symptoms, physical findings and radiographic changes of type II injuries in the two large series reported above are compared in Table 5.3. Persistent symptoms at follow-up were noted in 54%, of which 24% were major symptoms. Their symptoms and positive physical findings were as for type I injuries. Walsh et al (1985) assessed the residual shoulder weakness using the Cybex II in eight patients with type II injuries. The average time from

Table 5.1 The incidence of acromioclavicular joint injuries by type

Reference	Type I	Type II	Type III	Total
Rowe & Marble (1958)	8	17	27	52
Weaver & Dunn (1972)	16	16	15	47
Tossy et al (1963)	12	6	23	41
Allman (1967)	29	55	36	120
Total	65 (25%)	94 (36%)	101 (39%)	260

Table 5.2 A comparison of symptoms, physical findings and radiographic changes in type I injuries

	Bergfield et al (1978) No. of cases	%	Cox (1981) No. of cases	%	Total No. of cases	%
Symptoms	38/97	39	36/99	36	74/196	38
Nuisance	29/97	30	28/99	28	57/196	29
Major	9/97	9	8/99	8	17/196	9
Physical findings	42/97	43	43/99	43	85/196	43
Radiographic changes	29/97	29	69/99	70	98/196	50

Table 5.3 A comparison of symptoms, physical findings and radiographic changes in type II injuries

| | Bergfield et al (1978) | | Cox (1981) | | Total | |
	No. of cases	%	No. of cases	%	No. of cases	%
Symptoms	20/31	65	25/52	48	45/83	54
Nuisance	7/31	23	18/52	35	25/83	30
Major	13/31	42	7/52	13	20/83	24
Physical findings	22/31	71	40/52	77	62/83	75
Radiographic changes	15/31	48	39/52	75	54/83	65

injury to follow-up was 33.4 months. There was no significant deficit in the strength of the injured as compared with the uninjured shoulder, apart from a 24.3% deficit in strength when measured in horizontal abduction at a faster speed. The poor results tend to occur more readily in elderly patients, and this is probably related to the development of degenerative changes. Indeed, Cook & Tibone (1991) reported 23 athletes who developed degenerative changes after type I or type II injuries who were treated by distal clavicular excision. The average interval between injury and surgery was 31 months. However, the degree of arthritis does not necessarily correlate with the end functional result. This point will be discussed later.

Acute superior dislocation (type III injuries)

Controversy rages over whether type III acromioclavicular injuries should be treated operatively or non-operatively. Numerous operations and orthoses have been designed and reported upon. It is not the purpose of this volume to promulgate any particular treatment regime, but to give an overview of the results as reported in the English language literature.

Conservative treatment The results of conservative treatment vary from series to series (Table 5.4). Direct comparisons are difficult, as authors report their results in different ways. However, those factors which appear to be reported in comparable fashion are listed. All untreated grade 3 dislocations have a prominent lateral end of clavicle, but this prominence was considered significant in only three of 17 patients (18%) in Dawe's series (1980) and three of 35 patients (9%) reported by Glick et al (1977). Calcification of the coracoclavicular ligament was seen in 26 of 44 patients (59%) in Dias' 1987 series and 21 of 33 patients (64%) in Bjerneld's 1983 series. Dias reviewed his patients again at an average follow-up of 12.5 years after injury (Rawes and Dias 1996). Of the 35 patients contacted

34 had no or mild pain only. Two patients had noticed improvement in their pain from moderate to mild, whilst the patient with moderate pain had deteriorated. Calcification of the cocacoclavicular ligament was now present in 21 of 30 patients (70%) who had a follow-up radiograph. The question of the significance of soft tissue calcification in this injury will be discussed later.

Conservative versus operative treatment A number of papers make comparisons between different conservative and operative treatments, although there is no uniform method of presenting results (Table 5.5). These papers suggest that the percentage of satisfactory results is marginally better with conservative treatment. The results for Larsen et al's 1986 paper provided a 13 month follow-up. Their figures for excellent/good results at 3 months suggest that conservatively treated patients achieve this result more quickly. Certainly, Galpin et al (1985) reported that their conservatively treated patients returned to work at an average of 2.6 weeks post injury, as compared to 6.8 weeks for their operative group. Similarly, their conservative group of patients returned to sport at 1.7 months, compared to 2.2 months for their operative group. Bannister et al (1989) also found that their conservatively treated group of patients returned to work earlier than their operative group (4 weeks compared to 11 weeks for manual workers and 1 week as compared to 4 weeks after surgery for clerical workers). Return to sport was also noticed earlier in the conservatively treated group (7 weeks as compared to 16 weeks). Other factors in this group of patients are compared in Table 5.6. Conservatively treated groups had a higher percentage of patients with a full range of motion (90%) and full strength (91%) as compared to the operative group (79% full motion, 88% full strength). Walsh et al (1985) compared the residual shoulder weakness of nine type III patients treated surgically with that of eight treated conservatively using a Cybex II. They found that type III injuries treated

Table 5.4 Results of conservative treatment of type III acromioclavicular dislocations

Reference	No. of cases
No or minimal pain	
Glick et al (1977)	35/35
Bjerneld et al (1983)	30/33
Anzel & Streitz (1973)	18/20
Dias et al (1987)	42/44
Total	125/132 (95%)
Return to sport	
Glick et al (1977)	32/35
Dias et al (1987)	40/44
Dawe (1980)	12/17
Total	84/96 (87%)
Return to original work	
Bjerneld et al (1983)	30/33
Dias et al (1987)	44/44
Dawe (1980)	14/17
Total	88/94 (94%)
Full range of movement	
Glick et al (1977)	35/35
Dias et al (1987)	39/44
Wojtys & Nelson (1991)	22/22
Total	96/101 (95%)

non-operatively showed no significant strength deficits, but those treated surgically had a significant strength deficit in vertical abduction at fast speeds. MacDonald et al (1988) evaluated 20 male patients (10 treated operatively) for recovery of shoulder strength and function 13 months after treatment. The majority of the strength and flexibility tests showed no significant difference between the two groups. However, the non-surgical group was statistically superior to the surgical group in abduction, fast external rotation and flexibility in external rotation. The degree of calcification in the coracoclavicular ligament was marginally higher in the operative group (67% as compared to 64%). As would be expected, almost 100% of conservatively treated patients had a prominence of the lateral end of the clavicle. However, a surprisingly high number (28%) of the operated groups also had some deformity. At review at an average of over 9 years post injury, Taft et al (1987) found that 32 of 75 (43%) of non-

operatively treated patients had developed post-traumatic arthritis as compared to 13 of 52 (25%) surgically treated patients. However, only eight (25%) of those treated non-operatively and four (31%) of those treated operatively had significant symptoms. They found that post-traumatic arthritis developed in 39 of 87 patients (45%) in whom the anatomy was not maintained and in six of the 40 patients (15%) in whom the anatomy was maintained. They found that most poor results would be evident within 6 months of injury, with little or no further progression of symptoms thereafter.

Operative treatment Numerous operative techniques are reported for type III acromioclavicular injuries. Only the larger reported series are shown in Table 5.7, but it must be stressed that many different techniques are reported in these papers.

Excision of the outer end of the clavicle is often used in treating the symptomatic chronically dislocated

Table 5.5 A comparison of results between conservatively and surgically treated groups

Reference	Rating	Number of cases	
		Conservative	Operative
Baker & Stryker (1965)	Excellent/good	4/7	18/25
Bannister et al (1989)	Perfect/good	33/33	23/27
Powers & Bach (1974)	Good	24/28	12/18
Galpin et al (1985)	Pain-free	15/21	12/16
Jacobs & Wade (1966)	Asymptomatic	21/43	23/51
Larsen et al (1986)	Excellent/good	39/43	38/41
Larsen & Hede (1987)	Excellent	50/55	21/23
Taft et al (1987)	Satisfactory	69/75	49/52
Aggregated total of satisfactory results		255/305 (84%)	196/253 (77.5%)

Table 5.6 A comparison of results between conservatively and surgically treated groups

Reference	Number of cases	
	Conservative	Operative
Full range of motion		
Jacobs & Wade (1966)	34/43	35/51
Larsen et al (1986)	43/43	38/41
Total	77/86 (90%)	73/92 (79%)
Full strength		
Galpin et al (1985)	15/21	12/16
Larsen et al (1986)	43/43	38/41
Total	58/64 (91%)	50/57 (88%)
Calcification of coracoclavicular ligament		
Larsen & Hede (1987)	38/55	16/23
Larsen et al (1986)	25/43	27/41
Total	63/98 (64%)	43/64 (67%)
Prominent lateral end of clavicle		
Larsen & Hede (1987)	52/55	10/23
Galpin et al (1985)	21/21	3/16
Jacobs & Wade (1966)	39/43	22/51
Larsen et al (1986)	43/43	2/41
Total	155/162 (96%)	37/131 (28%)

acromioclavicular joint. Gillespie (1964) reported results following excision of the outer end of the clavicle in 30 patients. Five patients had to change to lighter employment. Overall, 13 patients (43%) were felt to have an unsatisfactory result. It was found that advancing age influenced the results unfavourably, and 70% of patients aged

Table 5.7 Results of operative treatment of type III acromioclavicular dislocations

Reference	Number of cases good/excellent*	Total	Percentage (good/excellent)
Roscoe & Simmons (1984)	151†	168	90
Bargren et al (1978)	43	63	68
Lancaster et al (1987)	87	90	97
Eskola et al (1987a)	82	86	95
Smith & Stewart (1979)	77	86	89
Eskola et al (1991)	67	70	96
Dumontier et al (1995)	37	56	66
Broos et al (1997)	52	87	60
Aggregated total	596	706	84

* Individual authors' assessment.
† This figure is calculated from data given in the cited paper.

50 years or more had unsatisfactory results. Seventy-three patients who had the outer end of the clavicle excised because of painful conditions of the acromioclavicular joint were reported by Eskola et al (1996). Thirty-two patients had a chronically dislocated acromioclavicular joint, eight had a fracture of the lateral end of the clavicle and 33 had primary acromioclavicular osteoarthrosis. The patients were evaluated at an average of nine years post operation. A good result was reported in 21 patients, with 29 satisfactory and 23 (32%) with a poor result. Of the 32 patients with a chronically dislocated acromioclavicular joint, nine (28%) had a good result, 13 (41%) a satisfactory result and 10 (31%) a poor result. Twenty-one patients (54%) in this subgroup had pain with exertion. Six patients (19%) had an average decrease in the abduction strength of the involved upper extremity of more than 30% compared with that of the contralateral arm. Pain was noted significantly more often in those patients who had elevation of the lateral end of the remaining part of the clavicle as compared with the scapula, and in those who had more than 10 millimetres of clavicle resected. However, Cook & Tibone (1991) reported on 23 athletes who had the lateral end of the clavicle excised for degenerative changes after a grade 1 and grade 2 dislocation. They were assessed at an average of 3.7 years after the operation. All but one were satisfied with the surgery, and 16 returned to the same level of sporting activity. Seventeen patients were assessed by Cybex testing. While slow speed Cybex testing demonstrated some weakness, faster speed testing showed little or no weakness of the involved shoulder.

Type IV, V and VI injuries

Posterior dislocation of the acromioclavicular joint has occasionally been described. Interposition of soft tissues such as meniscus and capsule prevents correction of the posterior displacement, and operative reduction is invariably required. Of the five patients described by Tsou (1989), treated by a percutaneous coracoclavicular fixation, two showed redisplacement after screw removal due to initial inadequate reduction of the dislocation. However, all patients regained full motion by 3 months post surgery. Gerber & Rockwood (1987) reported four cases of subcoracoid dislocation of the lateral end of the clavicle. Three patients had a transient neurological lesion which recovered. As all three of these patients suffered multiple injuries, these neurological lesions may not have occurred as a direct result of the dislocation. All required open reduction and all made a full functional recovery.

Complications of acromioclavicular dislocations

The main complications of acromioclavicular dislocations are calcification in the coracoclavicular space, post-traumatic arthritis of the acromioclavicular joint and osteolysis of the distal end of the clavicle.

Calcification of the coracoclavicular space Calcification of the coronoid and trapezoid ligaments is relatively common after dislocation of the acromioclavicular joint, in patients treated both conservatively and surgically (Table 5.8). The incidence appears to be slightly less in those cases treated operatively (42%) compared to those treated conservatively (54%), but is higher in complete dislocations when compared with type I and II injuries. Bergfield et al (1978) reported that only 41 of 128 midshipmen (32%) with type I and II acromioclavicular injuries treated conservatively had radiographic changes of calcification in the area of the coracoclavicular ligament. Similar results were reported by Bjerneld et al (1983), who found that 8% of 37 patients with partial separation and 64% of 33 patients with complete separations had calcification of the coracoclavicular space. The majority of authors have found that this calcification did not influence the final clinical or functional outcome. Larsen et al (1986) found that only two of their 52 patients (3.8%) with coracoclavicular calcification had a fair or poor result. Excessive calcification may cause slight restriction of abduction in the affected shoulder, however.

Post-traumatic arthritis Degenerative arthritis of the acromioclavicular joint may occur without a clear history of trauma, as was the case with 56 (67%) of the 83 patients reported by Worcester & Green (1968). They pointed out that the degenerative changes began during the second decade.

Taft et al (1987) found that most poor results due to degenerative changes would be evident within 6 months of injury, with little or no further progression of symptoms thereafter. Smith & Stewart (1979) also showed that the time of onset of the first degenerative changes showed a peak developing within 1 year. However, they showed a second peak occurring at 5–6 years. The incidence of post-traumatic arthritis reported in the literature is shown in Table 5.9. Most authors have found little positive correlation between the presence of arthritis and symptoms. However, 12 of the 45 patients (27%) with post-traumatic arthrosis reported by Taft were symptomatic, and Jacobs & Wade (1966) found that 65% of their patients with traumatic arthritis were symptomatic.

Osteolysis of the distal clavicle   Osteolysis of the lateral end of the clavicle has been described following dislocation or subluxation of the acromioclavicular joint. However, the incidence remains uncertain. Eskola et al (1991) reported 13 cases of osteolysis of the lateral head of the clavicle in 86 patients (15%) treated surgically for a complete dislocation. Bergfield et al (1978) noted these changes in 10 of

Table 5.8 The incidence of calcification after acromioclavicular dislocation

Reference	Number of cases	
	Non-operative	Operative
Larsen et al (1986)	25/43	27/41
Bjerneld et al (1983)	24/70	
Dias et al (1987)	26/44	
Larsen & Hede (1987)	39/56	16/23
Eskola et al (1987a)		23/86
Broos et al (1997)		34/87
Aggregated total	114/213 (54%)	100/237 (42%)

Table 5.9 The incidence of post-traumatic arthritis after acromioclavicular injuries

Reference	Number of cases	
	Conservative	Operative
Jacobs & Wade (1966)	5/43	12/35
Taft et al (1987)	32/75	13/52
Arner et al (1957)	20/39	10/17
Broos et al (1997)		36/87
Aggregated total	57/157 (36%)	71/191 (37%)

128 midshipmen (8%) treated conservatively for grade 1 and 2 injuries. The changes may occur very early after trauma. Stahl (1954) described two patients, one of whom showed early radiographic changes at 3 weeks. Levine et al (1976) stated that the onset may occur several years after the injury. While not all cases are necessarily symptomatic, Jacobs (1964) described the symptoms as pain and a sense of weakness during abduction and flexion of the arm, and he stated that these symptoms may persist for up to 2 years. He also stated that the symptoms may recur after further trivial trauma. However, not all cases are due to trauma. Cahill (1982) reported on 46 male athletes with osteolysis of the distal part of the clavicle. None had a history of acute injury to the acromioclavicular area, but all were athletes and 45 lifted weights as part of their training. Twenty-one of his patients underwent excision of the distal end of the clavicle, with relief of symptoms in the 19 patients followed up. He states that no case has been reported in a woman.

Summary

- Of the reported acromioclavicular joint injuries, 25% are type I injuries, 36% type II and 39% type III injuries.
- 38% of patients sustaining type I injuries have residual symptoms, but these are significant in only 9%.
- 54% of patients sustaining type II injuries have residual symptoms and in 24% these symptoms are rated as significant. Poor results tend to occur in elderly patients.
- 95% of patients with type III acromioclavicular injuries treated conservatively had minimal or no pain, and 95% had no restriction of movement.
- 87% of patients with type III injuries resumed sporting activities and 94% returned to their original work.
- The prominent lateral end of clavicle was a cosmetic problem in 9–18% of patients with type III injuries treated conservatively.
- 77–84% of conservatively or operatively treated patients had excellent/good results.
- Conservatively treated type III patients returned to work earlier, and resumed sport sooner than operated patients. They also had a better return to full power and a better range of motion.
- Deformity of the lateral end of the clavicle is inevitable after the conservative treatment of patients and occurred in 28% of those treated surgically.
- Calcification of the coracoclavicular ligament occurred in 54% of conservatively treated patients and 42% of those operated on.
- 8–32% of type I and II injuries have calcification as compared with 64% of type III injuries.

- Calcification has an adverse affect on the result in 4% of patients.
- Post-traumatic arthritis occurred in 36–37% of acromioclavicular dislocations. Its effect on the overall result in uncertain.
- The incidence of osteolysis of the lateral end of the clavicle is 8–15%. It may occur within 3 weeks or after several years. Symptoms usually settle within 2 years.

Clavicle
Introduction

Fractures of the clavicle are common, Robinson (1998) estimating their incidence in adults as 29.14 fractures per 100 000 population per year. Another major epidemiological review carried out in Malmo (Nordqvist et al 1995) found an overall incidence of 65 per 100 000 population per year. This Swedish study included children, and in the age group 0–14 years the overall incidence was 198 per 1000 000 population.

Clavicular fractures are usually classified according to their anatomical location:

- group I—fractures of the middle third
- group II—fractures lateral to the coracoclavicular ligament
- group III—fractures of the proximal end

Neer (1968) further subdivided group II fractures into:

- type I—with the coracoclavicular ligaments intact
- type II—with these ligaments detached from the medial segment
- type III—intra-articular fractures

Robinson (1998) produced a more detailed classification which allowed an accurate description of displacement, instability and comminution in relation to the outcome and prognosis. Readers are referred to the original article for a more detailed description of the subtypes.

The incidence of these various clavicular fractures is shown in Table 5.10. Seventy-three percent of these fractures occur in the middle third, 23% in the lateral third and 4% in the medial third.

Conservative treatment

Eskola et al (1986a) reported the results of 85 patients whose fractured clavicles were initially treated conservatively and followed up for 2 years. Two patients subsequently had internal fixation for delayed union and two went on to asymptomatic non-union. Their average period of incapacity was 34 days, and they all returned to their previous occupation. The subjective outcome in the 83 patients treated conservatively was that 59 patients (71%) were asymptomatic—including the two patients with non-union. A satisfactory outcome meant slight pain on exercise or restricted movement (20 patients, 24%), and a poor outcome was seen in four patients (5%). They found that patients with a primary displacement of the fracture of more than 15 mm, or with shortening observed at the follow-up examination, had more statistically significant pain than patients without these findings (see later).

In a separate study Stanley & Norris (1988) reported on a consecutive series of 140 patients with fractures of the clavicle treated conservatively and reviewed a minimum of 3 months after injury. They found that healing was complete at an average of 4.5 weeks for patients aged under 10 years, an average of 6.7 weeks for those aged 10–20 years and an average of 11 weeks for those aged over 20 years. Indeed, a third of those patients aged over 20 years still had symptoms related to their fracture 3 months after the injury, with major complaints being an inability to sleep on the affected side, an inability to carry shopping and aching in the shoulder, particularly during cold weather.

The average incidence of non-union quoted in the literature (Table 5.11) is 1.5% (range 0–4.8%).

The reported results for the different groups are as follows.

Middle third fractures

Although middle third fractures of the clavicle are by far the commonest type, there are few papers which discuss the results of conservative treatment. The usual healing period of a fracture of the middle third of the clavicle is 4–6 weeks in young adults and 6 weeks or more in older people. Full recovery is usually achieved by 4 months. Nordqvist et al (1998) reviewed 225 midclavicular fractures treated conservatively at an average of 17 years after injury. At follow-up 185 shoulders (82%) were asymptomatic, 39 (17%) had moderate pain and were rated as fair, and one patient was rated as poor. One hundred and twenty five of the fractures had healed normally, 53 were malunited and seven were non-unions. Forty of the malunited fractures and three non-unions were rated as good. They concluded that few patients with fractures of the mid part of the clavicle required operative treatment. However, a number of recent papers have reported poor results following the closed treatment of displaced middle third fractures.

Table 5.12 shows that the incidence of non-union after the conservative treatment of these displaced fractures averages 6.9% (range 5.8–15%). Bowditch and Stanley (1999) reported that 80% of their 38 patients who attended for clinical review had a good/excellent shoulder function score. Hill et al (1997), however, reported that only 36 of

Table 5.10 The reported incidence of various clavicular fractures

Reference	Total	Lateral third	Middle third	Medial third
Rowe (1968)	690	83 (12%)	566 (82%)	41 (6%)
Stanley & Norris (1988)	140	60 (43%)	76 (54%)	4 (3%)
Robinson (1998)	1000	280 (28%)	692 (69%)	28 (3%)
Aggregated total	1830	423 (23%)	1334 (73%)	73 (4%)

Table 5.11 The incidence of non-union after conservative treatment of fractures of the clavicle

Reference	Total number of patients	Number with non-union	Incidence (%)
Neer (1960)	2235	3	0.1%
Rowe (1968)	680	5*	0.8%
Nordqvist et al (1998)	225	7	3%
Stanley & Norris (1988)	140	0	0
Robinson (1998)	1000	48	4.8%
Aggreated total	4270	63	1.5%

* This figure is calculated from data given in the cited paper

Table 5.12 The incidence of non-union after conservative treatment of displaced fractures of the middle third of the clavicle

Reference	Total number of patients	Number with non-union	Incidence (%)
Robinson (1998)	503	29	5.8%
Bowditch & Stanley (1999)	52	5*	10%
Hill et al (1997)	52	8	15%
Aggregated total	607	42	6.9%

* This figure is calculated from data given in the cited papers.

their 52 patients surveyed (69%) were satisfied with the final result. Thirty-nine (75%) had no pain and 13 had mild to moderate pain which required analgesic medication. Nineteen patients (37%) reported difficulty in lifting objects of more than 20 lb (9 kg) above shoulder level and 23 (44%) had some discomfort when lying on the affected side. The clavicle is a subcutaneous bone and a healed fracture of the middle third will often produce an obvious bony swelling which may be a source of cosmetic embarrassment, especially to females, and may cause irritation to people who carry packs and webbing (as in the armed services).

Lateral third fractures

Type I fractures of the lateral third of the clavicle heal promptly with minimal treatment. All 30 stable distal third fractures in the series of Hessman et al (1997) had a good to excellent result after conservative treatment. Robinson (1998) recorded one case of non-union (0.6%) in 181 undisplaced distal third fractures. Only rarely, when the fracture enters and distorts the joint surface, do symptoms persist. These symptoms are due to traumatic arthritis of the acromioclavicular joint. Neer found only two out of 75 patients (2.6%) with persistent symptomatology after this type of fracture. Robinson (1998), however, found that symptomatic osteoarthritis of the acromioclavicular joint was seen only after type III intra-articular fractures of the lateral end and was diagnosed in 15.2% of these cases. However, this complication occurred in only 1.8% of the total distal third fractures. Late excision of the outer end of the clavicle (leaving the coracoclavicular ligament intact) has generally given good results in these cases, but Eskola et al (1996) included eight patients with type I fractures in their operative resection of the lateral end of the clavicle series. Four of these patients had a poor result.

Kavanagh et al (1985) reported on 30 patients with type II fractures; 15 were treated non-operatively and 15 surgically. Neer (1968) reported on 23 similar patients, 12 treated conservatively, four with excision of the outer end of the clavicle and seven by surgical stabilisation. The results, shown in Table 5.13, show a high incidence of delayed union and non-union (20% and 22% respectively) in the patients treated conservatively. Neer pointed out that the eventual functional results in the conservative group were satisfactory in seven out of 12 patients, although when union occurred it was with excessive callus and posterior angulation, and never before 16 weeks.

Of the 23 patients with type II injuries treated operatively and reported by Eskola et al (1987) at an average of 4–5 years' follow-up, only one went on to non-union; 19 patients were asymptomatic, three satisfactory with slight pain on exercise or disabling restriction of movement, and only one had a poor result. Three patients lost some movement and two had pain on exercise and rest. Two patients had osteoarthrosis of the acromioclavicular joint, of whom only one was symptomatic. The average time of incapacity for work was 68 days.

Hessman et al (1996) were able to review 27 patients who had surgery for unstable distal clavicular fractures. Fracture healing was reported in all cases. Only one patient had a poor functional result due to pain and a restricted range of motion. They also noted that an associated lesion of the acromioclavicular ligament occurred in 20% of their cases.

Medial third fractures

Medial third fractures are not reported in detail but generally heal well with minimal treatment. In Robinson's (1998) series there were 28 medial third fractures which all united with few complications. Brinker and Simon (1999), however, presented two cases of medial clavicle fracture non-union that were initially thought to be chronic anterior sternoclavicular dislocations.

Primary operative treatment

A number of papers report the results of primary internal fixation of clavicular fractures. Some of these papers, it will be seen, report 100% union rates with their surgical techniques, but it should be stressed that none of the authors advocated routine internal fixation. They suggest that it should be reserved for complicated fractures or those with skin or neurovascular complications. Neer (1960) reported an incidence of non-union of 4.6% following primary open reduction and internal fixation, and Rowe's 1968 non-union rate after surgery was 3.7%; their non-union rates for conservatively treated fractures of the middle third of the clavicle were 0.1% and 0.8% respectively.

The results of internal fixation via intramedullary techniques or ASIF plates, as reported in the literature, are shown in Table 5.14. In the series of Paffen & Jansen (1978) a 6.8% non-union rate was reported. Zenni et al (1981) found that six patients (24% of their series) had minor

Table 5.13 Healing in type II fractures of the lateral third of the clavicle

Reference	Total number of patients	Delayed union	Non-union
Conservative treatment			
Neer (1968)	12	8 (66%)	4 (33%)
Kavanagh et al (1985)	15	6 (40%)	6 (40%)
Robinson (1998)	99	11 (11%)	18 (18%)
Total	126	25 (20%)	28 (22%)
Excise outer end of clavicle			
Neer (1968)	4	Only one satisfactory result achieved	
Open reduction and internal wire fixation			
Neer (1968)*	7	0	0
Kavanagh et al (1985)*	15	0	0
Eskola et al (1987)	23	0	1
Hessman et al (1996)	27	0	0

* All patients in these series healed in 6–10 weeks.

Table 5.14 The results of primary internal fixation of clavicular fractures

Reference	Number of patients	Union	Average time to union (weeks)
Intramedullary techniques			
Ngarmukos et al (1998)	99	99	8 weeks
De Beer & Rossouw (1997)	31	30	—
Bonnet (1975)	25	25	—
Zenni et al (1981)	25	25	12
Paffen & Jansen (1978)	73	68	5.5–9
Plating techniques			
Khan & Lucas (1978)	19	19	—
Bostman et al (1997)	103	101	—

aching pain at the fracture site during changes in the weather. All the 31 patients in de Beer and Rossouw's 1997 series had excellent function, pain was said to be minimal in most, and patient satisfaction was reported to be 96%. The time to union ranged between 5.5 and 12 weeks for normal healing, and return to full function occurred in 7.5–11 weeks.

The role of plate fixation in the management of fresh displaced mid clavicular fractures was evaluated by Bostman et al (1997). One hundred and three consecutive adult patients with severely displaced fresh fractures of the middle third of the clavicle were treated by open reduction and internal fixation using AO/ASIF plates. Seventy-nine patients (77%) had an uneventful recovery whereas 24 suffered one or several complications, the major ones including deep infection (7.8%), plate breakage, non-union (two patients) and refracture after plate removal. The most common of the minor complications was plate loosening resulting in malunion. Patient noncompliance with the postoperative regimen was felt to be a major cause of the failures.

The external fixation technique was used on 15 patients with fresh fractures of the clavicle by Schuind et al (1988); seven had compound injuries and five had multiple injuries. All the fractures united without a secondary refracture, with full motion at the shoulder. The average time that the external fixator was retained was 51 days.

Malunion

Function of the shoulder after fractures of the clavicle is surprisingly good considering how frequently malunion occurs. However, malunion can lead to shoulder dysfunction and yet few investigators have identified the parameters of malunion leading to a poor result. Eskola et al (1986) found that patients with shortening of the fracture by more than 15 mm had more statistically significant pain, and in some cases dysfunction. Hill et al (1997) reported similar observations in cases with at least 20 mm of shortening. However, Nordqvist et al (1997) evaluated the incidence and clinical significance of post fracture shortening of the clavicle in 85 patients re-examined five years after fracture. Thirty-five clavicles had healed with at least 5 mm of shortening but this had no deleterious effect on mobility, strength or function of the shoulder. The follow-up in Nordqvist's paper was longer than in Eskola's (2 years) and Hill's (mean 36 months), so the effects of malunion on function may improve with time. Bosch et al (1998) and Chan et al (1999) both reported on four patients in whom a malunited fracture of the clavicle was believed to be a contributing factor to shoulder girdle dysfunction. Seven of these eight patients had improvement of the functional status of the involved limb after surgery; the eighth patient had only had a review at 6 weeks post surgery.

A case of malunion of the lateral end of the clavicle resulting in signs of rotator cuff impingement was reported by Naert et al (1998). A full pain free range of movement was obtained 3 months after removing the prominent fragment.

The treatment of non-union

Most clavicular non-unions occur in the middle third of the bone, Johnson & Collins (1963) found that this was the case in 68% of their patients with non-union. The incidence of the various symptoms, when reported, is shown in Table 5.15. As may be seen from this table, not all clav-

Table 5.15 The symptoms of clavicular non-union

	Taylor (1969)	Wilkins & Johnston (1983)	Boehme et al (1991)	Eskola et al (1986b)	Johnson & Collins (1963)
Number of patients	31	33	50	24	69
No or minimal symptoms	3 (9.6%)	11 (33%)	12 (24%)	0	28 (40.5%)
Pain	28 (90%)	24 (73%)	18 (86%)*	24 (100%)	33 (48%)
Crepitation	—	9	—	—	—
Paraesthesiae	—	2	5	2	10
Cosmetic	—	5	1	—	2
Severe weakness	—	4	7	10	7
Loss of movement	—	—	—	8	3
Inability to work	—	—	2*	6	—

* Symptoms reported from only 21 of their cases.

icular non-unions are symptomatic. The incidence varies between 0% (Eskola et al 1986b) and 40.5% (Johnson & Collins 1963). This wide variation may well be due to the authors' interpretation of 'minimal symptoms'. Taking the five reported papers as a whole, the incidence of clavicular non-unions with no or minimal symptoms is 26%. Significant pain from clavicular non-union occurs in 71% of patients.

The surgical treatment of non-union varies from the use of intramedullary fixation, internal compression plates or external fixators. All authors agree on the necessity for additional bone grafting. The results of the surgical treatment of non-union of the clavicle are shown in Table 5.16. The incidence of bony union varied between 83% and 97% (average 92.5%). Symptomatic recovery usually occurred within 4 months and radiographic union within 6 months. The number of asymptomatic patients in these series varied from 71% to 86% (average 80%). When reported, a full range of motion was seen in 86%. The five cases of delayed union and non-union treated by external fixation and bone grafting by Schuind et al (1988) all united with a normal range of motion.

Middleton et al 1995 reported on the problem of clavicular non-union in National Hunt jockeys. They excised the clavicular fragment distal to the fracture in six jockeys, all of whom rated the procedure as very satisfactory, allowing an early return to work and no recurrent injury to the shoulder.

Other complications

The most commonly reported complication of clavicular fractures, other than non-union, is compression of the neurovascular bundle. Early complications involving the subclavian artery, vein and brachial plexus are invariably due to direct trauma. The prognosis depends upon the success of the vascular repair or upon the relief of compression on these vessels achieved by internal fixation of the fracture. The results of the vascular repair are outside the scope of this volume, and the results of internal fixation of fresh clavicular fractures have been previously discussed.

Many authors, however, point out that compression can occur as a late event due to malunion or non-union. It is impossible to predict the frequency of this late complication, other than to state that it is rare. Howard & Schafer (1965) reported, amongst their cases, a patient with a brachial plexus compression injury, occurring 2 years after the original fracture. Penn (1964) stated that vascular complications have manifested themselves 20–48 years after the clavicular injury.

Penn also quoted a case of chylothorax from a thoracic duct injury occurring 6.5 years after the original fracture.

Table 5.16 Results of the surgical treatment of non-union of the clavicle

	Ballmer et al (1998)	Wu et al (1998)	Bradbury et al (1996)	Eskola et al (1986b)
Number of cases	37	27	32	24
Type of fixation	various	plate and bone graft	IM nail or plate and bone graft	plate and bone graft
Number united	35	25	31*	20
Length of incapacity	11 weeks av.; by 6 months if intercalary graft	4 months	—	86 days av.
Asymptomatic	32	—	—	17
Mild symptoms	3	—	—	6
Severe symptoms	2	—	—	1
Full range of movement	32	—	—	—
Weakness	—	—	—	9
Return to previous job	—	—	—	23

* One after replating.

Reflex sympathetic dystrophy has been reported to occur after clavicle fracture (Ivey et al 1991).

A case of transitory osteonecrosis of the head of the humerus and anterior instability of the glenohumeral joint after fracture of the clavicle was reported by Caira and Melanotte (1997). Full recovery occurred in five months after core decompression and anterior stabilisation.

Symptomatic osteoarthrosis of the acromioclacicular joint following intra-articular fractures of the lateral end of the clavicle have already been discussed. Edelson (1996) examined 300 scapuloclavicular bone specimens, nine of which had healed fractures of the clavicle, and in no instance did the adjacent acromioclavicular joint display significant arthritic changes. He speculated that the clavicular shortening that occurred spared the adjacent acromioclavicular joint from arthritic change.

Goddard et al (1990) reported on five children who had an atlanto-axial rotatory fixation in association with a fracture of the clavicle. They stressed the importance of early diagnosis to avoid chronic deformity.

Pulmonary complications can also occur as an early complication of clavicular fractures. In his series of 690 clavicular fractures, Rowe (1968) reported that pneumothorax occurred in 3% of patients, haemothorax in 1% and refracture of the clavicle in 2% of patients.

Fractures in childhood and adolescence

Fractures of the clavicle during childbirth are well documented and these fractures heal with no problems in 2–3 weeks. The incidence is variably reported as occurring in 0.4% (Roberts et al 1995) to 1.5% of total vaginal births (Many et al 1996). Various factors associated with an increased risk of fracture were heavy neonates and shoulder dystocia, older maternal age, a prolonged second stage of labour in primiparous patients, and instrumental deliveries (Many et al 1996). Erb's palsy occurred in 2% (Gilbert & Tchabo 1988) to 5% (Oppenheim et al 1990) of cases and was usually fully recovered by 3 months. Fractures in children from 2–12 years of age unite in 2–4 weeks. The prognosis for children who have had a fracture of the clavicle, excluding those complicated by a neurovascular injury, is excellent. Non-union is rarely reported (Nogi et al 1975) and its differentiation from congenital pseudarthrosis is important. No callus is seen in cases of congenital pseudarthrosis.

Epiphyseal separation of the medial end of the clavicle may simulate sternoclavicular dislocation, and has been discussed previously. Curtis et al (1991) recommend conservative treatment, and claim that remodelling from the periosteum and the remaining epiphysis occurs quite rapidly, with no long-term disability.

Similarly, Curtis et al (1991) recommended conservative treatment for all but severe epiphyseal separation of the lateral end of the clavicle simulating acromioclavicular dislocation, as they felt that rapid remodelling occurred. However, Ogden (1984), while reporting excellent results with either conservative or surgical treatment, did report partial duplication of the clavicle which caused a painful, tender, palpable lump, requiring resection of the original clavicle back to the beginning of the duplication.

Of the 10 patients with distal clavicular epiphyseal injuries reported by Havránek (1989), nine were treated conservatively and one surgically. Regardless of the type of treatment, all patients healed without functional sequelae, although seven of the conservatively treated patients had a deformity of the injured shoulder.

Summary

- The average period of incapacity following fracture of the clavicle is 5 weeks, and healing is complete by 11 weeks.
- At 3 months 33% remain symptomatic, and 5% have a poor result at 2 years.
- The average incidence of non-union after a fractured clavicle is 1.5%.
- 82% of patients are asymptomatic after the conservative treatment of mid clavicular fractures and 17% have some pain.
- Non-union occurs in 6.9% of severely displaced mid clavicular fractures.
- Type I lateral third fractures heal well, with a 2–3% incidence of persistent symptoms from damage to the acromioclavicular joint. This incidence increases to 15% with intra-articular fractures.
- Type II lateral third fractures treated conservatively have a 22% non-union rate and 20% delayed union beyond 16 weeks, although function is eventually satisfactory if healing occurs.
- Type II lateral third fractures treated surgically have a 4% non-union rate and an unsatisfactory result.
- The non-union rate for internal fixation of fresh clavicular fractures is 0–7%. The time to union is from 5.5–12 weeks, and full function occurs in 7.5–11 weeks.
- 23% of patients had some complication following internal fixation of fresh clavicular fractures.
- 24% of surgically treated patients may experience minor aching pain at the fracture site with weather changes.
- Malunion with more than 15–20 mm of shortening may contribute to a poor result after healing of clavicular fractures.

- Approximately 26% of clavicular non-unions are asymptomatic, and significant pain occurs in 71%.
- The incidence of union in the surgically treated and bone grafted clavicular non-union is 83–97%.
- The average time to radiographic union is 6 months and full function returns in an average of 4 months.
- Late brachial plexus lesions have been reported 2 years after the initial injury, and late vascular lesions have occurred 48 years later.
- Refracture of the clavicle is reported in 2% of cases.
- Clavicle fracture in neonates occurs in up to 1.5% of vaginal births. Erb's palsy occurs in 2–5% but recovery usually occurs in 3 months.
- Fracture of the clavicle in children heals with no problem. Non-union is very rare and must be differentiated from congenital pseudarthrosis.
- Fracture–separation of the medial clavicular epiphysis may be treated conservatively with excellent results.
- Untreated fracture–separation of the lateral clavicular epiphysis usually heals with excellent results and rapid remodelling. However, reduplication of the clavicle may occur and cause a tender lump which requires excision.

Fractures of the scapula
Introduction
Scapular fractures are relatively rare, constituting 1% of all fractures (Zdravkovic & Damholt 1974) and 2.8% of shoulder-girdle injuries (Norqvlst & Petersson 1995). They are best classified from a prognostic point of view into three types (Zdravkovic and Damholt):

- type I—fractures of the body
- type II—fractures of the apophysis (acromion, spine and coracoid process)

- type III—fractures through the superior lateral angle (glenoid rim, glenoid fossa, anatomical neck and surgical neck)

Intra-articular glenoid fractures have been classified into five types (Butters 1991)—see later.

Over 50% of these fractures of the scapula occur in the body (Table 5.17).

Patients with scapular fractures often have other injuries—some serious—which may have significant effects on the functional outcome of the injury (Table 5.18). For example, McLennan & Ungersma (1982) reported a 53% incidence (16 of 30 patients) of pneumothorax also occurring. In six patients it occurred on presentation and in 10 it was delayed for 1–3 days. In only two patients out of the 16 was the pneumothorax associated with rib fractures.

Unfortunately, scapular fractures are often missed. Harris & Harris (1988) performed a retrospective analysis of 100 patients with major blunt chest trauma who were discharged with the diagnosis of scapular fracture. In only 57 of these patients was it diagnosed on the initial chest radiograph. The fracture was visible but overlooked in 31 patients and excluded from the radiograph or obscured by superimposed structures or artefacts in the other 12.

Type I: fractures of the body
Fractures of the scapular body can usually be treated conservatively. The muscles covering the body prevent significant displacement of the fragments. These fractures require up to 5 weeks of treatment with slings and physiotherapy. Wilber & Evans (1977) found that all 27 patients with isolated fractures of the body of the scapula recovered full glenohumeral motion regardless of the type of treatment. Full recovery of glenohumeral movement also occurred in the 35 patients with fractures of the body

Table 5.17 The incidence of the different scapular fractures

Reference	No.	Type I	Type II	Type III
Armstrong & Van der Spuy (1984)	64	35	12	17
Thompson et al (1985)	56	30	7	19
McGinnis & Denton (1989)	40*	26	13	22
Wilber & Evans (1977)	40*	30	8	14
Stephens et al (1995)	92	53	18	21
Aggregated total	325†	174 (54%)	58 (18%)	93 (28%)

* More than one fracture location per patient recorded.
† Total number of fractures recorded.

Table 5.18 Injuries associated with scapular fractures

	Armstrong & Vander Spuy (1984)	Thompson et al (1985)	McGinnis & Denton (1977)	Stephens et al (1995)
Number of patients	62	56	39	92
Deaths	6	8	0	0
Rib fracture	27	30	20	45
Haemo- or pneumothorax	24	30	13	24
Brachial plexus	2	7	2	—
Subclavian vessels	1	7	0	—
Head injury	7	32	11	22
Clavicle fracture	24	17	10	17
Spinal fracture	4	12	7	—

reported by Armstrong & Van der Spuy (1984). The condition of so-called 'pseudo-rupture of the rotator cuff' can occur. Haemorrhage into the muscle bellies of supraspinatus, infraspinatus and subscapularis muscles produces signs typical of a rotator cuff rupture. As the haematoma formation absorbs, rotator cuff power returns.

Type II: fractures of the apophysis
Acromion and scapular spine

Ogawa and Naniwa (1997) studied 37 fractures lateral to the spinoglenoidal notch and classified them into two types. Type I comprised fractures of the anatomic acromion and the extremely lateral scapular spine, while Type II fractures were located in the more medial spine and descended to the spinoglenoidal notch. Type I fractures were frequently associated with fracture of the coracoid base and acromioclavicular joint injuries while Type II fractures were seldom accompanied by associated injuries. Twenty-eight fractures were classified as Type I, nine as Type II. Thirty-three cases were seen acutely whilst four were classified as chronic on examination 2 or more months after injury. Of the acute cases follow-up over a 1 year period was available in 14 cases treated conservatively and in 12 cases treated surgically. Two of the Type I fractures treated conservatively had an unsatisfactory result (one non-union and one brachial plexus palsy). Three of the four chronic cases had surgery. All chronic cases had a satisfactory result. The authors recommended conservative therapy in isolated and undisplaced fractures in the expectation of an excellent result. If significant downward displacement occurred in Type I fractures they recommended surgical reduction and fixation to prevent subacromial impingement and pseudoarthrosis. Open

reduction and internal fixation was also recommended with marked displacement in Type II fractures.

The three cases of scapular spine fracture reported by Wilber & Evans (1977) all regained full glenohumeral movement after conservative treatment.

Coracoid process

Fractures of the coracoid process are well documented. They may occur in isolation or in association with acromioclavicular dislocation, avulsion fractures of the superior border of the scapula, dislocation of the shoulder, or clavicular fractures (Ogawa et al 1997).

Ogawa et al (1997) reviewed 67 patients with fractures of the coracoid process and classified them by the relationship between the fracture site and the coracoclavicular ligament. Type I fractures were located behind the ligament and Type II were in front of them. There were 53 Type I fractures, 36 being at the base of the process and 17 involving the upper third of the glenoid. Eleven were Type II fractures and three were unclassified. Sixty of the 67 patients had an associated lesion (acromioclavicular dislocation 39, fracture of the superior scapular margin 24, clavicular fracture 14, anterior shoulder dislocation three). Thirty-five patients had some form of surgical stabilisation. Forty-five patients were reviewed at a mean of 37 months; 39 (87%) had an excellent result and the remaining six a fair result. The authors found no statistical difference in the results between the operative and non-operative groups or between the Type I and Type II fractures.

When the fracture occurs in isolation and is minimally displaced, conservative treatment is indicated. In the 10 patients reported by Froimson (1978) and Zilberman & Rejovitzky (1981) the fractures united in 2–4 months.

Patients were able to resume full work from 6 weeks to 3 months after the injury, and a full range of movement was restored by 4 months. Two (20%) of these patients had slight pain after heavy work and one had minimal limitation of abduction and internal rotation at 4 months. Nonunion has occasionally been reported, (De Rosa & Kettelkamp 1977).

Type III: fractures through the superior lateral angle

Scapular neck fractures are classified into anatomical or surgical (Hardegger et al 1984). The surgical neck of the scapula is medial to the base of the coracoid process. If the clavicle or coracoclavicular ligaments are disrupted in association with this fracture then it is unstable. The anatomical scapular neck is lateral to the base of the coracoid process and fractures at this site tend to be unstable.

Wilber & Evans (1977) reported the results of eight patients with fractures of the neck of the scapula, treated conservatively: all eight regained a full range of motion.

Six of the 11 patients with fractures of the neck of the scapula reported by Armstrong & Van der Spuy (1984) had residual stiffness at 6 months post injury, but in none did this constitute a functional disability.

Intra-articular glenoid fractures are classified into five types (Butters 1991). Type I is an anterior avulsion fracture which must be distinguished from a small glenoid rim or labrum avulsion fracture commonly seen with traumatic anterior shoulder instability. Type II is a transverse fracture through the glenoid fossa, with an inferior triangular fragment displaced with the humeral head. Type III fracture involves the upper third of the glenoid and includes the coracoid. Type IV is a horizontal glenoid fracture extending all the way through the body to the axillary border and Type V combines a Type IV fracture with a fracture separating the inferior half of the glenoid.

Type I fractures, if displaced, may predispose to instability. Wiedemann et al (1999) reported satisfactory results in all 21 anterior glenoid rim fractures treated by open reduction and internal fixation.

Good functional results are possible in Type III fractures without internal fixation (Ogawa et al 1997). A good result has been reported as occurring in 75% of Type II to V fractures treated with early mobilisation (Butters 1991). Surgery is reserved for cases in which the humeral head appears subluxed or whenever multiple shoulder injuries have destroyed the scapuloclavicular connection.

Wilber & Evans (1977) reported that six patients with glenoid fractures all had some loss of mobility. Three of these patients were seen 1–12 years after the injury. Two had slight pain and less than 25% loss of abduction and

flexion (a fair result according to the authors); the third patient had moderate pain but greater than 25% loss of abduction and flexion (a poor result).

Armstrong and Van der Spuy (1984) found that three of their six patients with fractures of the glenoid had markedly restricted and painful movements of the shoulder. In these three the average movements at 6 months were as follows: rotation 40°, elevation 100° and abduction 80°. All of these patients had been treated conservatively.

Zdravkovic & Damholt (1974) reviewed 40 patients with fractures through the superior lateral angle. Only seven had their fractures extending into the glenoid cavity. Of the 28 patients who were followed up, 17 (61%) had mild degenerative changes in the glenohumeral joint and one (3.6%) had severe changes. However, only nine patients (32%) had symptoms, of whom four (14%) had pain at rest. Ten patients (35.7%) had grating from the glenohumeral joint on movement, but all had full strength. Abduction with unrestricted scapulo-thoracic movement was limited in eight patients (28.6%) by an average of 30°. However, abduction with a fixed scapula was restricted in more patients, although the precise figure is not clear from this paper.

Only three glenoid fractures were reviewed long term. All were asymptomatic, but only one had a full range of motion.

Summary

- Scapular fractures constituted 1% of all fractures and 2.8% of shoulder-girdle injuries.
- Other injuries were commonly seen in association with scapular fractures—some of these injuries had profound effects on the late functional result.
- Pneumothorax was reported to occur in 53% of scapular fractures and their presentation was sometimes delayed.
- Fractures of the body of the scapula invariably result in full return of function.
- Undisplaced fractures of the acromion heal in 3–4 weeks with full return of function, but displaced fractures may cause persistent symptoms. 4% went on to non-union.
- Fractures of the scapular spine should recover full function.
- Coracoid process fractures should return to full function with conservative measures within 6 weeks to 4 months. 87% have an excellent result and 13% a fair result. Painful non-unions have been reported.
- 32–55% of patients with fractures of the superior lateral angle had persistent symptoms, of whom 14% had pain at rest. Degenerative change occurred in 61%.

- Movement was reduced in about 30–55% of patients in cases with a fracture of the superolateral angle.

Rupture of the biceps brachii muscle or its tendons

Rupture of the biceps brachii may occur at four sites:

- at the long head of biceps
- at the short head of biceps
- through the muscle belly
- at the distal tendon

Of the 102 cases reported by Gilcrest (1934), 77 (75.5%) occurred in the long head of biceps, two (2%) were found in the short head, 17 (16.5%) were through the muscle and six cases (6%) through the distal tendon. Waugh et al (1949) found that 10% of the ruptures in their series occurred in the distal tendon, whereas Cassels & Hamilton (1967) found the incidence of distal rupture to be 26.5%. In many cases of rupture of the long head of biceps the event occurred after relatively trivial injury secondary to degenerative changes in the bicipital groove.

A recent histological assessment of 104 cadaver biceps tendons and the glenoid origin (Refior & Sowa 1995) was undertaken. It suggests that histological changes indicative of degeneration of the tendon occur most commonly at the distal exit of the tendon from the sulcus. However, acute rupture can occur in the young athlete, usually due to a very forceful muscular contraction during athletic activity. Soto-Hall & Stroot (1960) found that after recent rupture, the power of flexion of the elbow was about 20% less than that on the opposite side, and the power of shoulder abduction with the arm in external rotation was about 17% less than the opposite side. However, in late ruptures no appreciable weakness was noted. Cassels & Hamilton (1967) found that 1 year after injury, weight-lifting ability was equal to that of the uninjured side and

loss of supination was not present. These patients returned to work at an average of 4 weeks after injury.

Warner and McMahon (1995) studied seven patients with rupture of the long head of biceps. They noted that in each patient 2–6 mm of superior translation of the humeral head occurred in all positions of humeral abduction except 0°. They felt that this might contribute to the development of impingement syndrome in patients who had a Type II or III acromion. After traumatic closed transection of the muscle of biceps brachii in military parachutists, Heckman & Levine (1978) found that in 28 untreated patients, 25 (89%) had weakness of the arm and easy fatiguability with activities requiring rapid, repetitive elbow flexion, and 12 patients (43%) had pain in the area of the defect. The range of elbow flexion in these young, fit men was excellent, but the maximum flexion power at 90° of elbow flexion was only 53% of normal. This maximum flexion power was increased to 76.5% in the nine patients reviewed following early surgical repair, and to 77% in the 10 cases treated by aspiration of the haematoma and plaster immobilisation.

The treatment of distal avulsion of the biceps tendon remains controversial. Cassels & Hamilton (1967) had 10 cases of distal avulsion treated non-operatively in their series of 100 patients, and at 1 year weight-lifting ability and supination equalled that of the uninjured side. Norman (1985) reported on 15 cases of distal rupture. One patient was reviewed 11 years after conservative treatment and had a severe loss of flexion power and of supination of the forearm but a full range of motion.

Most authors advocate surgical repair of these distal lesions, as there is rarely any underlying problem of degenerative change and the injury tends to occur in younger, more athletic patients.

The overall results of the surgical repair of distal biceps tendon ruptures is shown in Table 5.19. Ninety-four percent of patients achieved an excellent/good result.

Table 5.19 The results of the surgical repair of distal biceps tendon rupture

Author	Number of patients	Excellent	Good	Fair	Poor
Karunakar et al (1999)	20	14	5	1	0
Martens (1997)	18	10	8	0	0
Norman (1985)	14	3	10	1	0
Boucher & Morton (1968)	13	8	3	0	2
Aggregated total	65	35 (54%)	26 (40%)	2 (3%)	2 (3%)

Karunakar et al (1999) reported that 19% of their patients lost some forearm rotation (less than 100° combined pronation-supination). One patient had a 15° fixed flexion deformity. Isokinetic testing revealed that 10 patients (48%) had some weakness of supination while three (14%) had some weakness for flexion. Deficits in endurance were noted in eight patients (38%) for supination and seven (33%) for flexion.

In Martens' 1997 group of 18 patients, five lacked 5–10° of extension, two lacked 10–20° of supination and one patient had a pronation deficit of 10°. Five patients complained of a slight loss of supination strength.

A partial rupture of the distal biceps tendon can occur. In the patient of Rokito et al (1996), there was pain with resisted elbow flexion and forearm supination.

A few cases of isolated rupture of the short head of biceps have been reported (Postacchini & Ricciardi-Pollini 1977).

Summary

- Rupture of the long head of biceps usually occurs secondary to degenerative changes. At 1 year's follow-up no appreciable weakness has been reported in the injured side as compared with the uninjured limb. However, this may not be true in the younger, athletic patient.
- Superior translation of the humeral head occurs and this may contribute to the development of an impingement syndrome.
- Untreated closed rupture of the biceps brachii muscle in young men resulted in weakness and easy fatiguability in 89% and residual pain in 43%. The range of elbow flexion remained good, but maximum flexion power at 90° of elbow flexion was 53% of normal. This increased to 77% in surgically repaired lesions and in

those treated with closed reduction and plaster immobilisation.
- Distal avulsions of the biceps tendon treated surgically achieved 94% excellent/good results, 16–19% lost some forearm rotation, 5–28% lost some elbow movement, up to 48% lost some strength and endurance.

Winging of the scapula

Winging of the scapula occurs secondary to injury to the long thoracic nerve of Bell. This can be as part of a more widespread brachial plexus lesion, but can also occur in isolation.

Trauma is the chief cause of paralysis of serratus anterior. It may come on immediately after a hard blow or after heavy lifting or by sudden or prolonged exertion of the shoulder. Other non-traumatic causes include neuralgic amyotrophy.

The most prominent symptom of isolated paralysis of the long thoracic nerve and the serratus anterior is pain. The pain usually extends along the base of the neck and down over the scapular and deltoid regions on the affected side. It may extend upwards to the back of the head or into the forearm and hand. This pain is often described as burning in quality. It is usually associated with fatigue on elevating the arm or an inability to elevate the arm fully. There is also an abnormal prominence of the scapula.

Treatment for lesions in continuity is conservative, the results are shown in Table 5.20. It can be seen that, overall, 43 of the 58 patients (74%) for which recovery was recorded made a full recovery, 11 (19%) made a partial recovery, and four (7%) made no recovery. Recovery is variably reported to occur by 6 months (Johnson & Kendall 1955), 9 months (Gregg et al 1979) and 2 years (Foo & Swann 1983).

Table 5.20 The results of conservative treatment for serratus anterior paralysis

Reference	Number	Recovery			
		Full	Partial	Nil	Not known
Foo & Swann (1983)	20	14	—	—	6
Overpeck & Ghormley (1940)	15	7	4	3	1
Gozna & Harris (1979)	14	7	3	—	4
Gregg et al (1979)	10	9	1	—	—
Fardin et al (1978)	10	6	3	1	—
Total	69	43	11	4	11

Johnson & Kendall (1955) assessed the strength of the serratus anterior muscle at 45–60% (average 50%) at 3 months, and 70–100% (average 85%) at 6 months.

For those patients with significant residual incapacity surgery can be undertaken. Perlmutter & Leffert (1999) reported the results of transferring the pectoralis major tendon with a fascial graft to the scapula in 16 patients, 13 having a satisfactory result.

Summary

- Pain, fatigue or an inability to elevate the arm, and winging of the scapula, are symptoms of isolated paralysis of serratus anterior.
- After conservative treatment 74% have full recovery, 19% partial recovery and 7% no recovery.
- Recovery occurs between 6 months and 2 years. Muscle strength is 50% recovered at 3 months and 85% recovered at 6 months.

Rupture of Pectoralis Major

Rupture of the pectoralis major is an uncommon injury although individual cases are described. Cameron & Henderson (1998) reported on 80 patients following a literature review and an assessment of their three patients. Fifty-six (70%), had been treated surgically with the site of rupture being recorded as insertional in 39 (70%), musculo-tendinous in 13 (23%), intratendinous in two (3.6%), intramuscular in one, and the final case being an avulsion fracture at the humeral insertion. The mean age of rupture was 32 years. Weight training was the cause of rupture in 52% of patients, a work injury in 16%. Results were satisfactory for both conservative and surgical management. A musculotendinous disruption had a greater tendency to a fair result. The authors concluded that insertional tears should be treated by primary repair, particularly in athletic individuals, and that musculo tendinous tears be treated conservatively.

Impingement and rotator cuff tears

Disorders of the rotator cuff tendons are usually grouped under the diagnostic phrase of impingement syndrome. Neer (1983) described three stages of impingement lesions:

- Stage I consists of oedema and haemorrhage, and this may result from excessive overhead use in sport or at work. It tends to be observed in patients younger than 25 years and is usually a reversible lesion.
- Stage II consists of fibrosis and tendonitis and is typically seen in patients ranging from 25–40 years of age.

The shoulder functions satisfactorily for light activity but becomes symptomatic after vigorous overhead use.

- Stage III is the stage of tendon degeneration, bony changes and tendon ruptures. There is usually a prolonged history of shoulder problems.

Stage I impingement occurs in the younger age group and, as indicated above, may result from excessive sport. It is, however, imperative to rule out underlying glenohumeral instability as the primary source of the problem in the younger age group. Gartsman (1990) further classified Stage II impingement as Stage IIa, equivalent to Neer's original description, and Stage IIb, characterised by more severe lesions including partial thickness, but not full-thickness, tears.

There is controversy as to whether trauma or intrinsic problems cause impingement. However, it is probable that the interactions of four elements—vascular, degenerative, traumatic and mechanical or anatomic factors—combined are the cause, and it is unlikely that any one element is solely responsible for cuff lesion. Bigliani & Levine (1997), in a review article on subcromial impingement syndrome, suggested that its causes could be broadly classified as intrinsic (intratendinous) or extrinsic (extratendinous). They further characterised the causes as primary, or secondary (such as instability or neurological injury).

Intrinsic factors were: muscle weakness
overuse of the shoulder
degenerative tendinopathy
Extrinsic factors were: acromial morphology
glenohumeral instability
degeneration of the acromio-clavicular joint
impingement by the coracoacromial ligament
coracoid impingement
os acromiale
impingement on the postero-superior aspect of the glenoid

Weakness of the muscles of the rotator cuff, with eccentric contraction of the supraspinatus, increases tension on the tendon with resulting injury and degenerative change. It could occur in carpenters, mechanics, plumbers and other manual workers who use overhead motion in their work. Thus muscle strengthening exercises are important in the conservative treatment of impingement. Rathbun & MacNab (1970) showed a constant zone of avascularity in the supraspinatus tendon. They also noted that constant pressure from the humeral head wrings out the blood supply to these tendons when the arm is held in the resting position of adduction and neutral rotation. They felt that a zone of avascularity preceded the degenerative changes, which were always most extensive in the areas of avascularity. Degeneration of the tendons of the rotator cuff associated with ageing is also noted.

It is a controversial question as to whether trauma is a major cause of cuff lesions. Significant trauma either in association with an anterior dislocation or in isolation can rupture the cuff, especially in older patients. Overuse or repeated stressful use in the overhead position is also recognised as a cause of rotator cuff disease. It is felt that soft tissue inflammation resulting from overuse of the shoulder increases the area occupied by the soft tissues in the subacromial space and leads to friction and wear against the coracoacromial arch. Frost & Andersen (1999), in a study of slaughterhouse workers, showed an association between cumulative exposure to shoulder intensive work and impingement syndrome of the shoulder. Neer (1983) believed that 95% of tears of the rotator cuff were initiated by impingement.

Seventy to 80% of cuff tears are said to be associated with a hooked acromion (Toivonen et al 1995). Three anatomical types of acromion have been identified: type I, flat; type II, curved; and type III, hooked. Degeneration of the acromioclavicular joint may contribute to subacromial impingement. Cuomo et al (1998) implicated the presence of major inferior osteophytes on this joint as one of the causative factors in rotator cuff tears, major osteophytes being found in 62.5% of the rotator cuff tear group as compared with 12.5% in the intact group.

The coracoacromial ligament has also been implicated as a source of impingement, but underlying glenohumeral instability must be ruled out as the primary source of the problem in young athletic patients who display the symptoms.

From a medico-legal point of view, it can be seen that the relevance of trauma to these rotator cuff lesions is uncertain and variable. It would seem certain that 'trivial injury' may cause an abnormal tendon finally to tear, but is trauma alone the major factor in other cases in which the patient has not experienced previous shoulder symptoms? As Brems (1988) pointed out, biomechanical studies tell us that the tensile strength of normal tendon exceeds the tensile strength of bone. Therefore most truly acute, violent injuries to normal rotator cuffs would be expected to result in fractures about the shoulder rather than in tendon tears. It can be seen that each case must be assessed on its own merits as to the significance of the traumatic episode.

Impingement lesions (stages I and II)

It is generally felt that the majority of patients with impingement lesions settle with time, although those involved in some manual occupations or certain sports may be prone to recurrent pain. Chard et al (1988) reviewed 137 patients, 6 or more months after their first attendance at a shoulder clinic. They found that 35 (26%) had active tendonitis at a mean of 19 months after presentation (with symptoms for 2.5 years), making spontaneous resolution appear unlikely. In addition, 40 patients (29%) had mild residual pain. In a larger study Morrison et al (1997) reported the results of non-operative treatment in 616 patients who had subacromial impingement syndrome. The average duration of follow-up was 27 months. Four hundred and thirteen patients (67%) had a satisfactory result, 172 (28%) had an unsatisfactory result and went on to have arthroscopic subacromial decompression, and 31 (5%) had an unsatisfactory result but declined surgery. Seventy-four (18%) of the 413 patients who had a successful result had a recurrence of symptoms during the follow-up period, although the symptoms subsequently resolved with rest or the resumption of an exercise programme. Thirty-two (91%) of the 35 patients who had a type I acromion had a successful result compared with 173 (68%) of the 256 who had a type II acromion and with 208 (64%) of the 325 who had a type III acromion.

Brox et al (1999) compared the effectiveness of arthroscopic surgery, supervised exercises and placebo in 125 patients with Type II rotator cuff disease in a randomised clinical trial. At 2.5 year follow-up an excellent/good result was reported in 68% of those patients treated by arthroscopic surgery, 61% of those treated with supervised exercises and 25% of the placebo group.

For patients failing to resolve with conservative treatment, surgery is undertaken, usually involving a decompression by an anterior acromioplasty. The results of these operations performed via open surgical techniques (Table 5.21) or arthroscopic techniques (Table 5.22) are presented. Both techniques results in an 82–84% satisfactory surgical result. The results are worse in patients involved in some form of workers' compensation and in those whose symptoms developed after trauma.

Subcoracoid impingement has also been reported, with pain due to encroachment of the lesser tuberosity on the coracoid process. These patients complain of anterior shoulder pain made worse by forward flexion and medial rotation combined with horizontal adduction. Of the 23 patients reported by Russo & Togo (1991), 20 were treated conservatively. In 22% of these patients the same symptoms returned upon resumption of activity, although they were easier to endure. Their three patients who

Table 5.21 The results of open operation for impingement syndrome

	Hawkins et al (1988)	Post & Cohen (1985)	Björkenheim et al (1990)	Frieman & Fenlin (1995)	Dodenhoff et al (1997)
Number of shoulders	108	72	60	75	63
Follow-up	5.2 years	2 years	4 years	16.9 mths	20.8 mths
Satisfactory	94 (87%)	64 (89%)	44 (73%)	64	53
Unsatisfactory	14 (13%)	8 (11%)	16 (27%)	11 (15%)	10 (16%)
Workers' compensation	35	40	—	37	—
unsatisfactory	8 (23%)	7 (17.5%)	—	9 (24%)	—
Trauma	62				
Unsatisfactory with trauma	11 (18%)				
Satisfactory					
< 40 years		91%			
> 40 years		70%			
Total	378 Satisfactory 319		(84%) Unsatisfactory (16%)		

Table 5.22 The results of arthroscopic operations for impingement syndrome

	Esch (1989)	Patel et al (1999)	Roye et al (1995)	Stephens et al (1998)	Esch et al (1988)
Number of shoulders	67	114	90	83	45
Follow-up	1–3 years	19 mths	41 mths	8 years 5 mths	1.5 years
Satisfactory	56 (84%)	85 (75%)	84 (93%)	67 (81%)	37 (82%)
Unsatisfactory	11 (16%)	29 (25%)	6 (7%)	16 (19%)	8 (18%)
Total 399	329 (82.5%)	satisfactory	70 (17.5%)	unsatisfactory	

underwent surgical decompression had almost immediate relief of symptoms. Of the 14 shoulders decompressed for subcoracoid impingement reported by Dumontier et al (1999), all improved clinically after operation although three patients still had moderate pain and seven reported shoulder weakness.

There may be an association between an os acromiale and impingement syndrome. Impingement of the rotator cuff on the postero-superior aspect of the glenoid has been described in athletes engaged in overhead activities when the arm is in the throwing position (extension, abduction and external rotation) (Bigliani & Levine 1997).

Partial thickness tears of the rotator cuff occur mainly on the articular surface of the cuff and may be secondary to the impingement process, glenohumeral instability or an episode of trauma. Wright and Cofield 1996 reported that eight of their 39 (20.5%) patients had a bursal side partial thickness tear, 21 (54%) had a partial thickness articular surface tear while in 10 patients it was entirely interstitial. Budoff et al (1998), reporting on 79 shoulders, found that 51 partial thickness tears were articular (64.5%), one was on the bursal surface and 27 were on both surfaces.

Gartsman & Milne (1995) found that the partial thickness tear was attributable to impingement in 85 (77%) of 111 patients, to glenohumeral instability in 14 (13%) and to direct trauma in 12 (11%). Payne et al (1997) noted that 14 of their 43 athletes (33%) under the age of 40, with partial thickness tears of the rotator cuff, gave a history of an acute traumatic injury.

An operation is indicated for persistent pain that interferes with the activities of daily living, work or sports and is unresponsive to a 6–12 month course of non-operative treatment. Arthroscopic debridement alone, or combined with subacromial decompression and open repair, has been advocated for the treatment of partial thickness tears, and anterior reconstruction may be required for those patients whose tears are associated with instability. The results of the operative treatment of partial thickness tears are shown in Table 5.23. Eighty-five percent had a satisfactory outcome.

Rotator cuff tears usually fall into one of four categories:

1. Those due to a fracture of the greater tuberosity as the result of a single major injury. This type will be dealt with in a later section of this chapter.
2. Acute massive avulsions without fracture. These also occur as the result of a single major injury with or without anterior dislocation of the shoulder. They tend to be found in the younger, athletic patient, and can result from direct trauma to the shoulder after a fall or indirect or repetitive trauma transmitted up the outstretched arm.
3. Acute-on-chronic ruptures.
4. Chronic ruptures.

The last two categories are seen more typically in the elderly patient.

Acute tears

Acute rotator cuff tears tend to occur after severe trauma through relatively healthy tendinous tissue or as the result of acute anterior dislocation of the shoulder. Reeves (1969) reported the results of arthrograms performed on 47 patients with acute anterior dislocation of the shoulder; 26 of the patients had an associated capsular rupture and he found this to be the predominant injury sustained at the time of dislocation in patients over 50 years of age. When the arthrogram was repeated 7–10 days later, five patients showed rotator cuff defects.

Berbig et al (1999) recently reported similar findings based on the early ultrasonagraphic evaluation of the rotator cuff in 167 patients with primary traumatic anterior shoulder dislocation. They found 53 (31.7%) full-thickness tears in this group. Women ruptured the cuff more often than men.

Wallace & Wiley (1986) reported the long-term results of the conservative management of 36 manual workers with 37 acute shoulder injuries. Twenty-eight were stated to have definite full-thickness tears. After a mean follow-up of 5 years, 30 patients (81%) had significant pain, and 28 (76%) stated that they were the same or worse than at the 6 months review. All of the patients had a diminished range of motion, there was a marked reduction of power (by more than 60% measured on Cybex equipment), and only 13 of 24 patients (54%) under 65 years old were able to work.

Surgery is probably indicated in the young adult with a complete avulsion of the cuff. Basset & Cofield (1983) reported the results of 37 acute rotator cuff repairs performed within 3 months of injury. Pain relief was good despite any delay in surgery from the time of injury, but the range of active abduction achieved postoperatively was diminished by such a delay. Thus an average 168° of abduction was obtained in the 12 cases repaired within 3 weeks of injury, decreasing to 129° in the 19 cases repaired after 6 weeks. They found no correlation between the result and the size of the defect. Thirteen patients (35%) had no pain and the remaining 24 (64%) only slight pain. Just four patients (11%) did not feel that surgery had achieved any improvement.

Tibone et al (1986) reported 10 good results (67%) in 15 athletes treated by surgery for complete rotator cuff tears.

Chronic tears

Chronic tears are not necessarily symptomatic and should be regarded as part of the normal ageing process. Jerosch

Table 5.23 The results of surgery for partial thickness tears of the rotator cuff

	Gartsman & Milne (1995)	Budoff et al (1998)	Wright & Cofield (1996)	Payne et al (1997)
Number of shoulders	111	79	39	43
Follow-up	32.3 mths	53 mths	55 mths	24 mths
Satisfactory	98 (88%)	69 (87%)	33 (85%)	31 (72%)
Unsatisfactory	13 (12%)	10 (13%)	6 (15%)	12 (28%)
Total 272	231 (85%) satisfactory	41 (15%) unsatisfactory		

et al (1991) examined 122 autopsy specimens of the shoulder and found the incidence of partial tears to be 28.7% and of complete rupture 30.3%. The frequency of rupture increased with age. There was no information available on whether any of these patients had a history of shoulder complaints. However, Tempelhof et al (1999) were able to determine the prevalence of rotator cuff tears in the asymptomatic shoulder using ultrasonographic studies of 411 volunteers. Evidence of a rotator cuff tear was found in 23%; in patients aged 50–59 years, 13% (22 of 167) had tears; in those aged 60–69 years 20% (22 of 108) had tears; between 70 and 79 years, 31% (27 of 87) had tears; while in those aged over 80 years 51% (25 of 49) had tears. It is not clear what parameters convert an asymptomatic tear into a symptomatic tear. Takagishi (1978) reviewed the conservative treatment of 39 patients with arthrographically proven symptomatic rotator cuff tears. Overall, 17 patients (44%) achieved satisfactory recovery, 16 (76%) of 21 patients with small tears and only 1 (5%) of 18 patients with large tears.

Itoi et al (1997) measured the isokinetic strength in abduction and external rotation in 10 patients with full-thickness tears of the supraspinatus and 10 with partial thickness tears, after pain block with local anaesthetic. While there was no significant difference in the strength between the involved and uninvolved side in patients with partial thickness tears, decreases in strength of 19 to 33% in abduction and 22 to 33% in external rotation occurred in patients with full-thickness tears.

There are many reports of the surgical treatment of these chronic tears, utilising a variety of methods. Unfortunately, there is no standard method of classifying the size of the rupture or the quality of functional recovery. A few of the larger series reporting functional improvements are shown in Table 5.24.

The criteria for the assessment of functional improvement differ widely. However, from Table 5.24 it can be seen that on average 81% of patients will achieve a satisfactory functional outcome, although some residual disability will persist, especially in prolonged use of the arms above shoulder level.

Increasingly, the results of arthroscopic and arthroscopic assisted mini-open repairs are being reported. Gartsman et al (1998) presented their results of arthroscopic repair of full-thickness tears of the rotator cuff in 73 patients; 66 (90%) rated the result as good or excellent at an average 30 months' follow-up.

There is no agreement on the results of surgery in relation to the size of the defect, or to the timing of surgery. Hawkins et al (1985) found that the size of the tear did not significantly affect the results, although they did say that patients with a smaller tear tended to fare slightly better. However, Hattrup (1995) found that excellent results decreased from 89.2% in small or medium tears to 80.4% in large or massive tears. Harryman et al (1991) studied 105 surgically repaired rotator cuff tears. They found that the function of patients with intact surgically repaired large tears was as good as that in intact small tears. It was the integrity of the rotator cuff at follow-up, and not the size of the tear at the time of surgical repair, which was the major determinant of the outcome. However, patients with larger pre-operative tear sizes were much more likely to demonstrate recurrent cuff tears at follow-up.

The effect of the pre-operative cuff size to the postoperative function was also noted by Lannotti et al (1996). They evaluated 40 patients who underwent surgery for full-thickness cuff tears, at a 2 year follow-up. Patients with a satisfactory postoperative outcome had an average cuff tear size of 9 cm^2, while those with an unsatisfactory score had an average cuff size of 18 cm^2. Wülker et al (1991) found that older patients generally had a less favourable clinical result than younger patients. Hattrup (1995), in his study of 88 patients who had rotator cuff repairs, reported that 31 (88.6%) of 35 patients younger

Table 5.24 Satisfactory function following rotator cuff repair

Reference	No. of cases	Satisfactory function	Percentage
Hawkins et al (1985)	100	92	92
Wulker et al (1991)	97	74	76
Watson (1985)	89	62	70
Cofield et al (1985)	88	73	83
Misamore et al (1995)	107	89	83
Overall	481	390	81

than 65 years had an excellent result, whilst three (8.6%) had a satisfactory result and one (2.9%) an unsatisfactory result. Of the 53 patients aged over 65 years, 41 (77.4%) had an excellent result, seven (13.2%) were satisfactory and five (9.4%) had an unsatisfactory result. Watson (1985) found that maximal improvement occurred up to 2 years postoperatively, but that with longer follow-up patients over 60 years of age tended to deteriorate.

A number of studies have looked at muscle strength after rotator cuff repairs. These studies found that the average strength of abduction measured 80 to 87% of normal. The isokinetic strength of flexion was 75 to 84% of normal and for external rotation was 90% of normal (Rokito et al 1996). These studies reported that small tears generally had greater strength than larger tears. The strength of the muscles continued to improve from 6 months to 1 year after the repair, although greatest improvement occurred in the first 6 months. It is therefore recommended that rehabilitation continue beyond 6 months.

Wallace et al (1999) reported that the median time taken to return to driving after rotator cuff repair in 80 patients was 12 weeks.

Hawkins et al (1985) stated that it was their impression that patients involved in litigation achieved worse results than other patients, the compensation patients taking twice as long to return to work.

Misamore et al (1995) divided their 107 shoulders into two groups. One group (24 patients) were receiving Workers Compensation and the second group (79 patients) were not. Of the 24 shoulders of patients receiving Workers Compensation, 13 (54%) were rated good or excellent, compared with 76 (92%) of the 83 shoulders of patients not receiving Workers Compensation.

Summary

- There are three stages of impingement: stage I, oedema and haemorrhage; stage IIa, fibrosis and tendonitis, stage IIb partial tear, and stage III, degeneration, bony change and tendon rupture.
- Vascular, degenerative, traumatic and mechanical or anatomic factors are all implicated in the aetiology of rotator cuff lesion.
- 26–39% of patients with impingement lesions fail to respond to conservative treatment, and 29% have mild residual symptoms.
- 82–84% of patients with stage II impingement lesions have a satisfactory result with surgery.
- 22% of patients with subcoracoid impingement treated conservatively have continued symptoms, and 75–100% improve with surgery.

- 11–33% of partial thickness tears may have an acute traumatic origin.
- 85% of patients with partial thickness tears have a satisfactory result after surgery.
- The conservative treatment of acute rotator cuff injuries in manual workers resulted in 81% of patients having significant residual pain, loss of motion and a 60% reduction in strength.
- 67–89% of patients with acute tears had a satisfactory result from surgery.
- Up to 51% of chronic tears may be asymptomatic, although the incidence does increase with age.
- 44% of patients with chronic rotator cuff tears achieved satisfactory results with conservative treatment.
- A decrease in strength of 19–33% in abduction and 22–33% in external rotation occurs in isolated rupture of the supraspinatus tendon.
- 81% of surgically treated patients with chronic tears had satisfactory pain relief, and 79% achieved a satisfactory functional result.
- Improvement after surgery continued to occur over 2 years. However, in patients over the age of 60 years there may be some deterioration of the initial functional recovery obtained after surgery.
- Results of surgery are worse in those receiving Workers Compensation.

Anterior dislocation and subluxation of the glenohumeral joint

Incidence and classification

Despite the frequency with which anterior dislocations of the shoulder occur, there are very few data concerning the incidence of shoulder dislocations in the general population. In a small random sample in Sweden, Hovelius (1982) found that 1.7% of people between the ages of 18 and 70 had reported such an occurrence.

The overall incidence of initial anterior shoulder dislocation is 8.2 (Simonet et al 1984) to 24.5 (Nordqvist & Petersson 1995) per 100 000 per year.

Rowe (1980) suggested the following classification of anterior shoulder dislocations:

- traumatic anterior dislocation
  — primary anterior dislocation
  — transient anterior dislocation
  — recurrent anterior dislocation
  — chronic anterior dislocation
- atraumatic anterior dislocation
  — primary and recurrent anterior dislocation
  — recurrent voluntary anterior dislocation

To this list should be added congenital or developmental dislocations. Only the first group, which is likely to result in medico-legal action, will be considered further.

Primary anterior dislocation

Many factors play a part in determining the prognosis after primary anterior dislocation of the shoulder, of which the age of the patient is probably the most important. These factors, as they relate to the risk of recurrent dislocation, will be discussed later. Conservative treatment following primary anterior dislocation has been the rule, and with the development of arthroscopic techniques an increasing number of papers discuss the role of surgery in the treatment of acute primary dislocation.

Aronen & Regan (1984) treated 20 young American midshipmen for 3 weeks using a sling, followed by an intensive rehabilitation programme, and reported their patients back to full unrestricted activity at 3 months. Recovery time will be longer in the older age group who have an increased incidence of rotator cuff tear associated with their primary dislocation.

Kiviluoto et al (1980) found that 42 patients out of a total of 226 (19%) had some residual stiffness of the affected shoulder 1 year after treatment. Only one in four patients in this series were aged under 30. Only one (4%) of the 26 patients under the age of 30 had residual stiffness compared with 40 (26%) of the 154 patients aged over 30 years, after a comparable period of immobilisation of 1 week. The other patients in this series had different periods of immobilisation.

Studying this same group of patients, Pasila et al (1980) found that 38 (25%) of those over 50 years of age failed to attain normal mobility of the shoulder after 1 year. The corresponding figures for those aged under 50 years was four out of 99 patients (4%). The median time to recovery of normal mobility was 3 weeks after 1 week's immobilisation, increasing to 5 weeks after 3 weeks' immobilisation. This recovery period increased to 7 weeks in those patients over 50 years of age regaining normal mobility.

If the dislocation had been present for longer than 12 hours, the median period for recovery of normal mobility was 4–5 months (compared to 30 days for the study group taken as a whole).

Recovery time was also related to the degree of violence initiating the dislocation. Shoulders dislocating as the result of torsion recovered full mobility in a mean period of 24 days, compared to the 60 days required after a fall from a height.

In this group Pasila et al (1980) also found that out of 108 patients attaining normal mobility within 1 month, 25 (23%) redislocated. Residual stiffness present after 1 year tended to

be permanent, and only four out of 42 patients (9.5%) with this problem improved their mobility after 1 year.

Kazár & Relovszky (1969) evaluated 408 cases of acute anterior dislocation, after treatment by immobilisation (the duration of which did vary from patient to patient). They, too, noted the detrimental effect that the age of the patient had on the recovery of function. In their under-30 age group, one patient out of 48 (2%) had at least 90° limitation of movement as compared with 16 of 110 patients (14.5%) aged 31–50, and 94 of 250 (37.6%) aged over 50 years.

Rowe (1956) reported the functional recovery in those patients whose dislocation did not recur. Of 110 shoulders, 69 (63%) were normal with regard to function and comfort, 24 (22%) had mild limitation of activity, while 14 (13%) had moderate limitation of activity (inability or unease at work or in sport when using the arm in an elevated or overhead position). Three patients (3%) had marked limitation of usefulness and function. Rowe felt that the moderate and poor results reflected those patients with associated rotator cuff tears.

Pevny et al (1998) studied 125 patients aged 40 years or older who sustained a traumatic first-time anterior shoulder dislocation ski-ing, and reviewed them at a minimum 2 year follow-up. Of the 52 patients available for interview 32 (62%) had an excellent result, nine (17%) a good result, eight (15%) a fair result, and three (6%) a poor result. Eighteen (35%) rotator cuff tears were identified, and only 11 (61%) of these patients achieved an excellent or good outcome. Seven (64%) of the 11 patients with a fair or poor result had a rotator cuff tear. Gumina and Postacchini (1997) reviewed 95 patients aged 60 years or more at the time of primary traumatic anterior dislocation. After a mean follow-up of 7.1 years a decreased range of active movement of the involved shoulder was seen in 63 (66%) of patients, with clinical signs of a rotator cuff tear in 58 (61%). Forty-four of these 58 (76%) patients had subacromial and deltoid pain at night or on active abduction and forward flexion or both.

O'Driscoll & Evans (1991) reported that 47 of 188 patients (25%) who had surgery for anterior shoulder instability were subsequently shown to have developed bilateral involvement at a mean of 5.7 years after anterior repair of the operated shoulder. This incidence was significantly higher in those under 15 years at the time of initial dislocation, or under 18 at the time of surgery. Other predisposing factors included having sustained the initial injury to the operated shoulder as a result of minimal trauma.

Hovelius et al (1996) reported dislocation of the contralateral shoulder in 31 (12.5%) of 247 primary anterior dislocations. It occurred in 16% of those patients who were aged 12–22 years at the time of primary dislocation, 21% of those aged 23–29 years and only 3% of those aged 30–40 years at initial dislocation. They also noted that 24 (22%) of the 107 shoulders that had had recurrent dislocation within the first 5 years had stabilised at the 10 year follow-up without any surgical intervention.

Surgical treatment of traumatic primary anterior dislocation of the shoulder

Wintzell et al (1999) compared non-operative treatment of primary anterior shoulder dislocation with arthroscopic lavage in 60 patients. At 1 year follow-up four of 30 patients (13%) in the lavage group had redislocated compared with 13 of 30 (43%) in the group treated non-operatively. The functional outcome was also better in the lavage group. One hundred and twenty seven patients from West Point Military Academy who had acute anterior dislocations of the shoulder were reported by De Berardino et al (1996). Of the 55 patients treated non-operatively, 47 (85%) had a recurrence of instability, while of the 60 treated operatively, the number was only seven (12%).

Kirkley et al (1999) compared rehabilitation or immediate arthroscopic stabilisation in 40 patients under 30 years of age. At a minimum of 24 months' follow-up, three of the 19 patients (16%) treated surgically sustained a redislocation as compared with nine of the 19 (47%) treated with rehabilitation.

Inferior glenohumeral dislocation (luxatio erecta) involves less than 1% of glenohumeral dislocations. Either a fracture of the greater tuberosity or a rotator cuff tear was associated with this injury in 80% of patients, and 60% sustained some degree of neurological injury, most commonly to the axillary nerve; the injuries usually resolved, the recovery time varying from 2 weeks to 1 year

(Mallon et al 1990). Patients with an abducted position of the arm when the primary dislocation occurred (luxatio abducta) forms a subgroup of this type of dislocation (Hovelius et al 1996).

Factors related to recurrence of dislocation

Numerous published series quote recurrence rates following anterior dislocation, but the many variable factors between each series makes a direct comparison of doubtful value. However, the figures in the larger series shown in Table 5.25 reveal a 27% recurrence rate.

The length of follow-up is important when considering the incidence of recurrent dislocation. Hoelen et al (1990) noted that 83% of their patients had their first recurrence within 2 years, and 98% within 3 years. In Rowe's 1956 series, out of 151 recurrences 70.5% had occurred by 2 years, a further 19% by 2–5 years, 6% by 5–10 years, and 4.5% did not recur until more than 10 years after the initial dislocation.

As stated previously (Hovelius et al 1997), 22% of shoulders with recurrent dislocation may stabilise over 10 years.

The various factors that affect the prognosis relating to the recurrence of dislocation are:

- the age of the patient
- the length of immobilisation
- the severity of the initial trauma
- the sex of the patient
- the presence of associated fractures
- the effect of rehabilitation

The age of the patient
The age of the patient at the time of initial dislocation would appear to play an important part in whether recurrence will occur. The variation in recurrence rates as

Table 5.25 The incidence of recurrent dislocation after primary anterior dislocation

Reference	Total primary anterior dislocation	Recurrence	Percentage
Kazár & Relovszky (1969)	566	48	8.5
Rowe (1956)	398	151*	38
Rowe & Sakellarides (1961)	324	136	42
Hovelius et al (1997)	247	118	48
Kiviluoto et al (1980)	226	30	13
Hoelen et al (1990)	168	44	26
	1929	527	27

* Estimated from data given in the paper.

compared with age in the major series reviewed is reported in Table 5.26. Again, although the figures vary from series to series, patients under the age of 20 have a significantly higher risk of redislocation (46–94%) compared with those aged over 40 (4.5–14.5%).

The length of immobilisation

The recurrence rate compared to the length of immobilisation is recorded in Table 5.27. Thus it would appear that in those papers reviewing treatment of the general population (Rowe 1956, Rowe & Sakellarides 1961, Kiviluoto et al 1980) the figures for recurrent dislocation were improved by a period of up to 3 weeks' immobilisation,

whereas immobilisation beyond 3 weeks was of questionable value. On the other hand, Hovelius et al (1983) suggested that, in a group excluding patients over 40 years of age, immobilisation had no effect on the incidence of recurrence of dislocation. This conclusion was supported by Hoelen et al (1990).

The severity of the initial trauma

In their series of 247 primary anterior dislocations in the under-40 age group, Hovelius et al (1997) reported that the severity of the initiating trauma had no influence on the rate of recurrence of the dislocation. Rowe (1956) suggested that the recurrence rate was significant when

Table 5.26 The incidence of recurrent dislocation compared with age at the time of primary dislocation

Reference	>20			20–40			40+		
	No.	Recur	%	No.	Recur	%	No.	Recur	%
Hovelius et al (1997)*	99	65	66	148	53	36			
Rowe (1956)	57	47†	83	77	49†	63	220‡	26†	12
Rowe & Sakellarides (1961)	53	50	94	80	59	74	186	27	14.5
Kazár & Relovszky (1969)	28	13	46	97	15	15.5	441	20	4.5
Kiviluoto et al (1980)	18	10	55.5	65	11	17	143	9	6
Simonet & Cofield (1984)	32	27	84	43	21	49	41	4	10

* Age ranges 0–22 and 23–40.
† Estimated from data given in the paper.
‡ Figures for 50 years and over.

Table 5.27 The incidence of recurrence compared with length of immobilisation

Reference	Immobilisation time											
	None			1 week			2–3 weeks			3–6 weeks		
	Recur	No.	%	Recur	No.	%	Recur	No.	%	Recur	No.	%
Hovelius et al (1997)*	49	99	49.5							54	112	48
Rowe (1956)	52	63	82.5	29	46	63	–41	98	42	35	66	53
Rowe & Sakellarides (1961)	46	66	70				–61†	176	35	26	76	34
Kiviluoto et al (1980)		13	26	50	–6	27	22					

* Patients less than 40 years old.
† Group immobilised for 1–3 weeks.

compared with the type of initiating trauma, but cautioned that this must also be interpreted with respect to the age of the patient. Rowe & Sakellarides (1961), Kazár & Relovszky (1969) and Kiviluoto et al (1980) all suggested that there was a decreasing incidence of recurrent dislocation with increasing severity of initiating trauma. Again, direct comparison between these series is difficult.

The sex of the patient

There is some controversy as to whether the sex of the patient has any bearing on the likelihood of recurrent dislocation. Rowe (1956) found that the incidence of recurrence was twice as common in males as in females. However, both Hovelius et al (1997) and Simonet & Cofield (1984) reported that the incidence of recurrence was not increased in either sex when the patients were age-matched.

The presence of associated fractures

The presence of a fractured greater tuberosity decreases the likelihood of recurrent dislocation. Hovelius et al (1997) reported that only four of his 31 patients (13%) with this fracture had a recurrence of dislocation, compared with 114 of 216 patients (53%) without this fracture. Rowe (1956) reported recurrence occurring in three of 44 patients (6.8%) with fracture of the greater tuberosity, as compared with a recurrence rate of 38% in his study group as a whole. When Rowe & Sakellarides (1961) increased the number of patients in Rowe's 1956 series, the incidence fell to three recurrences in 66 patients (4.5%).

Humeral head defects may be seen in shoulders with no history of dislocation. Rowe (1956) examined the radiographs of 200 patients with no history of dislocation and found humeral head defects in 10%. Thirty-eight percent of their patients with primary dislocations had evidence of these defects, as compared with 57% with recurrent dislocation. Hovelius et al (1997) found that the rate of recurrence in their patients was related to the presence or absence of a humeral head defect. Of the 185 shoulders evaluated radiographically at the time of the primary dislocation and followed up for ten years, 99 (54%) had a posterior defect of the humeral head. Of these 99 shoulders, 60 redislocated at least once compared with 38 (44%) of the 86 that did not have such a lesion.

Hovelius et al (1983) reported that 8% of their patients with an anterior dislocation had a fracture of the glenoid rim, although they felt that the real incidence was higher. They found that the incidence increased with the age of the patient but that it bore no relation to the incidence of later redislocation. The absence of the influence of anterior glenoid rim fractures in the recurrence rate of dislocation was confirmed by Hoelen et al (1990) in 7% of their

patients with this fracture. This was contrary to Rowe's 1956 findings, where the incidence of glenoid rim fracture was 5.4%, but 13 of 21 patients (62%) with this associated fracture had a recurrence of dislocation.

Bigliani et al (1998) described 25 shoulders with recurrent instability and associated anterior glenoid rim lesions. Their classification system was: Type I, a displaced avulsion fracture with attached capsule (16 cases); Type II, a medially displaced fragment malunited to the glenoid rim (five cases); Type III, erosion of the glenoid rim with less than 25% (Type IIIA—three cases) or greater than 25% (Type IIIB—one case) deficiency. Various surgical procedures were undertaken depending on the type of lesion. At an average follow-up of 30 months, 22 shoulders (88%) had satisfactory results without recurrent instability, whereas three (12%) had postoperative redislocations.

The effect of adequate rehabilitation

In 20 midshipmen with an average age of 19.2 years, Aronen & Regan (1984) reported a recurrence of dislocation or subluxation in 25% after 3 weeks' immobilisation and an intensive rehabilitation programme.

Yoneda et al (1982) reported on 104 male patients with an average age of 21.5 years and whose shoulders were immobilised for 5 weeks followed by 6 weeks of graduated exercises. Their recurrent dislocation rate was 17.3%.

Rotator cuff tears in association with anterior dislocation

Rotator cuff tears are well documented in association with anterior dislocation of the shoulder and tend to occur with increasing frequency in the older patient. However, their incidence is difficult to assess accurately, because many authors' diagnoses are based on clinical impression rather than proven arthrogram.

Reeves (1969) reported the results of arthrograms performed on 47 patients with acute anterior dislocation of the shoulder, and found ruptures of the rotator cuff in 26 of them (55%). He found it to be the predominant shoulder injury sustained at the time of dislocation in patients over 50 years of age. The arthrograms were repeated after 7–10 days, and five patients still showed rotator cuff defects. Two of these five had disability severe enough to warrant surgical exploration, at which time the diagnosis was confirmed. Only one patient in this group of 26 developed recurrent dislocation.

In a study referred to previously, Berbig et al (1999) performed ultrasound examination on 167 patients with primary traumatic anterior shoulder dislocations. They found 53 (31.7%) full-thickness tears in this group. In patients aged under 50 years one rotator cuff tear (1.5%)

was found in 66 patients. In the age group 50–59 there were six tears (31.6%) in 19 patients; in the group 60–69 there were 11 tears (47.8%) in 23 patients; and in those aged 70 years and over there were 35 (59%) in 59 patients.

Pevny et al (1998) identified 18 (35%) rotator cuff tears in 52 patients aged 40 years or older, with only 11 (61%) of these 18 patients obtaining an excellent or good outcome.

In patients aged 60 years and older, Gumina and Postacchini (1997) diagnosed 58 tears (61%) in 108 patients. The cuff tear was symptomatic in only 76% of the patients in whom the condition was diagnosed.

Pasila et al (1980) found that 23 of their 26 patients with rotator cuff tears (88.5%) had permanent stiffness of the shoulder and in 14 of these the limitation was up to 40° in flexion. However, they stated that no patient had spontaneous pain or pain on movement of such severity as to indicate surgical treatment for rotator cuff rupture.

The treatment of patients with rotator cuff ruptures in association with recurrent anterior dislocation of the shoulder is difficult. Neviaser and Neviaser (1995) reported on 12 patients who had surgery for recurrent instability in this situation. All 12 had a stable shoulder after a 2–13 year follow-up, although one patient required a re-operation.

Other complications
Nerve injury
The reported incidence of nerve injury following acute anterior dislocation is quite variable. Rowe (1956) quoted an incidence of 5.4% in 500 dislocations, while Pasila et al (1978) had a 21% incidence, of which 29 were brachial plexus injuries and 21 axillary nerve injuries. This incidence of nerve injury rises to 60% in the case of luxatio erecta (Mallon et al 1990).

Visser et al (1999) investigated the incidence and the clinical consequences of nerve lesions in a prospective study by clinical and electrophysiological examination of 77 patients. Thirty-seven patients (48%) had denervation (axonal loss). The mean number of nerves involved was 1.8, with the axillary nerve featuring most frequently (42%). The numbers of the other nerve lesions were: suprascapular (14%), radial (7%), musculocutaneous (12%), median (4%) and ulnar (8%). A solitary nerve lesion was present in 51%. The probability of nerve injury increased by a factor of 1.3 for every 10 year period of the age of the patient. The severity of the lesion also increased with age. Bruising about the shoulder was associated with a 4.4 times greater probability of nerve injury, and it doubled in the presence of an associated fracture.

In Rowe's series 15% failed to recover, and Pasila et al (1978) reported that 30% of the patients in their series had not recovered completely at 1 year. However, all of the patients aged under 51 years recovered, compared to 58% of those aged over 51 years. Pasila et al further stated that recovery occurred for up to 1 year after injury, but quoted Assmus & Meirel who reported a poor prognosis in those patients showing no recovery by 8–10 weeks after injury.

Travlos et al (1990) reviewed 28 patients with brachial plexus lesions caused by anterior shoulder dislocation. They found that the neurological lesions involved the infraclavicular and the supraclavicular brachial plexus and most made a good functional recovery. With suprascapular lesions the involvement was always of the suprascapular nerve, and all of their six patients with this lesion had recovered fully at 14 months. Only two of their five patients with isolated axillary nerve lesions recovered, however. They noted that all those patients who recovered to grade 4 or 5 (see Medical Research Council 1943) did so by 18 months. All these had shown at least grade 1 power at 2 months and at least grade 3 by 6 months.

Four of the 32 patients (12.5%) with axillary nerve injury reported by Visser et al (1999) had persistent abnormalities of the EMG. The duration of recovery from axillary nerve injury was prolonged, lasting up to 35 weeks. Restricted movement of the shoulder was closely related to a lesion of the axillary nerve.

A neurological deficit was noted in 23 (8.2%) of 282 patients who underwent anterior reconstructive surgery for recurrent glenohumeral instability (Ho et al 1999). Complete resolution occurred in 18 (78%) of the patients. Three had a persistent sensory disturbance and one had permanent biceps weakness.

Vascular damage
Damage to the axillary artery has been reported frequently enough in the literature to substantiate its place as an uncommon but grave complication of anterior dislocation. Only one patient with an injury to the axillary artery was found in the 216 shoulder dislocations reported by Kroner et al (1989). Gates and Knox (1995) reported a case of axillary artery injury secondary to anterior dislocation and reviewed 22 reported cases. They found that 86% occurred in patients older than 50, 86% of the injuries are in the third part of the axillary artery, and 68% presented with an axillary mass. The injury increases in incidence with the attempted closed reduction of chronic dislocations. The long-term prognosis depends on the result of arterial repair.

Summary

- The younger patient with a treated primary anterior dislocation of the shoulder should have returned to full function by 3 months after injury.

- 2–4% of patients aged under 30 had some residual stiffness after primary anterior dislocation.
- 62% of patients aged over 40 had an excellent result after anterior dislocation. 35% in this age group have an associated rotator cuff tear.
- 66% of patients aged over 60 had a decreased range of motion after primary anterior dislocation.
- Recovery time was increased by a factor of four when the dislocation persisted for over 12 hours.
- Stiffness present after 1 year tended to be permanent.
- 12.5–25% of patients with anterior dislocation of the shoulder subsequently develop instability on the opposite side
- 13–16% of patients undergoing arthroscopic surgery for primary traumatic anterior shoulder dislocation had recurrence of dislocation.
- Luxatio erecta results in a greater tuberosity fracture or rotator cuff rupture in 80% of cases, and neurological injury in 60% of patients.
- 8.5–44% (average 27%) of patients had a recurrence after primary anterior dislocation.
- 70–83% of recurrences occurred within 2 years and a further 15–19% within 5 years.
- 22% of shoulders with recurrent dislocation may stabilise over a 10 year period.
- 46–94% of patients under 20 years of age suffered a recurrence of their dislocation, compared to 4.5–14.5% of patients aged over 40.
- The length of immobilisation of the shoulder in young patients with anterior dislocation would not appear to affect recurrence of dislocation, although immobilisation for 3 weeks would seem to be beneficial in the older age group.
- There would appear to be a decreasing incidence of recurrent dislocation with increasing severity of trauma, although this relationship is less certain in younger patients.
- The sex of the patient with a primary anterior dislocation had an uncertain influence on the incidence of recurrence.
- 4.5–13% of patients with associated fractures of the greater tuberosity experienced recurrence of dislocation.
- The presence of a humeral head defect was associated with an increased incidence of recurrent dislocation.
- Fractures of the glenoid rim had an uncertain association with recurrent dislocation.
- An intensive period of rehabilitation decreased the incidence of recurrent dislocation in younger patients.

- The incidence of rotator cuff tear in association with anterior dislocation is 32–55%, but rises with increasing age.
- Permanent disability persisted in 39–88.5% of patients sustaining a rotator cuff tear in association with their anterior dislocation.
- Surgery for rotator cuff tear in association with anterior dislocation produced acceptable results in most patients.
- The incidence of nerve damage in anterior dislocation of the shoulder was 5.4–48%.
- 12.5–30% of nerve injuries failed to recover completely, although this incidence increased to 58% in patients aged over 50 years.
- Recovery of axillary nerve injuries occurred up to 18 months after injury, although failure of any recovery after 8–10 weeks suggested a poor prognosis.
- The incidence of neurologic complication after surgery for recurrent anterior glenohumeral instability is 8.2%.
- Axillary artery damage was more common in the elderly and after attempted closed manipulation of chronic dislocation. The overall functional recovery depended upon the response of the artery to surgical repair.

Recurrent anterior dislocation and subluxation of the gleno-humeral joint

Tsai et al (1991) published the results of their study of shoulder function in patients with unoperated anterior shoulder instability. Pain induced by activity was reported in 46% of the 26 patients, while 65% reported reduced strength and 73% subjective instability. Subjective decrease in shoulder mobility was reported in 88%. The majority of patients (65%) reported instability only during physical activity, while the remaining 35% also reported dislocations during sleep.

There is a group of patients, usually athletes, who undergo episodes of recurrent anterior subluxation with or without true dislocation, the so-called 'dead arm syndrome' (Rowe & Zarins 1981). This may be classified as either type I instability, which is present in the subluxating shoulder that has never been dislocated, or type II dislocation, which is present in those shoulders with definite recurrent dislocation and episodes of chronic subluxation in the intervals between dislocations.

The patients may or may not experience a sensation of the shoulder slipping out of place, especially with external rotation and abduction. Pain may be felt in the overhead position and on throwing. Of Rowe & Zarins' patients,

55% were unaware that the shoulder was dislocating. After the acute episode their patients were aware of numbnesss and tingling in the arm and hand, and the arm felt weak. They remained aware of weakness and a decreased range of motion for the next few hours. A period of intensive rehabilitation may be of benefit to these patients prior to consideration for surgical treatment, although Rowe & Zarins achieved improvement by physiotherapy in only 13% of their patients.

Although athletic activities are a frequent precursor to this injury, forceful external rotation and a direct blow were a cause of 86% of Rowe & Zarins' cases and these injuries may therefore be the subject of litigation.

The surgery of recurrent anterior instability of the shoulder is well documented. Many operations have been described, numerous modifications proposed and each operation has its proponents and critics. It is not the purpose of this section to select any particular operation as being ideal, but rather to tabulate the incidence of recur-

rence for those procedures as reported in the literature in order to assist in medico-legal reporting.

Rockwood (1991a) has already provided an extensive review of the literature and has shown that all of the reconstructions gave approximately 97% excellent results. His interpretation of 'excellent' would appear to imply no redislocation and does not take into account residual pain and restricted movement. The incidence of recurrence following various reconstructions for anterior instability of the shoulder is recorded in Table 5.28.

Failure to redislocate by no means implies an excellent result. Direct comparison between papers is impossible because of different criteria for assessing patients. Karadimas (1997) reported 97% excellent or good results with the Magnusson–Stack operation, with 13% of patients having more than 10° loss of external rotation. Kiss et al (1998) reported 83% of their patients as satisfied after the Putti–Platt procedure. Ninety percent had a loss of external rotation. The average loss of external rotation

Table 5.28 The incidence of recurrence following various reconstructions for anterior instability of the shoulder

Procedure	Reference	No. of cases	Follow-up	Excellent or good %	Recurrent dislocation or instability %
Magnusson-Stack	Karadimas (1997)	210	9 yrs. av	97%	1%
	Rockwood (1991)	571			4.1%
Coracoid transfer (Latarjet)	Nizard et al (1997)	220	4 yrs. av		4.5%
(Bristow)	Rockwood (1991a)	750			1.7% av
Bankart	McDermott et al (1999)	100	mean 1.5 yrs	96.5% (home activities) 91.5% (work activities) 75.6% (sport activities)	8%
	Rockwood (1991)	513			3.3%
Putti-Platt	Kiss et al (1998)	3890	9 yrs. av	83%	9%
	Rockwood (1991)	432			3% av
Du-Toit stapling	Sisk & Boyd (1974)	239			2.9%
Eden-Hybbinette	Gebhard et al (1997)	100	18 mths	61%	7%
	Rockwood (1991)	254			6%
Capsular imbrication	Wirth et al (1996)	142	5 yrs	93%	3.5%

with the arm at the side of the body was 24°, while with the arm in 90° abduction the average loss was 23°. Loss of external rotation is also recorded in the majority of other procedures, but to varying degrees.

Kiss et al (1998) found that redislocation following the Putti–Platt repair occurred twice as commonly in patients who were aged under 30 years at the time of operation.

The length of follow-up is also important when comparing series. Rowe (1956) stated that 52% of recurrences following operative procedures recur in the first 2 years, 17% within 2–5 years, 28% within 5–10 years and 3% within 10–20 years.

In recent years there has been an increasing interest in the arthroscopic treatment of glenohumeral instability. Table 5.29 records the results from the larger series. As before, the techniques and criteria for functional assessment do vary, but they are demanding with a long learning curve. While the results show a greater failure rate (6–17%) than with open repair (1–9%), they are none the less encouraging.

Chronic anterior dislocation of the gleno-humeral joint

Chronic anterior dislocation of the shoulder is less common today with the improved accident services, but may still be seen in the elderly patient or after unrecognised fractures of the glenoid (Schulz et al 1969). The major complaint in the elderly tends to be restriction of movement rather than pain. Younger patients are inclined to experience more in the way of pain due to the better condition of their muscles and ligaments. Not all patients necessarily require operation. Hejna et al (1969) treated eight of their 15 patients non-operatively and achieved an average total abduction rate of 82°. Of the 10 unreduced shoulder dislocations followed up in the series of Schulz et al (1969), nine were rated as 'satisfactory' by the patient;

seven were clinically rated as good, one was fair and two were poor.

Closed reduction may be successful, but this becomes increasingly difficult and hazardous after 3–4 weeks due to the adherence by scar tissue of the brachial plexus and axillary artery to the capsule. In the elderly an arteriosclerotic axillary artery is especially at risk.

Open reduction may be achieved with or without preservation of the humeral head.

Of the 13 shoulders with humeral head preservation available for end result evaluation in the series of Schulz et al (1969), 11 were rated as 'satisfactory' by the patients. Eight were clinically rated as good results, four fair and one poor. Of the five patients who had humeral head excision, four were rated as 'satisfactory', two were clinically rated as good, one was fair and two were poor. Neviaser (1963) reported on 16 patients who had operation for chronic dislocation (anterior and posterior). He did not indicate how many were anterior, but the two reported cases of chronic anterior dislocation achieved abduction of 90° and 135°, respectively.

Summary

- Of patients with unoperated anterior shoulder instability, 46% have pain with activity, 65% have reduced strength, and 73% have subjective instability.
- 88% have subjective decreased shoulder mobility and 35% report dislocations during sleep.
- 13% of recurrent subluxations may be 'cured' by intensive rehabilitation.
- Recurrent dislocation after operative stabilisation occurred in 1–9% of cases. Up to 31% of recurrences occur after 5 years.
- Excellent results occurred in 61–97% of patients after operative stabilisation, although external rotation was reduced to varying degrees by most procedures.

Table 5.29 The results of arthroscopic stabilisation for shoulder instability

Reference	No. of cases	Follow-up	Excellent/good result	Recurrent dislocation or instability
Torchia et al (1997)	150	mean 4.1 yrs	83%	17%
Savoie et al (1997)	161	av 58 mths	91%	9%
Resch et al (1997)	100	av 35 mths	83%	9%
Koenig et al (1999)	105	mean 18 mths	—	6%
De Beer & Thiart (1998)	104	mean 20 mths	—	8%

- Arthroscopic stabilisation of the shoulder has a 6–17% rate of recurrence of instability. Satisfactory results occur in 83–91% of patients.
- Elderly patients with chronic dislocation may be managed non-operatively and may achieve a reasonable range of active abduction.
- Closed reduction should not be attempted after 3–4 weeks, while open reduction produces variable return of function.

Posterior dislocation of the gleno-humeral joint

Incidence and classification

Posterior dislocation of the shoulder is much less common than anterior dislocation, Rowe (1956) reporting a 2% incidence, yet the incidence of chronic dislocations from missed diagnosis is much greater. Posterior dislocation may be classified as follows:

- traumatic
  — acute
  — chronic (or locked)
  — recurrent (dislocation and subluxation)
- voluntary and involuntary

Voluntary and involuntary dislocation need not be discussed further other than to emphasise the importance of distinguishing them from traumatic dislocation or subluxation. The voluntary dislocators respond poorly to surgery due to commonly associated psychiatric problems.

Acute posterior dislocation of the shoulder

Little appears to have been written about prognostic indicators in acute posterior dislocation of the shoulder.

Roberts & Wickstrom (1971) reviewed 14 cases of posterior dislocation treated conservatively. Delay in diagnosis in these patients was not mentioned but some may have been seen late. Nine (64%) achieved excellent or good results with slight limitation of movement: their average age was 38 years. Five (36%) had fair or poor results: their average age was 67 years. Thus functional results would appear to be good or excellent in patients under 40 years of age but diminished in quality in the over-40s. They also found that recurrence occurred in nine of 24 patients (37.5%), with five of these immobilised for less than 3 weeks. Rowe (1956) reported a recurrence rate of 60% for his 10 cases of posterior dislocation.

Roberts & Wickstrom (1971) found the incidence of associated fractures of the posterior glenoid and proximal humerus (including the humeral head) in their series to be 19 of 41 cases (46%). Of the 15 patients with adequate follow-up, nine (60%) achieved a good or excellent result. They also reported two cases (5%) of neurological complication in 41 patients (a transient radial nerve palsy and an axillary nerve palsy with partial recovery).

Chronic posterior dislocation

Considering the rarity of posterior dislocation of the shoulder, the incidence of late diagnosis is high, Rockwood (1991) stating that 60% were not diagnosed at initial assessment.

Kessel (1982) reported eight cases, and found the predominant complaint to be loss of movement. Some patients had been incorrectly labelled as 'frozen shoulder'. Pain was only significant in relatively recent dislocations. These patients were generally able to abduct to a right angle and one patient could abduct to 160°. Using a points system, Rowe & Zarins (1982) found that chronic posterior dislocation was less disabling than its anterior counterpart. Patients with minimal functional limitation could be managed non-operatively.

Hawkins et al (1987) reported closed manipulation successful in 25% of 12 patients in whom it was attempted less than 6 weeks from injury. They also found that transfer of the subscapularis muscle or lesser tuberosity into the humeral head defect was successful in maintaining reduction in all eight patients operated on at their units, with an average of 160–165° elevation, and internal rotation to the 12th thoracic vertebrae. However, they had also treated five failures of this procedure referred from other units.

Transfer of the lesser tuberosity or subscapularis muscle into the humeral head defect is not recommended for articular defects involving more than 40% of the articular surface. In these cases hemiarthroplasty or total shoulder arthroplasty must be considered. In Hawkins' series hemiarthroplasty was performed in nine shoulders, with good results in six 66%, ranges of motion similar to the group mentioned above being achieved. Failure occurred in those with degenerative changes of the glenoid.

Total arthroplasty was successful in 90% of 10 cases, the one failure dislocating and the patient refusing further treatment. Of the nine successes, one patient had moderate pain, but all were able to carry out the activities of daily living.

Gerber and Lambert (1996) reconstructed the shape of the humeral head with an allogenic segment of the femoral head in four patients, three of whom reported little or no pain, no or slight functional restrictions in the activities of daily living and considered the result to be satisfactory. The fourth patient developed avascular necrosis of the remaining portion of the humeral head.

In their more complicated points system, Rowe & Zarins (1982) achieved excellent or good results in 40% of surgical reductions. Of 10 patients treated by sugery (open reduction, hemiarthroplasty or excision arthroplasty), the six fair results had moderate pain, 50% of elevation and only moderate limitation with overhead work.

Recurrent posterior dislocation and subluxation

Many operations are available for the treatment of recurrent posterior dislocation and subluxation, but there is insufficient information on each procedure to allow an adequate assessment of prognosis. However, many patients with atraumatic posterior instability of the shoulder respond favourably to an exercise programme. Indeed Burkhead and Rockwood (1992) reported that 80% of their patients responded to such a programme. However, Fronek et al (1989) found that a physical therapy programme achieved a successful result in 63% of 16 patients with posterior subluxation of the glenohumeral joint. They reported a 91% success rate in the 11 patients treated by posterior capsulorrhaphy with or without a bone block. Tibone & Ting (1990), however, reported an unsatisfactory result in nine (45%) of 20 patients following posterior staple capsulorrhaphy. Six had a recurrence of the posterior instability and three still had moderate to severe pain. Hawkins et al (1984) reported on 50 cases of posterior instability of the shoulder, of which 80% had voluntary instability. Surgery was performed in 26 patients but recurrence occurred in 50%. It took 4 months post operation for the patients to return to daily living activities, and 6 months for those returning to sport.

Fifteen percent of the 20 shoulders with posterior subluxation reported by Fuchs et al (1999) had a recurrence of their subluxation following capsular reefing and a postero-inferior capsular shift.

Wilkinson & Thomas (1985) reported four recurrences (19%) in 21 glenoid osteotomies.

Arthritis after dislocation

The development of post-dislocation arthropathy was described by Samilson & Prieto (1983). They reviewed 74 shoulders with glenohumeral arthropathy after single or multiple dislocations of the shoulder. As these patients were seen in a secondary referral centre the authors were unable to comment on the incidence of arthritis after dislocation, although they quoted Hindmarsh & Lindberg as noting a 7% incidence of moderate or severe arthritis after recurrent dislocations treated non-operatively. They found that posterior dislocation had a much higher incidence of moderate and severe arthritis than anterior dislocation, possibly related to a delay in the diagnosis of dislocation. The frequency of dislocation and the presence of a humeral head or glenoid rim defect were not related to the severity of arthritis.

Hovelius et al (1996) prospectively reviewed 245 patients who had had 247 primary anterior dislocations of the shoulder at a 10 year follow-up. Radiographs were made for 208 shoulders; 23 (11%) had mild arthropathy and 18 (9%) had moderate or severe arthropathy. They found that shoulders that had had one recurrence had approximately the same degree of arthropathy as was noted in the shoulders that had had recurrent or operatively treated dislocations.

Table 5.30 shows the reported incidence of osteoarthritis after the long-term follow-up for surgery to stabilise anterior glenohumeral instability. It can be seen that the reported incidence is 20–62%. However, those papers with the longer follow-up reported the higher overall incidence.

It has been suggested that the restriction of external rotation after surgery may predispose the shoulder to degenerative changes. However, the limitation of external rotation may be secondary to the arthritic condition itself. Van der Zwaag et al (1999) found no correlation, in their study of Putti-Platt repair, between external rotation at 6 months after operation and the development of glenohumeral arthrosis. They did find that the number of dislocations before operation correlated with the severity of arthrosis but not with its incidence.

Mild arthritis was noted to be asymptomatic by Allain et al (1998).

Operations in which internal fixation devices intruded on the joint cartilage frequently resulted in moderate to severe arthritis.

Shoulder dislocation in children

Dislocation of the shoulder in children is exceedingly rare, Rowe (1956) noting just eight dislocations out of 500 patients under 10 years of age. Laskin & Sedlin (1971) reported a case of luxatio erecta in a child of 3 months with Erb–Duchenne brachial plexus palsy. Dunkerton (1989) reported four cases of posterior dislocation of the shoulder at birth in association with obstetric brachial plexus palsy. All were diagnosed late. Curtis et al (1991) quoted incidences of recurrence of 50 to 100%.

Kawam et al (1997) noted that the seven shoulders in six patients aged 9–17 who had surgical stabilisation for recurrent posterior shoulder dislocation were all painfree and clinically stable at long-term follow-up averaging 9.4 years. One child had required reoperation 3.5 years after the initial surgery.

Table 5.30 Incidence of osteoarthritis after surgery for anterior glenohumeral instability

Author	Procedure	Number of shoulders	Number with osteoarthritis	Length of follow-up
Gebhard et al (1992)	Eden-Hybinette-Lange	100	25 (25%)	minimum 18 mths
Kiss et al (1998)	Putti-Platt	70	21 (30%)	9 years
Krause et al (1997)	Eden-Hybinette-Large or rotational humeral osteotomy	134	27 (20%)	10–14 years
Van der Zwaag et al (1999)	Putti-Platt	66	40 (61%) mild 35% moderate 20% severe 6%	mean 22 years
Allain et al (1998)	Latarjet	58	36 (62%) mild 43% moderate 12% severe 7%	av 14.3 years
Rosenberg et al (1995)	Bankart	33	18 (54.5%) mild 42.5% moderate 9% severe 3%	av 15 years

Summary

- 2% of shoulder dislocations are posterior.
- In 64% of patients with acute posterior dislocations results were excellent or good, but increasing age mitigates against this outcome.
- Associated fractures occurred in about 46% of posterior dislocations.
- Recurrent posterior dislocation occurred in 37.5–60% of patients.
- Chronic posterior dislocation may cause minimal functional loss in the elderly.
- Surgery for chronic posterior dislocation may produce 40–80% good results depending on the operation and surgical expertise.
- Surgery for recurrent posterior instability produced variable results, with 9–50% recurrence of instability being reported. It may take 4 months to return to the activities of daily living after surgical reconstruction for recurrent posterior instability.
- The incidence of arthritis after anterior dislocation of the shoulder may be as high as 20%, but it is more common in posterior dislocation. Mild arthritis is asymptomatic.
- The incidence of glenohumeral arthrosis after the long-term follow-up of surgical stabilisation for instability is 20–62%.
- Dislocation of the shoulder in children is rare and may be associated with obstetrical paralysis.
- Recurrent shoulder dislocation occurred in 50–100% of children.

Fractures of the proximal humerus

Incidence and classification

Fractures of the proximal humerus account for 3 to 5% of all injuries involving bone. Seventy-five percent occur in patients (especially women) over the age of 60 years, and the incidence is increasing (Nordqvist & Petersson 1995, Kannus et al 1996).

Neer (1970a) proposed a classification based on the four basic anatomical segments, which took into account the presence or absence of *displacement* of one or more of these major segments. This classification will be used to assess prognosis in this section. The six groups are as follows:

1. Minimum displacement—no segment is displaced more than 1 cm or angulated more than 45°.
2. Anatomical neck fracture—a two-part fracture.
3. Surgical neck fracture—a two-part fracture with the fragment displaced more than 1 cm or angulated more than 45°.

4. Greater tuberosity displacement—a two-, three- or four-part fracture.
5. Lesser tuberosity displacement—a two-, three- or four-part fracture.
6. Fracture dislocation—a two-, three-, or four-part injury with anterior or posterior dislocation.

Minimally displaced fractures

Minimally displaced proximal humeral fractures are usually managed conservatively: union is invariably in 6 weeks and the complication of avascular necrosis, although it can occur (Gerber et al 1998), is very rare. However, function is not guaranteed to return to normal and recovery time may be quite slow. As can be seen from Table 5.31, the percentage of excellent/good results achieved (according to the various author's criteria) is 85–95% (average 89%), taking the five largest series as a whole. The disability time with these fractures is not insignificant. Some patients do recover motion and function within 2 months, but they are exceptional. Lingering stiffness, pain at the extreme of motion and 'weather ache' usually persist for at least 6 months. Strength and coordination return even more slowly. Poor mobility seems to cause prolonged disability rather than pain. Young & Wallace (1985) reported that with their 34 patients in this category, pain became insignificant with regard to interfering with sleep or activities of daily living by 6 months. They also found that it took 6 months to achieve maximum recovery of abduction, as compared with 3 months to recover maximal internal rotation.

Ekström et al (1965) reported the results of the treatment of 50 of their 100 patients with repeated procaine injections into the fracture and early mobilisation. Overall, 50% stabilised their movements by 3 months and 93% by 6 months, although 66% of the procaine-treated group had

stabilised at 3 months. Similarly, 63% were fit to return to work by the 3 month stage and 94% by 6 months, although 78% of the procaine-treated group returned to work at the 3 month stage.

Early functional exercise is important in the treatment of these patients. Clifford (1981) reported a significant relationship between the time spent in a sling, the duration of physiotherapy and the final result in minimally displaced fractures. However, Kristiansen et al (1989) found no advantage in conventional physiotherapy over patients performing their own independent exercises, and no correlation between the duration of immobilisation or duration of physiotherapy and the final result. They also reported that little further functional recovery was seen after 6 months.

Two-part fractures
Anatomical neck fractures

Anatomical neck fractures are uncommon. Post (1980) stated that separation of the tuberosities in this group was rare, while DePalma & Cantilli (1961) found that all of the five patients that they reported had an associated fracture of the greater tuberosity or surgical neck. Three of their five cases achieved a good subjective result, but only two were rated good objectively. They reported avascular necrosis in only one of these patients. However, Post (1980) stated that the incidence of late avascular necrosis was high and was usually sufficiently disabling to require prosthetic replacement.

Surgical neck fractures

The results of the treatment of displaced surgical neck fractures are variable, those of conservative treatment being shown in Table 5.32. Overall, 83% achieved a satisfactory result. The results of the various surgical techniques reported for the treatment of two-part surgical neck fractures are shown in Table 5.33. The overall

Table 5.31 Results following treatment of minimally displaced proximal humeral fractures

Reference	Number of patients	Number of excellent/ good results	Percentage
Mills & Horne (1985)*	57	54	95
Clifford (1981)*	46	43	94
Ekström et al (1965)	100	90	90
Kristiansen & Christensen (1987)	48	45	94
Stewart & Hundley (1955)	271†	231	85
Overall	522	463	89

* Neer's assessment system (Neer 1970a).
† The patient group probably includes some displaced fractures.

Table 5.32 The results of conservative treatment of displaced surgical neck fractures

Reference	Number of patients	Number of excellent/ good results	Percentage
Mills & Horne (1985)	19	13	68.5
Young & Wallace (1985)	15	12	80*
Kristiansen & Christensen (1987)	18	15	83
DePalma & Cantilli (1961)	28†	26	93
Overall	80	66	82.5

* Over 60° abduction was considered an acceptable (good) result.
† This includes one patient with operative fixation.

Table 5.33 The results of surgical treatment of displaced surgical neck fractures

Reference	Number of patients	Method	Number of excellent/ good results*	Percentage
Hessman et al (1998)	36	Buttress plate	29	88
Lentz & Meuser (1980)	98†	Rush pin	85	87
Olmeda et al (1987)	56	Kirschner wires	42‡	75
Ogiwara et al (1996)	34	Enders nails	33	97
Overall	224		189	84

* Assessed by Neer's numerical points system (1970a).
† Includes some group III patients.
‡ Results at 3 months.

percentage of patients achieving a satisfactory result was 84%, an identical proportion to those treated conservatively. Olmeda et al (1989), using percutaneous Kirschner wires, found that their fractures healed within 6–7 weeks, and that all patients under 40 years of age achieved full function within 2 months. In the elderly patients they noted a gradual improvement in terms of clinical results up to 6 months post surgery.

All but one of the 34 patients reported by Ogiwara et al (1996) treated by Ender nails went on to bony union. These fractures healed at an average of 5.9 weeks (range 4–10 weeks). The average range of motion of the shoulder at follow-up was 129.7° (range 90–170°) elevation and 43.2° (range 10–80°) external rotation. The average loss of elbow extension was 4.3° (range 0–25°).

Greater tuberosity fractures

The unstable variety of fracture of the greater tuberosity should be considered as an avulsion of the attached rotator cuff muscles (Kessel 1982). The retracted tuberosity may impair motion by impinging under the acromion. A 1 cm displacement of this type in an active patient is best treated by open reduction and cuff repair. If the anatomy is restored the results should be good, as Flatour et al (1991) found, with a 100% acceptable/satisfactory result in 12 patients. In this group active elevation of the arm averaged 170°. DePalma & Cantilli (1961) reported on 86% good results in 14 cases. Delayed displacement of the greater tuberosity can occur, and Macpherson et al (1983) noted this occurrence in 10 of 89 cases (11%) of this type of fracture.

Lesser tuberosity fractures

This type of fracture is rare. Kessel (1982) stated that because complete avulsion of the lesser tuberosity carries with it the insertion of subscapularis, it may lead to significant disability. A minimally displaced avulsion of the lesser tuberosity once healed will have normal function other than slight loss of internal rotation. Earwaker (1990) reported on two patients with isolated avulsion of the lesser tuberosity of the humerus and reviewed six others. Of the two treated conservatively, one patient had significant disability, while of the six treated surgically, only one patient had significant disability. Post (1980) recommended internal fixation for large fragments.

Three-part fractures

There is disagreement in the literature as to whether three-part fractures of the proximal humerus are better treated by conservative or operative means. The results of those series in which conservative treatment was used are listed in Table 5.34. It can be seen that while Neer (1970b) had no successes with conservative management, DePalma & Cantilli (1961) found that they had reasonable results (although two of these patients were operated upon, but their results were not removed from the overall figures).

The results of surgical treatment are shown in Table 5.35. Overall, there appeared to be better final functional results after surgical treatment, 80% of patients so treated obtaining satisfactory or better results, as compared with 59% of those conservatively treated. These poor results of conservative treatment are heavily weighted by Neer's

surprisingly poor results. If these are excluded, the results are slightly better with 72% satisfactory or better results. Zyto et al (1997) randomised 40 patients of mean age 74 years with displaced three-part (37 patients) or four-part (three patients) fractures to either conservative treatment or internal fixation with tension band wiring. After 1 year follow-up there was no functional difference between the two groups of patients, and optimal function was achieved within a year. Major complications occurred only in the surgically treated group. Kristiansen (1989) presented the results of 10 three-part fractures, treated by external fixation; 60% achieved excellent or satisfactory results when reviewed at 6–12 months post operation.

Avascular necrosis was seen in two of 33 patients (6%) in Neer's 1970b series. The overall incidence of avascular necrosis after three-part fractures is between 3 and 14% (Gerber et al, 1998).

Four-part fractures

The results of the conservative treatment of four-part fractures of the proximal humerus are generally poor. Some authors have found the incidence of avascular necrosis and

Table 5.34 The results of the conservative treatment of three-part fractures of the proximal humerus

Reference	Number of patients	Number of excellent/satisfactory results	Percentage
Neer (1970b)	20	0	0
Zyto et al (1995)	19	15	79
Rasmussen et al (1992)	17	8	47
Leyshon (1984)	34	24	70
DePalma & Cantilli (1961)	19	17*	89.5
Overall	109	64	59

* Two patients treated by internal fixation.

Table 5.35 The results of the surgical treatment of three-part fractures of the proximal humerus

Reference	Number of patients	Number of excellent/satisfactory results	Percentage
Hessman et al (1998)	35	28	80
Neer (1970b)	22	13	59
Hawkins et al (1986)	15	13	86
Pritsch et al (1997)	18	18	100
Overall	90	72	80

reabsorption of the humeral head so common after this type of fracture that they recommend primary replacement arthroplasty. Neer (1970b) reported a 100% failure rate in 12 patients with four-part fractures who were treated conservatively, as did Leyshon (1984) with his eight reported cases, of which six developed avascular necrosis.

Stableforth (1984) found that 11 of 17 patients (65%) with undisplaced four-part fractures had flexion to over 90°. Eleven (65%) were independent for activities of daily living by 6 months and six (35%) had no or only occasional pain, while only two (12%) had constant pain. Of 16 patients with displaced four-part fractures, only one (6%) had flexion beyond 90°, seven (44%) were independent for daily activities by 6 months and three (19%) had no or occasional pain, while nine (56%) had constant pain. In a retrospective series, four patients out of 32 (12.5%) had avascular necrosis.

A few reports of small series of these fractures treated by internal fixation suggest that surgery may produce better results. Sturzenegger et al (1982) reported four satisfactory results in five patients treated with a buttress plate, with only one case of avascular necrosis, and Kristiansen & Christensen (1987) achieved three satisfactory outcomes in five surgically treated patients. Avascular necrosis occurred in four of the nine patients (44%) with four-part fractures treated by either conservative or operative means.

Jakob et al (1991) described a special type of four-part valgus impacted fracture of the proximal humerus which had a better outcome than laterally or posteriorly displaced four-part fractures. They reported 19 fractures in 18 patients, of which five were treated by closed reduction and Kirschner wire fixation, and 14 by internal fixation. Fourteen shoulders (74%) had excellent or good results, with union occurring at between 6 and 8 weeks. All five poor results had avascular necrosis and this had always developed by 2 years post fracture.

Fracture–dislocation

Fracture–dislocations may be composed of two-, three- or four-part fractures in combination with either an anterior or posterior dislocation.

Two-part fracture–dislocations, whether anterior or posterior, have a better prognosis than more comminuted fracture–dislocations. DePalma & Cantilli (1961) reported 100% good results in six two-part fracture–dislocations, while Einarsson (1958) had 14 acceptable results from 17 patients (82%). Knight & Mayne (1957) noted a 56% acceptable result (nine of 16 patients) when large articular covered fragments remained intact. Nine cases of posterior shoulder dislocation associated with fracture of the anatomical neck were reported by Ogawa et al (1999). All but one patient were treated with closed reduction and complete recovery of function occurred in all but two cases.

Neer (1970b) reported 45% (nine of 11 patients) acceptable results in three-part anterior dislocations and 66% (four of six patients) in three-part posterior fracture–dislocations. He noted a 100% failure rate in nine cases of four-part anterior fracture–dislocations and three four-part posterior fracture–dislocations. Altay et al (1999), however, treated 10 patients with four-part posterior fracture–dislocations of the shoulder by limited open reduction and percutaneous stabilisation, and reported nine excellent results at an average of 3.2 years post operatively.

The results of the larger reported series of comminuted fracture–dislocations are shown in Table 5.36, between 36% and 82% being satisfactory. The variability of the results presumably reflects the number of severely comminuted fracture dislocations in each group.

The results of replacement arthroplasty

The use of a replacement arthroplasty has been recommended for four-part fractures and fracture-dislocations

Table 5.36 The results of the treatment of comminuted fracture–dislocations of the proximal humerus

Reference	Number of patients	Number of satisfactory results	Percentage
Knight & Mayne (1957)	9	5	55
Moda et al (1990)	11	9	82
Einarsson (1958)	13	5	38.5
DePalma & Cantilli (1961)	5	4	80
Mills (1974)	14	11	78.5
Sturzenegger et al (1982)	14	5	36

and some three-part injuries. The Neer prosthesis is widely reported in the literature. However, the results are somewhat variable. While pain relief is gratifying, occurring in all 16 patients of Tanner & Cofield (1983), and 11 of 16 patients (69%) of Stableforth's 1984 series, and independence in daily activities is good—in 14 of 16 (87.5%) of Stableforth's cases—the ability to use the arm at shoulder level is less effective, 75% (12 of 16 patients) achieving this result in Tanner & Cofield's series. As a rule, the range of movement is not especially restored by prosthetic replacement. Tanner & Cofield noted that the average active abduction in their series was 100°. Zyto et al (1998), sounded a note of caution in the use of hemiarthroplasty for these fractures. They reviewed 27 patients at a mean follow-up period of 39 months. Nine patients (33%) still had moderate or severe pain. The median range of movement for all the patients was flexion 70°, abduction 70°, internal rotation 50° and external rotation 45°. Eight patients (30%) had moderate or severe disability. The comparative results of the various series are shown in Table 5.37.

Most of the poor results reported are due to a failure of restoration of a good range of movement, rather than to poor pain relief or failure to achieve independence in the activities of daily living. The main complication appears to be pericapsular calcification, which occurred in 36% of Kraulis & Hunter's 1976 series and 14% of Neer's 1970b series. Neer points out that this tends to occur especially if surgery is delayed beyond 5 days after injury, and it causes a limitation in the range of movement.

The importance of prolonged rehabilitation following prosthetic replacement has been emphasised, and Stableforth stated that improvement occurs over a period of 18 months from surgery.

Non-union of proximal humeral fractures

Non-union of the proximal humerus is not often encountered, notwithstanding the reported incidence of 23% after certain types of fracture in this region (Neer 1970b). Although not all patients require treatment, non-union of the proximal humerus is usually associated with considerable morbidity. Patients complain of pain, stiffness and disability, in association with shoulder dysfunction. Treatment of non-union of fractures of the surgical neck has been recommended utilising bone graft and plate (Walch et al 1996) or Rush pins, screws or wires (Scheck 1982). More proximal non-unions can be treated by prosthetic replacement and bone graft (Duralde et al 1996). Walch et al (1996) treated 20 patients with non-union of the proximal humerus with an intramedullary bone peg and plate fixation. Union occurred in 19 patients. Active anterior elevation of the shoulder improved from an average of 60° to an average of 131°. However, Duralde et al (1996) reported less satisfactory results in their 20 non-union patients. Ten patients had bone graft combined with humeral head replacement and 10 had open reduction and internal fixation. In nine patients (45%) the results was unsatisfactory. Healy et al (1990) performed a retrospective review of 25 patients with non-union of the proximal humerus, 21 of whom had a surgical reconstruction. In only 57% (12 of 21 patients) treated surgically were good results achieved, and in none of the four treated conservatively.

Avascular necrosis

Gerber et al (1998) reviewed 25 patients with a partial (six patients) or complete (19 patients) collapse of the humeral head caused by post-traumatic avascular necrosis. Follow-up was at an average of 7.5 years. Only 10 (40%) of the patients had little or no pain. The subjective result was rated good or excellent by 67% of the patients with partial avascular necrosis and in 32% of those with complete collapse. In the 13 patients in whom their treatment resulted in an anatomic or nearly anatomic healing of the fracture, 62% had an excellent or good result. In

Table 5.37 The results of the Neer hemiarthroplasty for fractures and fracture–dislocations of the proximal humerus

Reference	Number of patients	Number of excellent/ satisfactory results	Percentage
Neer (1970b)	42	39	93
Desmarchais et al (1984)	30	18	60
Frich et al (1991)	42	13	31
Caniggia et al (1997)	35	31	89
Dimakopoulus (1997)	38	32	84
Overall	187	133	71

the other 12 patients in whom their avascular necrosis was associated with a malunion of one or more of the fracture fragments only 16% had a satisfactory result. Active anterior elevation averaged 125° in the anatomically united group and 80° in the malunion group, and abduction averaged 110° in the first group and 63° in the malunion group. Radiologic signs of advanced arthrosis were present in 20 patients. Huten & Fleure (1999) also noted that an anatomical reduction until healing and age under 60 years were factors for a favourable prognosis.

Other complications of proximal humeral fractures

Injuries to the brachial plexus are not uncommon after fractures and fracture–dislocations of the proximal humerus, and are usually associated with a good prognosis (Strömqvist et al 1987). Injuries to the axillary artery are less common and can result from direct injury from sharp bony fragments, violent over-stretching and intimal tears, and avulsion or arterial spasm (Ng et al 1990).

Whiplash-associated injuries of the shoulder

Wallace et al (1999) presented 30 patients who developed shoulder symptoms as a result of indirect trauma sustained in a car accident. All were wearing seat belts at the time and claimed a normal shoulder prior to the accident. The conditions identified were:

- acromioclavicular joint subluxation/dislocation (4)
- sternoclavicular joint subluxations (3)
- sternoclavicular joint pain (2)
- rotator cuff tears (5)
- subacromial impingement (8)
- anterior instability (2)
- posterior instability (2)
- post-traumatic capsulitis (3)
- 2-part fracture of the greater tuberosity (1)

- undisplaced fracture of the acromion (1)
- winged scapula (2)

While all the acromioclavicular and sternoclavicular pathologies occurred in the shoulder restricted by the seat belt, 75% of the rotator cuff tears occurred in the shoulder not restricted, and 63% of the impingement cases were found in the shoulder restrained by the seat belt.

Fractures in children

Lesions of the proximal humeral epiphysis represent 3% of epiphyseal injuries (Neer & Horwitz 1965). The majority (91%) are Salter–Harris type II fractures, although type I fractures may occur in babies and infants (Dameron & Reibel 1969). Salter–Harris types III (Slaa & Nollen 1987) and IV injuries are very rare and type V injuries probably never occur. From a prognostic point of view, the classification of Neer & Horowitz is more appropriate. They grade their fractures according to the displacement as follows:

- grade I—less than 5 mm
- grade II—to one-third of the width of the shaft
- grade III—to two-thirds of the width of the shaft
- grade IV—greater than two-thirds of the shaft including total displacement

All reported series are unanimous in recording excellent functional results and open reduction is rarely required (see Table 5.38).

Even if anatomical reduction is poor, functional results appear good and remodelling can occur over 6 years.

Humeral shortening is not uncommon, occurring in 90% of patients in Baxter & Wiley's 1986 series. However, in only 30% of cases was this shortening over 1 cm. In Dameron & Reibel's 1969 series, 14 of 46 patients (30.5%) had shortening, as did 23% (10 of 43 patients) in Smith's 1956 series. Neer & Horowitz (1965) found that shortening was rare under the age of 11 years, occurring in 11 of 67 cases (16.5%); they reported shortening in five of 45 grade

Table 5.38 The results of treating proximal humeral epiphyseal fractures

Reference	Number of patients	Number of good results	Percentage
Larsen et al (1990)	21	21	100
Davies & Walker (1987)	23	23	100
Neer & Horowitz (1965)	62	62	100
Nilsson & Svartholm (1965)	44	43	98
Smith (1956)	43	43	100
Baxter & Wiley (1986)	29	29	100

I and II injuries (11%), and Baxter & Willey (1986) found that in these grades the shortening averaged 3.5 mm. In grade III fractures the incidence of shortening was 25% (Neer & Horowitz) and averaged 7.7 mm (Baxter & Wiley). In grade IV injuries it occurred in 28% (Neer & Horowitz) and averaged 12 mm, but could be as great as 7 cm.

Ross and Love (1989) reported two cases of isolated avulsion fractures of the lesser tuberosity of the humerus in children. Both regained full function with conservative treatment. However, the two cases reported by Paschal et al (1995) were diagnosed 14 months and 3 years, respectively, after the initial injury and required open reduction and internal fixation.

Summary

- Minimally displaced fractures usually unite in 6 weeks, and avascular necrosis is rare, although functional recovery can take up to 6 months.

- Approximately 89% of minimally displaced fractures will achieve excellent/good results (minimal discomfort and abduction above 90°).

- 50% of minimally displaced fractures stabilise their movements by 3 months, and 93% do so by 6 months. 63% return to work by 3 months and 94% by 6 months.

- Anatomical neck fractures are rare, but the incidence of avascular necrosis may be high.

- 83% of conservatively treated displaced surgical neck fractures achieve satisfactory results. After surgical treatment 84% achieve a satisfactory result.

- Greater tuberosity fractures produce good results when not displaced under the acromion, thus blocking abduction, 86–100% being satisfactory.

- Approximately 11% of greater tuberosity fractures will displace with conservative treatment.

- Lesser tuberosity fractures are rare. Large avulsed fragments may impair internal rotation.

- Approximately 72–80% of patients with three-part proximal humeral fractures will achieve satisfactory or better results. The results of conservatively treated patients seem to be worse. External fixation may produce acceptable results.

- Avascular necrosis occurs in 3–14% of three-part fractures.

- Patients with conservatively treated undisplaced four-part fractures have a 65% chance of achieving independent daily activity, as compared with a 44% chance for those with displaced four-part fractures. Persistent stiffness, pain and functional disability are common.

- Internal fixation may yield better results, although only small series are reported.

- The prognosis for fracture–dislocations decreases as the degree of comminution increases.

- 82–100% of two-part fracture-dislocations have satisfactory results.

- 45% of three-part fracture–dislocations have satisfactory results.

- The results after four-part fracture–dislocations are variable.

- 67–100% of patients having prosthetic replacement achieve pain relief, and 70–90% achieve independent daily living.

- The overall results are disappointing, mainly due to an inability to restore full active movement. The active postoperative range of abduction averages 70–100°.

- 71% achieve excellent or satisfactory results after prosthetic replacement for proximal humeral fractures, and pericapsular calcification occurs in 14–36% of patients. Improvement in overall function occurs over 18 months after surgery.

- Almost all fractures of the proximal humeral epiphyseal fractures have good functional results.

- Anatomical malalignment rarely causes functional or cosmetic problems.

- Shortening in grade I and II fractures occurs in 11% of patients where it averages 3.5 mm, in 25% of grade III fractures where it averages 7.7 mm, and in 28% of grade IV fractures where it averages 12 mm.

▇ References

Allain J, Goutallier D, Glorion C 1998 Long term results of the Latarjet procedure for the treatment of anterior instability of the shoulder. Journal of Bone and Joint Surgery 80A: 841–852

Allman F L 1967 Fractures and ligamentous injuries of the clavicle and its articulations. Journal of Bone and Joint Surgery 49A: 774–784

Altay T, Ozturk H, Us R M, Gunal I 1999 Four-part posterior fracture–dislocations of the shoulder. Treatment by limited open reduction and percutaneous stabilization. Archives of Orthopaedic and Trauma Surgery 119: 35–38

Anzel S H, Streitz W 1973 Closed management of acromioclavicular separations and dislocations. In: Proceedings of the Western Orthopedic Association. Journal of Bone and Joint Surgery 55A: 420

Armstrong C P, Van der Spuy J 1984 The fractured scapula: importance and management based on a series of 62 patients. Injury 15: 324–329

Arner O, Sandahl U, Orling H 1957 Dislocation of the acromio-clavicular joint. Acta Chirurgica Scandinavica 113: 140–152

Aronen J G, Regan K 1984 Decreasing the incidence of recurrence of first time anterior shoulder dislocations with rehabilitation. American Journal of Sports Medicine 12: 283–291

Baker D M, Stryker W S 1965 Acute complete acromioclavicular separation. Journal of the American Medical Association 192: 105–108

Ballmer F T, Lambert S M, Hertel R 1998 Decortication and plate osteosynthesis for non union of the clavicle. Journal of Shoulder and Elbow Surgery 7: 581–585

Bannister G C, Wallace W A, Stableforth P G, Hutson M A 1989 The management of acute acromioclavicular dislocation. Journal of Bone and Joint Surgery 71B: 848–850

Bargren J H, Erlanger S, Dick H M 1978 Biomechanics and comparison of two operative methods of treatment of complete acromioclavicular separation. Clinical Orthopaedics 130: 267–272

Bassett R W, Cofield R H 1983 Acute tears of the rotator cuff. Clinical Orthopaedics 175: 18–24

Baxter M P, Wiley J J 1986 Fractures of the proximal humeral epiphysis. Journal of Bone and Joint Surgery 68B: 570–573

Berbig R, Weishaupt D, Prim J, Shahin O 1999 Primary anterior shoulder dislocation and rotator cuff tears. Journal of Shoulder and Elbow Surgery 8: 220–225

Bergfield J A, Andrish J T, Clancy W G 1978 Evaluation of the acromioclavicular joint following first- and second-degree sprains. American Journal of Sports Medicine 6: 153–159

Bigliani L U, Levine W N 1997 Subacromial impingement syndrome. Journal of Bone and Joint Surgery 79A: 1854–1868

Bigliani L U, Newton P M, Steinmann S P, Connor P M, McIlveen S J 1998 Glenoid rim lesions associated with recurrent anterior dislocation of the shoulder. American Journal of Sports Medicine 26: 41–45

Bjerneld H, Hovelius L, Thorling J 1983 Acromioclavicular separations treated conservatively. Acta Orthopaedica Scandinavica 54: 743–745

Björkenheim J M, Paavolainen P, Ahovuo J, Slätis P 1990 Subacromial impingement decompressed with anterior acromioplasty. Clinical Orthopaedics 252: 150–155

Boehme D, Curtis R J, Dehaan J K, Kay S P, Young D C Rockwood C A 1991 Non union of fractures of the midshaft of the clavicle. Journal of Bone and Joint Surgery 73A: 1219–1226

Bonnet J 1975 Fracture of the clavicle. Archivum Chirurgicum Neerlandicum 27: 143–151

Bosch U, Skutek M, Peters G, Tscherne H 1998 Extension osteotomy in malunited clavicular fractures. Journal of Shoulder and Elbow Surgery 7: 402–405

Bostman O, Manninen M, Pihlajamaki H 1997 Complications of plate fixation in fresh displaced mid clavicular fractures. Journal of Trauma-Injury Infection and Critical Care 43: 778–783

Boucher P R, Morton K S 1968 Rupture of the distal biceps brachii tendon. In: Proceedings of the Canadian Orthopaedic Association. Journal of Bone and Joint Surgery 50B: 436

Bowditch M G, Stanley D 1999 Shoulder function following non-operative management of displaced middle third clavicle fractures. Journal of Bone and Joint Surgery 81B: Supp III: 301

Bradbury N, Hutchinson J, Hahn D, Colton C L 1996 Clavicular non union. 31/32 healed after plate fixation and bone grafting. Acta Orthopaedica Scandinavica 67: 367–370

Brems J 1988 Rotator cuff tear: evaluation and treatment. Orthopaedics 11: 69–81

Brinker M R, Simon R G 1999 Pseudo-dislocation of the sternoclavicular joint. Journal of Orthopaedic Trauma 13: 222–225

Broos P, Stoffelen D, Van de Sijpe K, Fourneau I 1997 Surgical management of complete Tossy III acromioclavicular joint dislocation with the Bosworth screw or the Wolter plate. A critical evaluation. Unfallchirurgie 23: 153–159

Brown J E 1961 Anterior sternoclavicular dislocation: a method of repair. American Journal of Orthopedics 6: 184–189

Brox J I, Gjengedal E, Uppheim G, Bøhmer A S, Brevik J I, Ljunggren A E, Staff P H 1999 Arthroscopic surgery versus supervised exercises in patients with rotator cuff disease (stage II impingement syndrome): A prospective randomized, controlled study in 125 patients with a 2 1/2 year follow up. Journal of Shoulder and Elbow Surgery 8: 102–111

Buckerfield C T, Castle M E 1984 Acute traumatic retrosternal dislocation of the clavicle. Journal of Bone and Joint Surgery 66A: 379–385

Budoff J E, Nirschl R P, Guidi E J 1998 Debridement of partial-thickness tears of the rotator cuff without acromioplasty. Journal of Bone and Joint Surgery 80A: 733–748

Burkhead W Z, Rockwood C A 1992 Treatment of instability of the shoulder with an exercise programme. Journal of Bone and Joint Surgery 74A: 890–896

Butters K P 1991 Fractures and dislocations of the scapula In: Rockwood C A, Green D P, Bucholz R W (eds) Fractures in adults. J B Lippincott, Philadelphia

Cahill B R 1982 Osteolysis of the distal part of the clavicle in male athletes. Journal of Bone and Joint Surgery 64A: 1053–1058

Caira S F, Melanotte P L 1997 Transitory osteonecrosis of the head of the humerus after fracture of the calvicle. Chirurgia Degli Organi di Movimento 82: 419–422

Cameron E, Henderson I 1998 Pectoralis major rupture. Journal of Bone and Joint Surgery 80B: Supp II: 148–149

Caniggia M, Maniscalco P, Picinotti A 1997 What is the proper degree of retroversion of the humeral stem of shoulder prosthesis for 4 fragment fractures of the proximal humerus? Journal of Bone and Joint Surgery 79B: Supp II: 194

Cassels R E, Hamilton L R 1967 Rupture of the biceps brachii. In: Proceedings of the American Academy of Orthopedic Surgeons. Journal of Bone and Joint Surgery 49A: 1016

Chan K Y, Jupiter J B, Leffert R D, Marti R 1999 Clavicle malunion. Journal of Shoulder and Elbow Surgery 8: 287–290

Chard M D, Sattelle L M, Hazleman B L 1988 The longterm outcome of rotator cuff tendonitis—a review study. British Journal of Rheumatology 27: 385–389

Clark R L, Milgram J W, Yawn D H 1974 Fatal aortic perforation and cardiac tamponade due to a Kirschner wire migrating from the right sternoclavicular joint. Southern Medical Journal 67: 316–318

Clifford P C 1981 Fractures of the neck of the humerus: a review of the late results. Injury 12: 91–95

Cofield R H, Lanzer W L 1985 Rotator cuff repair, results related to surgical pathology. Orthopaedic Transactions 9(3): 466

Cook F F, Tibone J C 1991 The Mumford procedure in athletes. American Journal of Sports Medicine 16: 97–100

Cox J 1981 The fate of the acromioclavicular joint in athletic injuries. American Journal of Sports Medicine 9: 50–53

Cuomo F, Kummer F J, Zuckerman J D, Lyon T, Blair B, Olsen T 1998 The influence of acromioclavicular joint morphology on rotator cuff tears. Journal of Shoulder and Elbow Surgery 7: 555–559

Curtis R J, Dameron T B, Rockwood C A 1991 Fractures and dislocations of the shoulder. In: Rockwood C A, Wilkins K E, King R E (eds) Fractures in children (Vol. 3). J B Lippincott, Philadelphia

Dameron T B, Reibel D B 1969 Fractures involving the proximal humeral epiphyseal plate. Journal of Bone and Joint Surgery 51A: 289–297

Davies S J M, Walker G F 1987 Proximal humeral fractures in children: to treat or to manage? Journal of Bone and Joint Surgery 69B: 154

Dawe C J 1980 Acromioclavicular joint injuries. In: Proceedings of the New Zealand Orthopaedic Association. Journal of Bone and Joint Surgery 62B: 269

De Beer J F, Rossouw W C 1997 Medio-lateral pinning of clavicle fractures in adults—A safe method. Journal of Bone and Joint Surgery 79B: supp IV: 446

De Beer M A, Thiart C J 1998 Arthroscopic anterior capsular reconstruction of the shoulder using a combination technique with Mitek anchors and Suretac. Journal of Bone and Joint Surgery 80B: Supp II: 163

De Berardino T M, Arciero R A, Taylor D C 1996 Arthroscopic stabilization of acute initial anterior shoulder dislocation: the West

Point experience. Journal of the Southern Orthopaedic Association 5: 263–271

De Jong K P, Kaulesar Sukul D M K S 1990 Anterior sternoclavicular dislocation: a long-term follow-up study. Journal of Orthopaedic Trauma 4: 420–423

De Rosa G P, Kettelkamp D B 1977 Fracture of the coracoid process of the scapula. Journal of Bone and Joint Surgery 59A: 696–697

Denham R H, Dingley A F 1967 Epiphyseal separation of the medial end of the clavicle. Journal of Bone and Joint Surgery 49A: 1179–1183

DePalma A F, Cantilli R A 1961 Fractures of the upper end of the humerus. Clinical Orthopaedics 20: 73–93

Desmarchais J E, Mauriad G, Benazet J P 1984 Treatment of complex fractures of the proximal humerus by Neer hemiarthroplasty. In: Proceedings of the Canadian Orthopaedic Association. Journal of Bone and Joint Surgery 66B: 296

Dias J J, Steingold R F, Richardson R A, Tesfayohannes B, Gregg P J 1987 The conservative treatment of acromioclavicular dislocations. Journal of Bone and Joint Surgery 69B: 719–722

Dimakopoulos P, Potamitis N, Lambiris E 1997 Hemiarthroplasty in the treatment of comminuted intra-articular fractures of the proximal humerus. Clinical Orthopaedics and Related Research 341: 7–11

Dodenhoff R M, Howell G D, Thomas W G, Hughes P M 1997 Neer anterior acromioplasty. An MRI and clinical review of 63 procedures. Journal of Bone and Joint Surgery 79B: Supp II: 201–202

Dumontier C, Sautet A, Gagey O, Apoil A 1999 Rotator interval lesions and their relation to coracoid impingement syndrome. Journal of Shoulder and Elbow Surgery 8: 130–135

Dumontier C, Sautet A, Man M, Apoil A 1995 Acromioclavicular dislocations: Treatment by coracoacromial ligamentoplasty. Journal of Shoulder and Elbow Surgery 4: 130–134

Dunkerton M C 1989 Posterior dislocation of the shoulder associated with obstetric brachial plexus palsy. Journal of Bone and Joint Surgery 71: 764–766

Duralde X A, Flatow E L, Pollock R G, Nicholson G P, Self E B, Bigliani L U 1996 Operative treatment of non unions of the surgical neck of the humerus. Journal of Shoulder and Elbow Surgery 5: 169–180

Earwaker J 1990 Isolated avulsion fracture of the lesser tuberosity of the humerus. Skeletal Radiology 19: 121–125

Edelson J G 1996 Clavicular fracture and ipsilateral acromioclavicular arthrosis. Journal of Shoulder and Elbow Surgery 5: 181–185

Einarsson F 1958 Fractures of the upper end of the humerus. Acta Orthopaedica Scandinavica (suppl.) 32: 131–142

Ekström T, Lagergren C, von Schreeb T 1965 Procaine injections and early mobilisation for fractures of the neck of the humerus. Acta Chirurgica Scandinavica 130: 18–24

Esch J C 1989 Arthroscopic subacromial decompression. Orthopaedic Review 18: 733–742

Esch J C, Ozerkis L R, Helgager J A, Kane N, Lilliott N 1988 Arthroscopic subacromial decompression: results according to the degree of rotator cuff tear. Arthroscopy 4: 241–249

Eskola A 1986 Sternoclavicular dislocation: a plea for open treatment. Acta Orthopaedica Scandinavica 57: 227–228

Eskola A, Santavirta S, Viljakka T, Wirta J, Partio E, Hoikka V 1996 The results of operative resection of the lateral end of the clavicle. Journal of Bone and Joint Surgery 78A: 584–587

Eskola A, Vainionpää S, Korkala O, Rokkanen P 1987 Acute complete acromioclavicular dislocation. Annales Chirurgiae et Gynaecologiae 76: 323–326

Eskola A, Vainionpää S, Korkala O, Santavirta S, Grönblad M, Rokkanen P 1991 Four year outcome of operative treatment of acute acromioclavicular dislocation. Journal of Orthopaedic Trauma 5: 9–13

Eskola A, Vainionpää S, Myllynen P, Pätiälä H, Rokkanen P 1986a Outcome of clavicular fracture in 89 patients. Archives of Orthopaedics and Traumatic Surgery 105: 337–338

Eskola A, Vainionpää S, Myllynen P, Pätiälä H, Rokkanen P 1986b Surgery for ununited clavicular fracture. Acta Orthopaedica Scandinavica 57: 366–367

Eskola A, Vainionpää S, Vastamäki M, Slätis P, Rokkanen P 1989 Operation for old sternoclavicular dislocation. Journal of Bone and Joint Surgery 71B: 63–65

Fardin P, Negrin P, Dainese R 1978 The isolated paralysis of the serratus anterior muscle: clinical and electromyographical follow-up of 10 cases. Electromyography and Clinical Neurophysiology 18: 379–386

Ferrandez L, Yubero J, Usabiaga J, No L, Martin F 1988 Sternoclavicular dislocation: treatment and complications. Italian Journal of Orthopaedics and Traumatology 14(3): 349–355

Ferry A M, Rook F W, Masterson J H 1957 Retrosternal dislocation of the clavicle. Journal of Bone and Joint Surgery 39A: 905–910

Flatour E L, Cuomo F, Maday M G, Miller S R, Mälveen S J, Bigliani L U 1991 Open reduction and internal fixation of two part displaced fractures of the greater tuberosity of the proximal part of the humerus. Journal of Bone and Joint Surgery 73A: 1213–1218

Foo C L, Swann M 1983 Isolated paralysis of the serratus anterior. Journal of Bone and Joint Surgery 65B: 552–556

Frich L H, Sojbjerg J O, Sneppen O 1991 Shoulder arthroplasty in complex acute and chronic proximal humeral fractures. Orthopaedics 14: 949–954

Frieman B G, Fenlin J M 1995 Anterior acromioplasty: Effect of litigation and workers compensation. Journal of Shoulder and Elbow Surgery 4: 175–181

Froimson A I 1978 Fracture of the coracoid process of the scapula. Journal of Bone and Joint Surgery 60A: 710–711

Fronek J, Warren R F, Bowen M 1989 Posterior subluxation of the glenohumeral joint. Journal of Bone and Joint Surgery 71: 205–216

Frost P, Andersen J H 1999 Shoulder impingement syndrome in relation to shoulder intensive work. Occupational and Environmental Medicine 56: 494–498

Fuchs B, Jost B, Gerber C 1999 Posterior inferior capsular shift for repair of recurrent posterior shoulder subluxation Journal of Bone and Joint Surgery 81B: supp II: 204

Galpin R D, Hawkins R J, Grainger R W 1985 A comparative analysis of operative versus nonoperative treatment of grade III acromioclavicular separations. Clinical Orthopaedics 193: 150–155

Gartsman G M 1990 Arthroscopic acromioplasty for lesions of the rotator cuff. Journal of Bone and Joint Surgery 72A: 169–180

Gartsman G M, Khan M, Hammerman S M 1998 Arthroscopic repair of full-thickness tears of the rotator cuff. Journal of Bone and Joint Surgery 80A: 832–840

Gartsman G M, Milne J C 1995 Articular surface partial-thickness rotator cuff tears. Journal of Shoulder and Elbow Surgery 4: 409–415

Gates J D, Knox J B 1995 Axillary artery injuries secondary to anterior dislocation of the shoulder. Journal of Trauma-Injury Infection and Critical Care 39: 581–583

Gebhard F, Draeger M, Steinmann R, Hoellen I, Hartel W 1997 Functional outcome of Eden-Hybinette-Lange operation in post-traumatic shoulder dislocation. Unfallchirurg 100: 770–775

Gerber C, Hersche O, Berberat C 1998 The clinical relevance of post traumatic avascular necrosis of the humeral head. Journal of Shoulder and Elbow Surgery 7: 586–590

Gerber C, Lambert S M 1996 Allograft reconstruction of segmental defects of the humeral head for the treatment of chronic locked posterior dislocation of the shoulder. Journal of Bone and Joint Surgery 87A: 376–382

Gerber C, Rockwood C A 1987 Subcoracoid dislocation of the lateral end of the clavicle. Journal of Bone and Joint Surgery 69A: 924–927

Gilbert W M, Tchabo J-G 1988 Fractured clavicle in newborns. International Surgery 73: 123–125

Gilcrest E L 1934 The common syndrome of rupture, dislocation and elongation of the long head of the biceps brachii. Surgery, Gynaecology and Obstetrics 58: 322–340

Gillespie H S 1964 Excision of the outer end of the clavicle for dislocation of the acromioclavicular joint. Canadian Journal of Surgery 7: 18–20

Glick J M, Milburn L J, Haggerty J F, Nishimoto D 1977 Dislocated acromioclavicular joint: follow-up study of 35 unreduced acromioclavicular dislocations. American Journal of Sports Medicine 5: 264–270

Goddard N J, Stabler J, Albert J S 1990 Atlanto-axial rotatory fixation and fracture of the clavicle. Journal of Bone and Joint Surgery 72B: 72–75

Gozna E R, Harris W R 1979 Traumatic winging of the scapula. Journal of Bone and Joint Surgery 61A: 1230–1233

Gregg J L, Labosky D, Harty M et al 1979 Serratus anterior paralysis in the young athlete. Journal of Bone and Joint Surgery 61A: 825–832

Gumina S, Postacchini F 1997 Anterior dislocation of the shoulder in elderly patients. Journal of Bone and Joint Surgery 79B: 540–543

Hardegger F H, Simpson L A, Weber B G 1984 The operative treatment of scapular fractures. Journal of Bone and Joint Surgery 66B: 725–731

Harris R D, Harris J H 1988 The prevalence and significance of missed scapular fractures in blunt chest trauma. American Journal of Roentgenology 151: 747–750

Harryman D T, Mack L A, Wang K Y, Jackins S E, Richardson M L, Matser F A 1991 Repairs of the rotator cuff: correlation of functional results with integrity of the cuff. Journal of Bone and Joint Surgery 73A: 982–989

Hattrup S J 1995 Rotator cuff repair: Relevance of patient age. Journal of Shoulder and Elbow Surgery 4: 95–100

Hawkins R J, Bell R H, Gurr K 1986 The three-part fracture of the proximal part of the humerus. Journal of Bone and Joint Surgery 68A: 1410–1414

Hawkins R J, Brock R M, Abrams J S, Hobeika P 1988 Acromioplasty for impingement with an intact rotator cuff. Journal of Bone and Joint Surgery 70B: 795–797

Hawkins R J, Koppert G, Johnston G 1984 Recurrent posterior instability (subluxation) of the shoulder. Journal of Bone and Joint Surgery 66A: 169–174

Hawkins R J, Misamore G W, Hobeika P E 1985 Surgery for full thickness rotator cuff tears. Journal of Bone and Joint Surgery 67A: 1349–1355

Hawkins R J, Neer C S, Pianta R M, Mendoza F X 1987 Locked posterior dislocation of the shoulder. Journal of Bone and Joint Surgery 69A: 9–18

Healy W L, Jupiter J B, Kristiansen T K, White R R 1990 Nonunion of the proximal humerus. Journal of Orthopaedic Trauma 4: 424–431

Heckman J D, Levine M I 1978 Traumatic closed transection of the biceps brachii in the military parachutist. Journal of Bone and Joint Surgery 60A: 369–372

Heinig C F 1968 Retrosternal dislocation of the clavicle. In: Proceedings of the American Association of Orthopedic Surgeons. Journal of Bone and Joint Surgery 50A: 830

Hejna W F, Fossier C H, Goldstan T B, Ray R D 1969 Ancient anterior dislocation of the shoulder. In: Proceedings of the American Academy of Orthopedic Surgeons. Journal of Bone and Joint Surgery 51A: 1030–1031

Hessman M, Gotzen L, Gehling H, Baumgaertel F, Klingelhoeffer I 1998 Operative treatment of displaced proximal humeral fractures: two year results in 99 cases. Acta Chirurgica Belgica 98: 212–219

Hessman M, Gotzen L, Kirchner R, Gehling H 1997 Therapy and outcome of lateral clavicular fractures. Unfallchirurg 100: 17–23

Hessman M, Kirchner R, Baumgaertel F, Gehling H, Gotzen L 1996 Treatment of unstable distal clavicular fractures with and without lesions of the acromioclavicular joint. Injury 27: 47–52

Hill J M, McGuire M H, Crosby L A 1997 Closed treatment of displaced middle-third fractures of the clavicle gives poor results. Journal of Bone and Joint Surgery 79B: 537–539

Ho G, Cofield R H, Balm M R, Hattrup S J, Rowland C M 1999 Neurologic complications of surgery for anterior shoulder instability. Journal of Shoulder and Elbow Surgery 8: 266–270

Hoelen M A, Burgers A M J, Rozing P M 1990 Prognosis of primary anterior shoulder dislocation in young adults. Archives of Orthopaedic and Traumatic Surgery 110: 51–54

Hovelius L 1982 Incidence of shoulder dislocation in Sweden. Clinical Orthopaedics 166: 127–131

Hovelius L, Augustini B G, Fredin H, Johansson O, Norlin R, Thorling J 1996 Primary anterior dislocation of the shoulder in young patients. Journal of Bone and Joint Surgery 78A: 1677–1684

Hovelius L, Eriksson K, Fredin H 1983 Recurrences after initial dislocation of the shoulder. Journal of Bone and Joint Surgery 65A: 343–349

Howard F M, Shafer S J 1965 Injuries to the clavicle with neurovascular complications. Journal of Bone and Joint Surgery 47A: 1335–1346

Huten D, Fleure P 1999 Post traumatic necrosis of the humeral head. Journal of Bone and Joint Surgery 81B: supp II: 128

Iannotti J P, Bernot M P, Kuhlman J R, Kelley M J, Williams G R 1996 Postoperative assessment of shoulder function: a prospective study of full-thickness rotator cuff tears. Journal of Shoulder and Elbow Surgery 5: 449–457

Itoi E, Minagawa H, Sato T, Sato K, Tabata S 1997 Isokinetic strength after tears of the supraspinatus tendon. Journal of Bone and Joint Surgery 79B: 77–82

Ivey M, Britt M, Johnston R V 1991 Reflex sympathetic dystrophy after clavicular fracture: case report. Journal of Trauma 31: 276–279

Jacobs B, Wade P A 1966 Acromioclavicular joint injury. Journal of Bone and Joint Surgery 48A: 475–486

Jacobs P 1964 Post-traumatic osteolysis of the outer end of the clavicle. Journal of Bone and Joint Surgery 46B: 705–707

Jakob R P, Miniaci A, Anson P S, Jaberg H, Osterwalder A, Ganz R 1991 Four part valgus impacted fractures of the proximal humerus. Journal of Bone and Joint Surgery 73B: 295–298

Johnson E W, Collins H R 1963 Nonunion of the clavicle. Archives of Surgery 87: 963–966

Johnson J T H, Kendall H O 1955 Isolated paralysis of the serratus anterior muscle. Journal of Bone and Joint Surgery 37A: 567–574

Kannus P, Palvanen M, Niemi S, Parkkari J, Jarvinen M, Vuori I 1996 Increasing number and incidence of osteoporotic fractures of the proximal humerus in elderly people. British Medical Journal 313: 1051–1052

Karadimas J E 1997 Recurrent traumatic anterior dislocation of the shoulder. 218. Consecutive cases treated by a modified Magnusson-Stack procedure and follow-up for 2–18 years. Acta Orthopaedica Scandinavica (suppl.) 275: 69–71

Karunakar M A, Cha P, Stern P J 1999 Distal Biceps Ruptures A follow up of Boyd and Anderson repair. Clinical Orthopaedics and Related Research 363: 100–107

Kavanagh T G, Sarkar S D, Phillips H 1985 Complications of displaced fractures (Type II Neer) of the outer end of the clavicle. Journal of Bone and Joint Surgery 67B: 492–493

Kawam M, Sinclair J, Letts M 1997 Recurrent posterior shoulder dislocation in children: The results of surgical management. Journal of Pediatric Orthopaedics 17: 533–538

Kazár B, Relovszky E 1969 Prognosis of primary dislocation of the shoulder. Acta Orthopaedica Scandinavica 40: 216–224

Kennedy J C 1949 Retrosternal dislocation of the clavicle. Journal of Bone and Joint Surgery 31B: 74–75

Kessel L 1982 Fractures and dislocations: the head and neck of humerus. In: Clinical disorders of the shoulder. Churchill Livingstone, Edinburgh, pp 125–137

Khan A A, Lucas H K 1978 Plating of fractures of the middle third of the clavicle. Injury 9: 263–267

Kirkley A, Griffin S, Richards C, Miniaci A, Mohtadi N 1999 Prospective randomized clinical trial comparing the effectiveness of immediate arthrosopic stabilization versus immobilization and rehabilitation in first traumatic anterior dislocations of the shoulder. Arthroscopy 15: 507–514

Kiss J, Mersich I, Perlaky G Y, Szollas L 1998 The results of the Putti-Platt operation with particular reference to arthritis, pain and limitation of external rotation. Journal of Shoulder and Elbow Surgery 7: 495–500

Kiviluoto O, Pasila M, Jaroma H, Sundholm A 1980 Immobilisation after primary dislocation of the shoulder. Acta Orthopaedica Scandinavica 51: 915–919

Knight R A, Mayne J A 1957 Comminuted fractures and fracture–dislocations involving the articular surface of the humeral head. Journal of Bone and Joint Surgery 39A: 1343–1355

Koenig U, Imhoff A B, Burkart A, Roscher E 1999 Arthroscopic shoulder stabilization—a prospective comparison between Fastak and Suretac. Journal of Bone and Joint Surgery 81B: supp II: 204

Kraulis J, Hunter G 1976 The results of prosthetic replacement in fracture–dislocations of the upper end of the humerus. Injury 8: 129–131

Krause M, Karbowski A, Stratmann M 1997 Surgical treatment for recurrent dislocation of the shoulder. Clinical and radiological results after 10 years. Journal of Bone and Joint Surgery. 79B: supp II: 253

Kristiansen B 1989 Treatment of displaced fractures of the proximal humerus: transcutaneous reduction and Hoffmann's external fixation. Injury 20: 195–199

Kristiansen B, Angermann P, Larsen T K 1989 Functional results following fractures of the proximal humerus. Archives of Orthopaedic and Traumatic Surgery 108: 339–341

Kristiansen B, Christensen S W 1987 Proximal humeral fractures. Acta Orthopaedica Scandinavica 58: 124–127

Kroner K, Lind T, Jensen J 1989 The epidemiology of shoulder dislocations. Archives of Orthopaedic and Traumatic Surgery 108: 288–290

Lancaster S, Horowitz M, Alonso J 1987 Complete acromioclavicular separations. Clinical Orthopaedics 216: 80–88

Larsen C F, Kioer T, Lindequist S 1990 Fractures of the proximal humerus in children. Acta Orthopaedica Scandinavica 61: 255–257

Larsen E, Bjerg-Nielsen A, Christensen P 1986 Conservative or surgical treatment of acromioclavicular dislocation. Journal of Bone and Joint Surgery 68A: 552–555

Larsen E, Hede A 1987 Treatment of acute acromioclavicular dislocation. Acta Orthopaedica Belgica 53(4): 480–484

Laskin R S, Sedlin E D 1971 Luxatio erecta in infancy. Clinical Orthopaedics 80: 126–129

Lentz W, Meuser P 1980 The treatment of fractures of the proximal humerus. Archives of Orthopaedics and Traumatic Surgery 96: 283–285

Levine A H, Pais M J, Schwartz E E 1976 Post traumatic osteolysis of the distal clavicle with emphasis on early radiologic changes. American Journal of Roentgenology 127: 781–784

Leyshon R L 1984 Closed treatment of fractures of the proximal humerus. Acta Orthopaedica Scandinavica 55: 48–51

MacDonald P B, Alexander M J, Frejuk J, Johnson G E 1988 Comprehensive functional analysis of shoulders following complete acromioclavicular separation. American Journal of Sports Medicine 16(5): 475–480

Macpherson I, Crossan J F, Allister C A 1983 Unstable fractures of the greater tuberosity of the humerus. In: Proceedings of British Orthopaedic Association. Journal of Bone and Joint Surgery 65B: 225

Mallon W J, Bassett F H, Goldner R D 1990 Luxatio erecta: the inferior glenohumeral dislocation. Journal of Orthopaedic Trauma 4: 19–24

Many A, Brenner S H, Yaron Y, Lusky A, Peyser M R, Lessing J B 1996 Prospective study of incidence and predisposing factors for clavicular fracture in the newborn. Acta Obstetricia et Gynecologica Scandinavica 75: 378–381

Martens C 1997 Surgical treatment of distal biceps tendon ruptures: results of a multicentre BOTA study and review of the literature. Acta Orthopaedica Belgica 63: 251–255

McDermott D M, Neumann L, Frostick S P, Wallace W A 1999 Early results of Bankart repair with a patient-controlled rehabilitation program. Journal of Shoulder and Elbow Surgery 8: 146–150

McGinnis M, Denton J R 1989 Fractures of the scapula: a retrospective study of 40 fractured scapulae. Journal of Trauma 29: 1488–1493

McLennan J G, Ungersma J 1982 Pneumothorax complicating fracture of the scapula. Journal of Bone and Joint Surgery 64A: 598–599

Mehta J C, Sachder A, Collins J J 1973 Retrosternal dislocation of the clavicle. Injury 5: 79–83

Middleton S B, Foley S J, Foy M A 1995 Partial excision of the clavicle for non union in National Hunt jockeys. Journal of Bone and Joint Surgery 77B: 778–780

Mills H J, Horne G 1985 Fractures of the proximal humerus in adults. Journal of Trauma 25: 801–805

Mills K L G 1974 Severe injuries of the upper end of the humerus. Injury 6: 13–21

Misamore G W, Ziegler D W, Rushton J L 1995 Repair of the rotator cuff. A comparison of results in two populations of patients. Journal of Bone and Joint Surgery 77A: 1335–1339

Moda S K, Chadha N S, Sangwan S S, Khurana D K, Dahiya A S, Siwach R C 1990 Open reduction and fixation of proximal humeral fractures and fracture dislocations. Journal of Bone and Joint Surgery 72B: 1050–1052

Morrison D S, Frogameni A D, Woodworth P 1997 Non-operative treatment of subacromial impingement syndrome. Journal of Bone and Joint Surgery 79A: 732–737

Naert P A, Chipchase L A, Krishnan J 1998 Clavicular malunion with consequent impingement syndrome. Journal of Shoulder and Elbow Surgery 7: 548–550

Neer C S 1960 Nonunion of the clavicle. Journal of the American Medical Association 172: 1006–1011

Neer C S 1968 Fractures of the distal third of the clavicle. Clinical Orthopaedics 58: 43–50

Neer C S 1970a Displaced proximal humeral fractures, part 1: classification and evaluation. Journal of Bone and Joint Surgery 52A: 1077–1089

Neer C S 1970b Displaced proximal humeral fractures, part 2: treatment of three-part and four-part displacement. Journal of Bone and Joint Surgery 52A: 1090–1103

Neer C S 1983 Impingement lesions. Clinical Orthopaedics 173: 70–77

Neer C S, Horowitz B S 1965 Fractures of the proximal humeral epiphysial plate. Clinical Orthopaedics 41: 24–31

Nettles J L, Linscheid R L 1968 Sternoclavicular dislocations. Journal of Trauma. 8: 158–164

Neviaser J S 1963 The treatment of old unreduced dislocations of the shoulder. Surgical Clinics of North America 43: 1671–1678

Neviaser R J, Neviaser T J 1995 Recurrent instability of the shoulder after age 40. Journal of Shoulder and Elbow Surgery 4: 416–418

Ng K C, Singh S, Low Y P 1990 Axillary artery damage from shoulder trauma. Singapore Medical Journal 31: 592–595

Ngarmukos C, Parkpian V, Patradul A 1998 Fixation of fractures of the midshaft of the clavicle with Kirschner wires. Results in 108 patients. Journal of Bone and Joint Surgery 80B: 106–108

Nilsson S, Svartholm F 1965 Fracture of the upper end of the humerus in children. Acta Chirurgica Scandinavica 130: 433–439

Nizard R, Tamames M, Witvoet J 1997 Survival analysis of the Latarjet procedure. Journal of Bone and Joint Surgery 79B: supp II: 143

Noda M, Shiraishi H, Mizuno K 1997 Chronic posterior sternoclavicular dislocation causing compression of a subclavian artery. Journal of Shoulder and Elbow Surgery 6: 564–569

Nogi J, Heckman J D, Hakala M, Sweet D E 1975 Non union of the clavicle in a child. Clinical Orthopaedics 110: 19–21

Nordqvist A, Petersson C J 1995 Incidence and causes of shoulder girdle injuries in an urban population. Journal of Shoulder and Elbow Surgery 4: 107–112

Nordqvist A, Petersson C J, Redlund-Johnell I 1998 Mid-clavicle fractures in adults: end result study after conservative treatment. Journal of Orthopaedic Trauma 12: 572–576

Nordqvist A, Redlund-Johnell I, von Scheele A, Petersson C J 1997 Shortening of clavicle after fracture. Incidence and clinical significance, a 5 year follow up of 85 patients. Acta Orthopaedica Scandinavica 68: 349–351

Norman W H 1985 Repair of avulsion of insertion of biceps brachii tendon. Clinical Orthopaedics 193: 189–194

O'Driscoll S W, Evans D C 1991 Contralateral shoulder instability following anterior repair: an epidemiological investigation. Journal of Bone and Joint Surgery 73B: 941–946

Ogawa K, Naniwa T 1997 Fractures of the acromion and the lateral scapular spine. Journal of Shoulder and Elbow Surgery 6: 544–548

Ogawa K, Yoshida A, Inokuchi W 1999 Posterior shoulder dislocation associated with fracture of the humeral anatomic neck: treatment guidelines and long term outcome. Journal of Trauma-Injury Infection and Critical Care 46: 318–323

Ogawa K, Yoshida A, Takahashi M, Michimasa U 1997 Fractures of the coracoid process. Journal of Bone and Joint Surgery 79B: 17–19

Ogiwara N, Aoki M, Okamura K, Fukushima S 1996 Ender nailing for unstable surgical neck fractures of the humerus in elderly patients. Clinical Orthopaedics and Related Research 330: 173–180

Olmeda A, Bonaga S, Turra S 1989 The treatment of fractures of the surgical neck of the humerus by osteosynthesis with Kirschner wires. Italian Journal of Orthopaedics and Traumatology 15: 353–360

Omer G E 1967 Osteotomy of the clavicle in surgical reduction of anterior sternoclavicular dislocation. Journal of Trauma 7: 584–590

Oppenheim W L, Davis A, Growdon W A, Dorey F J, Davlin L B 1990 Clavicle fractures in the newborn. Clinical Orthopaedics 250: 176–180

Overpeck D O, Ghormley R K 1940 Paralysis of the serratus magnus muscle. Journal of the American Medical Association 114: 1994–1996

Paffen P J, Jansen E W L 1978 Surgical treatment of clavicular fractures with Kirschner wires: a comparative study. Archivum Chirurgicum Neerlandicum 30: 43–53

Park J P, Arnold J A, Coker T P, Harns W D, Becker D A 1980 Treatment of acromioclavicular separations. American Journal of Sports Medicine 8: 251–256

Paschal S O, Hutton K S, Weatherall P T 1995 Isolated avulsion fracture of the lesser tuberosity of the humerus in adolescents. Journal of Bone and Joint Surgery 77A: 1427–1430

Pasila M, Jaroma H, Kiviluoto O, Sundholm A 1978 Early complications of primary shoulder dislocations. Acta Orthopaedica Scandinavica 49: 260–263

Pasila M, Kiviluoto O, Jaroma H, Sundholm A 1980 Recovery from primary shoulder dislocation and its complications. Acta Orthopaedica Scandinavica 51: 257–262

Patel V R, Singh D, Calvert P T, Bayley J I L 1999 Arthroscopic subacromial decompression: Results and factors affecting outcome. Journal of Shoulder and Elbow Surgery 8: 231–237

Payne L Z, Altchek D W, Craig E V, Warren R F 1997 Arthroscopic treatment of partial rotator cuff tears in young athletes. A preliminary report. American Journal of Sports Medicine 25: 299–305

Peacock H K, Brandon J R, Jones O L 1970 Retrosternal dislocation of the clavicle. Southern Medical Journal 63: 1324–1328

Penn I 1964 The vascular complications of fractures of the clavicle. Journal of Trauma 4: 819–831

Perlmutter G S, Leffert R D 1999 Results of transfer of the Pectoralis Major tendon to treat paralysis of the Serratus Anterior muscle. Journal of Bone and Joint Surgery 81A: 377–384

Pevny T, Hunter R E, Freeman J R 1998 Primary traumatic anterior shoulder dislocation in patients 40 years of age and older. Arthroscopy 14: 289–294

Pierce R O 1979 Internal derangement of the sternoclavicular joint. Clinical Orthopaedics 141: 247–250

Post M 1980 Fractures of the upper humerus. Orthopedic Clinics of North America 11: 239–252

Post M, Cohen J 1985 Impingement syndrome—a review of late stage II and early stage III lesions. Orthopaedic Transactions 9: 48

Postacchini F, Ricciardi-Pollini P T 1977 Rupture of the short head tendon of the biceps brachii. Clinical Orthopaedics 124: 229–232

Powers J A, Bach P J 1974 Acromioclavicular separation. Clinical Orthopaedics 104: 213–223

Pritsch M, Greental H, Horoszowski H 1997 Closed pinning for humeral fractures. Journal of Bone and Joint Surgery 79B: supp III: 337

Rasmussen S, Hvass I, Dalsgaard J, Christensen B S, Holstad E 1992 Displaced proximal humeral fractures: results of conservative treatment. Injury 23: 4–43

Rathbun J B, MacNab I 1970 The microvascular pattern of the rotator cuff. Journal of Bone and Joint Surgery 52B: 540–553

Rawes M L, Dias J J 1996 Long-term results of conservative treatment for acromioclavicular dislocation. Journal of Bone and Joint Surgery 78B: 410–412

Reeves B 1969 Acute anterior dislocation of the shoulder. Annals of the Royal College of Surgeons of England and Wales 44: 255–273

Refior H J, Sowa D 1995 Long tendon of the biceps brachii: Sites of predilection for degenerative lesions. Journal of Shoulder and Elbow Surgery 4: 436–440

Resch H, Povacz P, Wambacher M, Sperner G, Golser K 1997 Arthroscopic extra articular Bankart repair for the treatment of recurrent anterior shoulder dislocation. Arthroscopy 13: 188–200

Roberts A, Wickstrom J 1971 Prognosis of posterior dislocation of the shoulder. Acta Orthopaedica Scandinavica 42: 328–337

Roberts S W, Hernandez C, Maberry M C, Adams M D, Leveno K J, Wendel G D 1995 Obstetric clavicular fracture: the enigma of normal birth. Obstetrics and Gynecology 86: 978–981

Robinson C M 1998 Fractures of the clavicle in the adult. Epidemiology and classification. Journal of Bone and Joint Surgery 80B: 476–484

Rockwood C A 1991 Fractures and dislocations of the shoulder. In: Rockwood C A, Green D P, Bucholz R W (eds) Fractures in adults. J B Lippincott, Philadelphia, pp 577–682

Rockwood C A, Groh G I, Wirth M A, Grassi F A 1997 Resection arthroplasty of the sternoclavicular joint. Journal of Bone and Joint Surgery 79A: 387–393

Rokito A S, McLaughlin J A, Gallagher M A, Zuckerman J D 1996 Partial rupture of the distal biceps tendon. Journal of Shoulder and Elbow Surgery 5: 73–75

Rokito A S, Zuckerman J D, Gallagher M A, Cuomo F 1996 Strength after surgical repair of the rotator cuff. Journal of Shoulder and Elbow Surgery 5: 12–17

Roscoe M A, Simmons E H 1984 The treatment of complete acromioclavicular dislocation. In: Proceedings of the Canadian Orthopaedic Association. Journal of Bone and Joint Surgery 66B: 304

Rosenberg B N, Richmond J C, Levine W N 1995 Long term follow up of Bankart reconstruction. Incidence of late degenerative glenohumeral arthrosis. American Journal of Sports Medicine 23: 538–544

Ross J G, Love M B 1989 Isolated avulsion fracture of the lesser tuberosity of the humerus. Radiology 172: 833–834

Rowe C R 1956 Prognosis in dislocations of the shoulder. Journal of Bone and Joint Surgery 38A: 957–977

Rowe C R 1968 An atlas of anatomy and treatment of midclavicular fractures. Clinical Orthopaedics 58: 29–42

Rowe C R 1980 Acute and recurrent anterior dislocations of the shoulder. Orthopedic Clinics of North America 11: 253–270

Rowe C R, Marble H C 1958 shoulder girdle injuries. In: Cave E F (ed), Fractures and other injuries. Year Book Publishers, Chicago, pp 250–289

Rowe C R, Sakellarides H T 1961 Factors related to recurrences of anterior dislocations of the shoulder. Clinical Orthopaedics 20: 40–48

Rowe C R, Zarins B 1981 Recurrent transient subluxation of the shoulder. Journal of Bone and Joint Surgery 63A: 863–872

Rowe C R, Zarins B 1982 Chronic unreduced dislocations of the shoulder. Journal of Bone and Joint Surgery 64A: 494–505

Roye R P, Grana W A, Yates C K 1995 Arthroscopic subacromial decompression: two to seven year follow up. Arthroscopy 11: 301–306

Russo R, Togo F 1991 The subcoracoid impingement syndrome: clinical, semeiologic and therapeutic considerations. Italian Journal of Orthopaedics and Traumatology 17: 351–358

Samilson R L, Prieto V 1983 Dislocation arthropathy of the shoulder. Journal of Bone and Joint Surgery 65A: 456–460

Sanders J O, Lyons F A, Rockwood C A 1990 Management of dislocations of both ends of the clavicle. Journal of Bone and Joint Surgery 72A: 399–402

Savastano A A, Stutz S J 1978 Traumatic sternoclavicular dislocation. International Surgery 63: 10–13

Savoie F H, Miller C D, Field L D 1997 Arthroscopic reconstruction of traumatic anterior instability of the shoulder: the Caspari technique. Arthroscopy 13: 201–209

Scheck M 1982 Surgical treatment of non unions of the surgical neck of the humerus. Clinical Orthopaedics 167: 255–259

Schuind F, Pay-Pay E, Andrianne Y, Donkerwolcke M, Rasquin C, Burny F 1988 External fixation of the clavicle for fracture or nonunion in adults. Journal of Bone and Joint Surgery 70A: 692–695

Schulz T J, Jacobs B, Patterson R L 1969 Unrecognized dislocations of the shoulder. Journal of Trauma 9: 1009–1021

Simonet W T, Cofield R H 1984 Prognosis in anterior shoulder dislocation. American Journal of Sports Medicine 12: 19–24

Simonet W T, Melton L J, Cofield R H, Ilstrup D M 1984 Incidence of anterior shoulder dislocation in Olmsted County, Minnesota. Clinical Orthopaedics 186: 186–191

Sisk T D, Boyd H B 1974 Management of recurrent anterior dislocation of the shoulder: Du Toit type or staple capsulorrhaphy. Clinical Orthopaedics 103: 150–156

Slaa R L, Nollen A G E 1987 A Salter type 3 fracture of the proximal epiphysis of the humerus. Injury 18: 429–431

Smith F M 1956 Fracture–separation of the proximal humeral epiphysis. American Journal of Surgery 91: 627–635

Smith M J, Stewart M J 1979 Acute acromioclavicular separations. American Journal of Sports Medicine 7: 62–71

Soto-Hall R, Stroot J H 1960 Treatment of ruptures of the long head of biceps brachii. American Journal of Orthopedics 2: 192

Stableforth P G 1984 Four part fractures of the neck of the humerus. Journal of Bone and Joint Surgery 66B: 104–108

Stahl F 1954 Considerations on post-traumatic absorption of the outer end of the clavicle. Acta Orthopaedica Scandinavica 23: 9–13

Stanley D, Norris S H 1988 Recovery following fractures of the clavicle treated conservatively. Injury 19: 162–164

Stephens N G, Morgan A S, Corvo P, Bernstein B A 1995 Significance of scapular fracture in the blunt-trauma patient. Annals of Emergency Medicine 26: 439–442

Stephens S R, Warren R F, Payne L Z, Wickiewicz T L, Altchek D W 1998 Arthroscopic acromioplasty: a 6 to 10 year follow up. Arthroscopy 14: 382–388

Stewart M J, Hundley J M 1955 Fractures of the humerus. Journal of Bone and Joint Surgery 37A: 681–692

Strömqvist B, Lidgren L, Norgren L, Odenbring S 1987 Neurovascular injury complicating displaced proximal fractures of the humerus. Injury 18: 423–425

Sturzenegger M, Fornaro E, Jakob R P 1982 Results of surgical treatment of multifragmented fractures of the humeral head. Archives of Orthopaedics and Traumatic Surgery 100: 249–259

Taft T N, Wilson F C, Oglesby J W 1987 Dislocation of the acromioclavicular joint. Journal of Bone and Joint Surgery 69A: 1045–1051

Takagishi N 1978 Conservative treatment of the ruptures of the rotator cuff. Journal of the Japanese Orthopaedic Association 52: 781–787

Tanner M W, Cofield R H 1983 Prosthetic arthroplasty for fractures and fracture–dislocations of the proximal humerus. Clinical Orthopaedics 179: 116–128

Taylor A R 1969 Non union of fracture of the clavicle. In: Proceedings of the British Orthopaedic Association. Journal of Bone and Joint Surgery 51B: 568–569

Tempelhof S, Rupp S, Seil R 1999 Age-related prevalence of rotator cuff tears in asymptomatic shoulders. Journal of Shoulder and Elbow Surgery 8: 296–299

Thompson D A, Flynn T C, Miller P W, Fischer R P 1985 The significance of scapular fractures. Journal of Trauma 25: 974–977

Tibone J, Ting A 1990 Capsulorrhaphy with a staple for recurrent posterior subluxation of the shoulder. Journal of Bone and Joint Surgery 72: 999–1002

Tibone J E, Elrod B, Jobe F W et al 1986 Surgical treatment of tears of the rotator cuff in athletes. Journal of Bone and Joint Surgery 68A: 887–891

Toivonen D A, Tuite M J, Orwin J F 1995 Acromial structure and tears of the rotator cuff. Journal of Shoulder and Elbow Surgery 4: 376–383

Torchia M E, Caspari R B, Asselmeier M A, Beach W R, Gayari M 1997 Arthroscopic transglenoid multiple suture repair: 2 to 8 year results in 150 shoulders. Arthroscopy 13: 609–619

Tossy J D, Mead N C, Sigmond H M 1963 Acromioclavicular separations: useful and practical classification for treatment. Clinical Orthopaedics 28: 111–119

Travlos J, Goldberg I, Boome R S 1990 Brachial plexus lesions associated with dislocated shoulders. Journal of Bone and Joint Surgery 728: 68–71

Tsai L, Wredmark T, Johansson C, Gibo K, Engstiom B, Tornqvist H 1991 Shoulder function in patients with unoperated anterior shoulder instability. American Journal of Sports Medicine 19: 469–473

Tsou P M 1989 Percutaneous cannulated screw coracoclavicular fixation for acute acromioclavicular dislocations. Clinical Orthopaedics 243: 112–121

Van der Zwaag H M, Brand R, Obermann W R, Rozing P M 1999 Glenohumeral osteoarthrosis after Putti-Platt repair. Journal of Shoulder and Elbow Surgery 8: 252–258

Visser C P J, Coene L N J E M, Brand R, Tavy D L J 1999 The incidence of nerve injury in anterior dislocation of the shoulder and its influence on functional recovery. A prospective clinical and EMG study. Journal of Bone and Joint Surgery 81B: 679–685

Walch G, Badet R, Nove-Josserard L, Levigne C 1996 Non unions of the surgical neck of the humerus: surgical treatment with an intramedullary bone peg, internal fixation and cancellous bone grafting. Journal of Shoulder and Elbow Surgery 5: 161–168

Wallace W A, Almeida I, Neumann L, Manning P A 1999 Whiplash associated injuries to the shoulder—evaluation of a previously unrecognized problem. Journal of Bone and Joint Surgery 81B: supp II: 214

Wallace W A, Riddell A M, Manning P A, Reese J M, Neumann L 1999 Evaluation of factors affecting the time taken to return to driving after a rotator cuff repair. Journal of Bone and Joint Surgery 81B: supp II: 239

Wallace W A, Wiley A M 1986 The long-term results of conservative management of full thickness tears of the rotator cuff. In: Proceedings of the British Orthopaedic Association. Journal of Bone and Joint Surgery 68B: 162

Walsh W M, Peterson D A, Shelton G, Neumann R D 1985 Shoulder strength following acromioclavicular injury. American Journal of Sports Medicine 13: 153–158

Warner J J P, McMahon P J 1995 The role of the long head of the biceps brachii in superior stability of the glenohumeral joint. Journal of Bone and Joint Surgery 77A: 366–372

Watson M 1985 Major ruptures of the rotator cuff. Journal of Bone and Joint Surgery 67B: 618–624

Waugh R L, Hathcock T A, Elliott J L 1949 Ruptures of muscles and tendons with particular reference to rupture or elongation of long tendon of biceps brachii. Surgery 25: 370–392

Weaver J K, Dunn H K 1972 Treatment of acromioclavicular injuries, especially complete acromioclavicular separations. Journal of Bone and Joint Surgery 54A: 1187–1194

Wiedemann G, Brunner U, Kalteis T, Kettler M, Schweiberer L 1999 Functional and radiologic results of open reduction and internal fixation of anterior glenoid rim fractures. Journal of Bone and Joint Surgery 81B: supp II: 134

Wilber M C, Evans E B 1977 Fractures of the scapula. Journal of Bone and Joint Surgery 59A: 358–362

Wilkins R M, Johnston R M 1983 Ununited fractures of the clavicle. Journal of Bone and Joint Surgery 65A: 773–778

Wilkinson J A, Thomas W G 1985 Glenoid osteotomy for recurrent posterior dislocations of the shoulder. In: Proceedings of the British Orthopaedic Association. Journal of Bone and Joint Surgery 67B: 496

Wintzell G, Haglund-Akerlind Y, Ekelund A, Sandstrom B, Hovelius L, Larsson S 1999 Arthroscopic lavage reduced the recurrence rate following primary anterior shoulder dislocation. A ramdomised multicentre study with one year follow up. Knee Surgery, Sports Traumatology, Arthroscopy 7: 192–196

Wirth M A, Blatter G, Rockwood C A 1996 The capsular imbrication procedure for recurrent anterior instability of the shoulder. Journal of Bone and Joint Surgery 78A: 246–259

Wojtys E M, Nelson G 1991 Conservative treatment of Grade II acromioclavicular dislocations. Clinical Orthopaedics 268: 112–119

Worcester J N, Green D P 1968 Osteoarthritis of the acromioclavicular joint. Clinical Orthopaedics 58: 69–73

Wright S A, Cofield R H 1996 Management of partial-thickness rotator cuff tears. Journal of Shoulder and Elbow Surgery 5: 458–466

Wu C C, Shih C H, Chen W J, Tai C L 1998 Treatment of clavicular aseptic non union: comparison of plating and intramedullary nailing techniques. Journal of Trauma-Injury Infection and Critical Care 45: 512–516

Wülker N, Melzer C, Wirth C J 1991 Shoulder surgery for rotator cuff tears. Acta Orthopaedica Scandinavica 62: 142–147

Yang J, al-Etani H, Letts M 1996 Diagnosis and treatment of posterior or sternoclavicular joint dislocations in children. American Journal of Orthopaedics (Chatham, N J) 25: 565–569

Yoneda B, Welsh R P, MacIntosh D L 1982 Conservative treatment of shoulder dislocation in young males. In: Proceedings of the Canadian Orthopaedic Association. Journal of Bone and Joint Surgery 64B: 254–255

Young T B, Wallace W A 1985 Conservative treatment of fractures and fracture–dislocations of the upper end of the humerus. Journal of Bone and Joint Surgery 67B: 373–377

Zdravkovic D, Damholt V V 1974 Comminuted and severely displaced fractures of the scapula. Acta Orthopaedica Scandinavica 45: 60–65

Zenni E J, Kreig J K, Rosen M J 1981 Open reduction and internal fixation of clavicular fractures. Journal of Bone and Joint Surgery 63A: 147–151

Zilberman Z, Rejovitzky R 1981 Fracture of the coracoid process of the scapula. Injury 13: 203–206

Zyto K, Ahrengart L, Sperber A, Tornkvist H 1997 Treatment of displaced proximal humeral fractures in elderly patients. Journal of Bone and Joint Surgery 79B: 412–417

Zyto K, Kronberg M, Brostrom L A 1995 Shoulder function after displaced fractures of the proximal humerus. Journal of Shoulder and Elbow Surgery 4: 331–336

Zyto K, Wallace A, Frostick S P, Preston B J 1998 Outcome after hemiarthroplasty for three- and four-part fractures of the proximal humerus. Journal of Shoulder and Elbow Surgery 7: 85–89

The humerus

Phillip S. Fagg

▓ Introduction

The shaft of the humerus is defined as that part below the surgical neck and above the level of the epicondyles. The classification of these fractures is based on their anatomical location and the fracture pattern.

Fractures of the shaft of the humerus are uncommon, Emmett & Breck (1958) stating that they had encountered only 166, approximately 1% of the 11 000 fractures seen in their practice.

Conservative management

In 1933, Caldwell introduced his concept of the hanging cast to produce dependent traction in the treatment of humeral shaft fractures. Prior to this, the humerus was the most common site of non-union. Many orthopaedic surgeons felt that the hanging cast was the treatment of choice for fractures of the humeral shaft at all anatomical levels; however, some authors considered that in certain circumstances it was implicated as a contributary factor in the causation of non-union.

Brachial U splints, sugar tong splints or humeral braces have been favoured by other surgeons because these stabilise the fractured bone without adding sufficient weight to cause distraction at the fracture site.

Lateral or overhead traction is not commonly used now, although it still has a place in the treatment of patients who have sustained other—often multiple—injuries, or who have associated medical problems which mitigate against ambulatory treatment.

Thoracobrachial body casts are reserved by those who use them for special circumstances, such as very comminuted, unstable fractures, although their use in the past was more widespread.

Although no single method of treatment is used for the conservative management of humeral shaft fractures, treatments that are employed do seem to fall into the aforementioned four main groups, which are described in greater detail below.

Hanging cast

The hanging cast gained widespread popularity in the USA after its introduction by Caldwell in 1933. In 1940,

Caldwell reported four cases of delayed union and one of non-union in a series of 59 humeral fractures treated by this method. Its acceptance in the UK was less enthusiastic, no doubt due to the comments of Watson-Jones in *Fractures and Joint Injuries* (as quoted by Thompson et al 1965), in which he described it as a heavy plaster cast from the wrist to the axilla, sometimes even weighted with lumps of lead, being slung and suspended from the neck. In *The Closed Treatment of Common Fractures*, Charnley (1961) observed that the hanging cast method was open to serious mechanical criticism and that it readily produced over- distraction of the humerus.

However, the published results of humeral shaft fractures treated by this method suggested that these pessimistic comments by the English authorities were misplaced. The incidence of delayed union and non-union after this method of treatment of humeral shaft fractures is recorded in Table 6.1. It shows that Laferte & Rosenbaum (1937) reported no case of non-union in 58 fractures. Mann & Neal (1965) recorded the highest incidence of non-union at 6.5%. Thompson et al (1965) noted fragment distraction in some of these cases, but found that these distracted fractures also healed solidly.

The average period of immobilisation varied between 6 weeks (Laferte & Rosenbaum 1937; Stewart & Hundley 1955; Mann & Neal 1965), and 10 weeks (Scientific Research Committee, Pennsylvania Orthopedic Society 1959). Mann & Neal reported that radiological union occurred in an average of 12.1 weeks.

Stewart & Hundley (1955) reported 81.3% excellent and 12.2% good results out of their 107 fractures. Excellent results had no pain or impairment of function and no radiological evidence of deformity. Good results had no pain or functional impairment for ordinary use, but 20% or less limitation of motion in the elbow or shoulder and angulation of not more than 10°. Laferte & Rosenbaum (1937) reported that 75% of their patients had an excellent functional result, and 82% had excellent radiological alignment.

Humeral splints or braces

The trend in the treatment of humeral shaft fractures has been away from hanging casts in favour of some form of humeral splinting, either by U-slab (Klenerman 1966), or by a functional humeral brace (Sarmiento et al 1977).

The incidence of delayed union and non-union by these methods of treatment is recorded in Table 6.2. Klenerman's 1966 definition of delayed union (defined as the absence of clinical union 8 weeks after fracture) has been used. The average incidence of delayed union by these methods of treatment is 3%, and the average non-union rate is 2.5%.

The average healing time reported in these papers was similar to that reported for the hanging cast method. Union usually occurs in an average of 6–8 weeks, Klenerman (1966) reporting that 76% of fractures healed in this time. Sarmiento et al (1977) quoted 8.5 weeks as the healing time following the use of his functional brace and Zagorski et al (1988) reported it as 10.6 weeks after using a functional brace.

A comparison of the functional end-results recorded in these papers is difficult due to the different criteria adopted by the authors to assess their results.

Klenerman (1966) reported that 70% of his patients had an excellent result and 20% had a good result (90% in total). Zagorski et al (1988) recorded 93% excellent and 5% good results (98% total) in their 170 fractures assessed for function; their good results lacked the final 15° of forward flexion of the shoulder or 5° extension of the elbow.

Table 6.1   The incidence of delayed union and non-union after the hanging cast treatment of humeral shaft fractures

Reference	Number of patients	Number with delayed union	Number with non-union
Laferte & Rosenbaum (1937)	58	–	0
Caldwell (1940)	59	4 (6.8%)	1 (1.7%)
Stewart & Hundley (1955)	107	–	3 (2.8%)
Pennsylvania Orthopedic Society (1959)	69	–	3 (4.3%)
Mann & Neal (1965)	77	–	5 (6.5%)
Thompson et al (1965)	103*	1 (1%)	2 (1.9%)

* This includes 41 surgical neck fractures and six supracondylar fractures.

Table 6.2   The incidence of delayed union and non-union with humeral splints and braces for humeral shaft fractures

Reference	Method	Number of patients	Number with delayed union	Number with non-union
Klenerman (1966)	U-slab	87	8 (9.2%)	0
Wallny et al (1997a)	Brace	79	–	5 (6%)
Zagorski et al (1988)	Brace	170	–	3 (1.8%)
Hosner (1974)	POP cast	100	7 (7%)*	2 (2%)
Sarmiento et al (1990)	Brace	85†		3 (3.5%)
Total		521	15 (3%)	13 (2.5%)

* Delayed union was not defined in this paper.
† Distal third fractures only

Wallny et al (1997a) classified 81% of their patients as achieving an excellent/good result, 15.2% a moderate result and 3.8% a poor result. Eighty-six percent of their patients showed no restriction in range of motion of their shoulder and elbow. Three patients (4%) exhibited a 10° limitation in elbow extension, and five patients (6%) displayed limited shoulder motion in abduction to 100°.

Sarmiento et al (1990) reviewed the function of the shoulder and elbow in 58 of their patients with distal third fractures treated by a functional brace. Thirty-one (55%) lost no external rotation, 19 (33%) lost 5–15°, and eight (12%) lost up to 45°. Shoulder abduction was limited by 10–60° in nine patients (15.5%), and shoulder flexion by 5–20° in eight (13%). Elbow flexion was reduced by 5–25° in 15 patients (26%), and extension was limited by 5–25° in 14 (24%). The follow-up time for these patients was not specified, but it was felt that they may have improved with a longer period.

Hosner (1974) reported an 8–12 year follow-up in 53 patients. Twenty-seven (51%) had occasional mild pain in wet and cold weather. Six patients (11%) had some shoulder limitation—three by less than 25%—and the average age for these patients was 64, 20 years above the average age for the series. Seven patients (13%) lost some elbow movement—four less than 30°. No patient with loss of elbow movement for over 2 months improved.

The average angulation of the fractures treated ranged from 5° (Zagorski et al 1988) to 9° (Sarmiento et al 1990). However, 29 out of 67 (43%) of the patients whose malunion was measured had more than 10° of varus or valgus angulation (Sarmiento et al 1990), and similar figures (28 of 53 patients, 53%) were noted by Zagorski et al (1988).

Shortening of the humerus averaged 4 mm (Zagorski et al 1988) to 5 mm (Sarmiento et al 1990).

Traction

The use of either skin or skeletal traction in the management of the fractured humeral shaft is reserved for those patients with complex, comminuted fractures or those who have alternative injuries which contraindicate ambulatory treatment.

Vichare (1974) reported on 32 patients with multiple injuries including humeral shaft fracture. Describing his technique of skin traction on five patients, he stated that they all united within 6 weeks with no deformity. Holm (1970) had two instances of non-union in his 12 patients with complex or compound humeral fractures treated by traction, and the Pennsylvania Orthopedic Society (1959) had one non-union out of 18 patients treated by either skin or skeletal traction.

Bleeker et al (1991) used traction for 115 patients with an isolated humeral fracture as well as for multiply injured patients. Twenty-six patients (23%) had delayed union (defined as union after 90 days).

Thoracobrachial cast

The use of a thoracobrachial cast is not favoured now in the routine treatment of humeral shaft fractures, but may still be used for complex injuries. The largest reported series appears to be that by Stewart & Hundley (1955), which described the use of the thoracobrachial cast in 53 cases. Of this number, 84.9% required a general anaesthetic during application, and the average period of immobilisation was 10.4 weeks. Of the nine cases described by Vichare (1974), 77.7% united in 10 weeks, and the Pennsylvania Orthopedic Group (1959) reported that the average healing time in 14 cases was 13 weeks. Stewart & Hundley (1955) and Vichare (1974) both recorded just one case of non-union, while the Pennsylvania Orthopedic Society (1959) had none. Stewart & Hundley (1955) found that 71.7% of their patients had an excellent or good result.

Results of conservative management related to compound injuries and anatomical site
Compound injuries

There is little in the literature on the results of the conservative management of compound fractures of the humeral shaft. Most series include compound fractures but fail to report the results separately, or to suggest any major problems in their treatment.

The Pennsylvania Orthopedic Society (1959) included 10% compound injuries in its total of 159 cases. The healing time for these conservatively treated compound injuries averaged 13 weeks, as compared with an average of 12 weeks for the group as a whole. Of the 13 non-unions in the whole series, three (18.75%) occurred in compound fractures.

Zagorski et al (1988) reported the use of a functional brace in 43 patients with compound injuries of the humeral shaft. Only one patient (2.3%) had a non-union. These fractures healed at an average of 13.6 weeks, as compared with 9.5 weeks for those humeral fractures not complicated by an open wound.

Mann & Neal (1965) reported one non-union and one wound infection out of 20 compound fractures.

Anatomical site

Holm (1970) found that all non-unions in his series developed in transverse or short oblique midshaft fractures in young adults. Laing (1956) reported the constancy of the arterial supply to the adult humerus at the junction of the middle and lower third, and suggested that fractures at this level would probably destroy the main nutrient artery at the time of injury. This would result in the proximal end of the lower fragment depending for its arterial blood supply on vessels entering from the periosteum and ascending from the epicondyles, and might prejudice the results of internal fixation at this level, but it might not be so significant in conservatively treated fractures.

Klenerman (1966) reported five examples of delayed union out of 44 middle third fractures (11.3%); two of these had been treated by internal fixation. However, there were also two delayed unions out of 22 proximal third fractures (11%), and one out of 17 (5.9%) in the distal third. Mann & Neal (1965) recorded non-union in five of 29 proximal fractures (17.2%), four of 52 middle third fractures (7.7%) and one of 15 distal third fractures (5.8%).

Bleeker et al (1991) found that no fracture location was specifically prone to delayed union in their 168 patients. Their figures revealed that delayed union occurred in six of 43 upper third fractures (14%), 21 of 94 middle third fractures (22%), and five of 31 lower third fractures (18%).

Radiological alignment and functional end-result in humeral shaft fractures

Reporting on his extensive experience of the conservative management of humeral shaft fractures, Bohler (1965) stated that 'attaining adequate shortening of 1–10 mm is the most important task in fracture treatment. In transverse humeral shaft fractures, lateral displacement the full width of the shaft and shortening are functionally and cosmetically of no importance'.

Klenerman (1966) reported that residual varus angulation occurred at the fracture site irrespective of its level, and that posterior bowing was found more often than anterior bowing. He found that anterior bowing of 20° or varus angulation of 30° could be present before deformity became clinically obvious, and even then the function of the limb was good.

Thus it can be seen that accurate alignment is not essential for a good functional end-result. Rotation is probably the most important deformity to correct, and Klenerman points out that it is prevented by supporting the hand on the lower part of the chest.

In a study of Royal Air Force personnel compiled in 1944, Doran reported that the power of the limb could be restored provided that the elbow permitted a total range of flexion and extension of about 70°. He stated that power did not recover with 'free use', even though the range of elbow movements was full. In the great majority of cases he found power to be restored to 75% of normal, or better in an average of 4–6 weeks by resistance exercises. Mast et al (1975) assessed 26 patients on a Cybex machine and only two of these had an unsatisfactory functional result.

Summary

- The incidence of non-union after the hanging cast treatment of humeral shaft fractures is between 2.8% and 6.5%. Immobilisation is required for 6–10 weeks and radiological union is seen at about 12 weeks.
- Excellent or near normal function is found in 75–85% of humeral shaft fractures treated by the hanging cast method.
- The average period of immobilisation of humeral shaft fractures by humeral splints is 6–8 weeks, and the incidence of non-union averages 2.5%.
- Excellent or near normal function is found in 80–93% of patients with humeral shaft fractures treated by humeral splints.
- After the use of a thoracobrachial cast for humeral shaft fractures the average period of immobilisation is 10–13 weeks. Excellent or good results occur in 71.7%. The non-union rate varies from 1.8% to 11% with more complex injuries.
- Compound humeral shaft fractures heal slightly more slowly than closed fractures and the incidence of non-union is higher, at 2.3–18.5%.
- The delayed and non-union rate of humeral fractures is not specifically related to the anatomical site.
- Anterior bowing of 20°, varus angulation of 30° and complete lateral displacement did not alter the final outcome.

Primary operative management

As the treatment of choice in humeral shaft fractures, primary operative management has not been championed by many. Early reports in the literature were almost unanimous in showing the inferior results of primary internal fixation compared with conservative treatment. The Scientific Research Committee of the Pennsylvania Orthopedic Society (1959) reported non-union rates of 9.4% after intramedullary fixation, 14.3% after screw fixation and 28.6% after the use of plates. The average healing time for this operative group as a whole was 17 weeks as compared with 12 weeks after closed treatment. Wallny et al (1997b) compared 44 humeral fractures treated conservatively with functional bracing and 45 treated by operation with a locking nail. The functional end-results were somewhat better in the conservatively managed group. Thirty-eight patients (86%) treated with the brace regained full shoulder movement as compared with 22 patients (47%) treated surgically. Ten percent of patients treated with the brace lost some elbow mobility. A similar number (50% treated with the brace and 54% treated surgically) were free of pain. Two patients treated with a brace went on to non-union. Two of the patients treated surgically required a second operation, one for infection and one to release a haematoma. The majority of closed humeral shaft fractures should be treated conservatively.

However, operative management does have its part to play in the treatment of humeral shaft fractures. The indications for open reduction and internal fixation of fractures of the humeral shaft include:

- multiply injured patients with humeral fracture
- compound fractures
- fractures with associated vascular or neural injury
- injuries of the shoulder, elbow or forearm in the same limb
- bilateral upper limb fractures
- pathological fractures
- failure of closed methods of treatment
- obesity

Jensen & Rasmussen (1995) reported four non-unions in nine overweight patients (defined as more than 120% of normal weight) treated non-operatively with a Sarmiento brace. They recommended operative treatment in these patients.

Operative fixation falls into three main groups:

- intramedullary fixation
- plate fixation
- external fixation

Intramedullary fixation

The results of the treatment of humeral shaft fractures by various types of intramedullary fixation are shown in Table 6.3. It can be seen that the reported incidence of non-union varies between 1% and 8.5% (5.4% average for these reported series). The average time to union varies between 7 and 14 weeks.

Of the 165 patients reported by Maffei et al (1997), 19 cases were pathological fractures and 12 were non-unions, but the results for these groups were not separated from the acute fractures. Overall, 68% had an excellent functional result with a full range of shoulder motion. Thirty-two percent, however, lost some shoulder mobility. Eighteen percent lost 10° of shoulder motion but had no pain while 14% had pain as well as restricted motion of the shoulder. Crates & Whittle (1998), on the other hand, reported full shoulder function returning at an average of 2.3 months post-surgery in 90% of their patients treated with an antegrade Russell–Taylor humeral nail.

Hall & Pankovich (1987) found that the range of shoulder and elbow motion of their 86 patients treated by Ender nails approached that of the uninjured limb. On average their patients lost 3° of elbow extension, 7° of elbow flexion, 16° of shoulder abduction, 7° of external rotation and 7° of internal rotation. Patients aged over 50 years consistently progressed more slowly and took 5 months from injury to recover their full movement.

Compression plate fixation

The results of the treatment of humeral shaft fractures by compression plates are shown in Table 6.4. Union occurred in 97 to 100% of reported cases and most fractures united within 16–20 weeks. In most of these series they were problem fractures, and in Bell et al's 1985 series all patients had multiple injuries.

In Bell's series, 34 fractures were followed up, with an average time to union of 19 weeks (defined as the time of the disappearance of the fracture line). Six fractures (17.6%) took 6 months or longer to unite, and one case (2.9%) went on to a non-union. They reported 26 patients (76.5%) with a full range of shoulder movements, and 33 (97%) with a fully functional shoulder. Thirty-one (91%) had full elbow movements, the remaining three having severe elbow injuries.

Table 6.3 The results of intramedullary nailing of humeral shaft fractures

	Zanasi et al (1990)	Hall & Pankovich (1987)	Crates & Whittle (1998)	Shazar et al (1998)	Maffei et al (1997)
Technique	Küntscher nail	Ender nail	Russell-Taylor nail	Retrograde Ender nails	Seidal nail
Number of fractures	98	86	73	94	165
Non-union	2 (2%)	1 (1%)	4 (5.5%)	8 (8.5%)	13 (8%)
Average time to union (weeks)	–	7.2	14	14	7
Excellent function	–	–	66 (90%)	74 (81%)	68%

Table 6.4 The results of compression plate fixation of humeral shaft fractures

	Chiu et al (1997)	Bell et al (1985)	Griend et al (1986)	Zinghi et al (1988)
Number of fractures	59	34	34	74
Non-union	5 (8.5%)	1 (3%)	1 (3%)	0
Average time to union	9.4 weeks (with bone graft)	19 weeks	20 patients in 4 months	–
	12.5 weeks (no bone graft)		8 patients in 6 months	
			5 patients in 12 months	
Infection	2 (3%)	1 (3%)	2 (6%)	1 (1%)
Iatrogenic radial nerve palsy	3 (5%)	1 (3%)	1 (3%)	2 (3%)
Significant loss of shoulder motion	–	3*	6*	1
Failure of implant		2 (6%)	–	–

* All had severe elbow injuries in addition to humeral shaft fractures.

In Griend et al's 1986 series of 34 patients, 20 (58.8%) were united in 4 months and 28 (81.8%) within 6 months. They also reported one case (2.9%) of non-union. Their results in 31 patients with adequate records showed 100% return of shoulder movement, but eight (25.8%) with up to a 20° loss of elbow extension and six (19.3%) with less than 50° movement at the elbow, although all of these had severe articular or soft tissue injury.

Iatrogenic radial nerve palsies occurred in 3 to 5% of fractures, and significant infection in 1 to 6%, mostly in compound injuries.

There were two failures of implants in Bell's series, both of which subsequently healed with secondary procedures.

Comparison of intramedullary and compression plate fixation

A number of studies have compared the results of intramedullary fixation devices and compression plates in the management of acute humeral shaft fractures. The results are shown in Table 6.5.

In all the quoted papers functional recovery following the intramedullary nailing and compression plating was similar. McPherson et al (1999) concluded that intramedullary nail stabilisation did not provide a clear advantage over dynamic compression plates for humeral shaft fractures. While functional recovery was similar, their intramedullary nail group had more cases of impinge-

ment, a higher incidence of transient radial nerve palsies, and were more likely to require further surgery. Similarily, Rodriguez-Merchan (1995) reported similar functional results between his two groups, but in all patients except one the nails were removed because the patients had discomfort that interfered with their function.

External fixators

Little has been published concerning the use of external fixators in humeral shaft fractures. Wisniewski & Radziejowski (1996), in a prospective study, assessed 38 consecutive gunshot fractures of the humeral shaft, stabilised with an external fixator. In 34 patients (89%) union occurred between 12 and 24 (average 16) weeks. Two patients with delayed union required bone grafting. Non-union occurred in two patients (5%). Superficial pintrack infection was present in five patients; two had deep wound sepsis and one had osteomyelitis.

Smith & Cooney (1990) treated nine patients with a high-energy humeral injury with external fixation. All had compound injuries. A good to excellent result was achieved in six (67%) of these fractures. Delayed union occurred in five (63%) of eight fractures, and chronic osteomyelitis in one (12%). Shoulder motion was normal or slightly impaired in seven (78%) of nine patients, and elbow motion in the eight salvaged limbs was normal.

Table 6.5 Comparison of intramedullary and compression plate fixation in humeral shaft fractures

	Intramedullary fixation	Compression plate fixation	
Chiu et al (1998)	Ender nail	DCP	DCP +bone graft
Number of patients	31	30	29
Non-union	3 (9.8%)	5 (16.7%)	0
Average time to union	9.9 weeks	12.5 weeks	9.4 weeks
Infection	1 (3.2%)	1 (3.3%)	1 (3.4%)
Iatrogenic radial nerve palsy	0	2 (6.7%)	1 (3.4%)
Complication rate	21.8%	30%	6.9%
Lin (1998)	Humeral locked nail	DCP	
Number of patients	48	25	
Non-union	0	1 (4%)	
Average time to union	8.6 weeks	9.2 weeks	
Infection	0	1 (4%)	
Iatrogenic radial nerve palsy	0	1 (4%)	
McPherson et al (1999)	IM nail	DCP	
Number of patients	19	22	
Shoulder impingement	6 (31.5%)	1 (4.5%)	
Complication rate	13 (68%)	3 (13.6%)	
Rodreguez-Merchan (1995)	Hackethal nail	DCP	
Number of patients	20	20	
Non-union	0	0	
Excellent/good result	16 (80%)	16 (80%)	

Costa et al (1991) treated 15 fractures of the humeral shaft by external fixation, with union occurring in an average of 10 weeks. Excellent to good results occurred in 87.5% of patients.

Summary

- After intramedullary fixation non-union occurs in 5.4% of patients, and union occurs on average in 7–14 weeks.
- Loss of shoulder movement occurs in 10–32% of patients with proximally inserted devices. Some restriction of elbow movement occurs with retrograde intramedullary fixation. Older patients take longer to recover their movements.
- Humeral shaft fractures treated by compression plating heal in an average of 10–20 weeks. There is a 3–8.5% non-union rate.
- After plating humeral fractures there is an almost 100% return of shoulder function, and a 75–90% chance of recovery of full elbow movement if there was no articular or severe soft tissue damage around the joint.
- Infection occurs in up to 6% of plated humeral fractures.
- There is little difference in the functional recovery between IM nails and compression plating, but IM nails have a higher complication rate.
- There is insufficient literature on the use of external fixators in the treatment of humeral shaft fractures to draw any conclusions, but the radial nerve may be at risk from this technique.

Results of treatment of delayed or non-union

Delayed or non-union of humeral shaft fractures is not a common problem and the techniques of management have varied. At present the main methods of treatment are either intramedullary nailing techniques or compression plating with or without bone graft.

The results of various techniques for the surgical treatment of non-union of the humeral shaft are summarised in Table 6.6. Union occurred in 92 to 100% of cases. The non-unions healed in an average of 5–7.2 months.

Although various techniques for securing union have been described, most emphasise the importance of supplementing the internal fixation with bone graft.

The return of function following these procedures for non-union is not well documented. Rosen (1990) stated that there was a 75 to 90% return of function in the limbs of the 32 patients he operated on. Healy et al (1987) reported that in their 26 patients the average postoperative range of elbow movement was 12–122°, and the average shoulder elevation 149°. Barquet et al (1989) were the only authors to grade their patients' functional recovery. Of their 25 patients, 21 (84%) had a good result (i.e. no pain, limitation of adjacent joint mobility less than 20°, and angulation less than 10°), three (12%) a fair result (pain after effort or fatigue, limitation of mobility ranging between 20–40° and angulation greater than 10°), and one (4%) a poor result.

Summary

- Union occurs in 92–100% of humeral shaft non-unions treated surgically, over a period of 5–7.2 months.
- Return of function is generally good following surgery for humeral shaft non-union.

Radial nerve palsy

Radial nerve injury complicates closed fracture of the humerus in a significant number of cases, and strong arguments can be found in the literature both for and against early exploration. Many review articles were based on patients' data collected over a long period of time, and the conclusions made by these authors were based on the accumulated results obtained over a period during which changes in the management of these lesions occurred. Modern techniques, such as microsurgical repair of nerve lacerations, are likely to affect the final outcome favourably.

The reported incidence of radial nerve palsy complicating humeral shaft fractures varies widely, from 1.8% (Holstein & Lewis 1963) to 17.6% (Branch 1955). The incidence of radial nerve palsy in those series which report 100 or more fractures of the humeral shaft is recorded in Table 6.7. Taking these figures as a whole, there was an average incidence of 9.8% of immediate radial nerve palsy following humeral shaft fracture. The wide variation in incidence is likely to be explained by population differences and the differing types of violence occurring in the catchment areas of the different reporting centres.

The true incidence of radial nerve palsy following open reduction and internal fixation is also difficult to ascertain. Garcia & Maeck (1960) reviewed 31 years of radial nerve palsies occurring in New York, and found 24 cases occurring after 102 cases of internal fixation—an incidence of 23.5%. The Scientific Research Committee of the Pennsylvania Orthopedic Society, reporting in 1959 on a 5 year study group from 1952 to 1956, found three cases of radial nerve palsy occurring after the internal fixation of 45 fractures (an incidence of 6.6%). However, Garcia & Maeck pointed out that over the last decade of their review there had been no cases of radial nerve palsy postoperatively, suggesting that the incidence was declining

Table 6.6   The results of surgery for non-union of the humeral shaft

	Rosen (1990)	Healy et al (1987)	Barquet et al (1989)	Leyes et al (1997)	Otsuka et al (1998)
Technique	Compression plate and bone graft	Compression plate with or without bone graft	Compression plate and bone graft	Various	Compression plate with bone graft
Number of fractures	32	26	25	69	21
Number united	31 (97%)	24 (92%)	24 (96%)	64 (93%)	21
Average healing time (months)	6.6	5.6	6	–	5 months

with modern surgical techniques. It is therefore appropriate to quote only recent papers for a realistic figure. An overall incidence of postoperative radial nerve palsy of 3 to 5% is shown in Table 6.4. The overall rate of radial nerve palsy post manipulation of fractures was about 2%, this figure being based on three papers, which quote incidences of 1.25% (Mast et al 1975), 1.4% (Kettelkamp & Alexander 1967) and 3.5% (Pennsylvania Orthopedic Society 1957).

The incidence of radial nerve palsy related to the site of the fracture is shown in Table 6.8. All of the reported series seem to agree that it occurs less commonly in the proximal third of the humerus. Holstein & Lewis (1963) found no radial nerve palsies in proximal shaft fractures out of 341 cases of humeral shaft fracture. However, when those papers quoting incidences of radial nerve palsy with total numbers of fractures are compared, there is an overall incidence of 6% of radial nerve palsy occurring with proximal humeral shaft fractures.

It is further shown in Table 6.8 that all of the quoted papers, except those of Holstein & Lewis (1963) and Pollock et al (1981), reported the highest percentage of radial nerve palsies as occurring after middle third fractures.

Whitson (1954) reported that in 25 cadaveric dissections the radial nerve, as it left the front of the long head of triceps, was separated from the humerus in the region of the spiral groove by fibres of the medial head of triceps. As the lateral supracondylar ridge of the humerus was

Table 6.7 The incidence of radial nerve palsy in humeral shaft fractures

Reference	Total number of fractures	Total number of palsies	Percentage
Holstein & Lewis (1963)	341	6	1.8
Caldwell (1940)	108	4	3.7
Pollock et al (1981)	383*	23	6
Bleeker et al (1991)	239	19	8
Pennsylvania Orthopedic Group (1959)	159	19	11.3
Garcia & Maeck (1960)	226	27	11.9
Kettelkamp & Alexander (1967)	216	27	12.5
Sonneveld et al (1987)	111	17	15.3
Mast et al (1975)	240	42	17.5
Branch (1955)	187	33*	17.6

* Indicates the number estimated from available figures.

Table 6.8 The incidence of radial nerve palsy with fracture site

Reference	Proximal third	Middle third	Distal third
Bleeker et al (1991)	1/43 fractures	12/94 fractures	5/31 fractures
Mast et al (1975)	6/72 fractures	29/93 fractures	7/75 fractures
Garcia & Maeck (1960)	4	21	6
Holstein & Lewis (1963)	0	1	6
Kettelkamp & Alexander (1967)	5	23	5
Pollock et al (1981)	2	5	14
Sonneveld et al (1987)	0	16	1
Samardzic et al (1990)	0	27	10

approached, he found that the radial nerve was in contact with the lower margin of the spiral groove for a variable distance, from 0–7 cm (average 3.3 cm). He felt that these observations offered an explanation for the fact that the radial nerve escapes injury in many fractures of the humerus in which nerve damage would be expected.

Holstein & Lewis (1963) described a fracture syndrome in the distal third of the humerus. A spiral fracture occurred in which the distal fragment was displaced proximally and the proximal fragment deviated radially. The radial nerve was caught in the fracture site, the nerve being fixed to the proximal fragment by the intermuscular septum. Nerve damage occurred from the distal end of the proximal fragment.

Recovery after radial nerve palsy

The role of operative or non-operative treatment in the management of humeral shaft fractures complicated by radial nerve palsy remains controversial.

Immediate radial nerve palsy

On reviewing those papers which recorded the results of more than 10 cases of immediate radial nerve palsy, it can be seen that between 64.5% and 100% of cases (average 83%) achieved full recovery (Table 6.9).

There is disagreement as to whether early or delayed surgical exploration influences the final result. In 1955 Branch treated all of his 33 cases of radial nerve palsy by the hanging cast technique and achieved a 100% recovery rate without the need for surgical intervention. Pollock et al (1981) reported that only two out of 24 of their cases required surgical intervention. They recommended that these patients should be observed for return of function over 3.5–4 months before considering surgery.

Kettelkamp & Alexander (1967) explored 13 cases out of 33, 11 of them within 2 weeks. They found interruption of the radial nerve in only two patients: one was caused by a gunshot wound, and the other was associated with an open fracture. They claimed that no surgically correctable nerve injury or mechanical impingement was found on exploration of the closed fractures. The authors recommended exploration of the radial nerve if there was no return of function after 8–12 weeks. Similarly, Sonneveld et al (1987) performed early operative exploration in 14 of their 17 cases of radial nerve palsy. In all but one case the nerves were undamaged, apart from one with contusion. They concluded that paralysis of the radial nerve associated with fractures of the shaft of the humerus was not an indication for early operative treatment. On the other hand, Garcia & Maeck (1960) reported the results of exploration in 23 of 31 cases. Only one was severed, and it recovered completely after suture. Eighteen recovered completely after surgical exploration, compared with three of the eight cases treated expectantly. The authors found that in patients with complete motor loss, the majority showed some visible sign of injury to the nerve at operation. They recommended that patients with

Table 6.9 The overall recovery rate of immediate radial nerve palsies

Reference	Radial nerve palsies	Recovery	Percentage
Shaw & Sakellarides (1967)	31	20	64.5
Garcia & Maeck (1960)	31	21	67.7
Packer et al (1972)	31†	21	67.7
Mast et al (1975)	35	25	71.4
Sonneveld et al (1987)	17	15	88
Postacchini & Morace (1988)	42*	35	83
Kettelkamp & Alexander (1967)	27	25	92
Pennsylvania Orthopedic Group (1959)	19	18	94
Pollock et al (1981)	24	24	100
Mann & Neal (1965)	16	16	100
Branch (1955)	33‡	33	100

* Indicates some late-onset radial nerve palsies.

† This includes five post manipulation of fracture.

‡ Figure estimated from the paper.

complete nerve injuries should undergo surgery as soon after injury as possible, to inspect the nerve and repair it if necessary, but also that patients with incomplete palsies should be treated expectantly. They felt that surgery should be performed at the first sign of progression of the paralysis or if there was no sign of improvement after 4 months.

Postacchini & Morace (1988) reported 42 cases of radial nerve palsy following fracture. All 18 patients subjected to early surgical exploration recovered and surgically remedial lesions were found in six of these patients. Twelve of the 14 patients (86%) treated conservatively recovered satisfactory function, but only five of the 10 patients in whom surgery was delayed did so. In open fractures that require debridement, or in those fractures that require an open reduction with a concomitant radial nerve palsy, the need to explore the nerve is obvious. The timing of surgery for closed humeral shaft fractures with radial nerve palsy has been recommended as being required immediately or with a delay of up to 4 months. The time at which radial nerve recovery commences may be as early as 24 hours. Pollock et al (1981) reported that in their slowest case recovery did not commence until 7 months post injury, although from their series the commencement of the return of function occurred at an average of 7 weeks. Postacchini & Morace (1988) reported the start of recovery being delayed by up to 9 months, but that commencement of recovery occurred at an average of 10–12 weeks.

The time taken for full recovery to occur varied between 4 months (Pollock et al 1981) and 22 months (Postacchini & Morace 1988).

Samardzic et al (1990) reported the results of 37 radial nerve injuries in which microsurgical reconstruction was performed. Twenty-four cases had an interfascicular neurolysis, and 13 had interfascicular grafting. Of the cases treated by nerve grafting, eight (62%) had an excellent or good recovery, while three (23%) had a fair result. The first signs of recovery appeared between 6 and 8 months. Nineteen of the 24 cases (79%) treated by neurolysis had an excellent or good recovery of function, while four (17%) had a fair result. In these cases the first signs of recovery usually appeared between 2 and 4 months after surgery.

A delay of 8–16 weeks in the exploration of an immediate radial nerve palsy after closed humeral shaft fracture would appear to be acceptable.

Radial nerve palsy after fracture manipulation

Little information is available concerning radial nerve palsy developing after manipulation of the fracture.

Fischer & Haine (1975) reported that nine of their 13 cases had full recovery by 8 weeks after injury, with a further two having partial recovery. Mast et al (1975) reported that two of their three cases recovered at 2 months, but the third did not recover. The three in Kettelkamp & Alexander's 1967 series all recovered. Shaw & Sakellarides (1967) found five cases, four occurring in the so-called Holstein–Lewis fracture, for which early operation was performed; in all cases the nerve was found to be trapped within the fracture. These cases recovered at an average of 9 months. Packer et al (1972) had three cases related to humeral shaft fractures. All three were explored and recovered fully.

It would appear that radial nerve palsy occurring after a Holstein–Lewis fracture is manipulated should be explored, but for those occurring after the other types of humeral shaft fractures expectant treatment is appropriate.

Radial nerve palsy after internal fixation

As mentioned earlier in this section, with improvement in techniques the incidence of radial nerve palsy following internal fixation has lessened. It is reported to occur on average in 3 to 5% of cases. The majority of reported cases recovered within a few weeks. Shaw & Sakellarides (1967) reported on nine cases of postoperative radial nerve palsy, six complete palsies and three partial palsies. All of these recovered; the average time for full recovery was 3 months for a partial palsy and 8 months for a complete palsy. Two cases required neurolysis for adherence within scar tissue.

Other neurovascular lesions

Injuries to the brachial artery, median nerve and ulnar nerve, singly or in any combination, have all been reported in the literature. The majority seem to occur with open fractures or gunshot wounds.

Gainor & Metzler (1986) reported the management of 10 patients with fracture of the humeral shaft, with concomitant brachial artery injury. They emphasised the importance of rigid skeletal stability to safeguard the repair, the debatable role of arteriography which did delay the transit time to surgery, and the fact that ligation of the brachial artery above the profunda brachii artery resulted in the loss of the limb in about 50% of cases, whereas if the level of ligation was profunda only, about 25% of the limbs required amputation. Branch (1955) reported a 3% incidence of ulnar nerve lesions in 187 humeral shaft fractures. Sarmiento et al (1990) noted two partial median nerve lesions in 85 cases.

Summary

- The incidence of radial nerve palsy occurring immediately after humeral shaft fractures is 1.8–17.6% (average 9.8%).
- The incidence of radial nerve palsy occurring after internal fixation is 3–5%.
- The incidence of radial nerve palsy occurring after manipulation of fractured humeral shafts is 1.25–3.5% (average 2%).
- Radial nerve palsy occurs after proximal third fractures in approximately 6% of cases. These fractures are least likely to result in this palsy.
- Radial nerve palsy occurs in an average of 22% of middle third fractures.
- Distal third fractures result in radial nerve palsy in 11% of fractures.
- Full recovery of immediate radial nerve palsies occurs in 64.5–100% (average 83%) of cases.
- A delay of 3–4 months between the time of injury and exploration of the radial nerve is acceptable.
- Recovery of nerve function commences at an average of 7–12 weeks after the initial injury, but the first sign of nerve recovery can be delayed by up to 9 months.
- Full nerve recovery usually occurs between 4 and 22 months.
- Radial nerve palsy occurring after fracture manipulation recovers in 66–100% of cases at an average of 9 months. Early exploration would appear to be indicated in radial nerve palsy occurring after manipulation of the Holstein–Lewis fracture.
- Radial nerve palsy occurring after internal fixation tends to be transient, with a good prognosis. Recovery is complete at 3 months for a partial radial nerve palsy and at 8 months for a complete palsy.

Humeral fractures in children

Little has been written about the results of the treatment of humeral shaft fractures in children. These fractures can occur as a result of direct trauma in birth injury, the battered baby syndrome and as the result of a fall on the outstretched limb.

Transverse or spiral fractures of the middle third of the shaft tend to occur almost invariably in breech deliveries during attempts to deliver the extended arm. They may also occur when trying to deliver impacted shoulders by axillary traction in vertex presentations. Union occurs rapidly, usually within 3 weeks.

Radial nerve palsy is common, but less so than in adults (Dameron 1985). Nerve recovery usually occurs within 8–12 weeks (Dameron 1985). Mal-union is also reported to be common, but lateral angulation will correct in the first 2–3 years of subsequent growth, even if up to 40°. If a humeral shaft fracture with complete separation is immobilised with the forearm across the trunk, some internal rotation of the distal fragment can occur. If this rotational deformity measures less than 12° it should not be evident clinically (Dameron 1985).

Fractures in infancy and childhood can be treated with U-slabs, gutter slabs or spicas, and union occurs in 4–6 weeks.

Summary

- Birth injury resulting in fracture of the humeral shaft heals rapidly in 3 weeks.
- Fractures in infancy and childhood heal in 4–6 weeks.
- Radial nerve palsy usually recovers in 8–12 weeks.

Fracture of the supracondyloid process

The supracondylar spur is said to occur in 1 to 3% of people (Kolb & Moore 1967). It is an occasional cause of median nerve and/or brachial artery compression.

The first English-language description of a case of fracture of the supracondyloid process of the humerus was by Lund (1930). Genner (1959) described a case with complete recovery after periosteal excision of the spur. Kolb & Moore (1967) described two cases: one in a 4-year-old boy settled without treatment, and their second case was a 12-year-old boy in whom regeneration occurred after subperiosteal resection of the spur. They also drew attention to a case reported by Mardruzzato in 1938 of a 55-year-old woman with paresthesia in the median nerve distribution of the hand, with an established non-union near the apex of the supracondylar process. Excision of the process relieved her symptoms.

Summary

- Supracondylar spurs are reported to occur in 1–3% of the population and fracture may occasionally occur.
- Symptoms may resolve with conservative treatment.
- If excision is required for local pain, or median nerve or brachial artery compression, extra periosteal excision is required, and full recovery is the rule.

References

Barquet A, Fernandez A, Luvizio J, Masliah R 1989 A combined therapeutic protocol for aseptic non-union of the humeral shaft. Journal of Trauma 29: 95–98

Bell M J, Beauchamp C G, Kellam J K, McMurtry R Y 1985 The results of plating humeral shaft fractures in patients with multiple injuries: the Sunnybrook experience. Journal of Bone and Joint Surgery 67B: 293–296

Bleeker W A, Nijsten M W N, ter Duis H J 1991 Treatment of humeral shaft fractures related to associated injuries. Acta Orthopaedica Scandinavica 62: 148–153

Bohler L 1965 Conservative treatment of fresh closed fractures of the shaft of the humerus. Journal of Trauma 5: 464–468

Branch H E 1955 Fractures of the humerus: ambulatory traction technique. American Medical Association section on orthopaedic surgery. Journal of Bone and Joint Surgery 37A: 1118

Caldwell J A 1933 Treatment of fractures in the Cincinnati General Hospital. Annals of Surgery 97: 161–176

Caldwell J A 1940 Treatment of fractures of the shaft of the humerus by hanging cast. Surgery, Gynaecology and Obstetrics 70: 421–425

Charnley J 1961 The closed treatment of common fractures. Churchill Livingstone, Edinburgh

Chiu F Y, Chen C M, Lin C F, Lo W H, Huang Y L, Chen T H 1997 Closed humeral shaft fractures: a prospective evaluation of surgical treatment. Journal of Trauma-Injury and Critical Care 43: 947–951

Costa P, Giancecchi F, Cavazzuti A, Tartaglia I 1991 Internal and external fixation in complex diaphyseal and metaphyseal fractures of the humerus. Italian Journal of Orthopaedics and Traumatology 17: 87–94

Crates J, Whittle A P 1998 Antegrade interlocking nailing of acute humeral shaft fractures. Clinical Orthopaedics and Related Research 350. 40–50

Dameron T B 1985 Fractures and dislocations of the shoulder. In: Rockwood C A, Wilkins K E, King R E (eds) Fractures in children. J B Lippincott, Philadelphia, pp 577–607

Doran F S A 1944 The problems and principles of the restoration of limb function following injury as demonstrated by humeral shaft fractures. British Journal of Surgery 31: 351–368

Emmett J E, Breck L W 1958 A review and analysis of 11,000 fractures seen in private practice of orthopaedic surgery 1937–1956. Journal of Bone and Joint Surgery 40A: 1169–1175

Fischer D A, Haine J H 1975 Proceedings of the American Academy of Orthopedic Surgeons. Journal of Bone and Joint Surgery 55A: 1307

Gainor B J, Metzler M 1986 Humeral shaft fracture with brachial artery injury. Clinical Orthopaedics 204: 154–161

Garcia A, Maeck B H 1960 Radial nerve injuries in fractures of the shaft of the humerus. American Journal of Surgery 99: 625–627

Genner B A 1959 Fracture of the supracondyloid process. Journal of Bone and Joint Surgery 41A: 1333–1335

Griend R V, Tomasin J, Ward E F 1986 Open reduction and internal fixation of humeral shaft fractures: results using A O plating techniques. Journal of Bone and Joint Surgery 68A: 430–433

Hall R F, Pankovich A M 1987 Ender nailing of acute fractures of the humerus. Journal of Bone and Joint Surgery 69B: 558–567

Healy W L, White G M, Mick C A, Brooker A F, Weiland A J 1987 Non-union of the humeral shaft. Clinical Orthopaedics 219: 206–213

Holm C L 1970 Management of humeral shaft fractures: fundamental nonoperative techniques. Clinical Orthopaedics 71: 132–139

Holstein A, Lewis G P 1963 Fractures of the humerus with radial nerve paralysis. Journal of Bone and Joint Surgery 45A: 1382–1388

Hosner W 1974 Fractures of the shaft of the humerus. Reconstruction Surgery and Traumatology 14: 38–64

Jensen A T, Rasmussen S 1995 Being overweight and multiple fractures are indications for operative treatment of humeral shaft fractures. Injury 26: 263–264

Kettelkamp D B, Alexander H 1967 Clinical review of radial nerve injury. Journal of Trauma 7: 424–432

Klenerman L 1966 Fractures of the shaft of the humerus. Journal of Bone and Joint Surgery 48B: 105–111

Kolb L W, Moore R D 1967 Fractures of the supracondylar process of the humerus. Journal of Bone and Joint Surgery 49A: 532–534

Laferte M D, Rosenbaum M D 1937 The 'hanging cast' in the treatment of fractures of the humerus. Surgery, Gynaecology and Obstetrics 65: 231–237

Laing P G 1956 The arterial supply of the adult humerus. Journal of Bone and Joint Surgery 38A: 1105–1116

Leyes M, Pedro M, Munoz G, Gamelas J, D'Angelo F, Valenti J R, Navarro A, De Salis J A, Adaminas A 1997 Surgical treatment of humeral shaft non-union: A multicentric study. Journal of Bone and Joint Surgery 79B: Supp II: 195

Lin J 1998 Treatment of humeral shaft fractures with humeral locked nail and comparison with plate fixation. Journal of Trauma-Injury and Critical Care 44: 859–864

Lund H J 1930 Fracture of the supracondyloid process of the humerus—a case report. Journal of Bone and Joint Surgery 12: 925

Maffei G, Calvosa G, Palomba M 1997 Seidal intramedullary nailing of humeral diaphyseal fractures: A multiple centre report. Journal of Bone and Joint Surgery 79B: Supp II: 195

Mann R J, Neal E G 1965 Fractures of the shaft of the humerus in adults. Southern Medical Journal 58: 264–268

Mast J W, Spiegel P G, Harvey J P, Harrison C 1975 Fractures of the humeral shaft: a retrospective study of 240 adult fractures. Clinical Orthopaedics 112: 254–262

McPherson H D, McCormack R G, McKee M, Powell J N, Buckley R E 1999 Prospective trial comparing intramedullary nail fixation and open reduction internal fixation in the treatment of humeral shaft fractures with surgical indications. Journal of Bone and Joint Surgery 81B: Supp I: 103

Otsuka N Y, McKee M D, Liew A, Richards R R, Waddell J P, Powell J N, Schemitsch E H, 1998 The effect of comorbidity and duration of non union on outcome after surgical treatment for non union of the humerus. Journal of Shoulder and Elbow Surgery 7: 127–133

Packer J W, Foster R R, Garcia A, Grantham S A 1972 The humeral fracture with radial nerve palsy: Is exploration warranted? Clinical Orthopaedics 88: 34–38

Pollock F H, Drake D, Bovill E G, Day L, Trafton P G 1981 Treatment of radial neuropathy associated with fractures of the humerus. Journal of Bone and Joint Surgery 63A: 239–243

Postacchini F, Morace G B 1988 Fractures of the humerus associated with paralysis of the radial nerve. Italian Journal of Orthopaedics and Traumatology 14: 455–464

Rodriguez-Merchan E C 1995 Compression plating versus Hackethal nailing in closed humeral shaft fractures failing nonoperative reduction. Journal of Orthopaedic Trauma 9: 194–197

Rosen H 1990 The treatment of non-unions and pseudarthroses of the humeral shaft. Orthopedic Clinics of North America 21: 725–742

Samardzic M, Grujicic D, Milinkovic Z B 1990 Radial nerve lesions associated with fractures of the humeral shaft. Injury 21: 220–222

Sarmiento A, Horowitch A, Aboulafia A, Vangsness C T 1990 Functional bracing for comminuted extra-articular fractures of the distal third of the humerus. Journal of Bone and Joint Surgery 72B: 283–287

Sarmiento A, Kinman P B, Galvin E G, Schmitt R H, Phillips J G 1977 Functional bracing of fractures of the shaft of the humerus. Journal of Bone and Joint Surgery 59A: 596–601

Scientific Research Committee, Pennsylvania Orthopedic Society 1959 Fresh midshaft fractures of the humerus in adults. Pennsylvania Medical Journal 62: 848–850

Shaw J L, Sakellarides H 1967 Radial nerve paralysis associated with fractures of the humerus: a review of forty-five cases. Journal of Bone and Joint Surgery 49A: 899–902

Shazar N, Brumback R J, Vanco B 1998 Treatment of humeral fractures by closed reduction and retrograde intramedullary Ender nails. Orthopaedics 21: 641–646

Smith D K, Cooney W P 1990 External fixation of high-energy upper extremity injuries. Journal of Orthopaedic Trauma 4: 7–18

Sonneveld G J, Patka P, van Mourik J C, Bruere G 1987 Treatment of fractures of the shaft of the humerus accompanied by paralysis of the radial nerve. Injury 18: 404–406

Stewart M J, Hundley J M 1955 Fractures of the humerus: a comparative study in methods of treatment. Journal of Bone and Joint Surgery 37A: 681–692

Thompson R G, Compere E L, Schnute W J, Compere C L, Kernahan W T, Keagy R D 1965 The treatment of humeral shaft fractures by the hanging cast method. Journal of the International College of Surgeons 43: 52–60

Vichare N A 1974 Fractures of the humeral shaft associated with multiple injuries. Injury 5: 279–282

Wallny T, Westermann K, Sagebiel C, Reimer M, Wagner U A 1997a Functional treatment of humeral shaft fractures: indications and results. Journal of Orthopaedic Trauma 11: 283–287

Wallny T, Sagebiel C, Westermann K, Wagner U A, Reimer M 1997b Comparative results of bracing and interlocking nailing in the treatment of humeral shaft fractures. International Orthopaedics 21: 374–379

Whitson R O 1954 Relation of the radial nerve to the shaft of the humerus. Journal of Bone and Joint Surgery 36A: 85

Wisniewski T F, Radziejowski M J 1996 Gunshot fractures of the humeral shaft treated with external fixation. Journal of Orthopaedic Trauma 10: 273–278

Zagorski J B, Latta L L, Zych G A, Finnieston A R 1988 Diaphyseal fractures of the humerus: treatment with prefabricated braces. Journal of Bone and Joint Surgery 70A: 607–610

Zanasi R, Romano P, Rotolo F, Galmarini V, Zanasi L 1990 Intramedullary osteosynthesis 3: Küntscher nailing in the humerus. Italian Journal of Orthopaedics and Traumatology 16: 311–322

Zinghi G F, Sabetta E, Bungaro P, Sabalat S 1988 The role of osteosynthesis in the treatment of fractures of the humerus. Italian Journal of Orthopaedics and Traumatology 14: 67–75

Chapter 7

The elbow

Phillip S. Fagg

Tennis elbow

Tennis elbow is a painful condition that classically produces pain in the region of the lateral epicondyle of the elbow. Some authors use the term to include pain over the medial epicondyle or the posterior elbow. The relationship of the condition to a variety of sports and occupations has resulted in a number of synonyms. A lateral tennis elbow includes carpenter's elbow, dentist's elbow, tiller's elbow in yachtsmen, potato picker's plight and politician's paw. A medial tennis elbow is also referred to as a golfer's elbow, pitcher's elbow or little league elbow (in children). It affects 1 to 3% of the population, commonly between the ages of 40 and 60 (Chard & Hazelman 1989).

The term 'tennis elbow' is used as a designation for a number of different conditions that cause lateral elbow pain and is attributed to a number of aetiological factors, e.g. bursitis, periostitis, tears of the extensor tendons, radiohumeral synovitis and a synovial fringe, stenosis of the orbicular ligament, chondromalacia of the radial head and capitellum, calcific tendonitis, irritation of the articular branches of the radial nerve and posterior interosseus nerve entrapment. There seems to be general agreement that the extensor carpi radialis brevis muscle (ECRB) and its origin are involved in its pathogenesis. Ljung et al (1999) obtained muscle biopsies of the proximal and distal portion of the ECRB in 20 patients with longstanding lateral epicondylitis. Morphological abnormalities were significantly more frequent in patients than controls and included moth-eaten fibres, fibre necrosis and signs of muscle fibre regeneration. Changes were equally distributed proximally and distally. They concluded that these changes, directly or indirectly, might reflect the cumulative effect of mechanical and/or metabolic overload. Kraushaar and Nirschl (1999) pointed out that tennis elbow as not an inflammatory condition but a tendinosis, tendinosis being the disruption of normally orderly tendon fibres by a characteristic pattern of invasion by fibroblasts and atypical granulation tissue.

The importance of these conditions in medico-legal reporting is that they may be associated with repetitive tasks at work. Dimberg (1987) found that the prevalence of tennis elbow in the Volvo Aircraft Engine Division was 7.4%. Work was thought to be the probable cause in 35%, tennis in 8%, other leisure activities in 27%, and no cause was found in the remaining 30% of patients. There was no statistically significant difference between its prevalence among white collar and manual workers. It was found that those workers with work-related epicondylitis had higher elbow stress jobs as compared with other sufferers and the workforce as a whole.

Kamien (1990) felt that tennis elbow had two distinct modes of onset of equal incidence. The first type of onset was gradual, with a history of recent unaccustomed repetitive rotatory movements of the hand and wrist, such as laying bricks, using a screwdriver etc. The second type of onset was acute, occurring with a sudden torque injury such as an electric drill jamming or a mechanic using maximum force in removing an obstinate screw or belt.

Barton et al (1992) reviewed the available literature relating to tennis elbow and occupational factors. They concluded that while the cause and nature of tennis elbow were still subjects for speculation, there was good evidence that it was not more common among manual workers and that it was not clearly associated with any particular working activity. When it did occur, however, it was more likely to be troublesome for those with manual work.

The majority of patients respond to various conservative treatments. Numerous non-operative modalities have been described for the treatment of lateral tennis elbow. These include acupuncture, extracorporeal shock wave therapy, ultrasonography, low energy laser, steroid injection, glycosaminoglycen injections, friction/massage, bracing, muscle stretching to name just some of the reported treatments. Boyer and Hastings (1999) have reviewed the published literature on the non-operative treatment of patients with lateral tennis elbow and note the poor quality of most of these studies. They felt that there was little scientific evidence that non-operative treatment modalities influenced the long-term natural history of this condition. They also suggested that 70 to 80% of cases resolve spontaneously within 1 year if left untreated. Of the 871 patients reported by Boyd & McLeod (1973), 834 (96%) responded to conservative therapy within 6–12 months. However, conservative treatment has been reported to fail in between 3.3% (Posch et al 1978) and 11.5% (Coonrad & Hooper 1973) of patients.

In those cases that fail to settle, several treatment options are available, from simple manipulation to surgical decompression, the exact nature of which will depend on the presumed underlying diagnosis.

The most common procedures performed for tennis elbow are modifications of the extensor release. The results are recorded in Table 7.1. Overall, 81% of patients achieve a satisfactory result. Limbers (1980) claimed that 28% of patients with tennis elbow were not improved whatever operative procedure was chosen. The average time to return to work after surgery was 5 (Goldberg et al 1988) to 6.7 weeks (Tan et al 1989), although Coonrad & Hooper (1973) felt that recovery could occur up to 1 year after surgery. Of Goldberg et al's (1988) 34 patients 91% regained full strength and a full range of movement. Four patients lacked the final 5° of elbow extension. However, Verhaar & Walenkamp (1986) reported that 57% of their 165 patients had some loss of muscular strength after surgery.

The results of the operative treatment of medial epicondylitis appear to be influenced by the presence of co-existing ulnar neuritis; Kurvers and Verhaar (1995) reviewed the results in 40 consecutive elbows at a mean of 44 months postoperatively. Eleven of the 16 patients (69%) who had isolated medial epicondylitis treated with a flexor release were free of symptoms at the time of follow-up, compared with only three of the 24 elbows (12.5%) that had co-existent ulnar neuritis. Similarly Gabel and Morrey (1995) reported that 24 of 25 elbows (96%) that had medial epicondylitis alone or in association with a mild ulnar neuropathy had a good or excellent result after surgery, as compared with two of the five elbows that had moderate or severe associated ulnar neuropathy. They also noted that nine elbows (out of 30) needed more than 6 months' recovery before maximum improvement was obtained.

Summary

- The relationship of tennis elbow to occupational factors is not certain.
- 70–80% of cases of untreated tennis elbow settle within one year.
- Conservative treatment fails in 3–11% of cases.
- Overall, 81% of patients with tennis elbow achieve a satisfactory result after surgery.
- Most patients return to work 5–7 weeks after surgery.
- Some loss of strength has been reported in 9–57% of patients.
- 69–96% of patients have a good result after surgery for medial epicondylitis, but if there is a concomitant ulnar neuropathy this drops to only 12.5–40%.

Distal humeral fractures in adults

Acute fractures of the distal humerus are not common, accounting for only 2% of all fractures, and 10 to 15% of all humeral fractures in adults, occurring mostly in elderly people. These are often severe injuries with comminution and displacement.

There is no generally accepted method of classification of these distal humeral fractures in adults, but from a prognostic point of view they can be classified into:

- supracondylar—extra-articular
- transcondylar—intra-articular
- monocondylar—intra-articular, including capitellum fractures
- bicondylar—intra-articular

Early reports favoured a non-operative management because of poor operative results (Riseborough & Radin 1969). The major complication is a loss of flexion and extension at the elbow. Other uncommon complications include pain, instability, avascular necrosis, non-union, deformity, weakness and decreased pronation and supination.

In patients with limited functional demands an adequately mobile painfree elbow may be achieved with the 'bag-of-bones' technique. The range of motion that can be

Table 7.1 The results of modifications of the extensor release for tennis elbow

Reference	Number of patients	Number excellent/satisfactory	Percentage
Verharr & Walenkamp (1986)	165	119	72
Posch et al (1978)	43	37	86
Nirschl & Pettrone (1979)	88	75	85
Goldberg et al (1988)	34	33	97
Tan et al (1989)	24	22	92
Overall	354	286	81

achieved by this technique ranges from 70–130° (average 98°). This is obviously not an appropriate treatment regime for younger patients or active, independent elderly patients (Ring & Jupiter 1999).

The range of motion in flexion and extension necessary to perform normal daily activities was measured by Morrey et al (1981a). They concluded that most activities could be accomplished with 100° of elbow flexion in an arc from 30° to 130°.

Supracondylar extra-articular fractures
These fractures are uncommon in adults and all series are small. Of the 16 supracondylar fractures without articular involvement reported by Horne (1980), all four patients treated by open methods did well, while three of 12 patients treated by closed methods did poorly. Two of the three poor results were in completely unreduced fractures.

Aitken & Rorabeck (1986) reported acceptable results in their six patients, four being treated closed and two by rigid internal fixation. An acceptable result had at least a 75° arc of flexion and slight pain, and yet an ability to perform the activities of daily living.

Soltanpur (1978) reported good results in the four adult patients with a flexion type of supracondylar fracture treated conservatively. Equally, operative treatment gave satisfactory results in all five patients reported by Browne et al (1986) and three of the four reported by Holdsworth & Mossad (1990).

Transcondylar intra-articular fractures
Transcondylar fractures of the distal humerus are characterised by a transverse fracture at the level of the olecranon and coronoid fossa. They tend to occur in older osteoporotic patients, and are difficult to stabilise by internal fixation because the distal fragments are small and their surface is covered by articular cartilage. Perry et al (1989) classified them into:

- undisplaced
- simple displaced
- T-type
- fracture–dislocation of the humeral condyles from the trochlear notch

Of the 11 patients that they followed up for a mean 28 months, functional elbow flexion was preserved, and yet loss of extension occurred in all patients (range 5–40°, mean 27°). Undisplaced fractures had the best prognosis with least loss of elbow motion. The two patients with fracture–dislocations developed radiographic signs of arthritis within 14–42 months.

Unicondylar intra-articular fractures
The unicondylar fracture can be subdivided into three types (Müller et al 1991):

- type B(1)—involving the medial condyle, including the trochlea
- type B(2)—involving fractures of the lateral condyle, including the capitellum
- type B(3)—referring to coronal fractures of either the trochlea or the capitellum

Jupiter et al (1988) reported that four of five patients undergoing internal fixation for medial condyle fractures had acceptable results. Holdsworth & Mossad (1990) with three fractures and Aitken & Rorabeck (1986) with two reported acceptable results in all cases, employing internal fixation.

Of the B(2) fractures of the lateral condyle including the capitellum, Jupiter et al (1988) reported acceptable results in 10 of their 12 patients (83%) treated by internal fixation, and Holdsworth & Mossad (1990) had eight acceptable results from their 11 patients (73%).

Kuhn et al (1995) described six cases of a divergent single column fracture of the distal part of the humerus. In all patients the fracture was initiated in the trochlear groove as a result of a direct impact on the olecranon which divided the trochlea and then split the two columns of the humerus divergently. This pattern of fracture appeared to occur exclusively in adolescents and young adults. There were three fractures of the medial column and three of the lateral column. They were all treated by closed reduction and percutaneous internal fixation, and all five elbows followed up regained full motion by 8 months.

Type B(3) coronal fractures of the capitellum are further divided into: Type I fracture involving the whole of the capitellum; Type II fracture involving a shell of articular cartilage with a thin layer of bone; and Type III fracture with comminution (Bryan and Morrey 1985).

The reported results of the treatment of these fractures has suggested that open reduction with or without internal fixation is superior to simple excision. Collert (1977) reported poor results in three of eight patients (37.5%) treated by removal of the displaced capitellar fragment, as compared with two poor results in the 12 patients (17%) treated by open reduction with or without internal fixation. No case of secondary osteoarthritis was seen up to 6 years' follow-up. Similarly, Grantham et al (1981) reported unacceptable results in one of six patients (17%) treated by closed reduction or open reduction and internal fixation. Of the 11 cases treated by excision of the capitellar fragment, seven (64%) had an unacceptable result.

Ma et al (1984) had eight good results in nine patients (89%) treated by percutaneous probe reduction. However,

Ochner et al (1996) reported the successful closed reduction of nine displaced coronal capitellar fractures. No fracture subsequently displaced, if successfully reduced. Following closed reduction the elbow was immobilised at 90° for 3 weeks before gentle active mobilisation was commenced.

Poynton et al (1998) compared open reduction with Kirschner wire fixation in six patients with open reduction and Herbert screw fixation in another six patients with Type I capitellar fractures. Eleven of the 12 patients (92%) had a good postoperative result with an excellent range of motion. The other patients developed a Kirschner wire pin tract infection. However, the Herbert screw group returned to previous activities more quickly at 5.5 weeks as compared to 9 weeks in the Kirschner wiring group.

The recommended treatment for the Type II capitellar fracture is excision which may be by open or arthroscopic techniques (Feldman 1997).

Isolated fractures of the humeral trochlea are very rare. Foulk et al (1995) reported a good functional result in a patient treated with open reduction and internal fixation.

Bicondylar intra-articular fractures

These injuries are often severe, with comminution and displacement. A number of classifications of the fractures are available (Riseborough & Radin 1969, Müller et al 1991), but from a prognostic point of view they will be considered as simple T or Y fractures, with or without displacement (Müller C1, Riseborough & Radin TI, II and III), or complex fractures with comminution of the metaphysis or articular surface (Müller C2, C3, Riseborough & Radin TIV).

Early reports of internal fixation of these intra-articular fractures suggested that internal fixation gave poor results (Riseborough & Radin 1969), but modern reports emphasise the superior results of operative treatment. The results in papers comparing conservative treatment with surgery are shown in Table 7.2. These papers do show a marked difference in the results reported. However, the more modern papers do suggest better results obtained by surgery as compared with the earlier papers.

Miller (1964) reported that the final range of motion after closed reduction was 58–105°, as compared with the average motion after open reduction of 25–136°.

A number of papers report the long-term follow-up of intra-articular fractures after internal fixation (Table 7.3). Overall, 69% of patients achieved a satisfactory result after internal fixation, although different assessment criteria were used in these series. The advantage of early stable fixation is the opportunity to start an early active exercise programme. Aitken & Rorabeck (1986) reported that 15 of their 16 patients (94%) who commenced physiotherapy within 4 weeks of injury had an acceptable result, as compared with seven patients out of 13 (54%) who did not commence mobilisation until after 4 weeks from injury. Waddell et al (1988) reported that the patients' range of motion and pain were the same at 6 months as at long-term follow-up.

Unfortunately, the patients' subjective assessment of their final result may not match the assessment of the clinicians. Wildburger et al (1991) reported that of their 72 patients classified clinically, 79% had an excellent result, 10% a good result and 11% a fair result. These same patients graded their subjective assessment as 54% excellent, 35% good and 11% fair to poor.

Management of the acute injury with total elbow arthroplasty has been considered for elderly patients with extremely comminuted fractures. Cobb and Morrey (1997)

Table 7.2 A comparison of conservative and operative treatment for intra-articular fractures of the distal humerus

	Riseborough & Radin (1969)	Horne (1980)	Aitken & Rorabeck (1986)	Zagorski et al (1986)
Total number of patients	29	24	17	42
Conservative				
Number of patients	22	6	7	13
Acceptable	18 (82%)	3 (50%)	4 (57%)	1 (8%)
Unacceptable	4	3	3	12
Operative				
Number of patients	7	18	10	29
Acceptable	3 (43%)	5 (28%)	6 (60%)	22 (76%)
Unacceptable	4	13	4	7

Table 7.3 The results of the internal fixation of intercondylar fractures of the distal humerus

Reference	Number of patients	Excellent/ good	Percentage	Fair/poor	Percentage
Wildburger et al (1991)*	72	57	79	15	21
Kundel et al (1996)	77	40	52	37	48
Waddell et al (1988)†	46	30	65	16	35
Papaioannou et al (1995)	54	42	78	12	22
Holdsworth & Mossad (1990)*	*38	29	76	9	24
Overall	287	198	69	89	31

* Excellent/good result: 30° extension to 120° flexion.
† Excellent/good result: at least 60° of extension–flexion.

reported their results of primary total elbow arthroplasty in 20 patients (21 elbows) with an acute fracture of the distal aspect of the humerus. Fifteen elbows had an excellent result and five had a good result. One patient had a revision total elbow arthroplasty.

Post-traumatic osteoarthritis

An important complication of these injuries is post-traumatic osteoarthritic changes which, in the course of time, can result in further painful limitation of movement. Jupiter et al (1988), after an average of 5.8 years' follow-up, reported a normal articular width on follow-up radiographs in 11 patients (32%), slight to moderate narrowing in 19 patients (56%), and extensive post-traumatic arthritis in four patients (12%). They felt that the clinical evaluation did not correlate with the follow-up radiograph. The rate at which these elbows deteriorate has not been adequately documented. Most individuals are often unable to hold down their usual job, and a frequent problem is limitation of some activities of daily living and sports activities.

Total elbow replacement can be used in the treatment of patients with disabling pain from post-traumatic osteo-arthritis. Schneeberger et al (1997) reported their results in 41 consecutive patients (38 post-traumatic osteoarthritis, three post-traumatic dysfunction from a flail elbow). At an average of 5 years 8 months' follow-up, 16 patients (39%) had an excellent result, 18 (44%) a good result, five (12%) a fair result and two (5%) had a poor result. The post-operative average arc of flexion was 27–131°. Eleven patients (27%), however, had a major complication and nine (22%) needed an additional operation.

Non-union

Mitsunaga et al (1982) reported on 32 patients who had a non-union about the elbow. Twenty-five elbows were treated by open reduction and internal fixation; 22 (88%) healed, although six needed a second procedure. Post-operatively the average range of motion was 71°, and the average score for pain was 2 points (maximum 4 points—no pain = 1 point). When utilising AO plates with or without bone graft, Ackerman & Jupiter (1988) achieved union in 17 of 18 patients (94%). However, function after an average of a 3.6 year follow-up was poor, with only 35% of patients achieving a satisfactory result, with extension–flexion from 30–120°.

Morrey and Adams (1995) reported the use of a semi-constrained elbow prosthesis for non-union of a distal humeral fracture. Of their 36 patients, 31 (86%) achieved an excellent or good result, three (8%) had a fair result and two (6%) had a poor result. The mean arc of motion after surgery was 16–127°.

Masada et al (1990) reviewed their results of surgery on 30 elbows with an established non-union of a fracture of the lateral humeral condyle of more than 5 years' duration. Fifteen of the patients had apprehension when using the elbow due to lateral instability or pain in the elbow, and 13 of the 15 were thus treated by osteosynthesis resulting in the pain and apprehension disappearing. However, most of these patients lost 19° of elbow motion (the pre-operative average range of motion was 119°). In no patient did the authors find marked arthritic changes on radiographs at follow-up (2–13 years postoperation).

Summary

- 69% of patients had a satisfactory result after internal fixation for intra-articular fractures of the distal humerus.
- Extensive post-traumatic arthritis occurred in 12% of patients with intra-articular distal humeral fractures at

6 years' follow-up, while mild to moderate radiographic changes were seen in 56%.

■ 35% of patients achieved a satisfactory functional result after surgery for non-union of the distal humerus, 86% after total elbow replacement.

Epiphyseal injuries of the distal humerus and supracondylar fractures in children

There are six secondary centres of ossification at the elbow in the developing child, and they can be useful in determining the skeletal age of the child. They appear in the following order: capitellum radial head, medial epicondyle, trochlea, olecranon and lateral epicondyle (Fig. 7.1).

Medial epicondyle

Fractures of the medial epicondyle represent up to 11% (Hines et al 1987) of all elbow fractures in children. They may be displaced to variable degrees, entrapped within the joint or associated with dislocation. These latter two groups are associated with elbow instability.

The results of the treatment of medial epicondyle fractures are equally good with conservative or operative treatment. Dias et al (1987) reviewed 20 displaced fractures, all associated with elbow dislocation managed non-operatively. All the fractures were significantly displaced (mean 10 mm), and none had radiological union at a mean time of 3.5 years' follow-up. However, only one had slight local tenderness and one slight functional impairment. Nine patients had a slight loss of extension but only one of these lost more than 20° of extension. Although all patients demonstrated laxity of the ulnar collateral liga-ment, this was not a source of functional instability. No patient had developed late-onset ulnar neuritis.

Hines et al (1987) reviewed 31 patients with displaced medial epicondyle fractures treated, at an average of 4 years after injury, by operative means. Twenty-seven patients had good results and all except one fracture united. Three of the seven patients with a fracture fragment trapped in the joint had a poor result. The one patient with a non-union had ulnar nerve symptoms. Wilson et al (1988) reviewed 43 children with a fracture of the medial epicondyle; 20 had non-operative treatment and 23 had operations. They confirmed that the final disability was slight, irrespective of the treatment used. Although surgery achieved bony union in 87% of the cases, as compared with 55% of those treated non-operatively, 95% of the non-operatively managed group were completely asymptomatic, as compared with 61% of those treated surgically. However, these residual symptoms were only minor, and all patients denied any symptoms of instability. No late neurological problems were noted at review (mean 4.6 years post injury).

However, a tardy ulnar nerve palsy may result from a compromised cubital tunnel. Josefsson & Danielsson (1986) reviewed 56 unreduced conservatively treated medial epicondyle fractures at an average of 35 years after injury. They reported a 55% incidence of non-union and 10% incidence of ulnar nerve symptoms in those patients with non-union.

Medial humeral condyle

This injury is rare, accounting for between 1.5% (Papavasilion et al 1987) and 2% (Bensahel et al 1986) of elbow fractures in children. The results of treatment are shown in

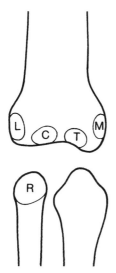 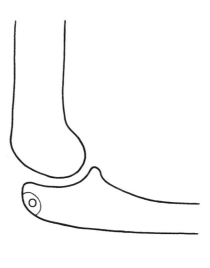

Fig 7.1 Secondary centres of ossification. M, medial epicondyle; T, trochlea; C, capitellum; R, radial head; L, lateral epicondyle; O olecranon.

Table 7.4. The results are invariably good if treatment is not delayed. Avascular necrosis of the medial condyle occurred in the two cases of displaced and rotated fractures treated by open reduction reported by Papavasilion et al, although this did not affect function.

Lateral humeral condyle

Fractures of the lateral humeral condyle constitute 10 to 20% of elbow fractures in children (Badelon et al 1988). These fractures are usually divided into three types: non- or minimally displaced (<2 mm), moderately displaced (>2 mm), and severely displaced with rotation. When these fractures are undisplaced or minimally displaced, they can be treated conservatively. Bast et al (1998) reported that in 98% of the 95 children with undisplaced or minimally displaced fractures of the lateral humeral condyle union occurred in 3–7 weeks. Two of the fractures displaced and required open reduction. Although these injuries are normally stable, further displacement and subsequent non-union can occur; therefore, review with repeat X-rays is required to check the position. Thonell et al (1988) reviewed 159 children with non-displaced or minimally displaced fractures. Subsequent displacement occurred in 18 fractures (11%).

Fractures displaced >2 mm should be openly reduced and pinned to prevent further displacement and non-union. The result of the treatment of these fractures are shown in Table 7.5, with 95% having an excellent or good result. The results are not so good if surgery is delayed, however.

Hirner et al (1998) reported the results of the surgical treatment of 10 patients with fracture of the lateral humeral condyle presenting 1–6 months after injury. Postoperatively all patients had pain relief. The preoperative range of flexion/extension was between 0° and 120°. Only four patients improved their range of movement. Premature fusion can occur between the capitellar epiphysis and the metaphysis, resulting in the 'fishtail' deformity of the distal humerus. This deformity occurred in eight of the 45 patients reported on by Badelon et al (1988), but it is of no consequence since it causes no symptoms, nor does it interfere with function (Flynn 1989).

Non-union is a problem of these fractures, resulting in a consequent valgus deformity, loss of movement and a tardy ulnar nerve palsy. Flynn (1989) reported the results of 14 cases of non-union of the lateral condyle, the final functional outcome of which was known. Eleven of these patients had a bone graft with internal fixation. Eight patients had an excellent result, one good, two fair and three poor. None of the three poor results had had surgical treatment. A further series of non-unions of the lateral humeral condyle in children treated by osteosynthesis was reported by Shimada et al (1997). They reviewed the results of osteosynthesis for the treatment of established non-union in 16 children with an average age of 9 years. The average interval between the injury and the operation was 5 years. Osseous union was achieved after the initial operation in 13 patients (81%) and after a second operation in a further two patients.

Table 7.4 The results of the treatment of medial condyle fractures in children

Reference	Fractures treated early				Fractures treated late			
	Number	Good	Fair	Poor	Number	Good	Fair	Poor
Bensahel et al (1986)	21	19	1	1	6	0	2	4
Papavasilion et al (1987)	13	13	0	0	2	0	0	2

Table 7.5 The results of the surgical treatment of lateral humeral condyle fractures

Reference	Number	Excellent	Good	Fair	Poor
Badelon et al (1988)	45	29	11	3	2
van Vugt et al (1988)	32	25	6	1	0
Jeffery (1989)	24	22	0	2	0
So et al (1985)	24	12	11	1	0
Sharma et al (1995)	37	36	1	0	0
Total	162	124 (77%)	29 (18%)	7 (4%)	2 (1%)

The result was rated excellent in eight patients (50%), good in seven (44%) and poor in one (6%). Tardy ulnar nerve palsy is a late complication of the cubitus valgus associated with a non-union. Miller (1924) reported that 47% of tardy ulnar nerve palsies in adults were associated with fractures of the lateral condyle, and the symptoms developed 30–40 years after the injury. Gaye & Love (1947) reported that the average time from injury to the development of symptoms was 22 years in 100 patients.

Cubitus varus can also occur after these fractures. So et al (1985) reported a loss of carrying angle in 10 out of 24 patients at a mean follow-up of 4.8 years. The deformity was mild, averaging 9–10° in most fractures.

T-shaped intra-articular fractures

These fractures are very uncommon, representing 0.7% of all elbow fractures in children. Papavasilion & Beslikas (1986) reported the results of six cases. All patients lost some extension (range 5–20°), and two had increased cubitus valgus. One patient demonstrated radiological evidence of avascular necrosis of the trochlea, but at a 2 year follow-up this did not appear to affect the patient's clinical function.

Fracture–separation of the distal humeral epiphysis

Fracture–separation of the distal humeral epiphysis is rare and may be misdiagnosed as a fracture of the lateral condyle or elbow dislocation. De Jager & Hoffman (1991) reported the results in 12 patients and reviewed the literature. Five of their 12 patients lost elbow flexion–extension by less than 25° and one untreated case had a flexion deformity of 55°. Cubitus varus was the most common complication, 5–15° occurring in 12 of 48 patients reported in the literature.

A higher incidence of cubitus varus deformity following fracture–separation of the distal end of the humeral epiphysis was reported by Abe et al (1995a). Fifteen of the 21 children in their study developed cubitus varus deformity, although eight of these were secondary referrals with an established deformity. However, seven of the 13 children (54%) treated from the time of injury, at their hospital, developed the deformity.

Supracondylar fractures

Supracondylar fractures account for 55% of all elbow fractures in children (Landin & Danielsson 1986). The majority are of the extension variety, with the lower humeral fragment displaced posteriorly. They may be graded into undisplaced, displaced but with an intact posterior cortex, or completely displaced.

Henrickson (1966) presented the results in 545 patients treated by immobilisation (224 patients), manipulation and immobilisation (232), open reduction and internal fixation (73) and traction (six patients). The criteria used in the evaluation of these cases are shown in Table 7.6. The end-results were excellent in 73%, good in 21% and poor in 6% of patients. There was a 3% incidence of poor results in the undisplaced fractures.

The major problem in treatment is with the severely displaced fracture, where all contact is lost between the lower humeral fragment and the metaphysis of the humerus. Several different treatments are available and the literature on the subject is voluminous.

Kurer & Regan (1990) reviewed the literature and found 1708 comparable displaced supracondylar fractures. They used the classification system of Mitchell & Adams (1961) (Table 7.7). Their comparative results of the different treatments are shown in Table 7.8. The worst results occurred with manipulation and splint immobilisation alone.

Table 7.6 The criteria used in the evaluation of the end-results of supracondylar fractures (from Henrickson 1966)

Criterion	Excellent	Good	Poor
Difference in carrying angle	±10°	±15–20°	±25° or more
Limited flexion, extension, pronation and/or supination	0–10°	15–20°	25° or more
Pain	None	On exertion or with change of weather	On exertion or with change of weather
Symptoms during work	None	Mild	Severe
Muscle contracture	None	None	Yes
Persistent nerve injury	No	No	Yes

Table 7.7 Mitchell & Adams' classification of elbow function following supracondylar fracture

Grade	Carrying angle	Range of movement
Excellent	<5° change	<10° change
Good	5–15° change	10–20° change
Unacceptable	>15° change	>20° change

Table 7.8 Comparative results of different treatment methods of supracondylar fractures (after Kurer & Regan 1990)

Treatment	Number of patients	Excellent (%)	Good (%)	Unsatisfactory (%)
MUA and splint	281	48.8	28.1	23.1
Skin traction	206	66.5	20.9	12.6
Olecranon traction	507	72	17.8	10.2
Percutaneous K-wires	455	62.4	24.4	13.2
Open reduction, K-wires	259	62.9	21.2	15.9

Olecranon screw traction for displaced supracondylar fractures of the humerus is a safe and reliable method of treatment which can be applied by an inexperienced surgeon. Chandratreya and Hunter (1999) reviewed the notes and radiographs of 166 children with completely displaced supracondylar fractures of the humerus treated by this means. The average duration of traction was 14 days and the screw was removed on the ward in 132 patients. Only three patients (2%) developed clinical cubitus varus deformity.

Neurovascular problems are not uncommon in association with supracondylar fractures, and these structures can become entrapped, preventing manipulative reduction of the fracture. Absent radial pulse on presentation is found in between 3.2% (Sabharwal et al 1997) and 11.9% (Shaw et al 1990) of patients and tends to occur in the more displaced fractures. If the vascular injury is untreated or unrecognised, Volkman's ischaemic contracture can occur. Muscle infarction principally involves the deep finger flexors and the long flexor to the thumb. The digits become clawed and sensation is impaired, particularly in the median nerve distribution. There is intrinsic muscle weakness in the hand and the end-result is a virtually non-functioning hand. The incidence of permanent ischaemic contracture is 0.4% (Henrickson 1966).

Nerve injuries occur in between 3% (Henrickson 1966) and 14% (Pirone et al 1988) of patients. In their review of 1708 cases, Kurer & Regan (1990) found that 45% of nerve injuries were to the radial nerve, 32% to the median nerve and 23% to the ulnar nerve. The anterior interosseous nerve can also be injured (Bamford & Stanley 1989). The majority of nerve injuries recover completely, although in the report of Culp et al (1990) only nine of 18 nerve lesions had recovered at a mean of 2.5 months. The other nine nerves were explored, but only one was found to be ruptured. Nerve injury can also occur iatrogenically. The ulnar nerve is especially vulnerable to injury during the insertion of the medial wire of the percutaneous cross Kirschner wire technique. Lyons et al (1998) reported 19 postoperative ulnar nerve palsies in 375 supracondylar fractures (5%) that had percutaneous pinning after closed or open reduction. All of the patients followed up had complete return of function, although five had return of function after 4 months (maximum 40 weeks). Unfortunately, full recovery cannot always be guaranteed. Of the six patients with postoperative ulnar nerve injury reported on by Rasool (1998), three achieved full recovery, while in two patients partial recovery occurred and one patient had no recovery.

Another complication of supracondylar fracture is varus and valgus deformity. The reported incidence of cubitus varus is variable. Ippolito et al (1986) reported an incidence of 7.5%, with the highest incidence in undisplaced or slightly displaced fractures, whereas Henrickson (1966) found a 20% incidence of varus over 10°. Wilkins (1990) emphasises that the effects of a cubitus varus are primarily cosmetic, resulting in a gunstock deformity. The functional effects are usually minimal. However, tardy ulnar nerve palsy can occur after a cubitus varus deformity. Abe et al (1995b) reported on 15 patients with tardy ulnar nerve palsy caused by cubitus varus deformity. The mean interval between fracture and onset of symptoms was 15 years. At exploration the main cause of the palsy was compression by a fibrous band running between the two heads of flexor carpi ulnaris. Abe et al (1995c) described recurrent posterior dislocation of the head of the radius occurring after further injury in four patients with a pre-existing cubitus varus deformity. The recurrent dislocation was eliminated by performing a supracondylar osteotomy of the humerus in association with tightening of the lateral ligament complex.

Cubitus valgus can also occur following supracondylar fractures, and the reported incidence is 0.9 to 8.6% (Ippolito et al 1986). Wilkins (1990) reports that cubitus valgus has more functional loss, with loss of extension and possibly the late development of tardy ulnar nerve palsy. De Boeck and De Smet (1997), on the other hand, felt that the main effect of cubitus valgus was cosmetic, but this cosmetic deformity was less obvious than that seen in cubitus varus. None of their 10 patients developed tardy ulnar nerve palsy but the average follow-up was only 5 years post injury. In none of their patients did they report any important functional incapacity. The average flexion lag for all 10 patients was 5°, none exceeding 12°, and the average extension lag was 7°, none exceeding 15°. The cosmetic effect is less significant. Ippolito et al (1986) reported that deformities could improve or worsen with time due to growth plate injury or stimulation by fracture callus.

Myositis ossificans is rarely reported and there is almost no increased risk of myositis after open reduction or percutaneous wiring (Kurer & Regan 1990). Initial ossification in the brachialis muscle at fracture healing can disappear at long-term follow-up (Ippolito et al 1986). Henrickson (1966) reported osteoarthritis as occurring in 11 patients (2% of cases).

Only 2.5 to 6% of supracondylar fractures in children are of the flexion type with anterior displacement of the lower humeral fragment (Williamson & Cole 1991). Of the 14 patients reported by Williamson & Cole, 10 had excellent or good results, while two had cubitus varus, and elbow stiffness was noted in the other two patients. Henrickson (1966) reported the incidence of cubitus varus and valgus as 5.5% and 3%, respectively, after these flexion-type fractures.

Capitellar fractures

Fractures of the capitellum are rare in children. Letts et al (1997) reported on seven children with this fracture. Five patients had open reduction and internal fixation and two were treated non-operatively. All had a good outcome although the authors recommended open reduction and internal fixation for the displaced capitellar fracture in children.

Occult fracture of the elbow

An elevated posterior fat pad present on a lateral radiograph of a child's elbow after injury is considered suggestive of an intracapsular fracture about the elbow. Skaggs and Mirzayan (1999) reported the results of a prospective study of 45 children who had an average age of $4\frac{1}{2}$ years, a history of trauma to the elbow and an elevated posterior fat pad sign. Thirty-four (76%) of the 45 patients had evidence of a fracture on a follow-up radiograph. Eighteen (53%) of the 34 had a supracondylar fracture of the humerus, nine (26%) a fracture of the proximal part of the ulna, four (12%) a fracture of the lateral condyle, and three (9%) a fracture of the radial neck.

Summary

- Fractures of the medial epicondyle, unassociated with elbow instability, do well irrespective of treatment. Non-union can occur in up to 55% of cases, but is usually asymptomatic. Ulnar nerve symptoms have been reported in 10% of patients at 35 years' follow-up.
- Medial humeral condyle fractures invariably do well if treatment is not delayed.
- 11% of minimally displaced lateral humeral condyle fractures displace. Surgical treatment of these fractures results in 95% satisfactory results. Premature fusion is asymptomatic. Non-union of lateral humeral condyle fractures results in cubitus valgus, loss of movement and tardy ulnar nerve palsy.
- Cubitus varus occurs as a complication of fracture–separation of the distal humeral epiphysis in 25–54% of patients.
- The end-results of supracondylar fractures are excellent or good in over 90% of patients. Nerve injury occurs in 3–14% of these fractures. Iatrogenic ulnar nerve palsy occurs in up to 5% of patients treated with percutaneous crossed wires.
- 76% of children with a positive fat pad sign are subsequently found to have a fracture.

Olecranon fractures

Olecranon fractures have been classified by Morrey (1995) as Type I, undisplaced, Type II, displaced but stable and Type III, displaced unstable fractures. Each type is further classified as either A, non-comminuted or B, comminuted.

The conservative treatment of Type I olecranon fractures yields good results if the fracture is displaced less than 2–3 mm. Operative surgery with internal fixation or primary excision produces better results with Type II and III fractures, as these are in effect disruptions of the extensor mechanism of the elbow. A number of different surgical techniques are available for the treatment of these fractures. Opinions vary as to whether better results are obtained with a screw plus wire combination, an intramedullary screw alone or an AO tension band wire or plate. However, Helm et al (1987) reported no difference in the final functional result regardless of whether a tension band or screw fixation was used.

Veras et al (1999) have suggested that conservative treatment of displaced fractures of the olecranon in the elderly is appropriate. They analysed the functional results of the conservative treatment in 12 patients with a mean age of 81.8 years. At a 15 months follow-up none of the patients was limited in daily activities; 67% were asymptomatic with an acceptable range of motion of their elbows. The clinical results were good in eight patients, fair in three and poor in one despite nine cases of non-union.

The results of the surgical treatment of olecranon fractures are shown in Table 7.9. The criteria for functional evaluations do vary between authors. Eighty-one percent of patients have an excellent/good result, meaning no pain, minimal loss or forearm rotation and less than 20° loss of flexion. A fair result has more than 45° of useful motion and 50% of forearm rotation and minimal pain.

Few patients complained of pain after their olecranon fracture was treated. Holdsworth & Mossad (1984) found that 73% of their 52 patients were asymptomatic, while 17% complained of pain only when the elbow was knocked. The remainder had occasional spontaneous pain. A slightly lower number of patients—61% of 33 patients—reported by Kiviluoto & Santavirta (1978) were symptom free, with the rest experiencing occasional pain.

It is typical for a patient to lose 10–15° of extension after these injuries. The loss of more than 10° of flexion is uncommon (Morrey 1995).

Extension was reported to be lost to some degree in between 50% (Eriksson et al 1957) and 75% (Holdsworth & Mossad 1984) of patients. Between 81% (Kiviluoto & Santavirta 1978) and 94% (Holdsworth & Mossad 1984) lost less than 30° of extension. Eriksson et al (1957) noted that only 3% of patients are consciously aware of any limitation of movement. Most patients recover final movement by 3 months (Gartsman et al 1981). The average time to return to work was 6.7 months in Wolfgang et al's 1987 series.

Holdsworth & Mossad (1984) measured extensor peak strength and reported that 38% of their patients had 75% or more strength than that of the contralateral side, while 78% of patients recovered more than 50% of the extensor peak strength of the contralateral limb. Worse functional results were seen in older patients in this series. Murphy et al (1987) also found that patients under 30 years of age had better results. Complications due to the backing out of tension band wires were common, occurring in 55% (Jensen & Olsen 1986) to 80% (Murphy et al 1987) of patients.

Of the 41 patients in Wolfgang et al's series (1987), 68% were healed by 3 months after tension band techniques, 85% by 4 months, and 98% were considered solid by 6 months. Very few papers consider the treatment of compound fractures of the olecranon. Tapasvi et al (1999) reported the use of an external fixator in the management of 21 open fractures of the proximal ulna. At 3 year follow-up all patients were rated clinically as good or excellent. All the fracture united well, the average time to union being 9 weeks.

There is the potential risk of progressive osteoarthritic change in future years, particularly if accurate reduction has not been accomplished. Although Helm et al (1987) report-

Table 7.9 The results of the surgical treatment of olecranon fractures

Reference	Number of patients	Excellent	Good	Fair	Poor
Wesley et al (1976)*	25	17	2	5	1
Kiviluoto & Santavirta (1978)†	35	13	7	13	2
Holdsworth & Mossad (1984)‡	52	34	15	0	3
Wolfgang et al (1987)‡	41	30	6	0	5
Total	153	94 (61%)	30 (20%)	18 (12%)	11 (7%)

* Zuelzer hook plate.
† Various techniques.
‡ AO tension band.

ed only one patient out of 48 (2%) showing evidence of degenerative changes after internal fixation of these fractures, both Kiviluoto & Santavirta (1978) and Gartsman et al (1981) reported a 20% incidence. The more severe the injury, the more likely it is to result in long-term degenerative changes. Such osteoarthritis will cause painful limitation of elbow movement, which can compromise activities of daily living, work and leisure pursuits.

Non-union can occur and it was reported in 2 to 5% of Wolfgang et al's 1987 series. However, even in the presence of a non-union good function can result. As stated previously, Veras et al (1999) reported that 67% of elderly patients with displaced olecranon fractures treated conservatively were asymptomatic and 11 of the 12 patients were satisfied with their outcome. McEachan et al (1998) reported that the average loss of extension in patients with united olecranon fractures was 10° compared to 27° in those with a non-union. The strength of elbow extension was not significantly different between the groups. Any weakness was asymptomatic and any persistent extension weakness responded well to physiotherapy. Simple excision of the olecranon fragment and triceps advancement seems to produce good results (Morrey 1995).

Olecranon fractures in children are rare. Fractures of the unfused olecranon epiphysis are more common in athletes and may require open reduction and internal fixation (Turtel et al 1995). Metaphyseal fractures of the olecranon are uncommon, 20% being associated with a fracture or dislocation of the proximal radius (Wilkins 1991). Gaddy et al (1997) reported their results after treating 35 children who had fractures of the olecranon. In 23 patients, displacement of the fracture was less than 3 mm. All were treated by closed methods and all had a satisfactory result at follow-up. They healed by 6 weeks after fracture (average 3.5 weeks). Twelve children with displaced fractures were treated by open reduction and internal fixation. All 10 who attended for follow-up had satisfactory results.

Summary

- 81% of patients achieve an excellent or good result after the surgical treatment of olecranon fracture.
- Most patients lose some extension of the elbow after these fractures.
- Not all patients with non-union have poor function.
- Degenerative changes have been reported in 2–20% of patients at long-term follow-up.

Fracture of the coronoid process of the ulna

Although fractures of the coronoid process of the ulna typically occur in association with posterior dislocation of

the elbow, isolated injuries may occur. Regan & Morrey (1989) reviewed 35 patients with this fracture and found three types:

- type I (14 patients)—avulsion of the tip of the process
- type II (16 patients)—a fragment involving 50% of the process or less
- type III (five patients)—a fragment involving more than 50% of the process

A concurrent dislocation or associated fracture was present in 14%, 56% and 80% of these patients respectively. A satisfactory result was achieved in 92% of patients who had a type I fracture, 73% of those with a type II fracture and 20% of those with a type III fracture.

Occasional complications can occur after type I injuries. Liu et al (1996) reported two complications occurring in this injury in athletes. One patient developed loose body formation and the other a fibrous non-union with mechanical blockage of elbow flexion. Both patients returned to full athletic activities after surgery.

Residual stiffness of the joint was most often present in patients who had a type III fracture, where the average arc of flexion was 39–100°. Post-traumatic degenerative changes were noted as absent in 19 elbows, mild in 11 and moderate in two. No radiographs showed severe degenerative changes of the elbow.

Summary

- Fractures of the coronoid process of the ulna usually occur in association with posterior dislocation of the elbow.

Radial head and neck fractures

Adult injuries

Fractures of the radial head are classified as follows (Mason 1954):

- type I—an undisplaced segmental fracture of the radial head
- type II—the fracture segment is displaced with a step in the articular surface at the radiohumeral joint
- type III—gross comminution of the whole radial head
- type IV—any of the above with elbow dislocation

The majority of radial head and neck fractures should be treated conservatively, which most often gives excellent results. Radin & Riseborough (1966) classified their results as follows:

- good—if there was less than 10° loss of motion in any direction and no symptoms

- fair—if there was up to 30° loss of motion in any direction, or minor complaints, or both
- poor—if there were major complaints or more than 30° loss of motion in any direction, or both

They found that 15 of 30 type I fractures had a good result, and 11 a fair result (87% satisfactory result). Thompson (1988) reported that all 20 adult patients in his series of undisplaced radial head fractures healed with no patient reporting any functional impairment. While only seven patients (35%) had no discernible loss of motion about the injured elbow, the loss of motion in the remaining 13 elbows was so small that it averaged only 1–2°. Two elbows lost 10° of extension.

Morrey (1995) felt that 90% of patients had a good result with early motion in these type I fractures. However, he suggested that 5% of type I injuries went on to develop non-union of the fracture.

Miller et al (1981) looked at the long-term follow-up of the conservative treatment of the type II fracture. Using the above criteria they reported that 29 of their 34 patients (81%) treated conservatively achieved satisfactory results. They further reported that there was only rarely a deterioration in the short-term result. Even better results were reported by Mathur & Sharma (1984). They used a plaster cast to immobilise the elbow and yet allow free rotation of the forearm. Of their 50 patients 43 returned to a full range of motion and a further six lost less than 10° of motion (96% good result).

Aspiration of the elbow soon after injury to remove the haemarthrosis is quite effective in significantly reducing pain. Fleetcroft (1984) suggested that the long-term functional result was permanently improved after aspiration of the haematoma. He reported that full flexion and extension was achieved in 83% of those patients aspirated, and rotation was full in all. On the other hand, in his non-aspirated group only 58% had full flexion and extension and 86% had full rotation.

However, Holdsworth et al (1987), while confirming that pain relief was immediate and lasting, were unable to show any long-term difference in the final outcome after aspiration of the haematoma. They found that the older the patient was, the worse the functional results were. They also noted that loss of extension of the elbow was the main disability after fracture of the radial head and that this loss correlated well with the residual symptoms.

Displaced segmental fractures may cause significant limitation of forearm rotation, and open reduction with internal fixation, or excision of the fragment, may be undertaken. Geel & Palmer (1992) reported the results of internal fixation in 19 patients with radial head fractures. Fourteen (74%) had an excellent result using a functional rating index assigning points for range of elbow and forearm motion, grip strength, stability and subjective assessment of pain. Five of the 19 patients (26%) had a fair result and no patient had a poor result. Four patients had limited movement with average loss of extension of 5°, average loss of flexion of 14° and average loss of pronation and supination of 8°. These four patients experienced mild to moderate pain after heavy lifting. One patient developed radial head necrosis, necessitating radial head excision. All returned to their pre-operative work status and the average period absent from work was 1.5 months.

Twenty-six fractures of the radial head treated by internal fixation were reported by Esser et al (1995). Eleven were type II fractures, nine type III fractures and six type IV fractures. All the 11 patients with type II fractures had a satisfactory result. Elbow flexion averaged 142° and the average loss of extension was only 1°. Excellent results were achieved in seven patients and good results in two patients with type III injuries. The average range of elbow flexion was 138° and the average loss of extension 3°. Four of the six patients with a type IV fracture dislocation had an excellent or good result. The average range of motion was 132° flexion, and 13° loss of extension, 70° supination and 85° pronation. Two patients underwent delayed excision of the radial head.

All 19 of the type II fractures reported by Pearce and Gallannaugh (1996) treated by open reduction and Herbert screw fixation had an excellent (16 patients) or good (three patients) result. All 19 patients had a mild loss of elbow extension (10–15°).

Morrey (1995) recommends early excision of the radial head in type III fractures within 48 hours of injury. Fuchs and Chylarecki (1999) reported the results of 151 patients who underwent radial head resection for comminuted fractures. Fifty-nine patients were operated on during the first 2 weeks after injury (primary treatment), 47 patients were operated on between 3 weeks and 6 months after injury (early secondary) and 45 patients were operated on more than 6 months after injury (late secondary). Follow-up of 108 patients was conducted at an average of 6 years after operation. Sixty-nine percent of patients treated by primary resection considered their results as satisfactory compared with 44% of those treated with secondary resection. The comparative data from this paper are shown in Table 7.10. Mikic & Vukadinovic (1983) reported that only 50% of their 60 patients had a satisfactory result after the radial head was excised. Broberg & Morrey (1986) reported the results of delayed excision of the radial head in 21 patients; 90% were functionally satisfied and 77% were rated objectively as having an excellent or good result. Grip strength was reduced by 7% after radial head excision (Coleman et al 1987).

Excision of the radial head in an otherwise intact elbow joint does alter the normal kinematics of the joint. Jensen et al (1999), using cadavaric elbow specimens, showed that while there was no increased laxity in forced valgus or internal rotation, the radial head did seem to act as a stabiliser to the elbow joint in forced varus and forced external rotation.

Radial head and neck fractures are associated with elbow dislocation in 10% of patients (Morrey 1995). The anterior band of the ulnar collateral ligament is the primary restraint to valgus instability with the radio-capitellar articulation providing an important secondary restraint. In the presence of ulnar collateral ligament rupture, radial head excision will produce gross instability. This is clearly demonstrated in the detailed case report of Liu and Henry (1995). In these situations the radial head must be reconstructed, replaced by a prosthesis or stabilised with an external fixator (Morrey 1995).

Frankle et al (1999) reported the results of 21 elbow dislocations with an associated radial head fracture. In all patients initial treatment involved closed reduction of the ulnohumeral joint and benign neglect (four patients), open reduction and internal fixation (nine patients), and immediate silicone head replacement (eight patients). All were treated with early range-of-motion exercises. Despite radial head treatment, six patients remained unstable, all with comminuted type III radial heads. Myositis ossificans occurred in five patients.

Gausepohl et al (1999) described the use of a unilateral external fixator in 16 patients with unstable fracture–dislocations of the elbow. The fixator remained in situ for 5–6 weeks. No acute re-dislocations or late instability were encountered. The functional arc in flexion and extension was greater than 100° in all patients, with pronation and supination being 80° and 70° respectively.

Subluxation of the distal radio-ulnar joint as a complication of excision of the radial head was reported to occur in 37 of 58 wrists (64%) by Taylor & O'Conner (1964), and 50% of the 58 patients had symptoms of weakness or pain at the wrist. McDougall & White (1957) reported that 12 of 44 patients (27%) with radial head excision had wrist symptoms, and Mikic & Vukadinovic (1983) reported the same in 30% of their 60 patients. However, Radin & Riseborough (1966) reported that although subluxation occurred in 14 of 36 wrists (39%), only three patients had mild symptoms, and they could find no correlation between the degree of subluxation at the distal radio-ulnar joint and symptoms.

A similar lack of correlation between proximal migration of the radius and wrist symptoms was reported by Morrey et al (1979) and Stephen (1981).

Table 7.10 Results of radial head excision (after Fuchs & Chylarecki 1999)

		Figures in percentages		
		Primary	Early secondary	Late secondary
Elbow pain:	Number	71	45	36
	moderate	22	31	33
	bad	7	24	31
Restriction of activities of daily living	Number	74	51	45
	moderate	19	18	34
	bad	7	31	21
Restriction at work	Number	64	30	27
	moderate	17	36	45
	bad	19	34	28
		Movements in degrees		
Extension deficit		16	27	22
Flexion deficit		13	29	12
Supination deficit		17	35	22
Pronation deficit		12	23	12

The results of the use of a silastic prosthesis after radial head excision have been variable. Mackay et al (1979) reported that 17 of their 18 patients (94%) had satisfactory results. Harrington et al (1999) reported on the use of a titanium metal radial head prosthesis in 20 patients with radial head fracture and gross instability of the elbow; 16 (80%) had a satisfactory result.

Carn et al (1986) found that only 70% of their 10 patients had a satisfactory result. Their patients had an average 8% loss of grip strength. Morrey et al (1981b) reported five failures out of 17 cases of silastic replacement (70% satisfactory results). They concluded that the indications for the use of the silastic radial head prosthesis after fracture are extremely limited.

Fracture of the prosthesis is not uncommon (Mackay et al 1979) and it may be the cause of symptoms.

The long-term complications of type II and III injuries of the radial head are osteoarthritis, with resultant painful limitation of elbow motion and forearm rotation. The risk is greater the worse the damage to the articular surface of the radial head. The reported incidence of degeneration at the elbow after radial head fracture varies between 52% of 60 patients (Mikic & Vukadinovic 1983) and 100% of 36 patients (Goldberg et al 1986). Although Mikic & Vukadinovic reported that 43% of the 60 patients had symptoms from the elbow, most authors report no correlation between the presence of radiographic degeneration and elbow symptoms (Morrey et al 1979, Carn et al 1986, Goldberg et al 1986).

In some cases, particularly where the radial head has been removed and not replaced by a prosthesis, there is a risk of cubitus valgus developing. This gives rise to the long-term possibility of compression ulnar neuropathy within the cubital tunnel, and this is because the ulna displaces outwards with approximation of the roof of the cubital tunnel to the floor. Mikic & Vakadinovic (1983) reported that 15 of their 55 adult patients (27%) developed increase of the cubitus valgus after radial head resection. This increase averaged 5° (Goldberg et al 1988) to 20° (Coleman et al 1987).

Ulnar nerve symptoms occurred in five (8%) of the patients of Mikic & Vukadinovic (1983) and in one (8%) of the 12 patients of Stephen (1981).

Fracture of the radial head can occur in association with acute dislocation of the distal radio-ulnar joint, although this is uncommon. Edwards & Jupiter (1988) reported seven cases. Three excellent results occurred in the patients who were diagnosed and treated early, with full restoration of radial length and stabilisation of the distal radio-ulnar joint. Two good and one fair result occurred in patients whose treatment was delayed

for 4–10 weeks, and the one poor result occurred in a patient who refused further treatment after radial head excision.

Isolated dislocation of the radial head is a rare injury in adults, but can occur in an anterior, lateral (Wiley et al 1991) or posterior (Jakim & Sweet 1990) direction. Closed reduction is usually successful, and if the correct diagnosis is made the long-term functional results are excellent. However, even if unrecognised, the loss of movement may be small (10° loss of flexion and 30° loss of supination in the case of Kadic & Bloem 1991).

Proximal radial epiphysis injuries

Fractures of the radial neck in children account for 4.5 to 21% of elbow injuries in children. Associated injuries occur in 30 to 50% of patients (Radomisli & Rosen 1998).

Radial neck fractures with little or no displacement require simple protection. No reduction is needed in fractures angulated less than 30° in younger children (Radomisli & Rosen 1998). Most authors recommend attempts to reduce angulation of over 30°.

The displaced fractures can be treated by closed reduction, percutaneous manipulation or open reduction.

Wilkins (1991) reviewed the literature and found an overall incidence of poor results in 15 to 33% of cases, despite apparently adequate treatment. Voke & Van Laer (1998) reviewed 38 children with displaced radial neck fractures 2–20 years after the initial accident. Although radial head deformity was present in 83%, a functional disorder was found in only four children (11%). On follow-up radiographs, all conservatively treated fractures with angulation up to 50° had corrected spontaneously. Merchan (1991) reported the results in 36 children with displaced radial head fractures who had open reduction and Kirschner wire fixation. Good results (full mobility with no pain) occurred in 18 patients (50%), fair results (loss of <20° of mobility) in eight (22%) and poor results (loss of >20° mobility in any direction, or definite pain) in 10 patients (28%). Dormans & Rang (1990) reported that 28 of their 48 patients (58%) had an essentially normal range of motion, while seven patients (15%) lost 45° or more of rotation.

Complications after the treatment of radial neck fractures occurs in 20 to 60% of patients (Radomisli & Rosen 1998). They record that the common complications involve loss of motion (0 to 79% of patients), pain (9.8 to 66% of patients), avascular necrosis (7 to 44% of patients), premature epiphyseal closure (0 to 31% of patients), and periarticular ossification (2.8 to 13% of patients). Non-union, increased carrying angle and overgrowth of the radial head also occur. Premature epiphyseal fusion is seldom a significant problem. Synostosis occurred in one patient in Merchan's 1991 series (2.7%), and it can occur after closed reduction. Heterotopic calcification occurred in five patients (13.9%) and is seen most commonly after open reduction. Avascular necrosis occurred in one patients (2.7%). The presence of avascular necrosis does not necessarily preclude a good result, but cubitus valgus with compression of the ulnar nerve in adult life may occur (Jeffrey 1972). Posterior interosseous nerve injury is mostly an operative complication. Non-union is also rare—one patient (2.7%, Merchan 1991)—and it can be disastrous, although good functional results have been reported.

Rarely, fracture of the neck of the radius can occur in association with an elbow dislocation, but good results can be achieved with closed reduction (Papavasilion & Kirkos 1991), although open reduction is usually required.

Summary

- Type I radial head fractures have an 87–100% satisfactory result. 5% develop non-union.
- Type II radial head fractures have an 81–96% satisfactory result.
- 50–90% of patients had a satisfactory result after radial head excision.
- Type IV radial head fractures are associated with a higher complication rate.
- Degenerative changes have been reported to occur in 52–100% of radial head fractures.
- Poor results occur in 15–33% of proximal radial epiphysis injuries.

Elbow dislocations
In adults

Elbow dislocations occur most commonly in young adults or the elderly. Acute elbow dislocations are usually classified according to the direction of dislocation. The majority of dislocations are posterolateral (up to 85%, Habernek & Ortner 1992). True posterior dislocations are the next most common, followed by posteromedial dislocations. Anterior, medial, lateral and divergent dislocations are rare.

Associated avulsion fractures of the medial and lateral epicondyles occur in 12 to 62% of elbow dislocations (Hotchkiss et al 1991). Protzman (1978) reported that these associated fractures did not prejudice the final result. However, Royle (1991) noted a 40% fair/poor result in elbow dislocations associated with fractures, compared with a 17% fair/poor result with simple elbow dislocation alone.

Following reduction of the dislocation, the elbow may be treated conservatively, or the ligaments may be repaired surgically. Josefsson et al (1987) reported the results of a prospective randomised study comparing surgical and non-surgical treatment in 30 patients with simple dislocation of the elbow. They found no evidence that the results were improved by surgical repair. The main movement to suffer some permanent loss following elbow dislocations is extension. The average loss of extension is 4° (Royle 1991) to 7° (Protzman 1978), increasing to 16° (Royle 1991) in those with fracture. Protzman (1978) noted a direct correlation between the duration of immobilisation, the loss of extension and the period of disability. The 27 patients immobilised for less than 5 days had an average 3° loss of extension and an average disability period of 6 weeks. Those seven patients immobilised for longer than 3 weeks lost an average of 21° extension and had a disability period averaging 24 weeks. Mehlhoff et al (1988) reported similar unsatisfactory results after prolonged immobilisation. They reported an average of 12° loss of extension in 52 patients, which was the same as the extension loss reported in 52 patients by Josefsson et al (1984).

Improvement in the range of movement normally occurs from 6 months to 1 year (Mehlhoff et al 1988).

Periarticular calcification occurred in 60% (Protzman 1978) to 95% (Josefsson et al 1984) of patients. However, this calcification does not appear to affect the final functional result. Some residual pain was noted in 45% of the 52 patients reported by Mehlhoff et al (1988) at an average of 34 months' follow-up.

Josefsson et al (1984) reported signs of early degenerative joint disease in 38% of 50 patients after an average follow-up of 24 years. A similar incidence of post-traumatic osteoarthrosis was reported by Eygendal et al (1999). Twenty-one patients out of 48 (44%), with a posterolateral elbow dislocation without associated fracture, followed up at an average of 9 years after simple closed reduction, had radiological evidence of degeneration in the elbow joint. Habernek & Ortner (1992) found only one of eight patients (12.5%) treated conservatively with moderate arthritis after 4 years, compared with seven patients (26%) treated surgically; severe arthritis occurred in three patients (11%) also treated surgically. In a long-term follow-up of 19 patients with dislocations of the elbow and radial head fractures, Josefsson et al (1989) reported severe osteoarthritis with reduced joint space in 12 patients (63%).

Chronic elbow instability without fractures in adults can be broken down to 1) valgus instability, 2) posterolateral rotatory instability or 3) isolated radial head instability. By far the most common is valgus instability. Of the 48 patients treated for simple posterolateral elbow dislocation by Eygendal et al (1999), 15 (31%) had instability to valgus stress at physical examination. Twenty-four patients (50%) demonstrated some medial instability. Despite this high level of instability on examination, 37 patients (77%) described their elbow function as good or excellent. Josefsson et al (1984) found that eight of their 52 patients (15%) had signs of valgus instability on examination, although none of these patients had symptoms related to this residual instability. Posterolateral rotatory instability is much less common and was first described by O'Driscoll et al (1991). They reported on five patients with 'recurrent dislocations' and a 'snapping sensation' present in the elbow during maximal supination of the forearm. It is diagnosed by the lateral pivot-shift test of the elbow and is usually the result of injury to the lateral collateral ligament complex. Surgical treatment is aimed at its reconstruction.

Isolated radial head subluxation in adults is extremely rare (see under radial head).

Complex fracture–dislocation of the elbow usually occurs as a result of high velocity injuries and has a higher risk of recurrent or chronic instability and arthrosis. The more bony structures are involved, the more complex is the injury which can include anterior or transolecranon fracture–dislocation of the elbow, posterior Monteggia lesions, and sideswipe injuries (Ring & Jupiter 1998). Such injuries can result in a variety of complex instabilities (Morrey 1997), but these can be successfully treated with hinged external fixators (Morrey 1997, McKee et al 1998). McKee and his co-workers described the use of their hinged external fixator in 16 patients with complex elbow instabilities. At final follow-up of 23 months the results were: one (6%) poor, three (19%) fair, 10 (63%) good and two (12%) excellent. The mean range of flexion-extension was 105°.

Old unreduced posterior dislocation of the elbow is uncommon. Oberli (1999) described the treatment of eight patients at an average of 21 weeks (range 6–84 weeks between injury and the commencement of treatment. In each case tissue distraction using an external fixator between the distal humerus and proximal ulna was utilised. One patient required lengthening of the triceps tendon. The average duration of external fixation was 71 days. The average arc of motion improved from 30° pre-operatively to 92° postoperatively. The average gain in maximal flexion was 80°.

Neurovascular complications are also associated with elbow dislocations. There have been many reports of injury to the brachial artery. Platz et al (1999) described four cases. The median nerve may be trapped in the joint (Hallett 1981). The radial nerve would appear to be the least vulnerable to injury.

In children

Dislocation of the elbow occurs in 3–6% of elbow injuries in children (Wilkins 1991). As in the adult, elbow dislocations in children are classified according to the direction of dislocation. However, the vast majority are true posterior dislocations. Most of these injuries can be treated by closed reduction with or without immobilisation in a plaster back slab. Occasionally, open reduction is required, especially if the medial epicondyle is trapped in the humero-ulnar articulation.

There is usually a loss of elbow extension of some 10–15° following these injuries. Fowles et al (1990) reported that 11 (58%) out of 19 children treated with closed reduction had normal elbows, while eight (42%) lost an average of 15° of flexion.

Wilkins (1991) reported a review of three large series of patients with elbow dislocation. In 285 patients there was an 11% incidence of nerve injury. The ulnar nerve was the most commonly injured, and there was usually a transient paraesthesia with rapid recovery. The median nerve is less commonly affected but can be trapped in the joint (Hallett 1981).

Arterial injuries are rare and three-quarters occur in open dislocations. The functional outcome following these injuries is related to their treatment. While good results have occurred following simple ligation of the artery, the collateral circulation is disrupted by the haematoma and soft tissue injury, and arterial repair is indicated.

True myositis following these injuries is also rare. As this involves ossification within the muscle sheath it can result in a significant loss of motion. Heterotopic calcification in the ligaments and capsules is more common but rarely results in loss of elbow function (Wilkins 1991). The incidence of true myositis ossificans is between 3% (Thompson & Garcia 1967) and 5% (Roberts 1969), increasing to 18% in dislocations associated with fractures (Thompson & Garcia 1967). Heterotopic calcification was reported by Linscheid & Wheeler (1965) as occurring in 28% of cases.

Recurrent dislocation of the elbow is rare. In the combined series of 285 cases reported by Wilkins (1991) the incidence was 0.7%.

Osteochondral fractures can occur, arising from the olecranon fossa or the trochlea (Blamoutier et al 1991). These injuries are rare and open surgery is required to reduce the fracture. When performed early this leads to excellent functional results.

Summary

- Loss of extension after simple dislocation of the elbow in the adult averages 7–12°. Improvement can occur over 1 year from injury.

- Degenerative changes were reported in 38–44% of patients at follow-up. This increased to 63% in dislocation of the elbow associated with a radial head fracture.

- There is usually some loss of elbow extension of 10–15° following elbow dislocation in children. 11% have a nerve injury which is usually transient.

The post-traumatic stiff shoulder

A flexion contracture of the elbow is fairly common after severe elbow trauma. This can result in a significant loss of function. The contracture usually results from scarring and thickening of the anterior elbow capsule. Currently the two most widely used surgical approaches are anterior and lateral. With the lateral approach care has to be taken not to damage the lateral collateral ligament and cause posterolateral instability. Cohen & Hastings (1998) reviewed 22 patients 26 months after operative release. The total humero-ulnar joint movement increased from a mean of 74° to 129°. Canadell et al (1997) reported an increase of motion from 45° pre-operatively to 92° postoperatively in 43 patients.

■ References

Abe M, Ishizu T, Nagaoka T, Onomura T 1995a Epiphyseal separation of the distal end of the humeral epiphysis: a follow-up note. Journal of Pediatric Orthopedics 15: 426–434

Abe M, Ishizu T, Shirai H, Okamoto M, Onomura T 1995b Tardy ulnar nerve palsy caused by cubitus varus deformity. Journal of Hand Surgery—American Volume 20: 5–9

Abe M, Ishizu T, Nagaoka T, Onomura T 1995c Recurrent posterior dislocation of the head of the radius in post-traumatic cubitus varus. Journal of Bone and Joint Surgery 77b: 582–585

Ackerman G, Jupiter J B 1988 Non-union of fractures of the distal end of the humerus. Journal of Bone and Joint Surgery 70A: 75–83

Aitken G K, Rorabeck C H 1986 Distal humeral fractures in the adult. Clinical Orthopaedics 207: 191–197

Badelon O, Bensahel H, Mazda K, Vie P 1988 Lateral humeral condylar fractures in children: a report of 47 cases. Journal of Pediatric Orthopaedics 8: 31–34

Bamford D J, Stanley D 1989 Anterior interosseous nerve paralysis: an under-diagnosed complication of supracondylar fracture of the humerus in children. Injury 20: 294–295

Barton N J, Hooper G, Noble J, Steel W M 1992 Occupational causes of disorders in the upper limb. British Medical Journal 304: 309–311

Bast S C, Hoffer M M, Aval S 1998 Nonoperative treatment for minimally and non displaced lateral humeral condyle fractures in children. Journal of Pediatric Orthopaedics 18: 448–450

Bensahel H, Csukonyi Z, Badelon O, Badaoni S 1986 Fractures of the medial condyle of the humerus in children. Journal of Pediatric Orthopaedics 6: 430–433

Blamoutier A, Klaue K, Damsin J P, Carlioz H 1991 Osteochondral fractures of the glenoid fossa of the ulna in children: review of four cases. Journal of Pediatric Orthopaedics 11: 638–640

Boyd H B, McLeod A C 1973 Tennis elbow. Journal of Bone and Joint Surgery 55A: 1183–1187

Boyer M I, Hastings H 1999 Lateral tennis elbow: 'Is there any science out there?' Journal of Shoulder and Elbow Surgery 8: 481–491

Broberg M A, Morrey B F 1986 Results of delayed excision of the radial head after fracture. Journal of Bone and Joint Surgery 68A: 669–674

Browne A O, O'Riordan M, Quinlan W 1986 Supracondylar fractures of the humerus in adults. Injury 17: 184–186

Bryan R S, Morrey B F 1985 Fractures of the distal humerus. In: Morrey B F (ed.) The elbow and its disorders. E B Saunders, Philadelphia

Canadell J, Santiago A, Conrado A 1997 Arthrolysis of post traumatic stiffness of the elbow. Journal of Bone and Joint Surgery 79B: supp II: 139

Carn R M, Medige J, Curtain D, Koenig A 1986 Silicone rubber replacement of the severely fractured radial head. Clinical Orthopaedics 209: 259–269

Chandratreya A P, Hunter J P 1999 Olecranon screw traction revisited. Journal of Bone and Joint Surgery 81B: supp III: 287

Chard M D, Hazelman B L 1989 Tennis elbow—a reappraisal. British Journal of Rheumatology 28: 186

Cobb T K, Morrey B F 1997 Total elbow arthroplasty as primary treatment for distal humeral fractures in elderly patients. Journal of Bone and Joint Surgery 79A: 826–832

Cohen M S, Hastings H 1998 Post-traumatic contracture of the elbow. Operative release using a lateral collateral ligament sparing approach. Journal of Bone and Joint Surgery 80B: 805–812

Coleman D A, Blair W F, Shurr D 1987 Resection of the radial head for fracture of the radial head. Journal of Bone and Joint Surgery 69A: 385–392

Collert S 1977 Surgical management of fracture of the capitulum humeri. Acta Orthopaedica Scandinavica 48: 603–606

Coonrad R W, Hooper W R 1973 Tennis elbow: its course, natural history, conservative and surgical management. Journal of Bone and Joint Surgery 55A: 1177–1182

Culp R W, Osterman A L, Davidson R S, Skirven T, Bora F W 1990 Neural injuries associated with supracondylar fractures of the humerus in children. Journal of Bone and Joint Surgery 72A: 1211–1215

De Boeck H, De Smet P 1997 Valgus deformity following supracondylar elbow fractures in children. Acta Orthopaedica Belgica 63: 240–244

De Jager L T, Hoffman E B 1991 Fracture separation of the distal humeral epiphysis. Journal of Bone and Joint Surgery 73B: 143–146

Dias J J, Johnson G V, Hoskinson J, Sulaiman K 1987 Management of severely displaced medial epicondyle fractures. Journal of Orthopaedic Trauma 1: 59–62

Dimberg L 1987 The prevalence and causation of tennis elbow (lateral humeral epicondylitis) in a population of workers in an engineering industry. Ergonomics 30: 573–580

Dormans J P, Rang M 1990 Fractures of the olecranon and radial neck in children. Orthopaedic Clinics of North America 21: 257–268

Edwards G S, Jupiter J B 1988 Radial head fractures with acute distal radioulnar dislocation. Clinical Orthopaedics 234: 61–69

Eriksson E, Sahlen O, Sandahl U 1957 Late results of conservative and surgical treatment of fracture of the olecranon. Acta Chirurgica Scandinavica 113: 153–156

Esser R D, Davis S, Taavao T 1995 Fractures of the radial head treated by internal fixation: late results in 26 cases. Journal of Orthopaedic Trauma 9: 18–23

Eygenda A L, Verdegaal S H M, Obermann W M, Van Vught A B, Rozing P M 1999 Results after posterolateral elbow dislocation related to valgus instability. Journal of Bone and Joint Surgery 81B: supp II: 191

Feldman M D 1997 Arthroscopic excision of type II capitellar fractures. Arthroscopy 13: 743–748

Fleetcroft J P 1984 Fractures of the radial head: early aspiration and mobilisation. Journal of Bone and Joint Surgery 66B: 141–142

Flynn J C 1989 Non-union of slightly displaced fractures of the lateral humeral condyle in children: an update. Journal of Pediatric Orthopaedics 9: 691–696

Foulk D A, Robertson P A, Timmerman L A 1995 Fracture of the trochlea. Journal of Orthopaedic Trauma 9: 530–532

Fowles J V, Slimane N, Kassab M T 1990 Elbow dislocation with avulsion of the medial humeral epicondyle. Journal of Bone and Joint Surgery 72B: 102–104

Frankle M A, Koval K J, Sanders R W, Zuckerman J D 1999 Radial head fractures associated with elbow dislocations treated by immediate stabilization and early motion. Journal of Shoulder and Elbow Surgery 8: 355–360

Fuchs S, Chylarecki C 1999 Do functional deficits result from radial head resection? Journal of Shoulder and Elbow Surgery 8: 247–251

Gabel G T, Morrey B F 1995 Operative treatment of medial epicondylitis. Influence of concomitant ulnar neuropathy at the elbow. Journal of Bone and Joint Surgery 77A: 1065–1069

Gaddy B C, Strecker W B, Schoenecker P L 1997 Surgical treatment of displaced olecranon fractures in children. Journal of Pediatric Orthopaedics 17: 321–324

Gartsman G M, Sculco T P, Otis J C 1981 Operative treatment of olecranon fractures. Journal of Bone and Joint Surgery 63A: 718–721

Gausepohl T, Pennig D, Mader K 1999 The early motion fixator concept for treatment of acute unstable fracture dislocation of the elbow. Journal of Bone and Joint Surgery 81B: supp II: 191

Gaye J R, Love J G 1947 Diagnosis and treatment of tardy palsy of the ulnar nerve. Journal of Bone and Joint Surgery 29: 1087–1097

Geel C W, Palmer A K 1992 Radial head fractures and their effect on the distal radioulnar joint. Clinical Orthopaedics 275: 79–84

Goldberg E J, Abraham E, Siegel I 1988 The surgical treatment of chronic lateral humeral epicondylitis by common extensor release. Clinical Orthopaedics 233: 208–212

Goldberg I, Peylon J, Yosipovitch Z 1986 Late results of excision of the radial head for an isolated closed fracture. Journal of Bone and Joint Surgery 68A: 675–679

Grantham S A, Norris T R, Bush D C 1981 Isolated fracture of the humeral capitellum. Clinical Orthopaedics 161: 262–269

Habernek H, Ortner F 1992 The influence of anatomic factors in elbow joint dislocation. Clinical Orthopaedics 274: 226–230

Hallett J 1981 Entrapment of the median nerve after dislocation of the elbow. Journal of Bone and Joint Surgery 63B: 408–412

Harrington I J, Barrington T W, Evans D C, Sekyi-Otu A, Tuli V 1999 Replacement of the radial head in the treatment of unstable elbow fractures: a long term review. Journal of Bone and Joint Surgery 81B: supp I: 106

Helm R H, Hornby R, Miller S W M 1987 The complications of surgical treatment of displaced fractures of the olecranon. Injury 18: 48–50

Henrickson B 1966 Supracondylar fracture of the humerus in children. Acta Chirurgica Scandinavica (suppl.) 369

Hines R F, Herndon W A, Evans J P 1987 Operative treatment of medial epicondyle fractures in children. Clinical Orthopaedics 223: 170–174

Hirner M, George J A, Eltringham J M, Erken E H W 1998 Delayed open reduction of lateral condylar fractures of the humerus in children. Journal of Bone and Joint Surgery 80B: supp II: 159

Holdsworth B J, Clement D A, Rothwell P N R 1987 Fractures of the radial head—the benefit of aspiration. Injury 18: 44–47

Holdsworth B J, Mossad M M 1984 Elbow function following tension band fixation of displaced fractures of the olecranon. Injury 16: 182–187

Holdsworth B J, Mossad M M 1990 Fractures of the adult distal humerus: elbow function after internal fixation. Journal of Bone and Joint Surgery 72B: 362–365

Horne G 1980 Supracondylar fractures of the humerus in adults. Journal of Trauma 20: 71–74

Hotchkiss R N, Green D P, Bucholz R W 1991 Fractures in adults, vol 1. J B Lippincott, Philadelphia

Ippolito E, Caterini R, Scola E 1986 Supracondylar fractures of the humerus in children. Journal of Bone and Joint Surgery 68A: 333–334

Jakim I, Sweet M B E 1990 Isolated traumatic posterior dislocation of the radial head. South African Medical Journal 78: 665–667

Jeffery R S 1989 Injuries of the lateral humeral condyle in children. Journal of the Royal College of Surgeons, Edinburgh 34: 156–159

Jeffrey C C 1972 Fractures of the neck of the radius in children. Journal of Bone and Joint Surgery 54B: 717

Jensen S L, Olsen B S, Sojbjerg J O 1999 Elbow joint kinematics after excision of the radial head. Journal of Shoulder and Elbow Surgery 8: 238–241

Jenson C M, Olsen B B 1986 Drawbacks of traction-absorbing wiring (TAW) in displaced fractures of the olecranon. Injury 17: 174–175

Josefsson P O, Danielsson L G 1986 Epicondylar elbow fracture in children: 35 year follow up of 56 cases. Acta Orthopaedica Scandinavica 57: 313–315

Josefsson P O, Gentz C-F, Johnell O, Wendeberg A B 1987 Surgical versus non-surgical treatment of ligamentous injuries following dislocation of the elbow. Journal of Bone and Joint Surgery 69A: 605–608

Josefsson P O, Gentz C-F, Johnell O, Wendeberg A B 1989 Dislocations of the elbow and intraarticular fractures. Clinical Orthopaedics 246: 126–130

Josefsson P O, Johnell O, Gentz C-F 1984 Long term sequelae of simple dislocation of the elbow. Journal of Bone and Joint Surgery 66A: 927–930

Jupiter J B, Neff U, Regazzoni P, Allgower M 1988 Unicondylar fractures of the distal humerus: an operative approach. Journal of Orthopaedic Trauma 2: 102–109

Kadic M A C, Bloem R M 1991 Traumatic isolated anterior dislocation of the radial head. Acta Orthopaedica Scandinavica 62: 288–289

Kamien M 1990 A rational management of tennis elbow. Sports Medicine 9: 173–191

Kiviluoto O, Santavirta S 1978 Fractures of the olecranon. Acta Orthopaedica Scandinavica 49: 28–31

Kraushaar B S, Nirschl R P 1999 Tendinosis of the elbow (Tennis elbow). Clinical features and findings of histological, immunohistochemical and electron microscopy studies. Journal of Bone and Joint Surgery 81A: 259–278

Kuhn J E, Louis D S, Loder R T 1995 Divergent single-column fractures of the distal part of the humerus. Journal of Bone and Joint Surgery 77A: 538–542

Kundel K, Braun W, Wieberneit J, Ruter A 1996 Intra-articular distal humerus fractures. Factors affecting functional outcome. Clinical Orthopaedics & Related Research 332: 200–208

Kurer M H J, Regan M W 1990 Completely displaced supracondylar fracture of the humerus in children. Clinical Orthopaedics 256: 205–214

Kurvers H, Verhaar J 1995 The results of operative treatment of medial epicondylitis. Journal of Bone and Joint Surgery 77A: 1374–1379

Landin L A, Danielsson L G 1986 Elbow fractures in children. Acta Orthopaedica Scandinavica 57: 309–312

Letts M, Rumball K, Bauermeister S, McIntyre W, D'Astous J 1997 Fractures of the capitellum in adolescents. Journal of Pediatric Orthopaedics 17: 315–320

Linscheid R L, Wheeler D K 1965 Elbow dislocations. Journal of the American Medical Association 194: 113–118

Liu S H, Henry M H 1995 Fracture of the radial head with ulnar collateral ligament rupture. Journal of Shoulder and Elbow Surgery 4: 399–402

Liu S H, Henry M, Bower R 1996 Complications of Type I coronoid fractures in competitive athletes: Report of two cases and review of the literature. Journal of Shoulder and Elbow Surgery 5: 223–227

Ljung B O, Lieber R L, Friden J 1999 Wrist extensor muscle pathology in lateral epicondylitis. Journal of Hand Surgery 24B: 177–183

Lyons J P, Ashley E, Hoffer M M 1998 Ulnar nerve palsies after percutaneous cross-pinning of supracondylar fractures in children's elbows. Journal of Pediatric Orthopaedics 18: 43–45

Ma Y-Z, Zheng C B, Zhou T L, Yeh Y C 1984 Percutaneous probe reduction of frontal fractures of the humeral capitellum. Clinical Orthopaedics 183: 17–21

Mackay I, Fitzgerald B, Miller J H 1979 Silastic replacement of the head of the radius in trauma. Journal of Bone and Joint Surgery 61B: 494–497

Masada K, Kawai H, Kawabata H, Masatomi T, Tsuyuguchi Y, Yamamoto K 1990 Osteosynthesis for old, established non-union of the lateral condyle of the humerus. Journal of Bone and Joint Surgery 72A: 32–40

Mason M L 1954 Some observations on fractures of the head of the radius with a review of one hundred cases. British Journal of Surgery 42: 123–132

Mathur N, Sharma C S 1984 Fracture of the head of the radius treated by elbow cast. Acta Orthopaedica Scandinavica 55: 567–568

McDougall A, White J 1957 Subluxation of the inferior radio-ulnar joint complicating fracture of the radial head. Journal of Bone and Joint Surgery 39B: 278–287

McEachan J, Meighan A, Rymaszewski L A 1998 Elbow function following a non union of an olecranon fracture. Journal of Bone and Joint Surgery 80B: suppl I: 106

McKee M D, Bowden S H, King G J, Patterson S D, Jupiter J B, Bamberger H B, Paksima N 1998 Management of recurrent complex instability of the elbow with a hinged external fixator. Journal of Bone and Joint Surgery 80B: 1031–1036

Mehlhoff T L, Noble P C, Bennett J B, Tullos H S 1988 Simple dislocation of the elbow in the adult. Journal of Bone and Joint Surgery 70A: 244–249

Merchan E C R 1991 Displaced fractures of the head and neck of the radius in children: open reduction and temporary transarticular internal fixation. Orthopaedics 14: 697–700

Mikic Z D, Vukadinovic S M 1983 Late results in fractures of the radial head treated by excision. Clinical Orthopaedics 181: 220–228

Miller E M 1924 Later ulnar nerve palsy. Surgery, Gynaecology and Obstetrics 38: 37–46

Miller G K, Drennan D B, Maylahn D J 1981 Treatment of displaced segmental radial head fractures. Journal of Bone and Joint Surgery 63A: 712–717

Miller W E 1964 Comminuted fractures of the distal end of the humerus in the adult. Journal of Bone and Joint Surgery 46A: 644–657

Mitchell W, Adams M D 1961 Supracondylar fractures of the humerus in children, a ten year review. Journal of the American Medical Association 175: 573–577

Mitsunaga M M, Bryan R S, Linscheid R L 1982 Condylar non-unions of the elbow. Journal of Trauma 22: 787–791

Morrey B F 1995 Current concepts in the treatment of fractures of the radial head, the olecranon, and the coronoid. Journal of Bone and Joint Surgery 77A: 316–327

Morrey B F 1997 Complex instability of the elbow. Journal of Bone and Joint Surgery 79A: 460–469

Morrey B F, Adams R A 1995 Semiconstrained elbow replacement for distal humeral non union. Journal of Bone and Joint Surgery 77B: 67–72

Morrey B F, Askew L J, Chao E Y 1981a A biomechanical study of normal functional elbow motion. Journal of Bone and Joint Surgery 63A: 872–877

Morrey B F, Askew L J, Chao E Y 1981b Silastic prosthetic replacement for the radial head. Journal of Bone and Joint Surgery 63A: 454–452

Morrey B F, Chao E Y, Hui F C 1979 Biomechanical study of the elbow following excision of the radial head. Journal of Bone and Joint Surgery 61A: 63–68

Müller M E, Allgower M, Schneider R, Willenegger H 1991 Manual of internal fixation, 3rd edn. Springer-Verlag, Berlin

Murphy D F, Greene W B, Dameron T B 1987 Displaced olecranon fractures in adults. Clinical Orthopaedics 224: 215–223

Nirschl R P, Pettrone F A 1979 Tennis elbow: the surgical treatment of lateral epicondylitis. Journal of Bone and Joint Surgery 61A: 832–839

Oberli H 1999 Tissue distraction by external fixation of old unreduced dislocations of the elbow. Journal of Bone and Joint Surgery 81B: supp I: 6–7

Ochner R S, Bloom H, Palumbo R C, Coyle M P 1996 Closed reduction of coronal fractures of the capitellum. Journal of Trauma-Injury Infection and Critical Care 40: 199–203

O'Driscoll S W, Bell D F, Morrey B F 1991 Posterolateral rotatory instability of the elbow. Journal of Bone and Joint Surgery 73A: 440–446

Papaioannou N, Babis G C, Kalavritinos J, Pantazopoulos T 1995 Operative treatment of type C intra-articular fractures of the distal humerus: the role of stability achieved at surgery on final outcome. Injury 26: 169–173

Papavasilion V, Nenopoulos S, Venturis T 1987 Fractures of the medial condyle of the humerus during childhood. Journal of Pediatric Orthopaedics 7: 421–423

Papavasilion V A, Beslikas T A 1986 T-condylar fractures of the distal humeral condyles during childhood: an analysis of six cases. Journal of Pediatric Orthopaedics 6: 302–305

Papavasilion V A, Kirkos J M 1991 Dislocation of the elbow joint associated with fracture of the radial neck in children. Injury 22: 49–50

Pearce M S, Gallannaugh S C 1996 Mason type II radial head fractures fixed with Herbert bone screws. Journal of the Royal Society of Medicine 89: 340–344

Perry C R, Gibson C T, Kowalski M F 1989 Transcondylar fractures of the distal humerus. Journal of Orthopaedic Trauma 3: 98–106

Pirone A M, Graham H K, Krajbich J I 1988 Management of displaced extension-type supracondylar fractures of the humerus in children. Journal of Bone and Joint Surgery 70A: 641–650

Platz A, Heinzelmann M, Ertel W, Trentz O 1999 Posterior elbow dislocation with associated vascular injury after blunt trauma. Journal of Trauma-Injury Infection and Critical Care 46: 948–950

Posch J N, Goldberg V M, Larrey R 1978 Extensor fasciotomy for tennis elbow: a long term follow-up study. Clinical Orthopaedics 135: 179–182

Poynton A R, Kelly I P, O'Rourke S K 1998 Fractures of the capitellum—a comparison of two fixation methods. Injury 29: 341–343

Protzman R R 1978 Dislocation of the elbow joint. Journal of Bone and Joint Surgery 60A: 539–541

Radin E L, Riseborough E J 1966 Fractures of the radial head. Journal of Bone and Joint Surgery 48A: 1055–1064

Radomisli T E, Rosen A L 1998 Controversies regarding radial neck fractures in children. Clinical Orthopaedics & Related Research 353: 30–39

Rasool M N 1998 Ulnar nerve injury after K-wire fixation of supracondylar humerus fractures in children. Journal of Pediatric Orthopaedics 18: 686–690

Regan W, Morrey B 1989 Fractures of the coronoid process of the ulna. Journal of Bone and Joint Surgery 71A: 1348–1354

Ring D, Jupiter J 1999 Complex fractures of the distal humerus and their complications. Journal of Shoulder and Elbow Surgery 8: 85–97

Ring D, Jupiter J B 1998 Fracture-dislocation of the elbow. Journal of Bone and Joint Surgery 80A: 566–580

Riseborough E J, Radin E L 1969 Intercondylar T fractures of the humerus in the adult. Journal of Bone and Joint Surgery 51A: 130–141

Roberts P H 1969 Dislocation of the elbow. British Journal of Surgery 56: 806–815

Royle S G 1991 Posterior dislocation of the elbow. Clinical Orthopaedics 269: 201–204

Sabharwal S, Tredwell S J, Beauchamp R D, Mackenzie W G, Jakubec D M, Cairns R, LeBlanc J G 1997 Management of pulseless pink hand in pediatric supracondular fracture of humerus. Journal of Pediatric Orthopaedics 17: 303–310

Schneeberger A G, Adams R, Morrey B F 1997 Semiconstrained total elbow replacement for the treatment of post-traumatic osteoarthritis. Journal of Bone and Joint Surgery 79A: 1211–1222

Sharma J C, Arora A, Mathur N C, Gupta S P, Biyani A, Mathur R 1995 Lateral condylar fractures of the humerus in children: fixation with partially threaded 4.0 mm AO concellous screws. Journal of Trauma-Injury Infection and Critical Care 39: 1129–1133

Shimada K, Masada K, Tada K, Yamanoto T 1997 Osteosynthesis for the treatment of non-union of the lateral humeral condyle in children. Journal of Bone and Joint Surgery 79A: 234–240

Skaggs D L, Mirzayan R 1999 The posterior fat pad sign in association with occult fractures of the elbow in children. Journal of Bone and Joint Surgery 81A: 1429–1433

So Y C, Fang D, Leong J C Y, Bong S C 1985 Varus deformity following lateral humeral condylar fractures in children. Journal of Pediatric Orthopaedics 5: 569–572

Soltanpur A 1978 Anterior supracondylar fracture of the humerus (flexion type). Journal of Bone and Joint Surgery 60B: 383–386

Stephen I B M 1981 Excision of the radial head for closed fracture. Acta Orthopaedica Scandinavica 52: 409–412

Tan P K, Lam K S, Tan S K 1989 Results of modified Bosworth's operation for persistent or recurrent tennis elbow. Singapore Medical Journal 30: 359–362

Tapasvi S, Diggikar M S, Joshi A P 1999 External fixation for open proximal ulna fractures. Injury 30: 115–120

Taylor T K F, O'Connor B T 1964 The effect upon the inferior radio-ulnar joint of excision of the head of the radius in adults. Journal of Bone and Joint Surgery 46B: 83–88

Thompson H C, Garcia A 1967 Myositis ossificans: aftermath of elbow injuries. Clinical Orthopaedics 50: 129–134

Thompson J D 1988 Comparison of flexion versus extension splinting in the treatment of Mason Type I radial head and neck fractures. Journal of Orthopaedic Trauma 2: 117–119

Thonell S, Mortersson W, Thomasson B 1988 Prediction of the stability of minimally displaced fractures of the lateral humeral condyle. Acta Radiologica 29: 367–370

Turtel A H, Andrews J R, Schob C J, Kupferman S P, Gross A E 1995 Fractures of unfused olecranon physis: a re-evaluation of this injury in three athletes. Orthopaedics 18: 390–394

Van Vugt A B, Severijnen R V S M, Festen C 1988 Fractures of the lateral humeral condyle in children: late results. Archives of Orthopaedic and Traumatic Surgery 107: 206–209

Veras D M L, Sirera V M, Busquets N R, Castellanos R J, Carrera C L, Mir B X 1999 Conservative treatment of displaced fractures of the olecranon in the elderly. Injury 30: 105–110

Verhaar J A N, Walenkamp G H I M 1986 Operative therapy of radial humeral epicondylitis. In: Proceedings of the Netherlands Orthopaedic Association. Acta Orthopaedica Scandinavica 57: 451

Vocke A K, Von Laer L 1998 Displaced fractures of the radial neck in children: long-term results and prognosis of conservative treatment. Journal of Pediatric Orthopaedics 7: 217–222

Waddell J P, Hatch J, Richards R 1988 Supracondylar fractures of the humerus: results of surgical treatment. Journal of Trauma 28: 1615–1621

Wesley M S, Barenfeld P A, Eisenstein A L 1976 The use of the Zuelzer hook plate in fixation of olecranon fractures. Journal of Bone and Joint Surgery 58A: 859–863

Wildburger R, Mohring M, Hofer H P 1991 Supraintercondylar fractures of the distal humerus: results of internal fixation. Journal of Orthopaedic Trauma 5: 301–307

Wiley J J, Loehr J, McIntyre W 1991 Isolated dislocation of the radial head. Orthopaedics Review 20: 973–976

Wilkins K E 1990 Residuals of elbow trauma in children. Orthopaedic Clinics of North America 21: 291–314

Wilkins K E 1991 Fractures and dislocations of the elbow region. In: Rockwood C A Jr, Wilkins K E, King R E (eds) Fractures in children. J B Lippincott, Philadelphia

Williamson D M, Cole W G 1991 Flexion supracondylar fractures of the humerus in children: treatment by manipulation and extension cast. Injury 22: 451–455

Wilson N I L, Ingram R, Rymaszewski L, Miller J H 1988 Treatment of fractures of the medial epicondyle of the humerus. Injury 19: 342–344

Wolfgang G, Burke F, Bush D et al 1987 Surgical treatment of fracture of the olecranon. Acta Chirurgica Scandinavica 113: 153–156

Zagorski J B, Jennings J J, Burkhalter W E, Uribe J W 1986 Comminuted intrarticular fractures of the distal humeral condyles. Clinical Orthopaedics 202: 197–204

Chapter 8

The forearm
Phillip S. Fagg

Fractures of both bones in the adult
Conservative treatment

Undisplaced fractures of the forearm in adults are adequately treated in an above-elbow plaster of paris, and union should occur in 6–8 weeks.

The results of the conservative treatment of displaced fractures would appear to be far from satisfactory (Table 8.1), the average non-union rate in these three series being 7.2%. In 60% of the patients reported on by Knight & Purvis (1949), a residual deformity of rotation from 25–60° was present. Only 12 of their 41 patients (29%) achieved a satisfactory result.

Of the 90 cases of adult forearm fractures reported by Bolton & Quinlan (1952), 56 (62%) healed in good anatomical alignment, 53 (59%) had good function and 61 (55%) had full or only minimal restriction of rotation. Acceptable rotation was achieved in 90% of lower third fractures, 57.5% of middle third fractures and 60% of proximal third fractures, 59% of patients returning to their former employment.

Bradford et al (1953) reported the results of manipulation in 19 displaced fractures, of which 12 (63%) achieved a satisfactory position. However, in seven of these 12 fractures (58%) the position was lost over the course of the next 3 weeks, leaving only five of the original 19 fractures (26%) in an acceptable reduced position.

On the other hand, when reporting the results of 45 fractures of forearm bones in 43 patients treated with a forearm functional brace, Sarmiento et al (1975) found only one non-union (2%) and two cases of malunion (4.5%). The healing time averaged 9.9 weeks for isolated ulnar fractures, 11 weeks for isolated radial fractures and 15.1 weeks for fractures of both bones. The average loss of pronation and supination in these fractures was less than 10°, only two cases losing more than 10° of rotation in pronation or supination.

The effect of various angular deformities of the forearm bones was investigated experimentally on cadaver forearms by Sarmiento and his co-workers (Table 8.2). They suggested that the amount of loss of rotational motion of the forearm that is functionally acceptable is 20% of the normal range of motion, and that only 50° of pronation and 50° of supination were necessary for most activities of daily living.

Intramedullary fixation

Many varieties of intramedullary fixation have been used in the treatment of forearm fractures. Smith and Sage (1957) reviewed 555 fractures, in 338 patients, treated by Rush pins, Kirschner wires, Steinman pins, Kuntschner nails or Lottes nails. They found an overall non-union rate of 20%. When the 38% of non-unions from the use of Kirschner wires were excluded, this rate fell to 14%. The rate of non-union in the larger reported series of intramedullary fixation for forearm fractures is recorded in Table 8.3. The overall non-union rate from these five series was 9.3%, while the average time to union varied between 10 and 20 weeks.

The functional results obtained by the use of the various fixation devices reviewed in Smith & Sage's paper showed that 82% achieved a satisfactory result. A satisfactory result implied less than a 20° reduction in elbow flexion/extension and less than a 60° reduction in pronation/supination. The functional results reported by the authors of five of the larger series are recorded in Table 8.4.

Table 8.1 The results of the conservative treatment of displaced forearm fractures in adults

Reference	Number of Fractures	Non-union	Delayed union	Malunion	Time to union (weeks)
Knight & Purvis (1949)	41	5 (12%)	–	–	18–20
Bolton & Quinlan (1952)	90	4 (4.5%)	–	2 (2%)	13
Matthews & Saunders (1979)	22	2 (9%)	4 (18%)	2 (9%)	–

Table 8.2 Angular deformities of forearm bones and forearm fractures

Site	Loss of forearm motion related to angulation					
	5° supination/pronation		10° supination/pronation		15° supination/pronation	
Radius alone*						
Proximal	N/S	N/S	2–12°	N/S	3–34°	N/S
Middle	7–13°	N/S	0–22°	N/S	6–49°	6–19°
Distal	N/S	6–17°	N/S	14–24°	3–17°	16–36°
Ulna alone*						
Proximal	N/S	N/S	N/S	N/S	N/S	8–11°
Middle	N/S	9–13°	N/S	10–17°	24–31°	15–33°
Distal	N/S	N/S	3–13°	N/S	9–23°	9–24°
Radius and ulna†						
Middle	6%	9%	17%	15%	42%	28%
Distal	5%	10%	8%	18%	11%	33%

N/S = not significant.
* Sarmiento et al (1992).
† Tarr et al (1984).

Table 8.3 The non-union rate after intramedullary forearm fixation

Reference	Number of fractures	Number of non-unions	Percentage	Nail
Caden (1961)	157	26	16.6	Rush pin
Street (1986)	137	10	7	Square
Cotler et al (1971)	125	8	6.4	Schneider
Sage (1959)	82	5	6.2	Sage
Moerman et al (1996)	70	4	6	Rush pin
Overall	571	53	9.3	

Table 8.4 The functional results after intramedullary forearm fixation

Reference	Number of patients	Number of satisfactory results	Percentage	Nail
Street (1986)	103	86*	83.5	Square
Cotler et al (1971)	87	82	94	Schneider
Michels & Weissman (1976)	80	67	84	Rush pin
Sage (1959)	39	27†	69	Sage
Moerman et al (1996)	70	58*	83	Rush pin
Overall	379	320	84.4	

* Less than 50% loss of pronation/supination.
† Pronation and supination each lacking less than 45°.

Thus, overall, 84.4% achieved a satisfactory functional result following intramedullary fixation although, as can be seen, these authors did vary in their interpretation of what constituted a reasonable result.

Plate fixation

In the series reported by Knight & Purvis (1949), there was a 20% non-union rate in the 20 cases of forearm fracture treated by plate fixation, and only 35% of these 20 patients had a satisfactory end-result. Using a rigid plate, Hicks (1961) was able to reduce the non-union rate to 6% in 66 fractures. Although earlier papers had shown a significant complication rate with plate fixation, Burwell & Charnley (1964), using Burns & Shermans plates on 218 forearm fractures, showed that failure was due to poor anatomical reduction and the use of inappropriately short plates. Their overall non-union rate was 9.6% in 218 fractures. However, in those patients in which fixation was intact this fell to 2.2%, whereas where fixation was inadequate this non-union rate rose to 44.7%.

The results of the treatment of forearm fractures with rigid plates in some of the larger series are recorded in Table 8.5. The overall union rate was 96.2%.

In view of the fact that primary bone union occurs after rigid plate fixation, it can be difficult to be sure at what point radiological union has occurred. That this depends on author interpretation probably explains why Anderson et al (1975) found the average time to union to be 7.4 weeks in their 330 fractures, while Langkamer & Ackroyd (1991) reported it to be 18.8 weeks.

Ability to use the arm freely occurred on average at 13.9 weeks after surgery, return to work at an average of 20.1 weeks, and full recovery took 10.3 months. The functional results achieved after forearm plating in the larger series are recorded in Table 8.6. Overall, 86.7% achieved a satisfactory result.

Langkamer and Ackroyd (1991) recommended bone grafting for comminuted diaphyseal forearm fractures, as have Hadden et al (1983) and Anderson et al (1975). Wright et al (1997), in their retrospective review, investigated the

Table 8.5 The results of compression plating of forearm fractures

Reference	Number of fractures	Number united	Percentage united
Anderson et al (1975)	330	321	97.3
Hadden et al (1983)	177	172	97.2
Langkamer & Ackroyd (1991)	156	140	87.7
Wright et al (1997)	183	175	95.6
Hertel et al (1996)	248	244*	98.4
Overall	1094	1052	96.2

* Figure estimated from paper.

Table 8.6 The functional results after compression plating of forearm fractures

Reference	Number of forearms	Number with satisfactory results	Percentage
Anderson et al (1975)	223	200*	89.7
Hadden et al (1983)	111	89†	80.2
Langkamer & Ackroyd (1991)	108	91*	84.3
Chapman et al (1989)	87	79*	90.8
Dodge & Cady (1972)	71	61‡	85.9
Overall	600	520	86.7

* Less than 50% loss of pronation/supination.
† Less than 30% loss of pronation/supination.
‡ Less than 20% loss of forearm rotation.

union rate of forearm fractures for which immediate bone grafting was recommended but not performed. They found that open reduction and internal fixation of comminuted diaphyseal forearm fractures without bone grafting produced union rates comparable to those reported for open reduction and internal fixation with immediate bone grafting. A similar conclusion was reached by Wei et al (1999) in their retrospective study of 64 diaphyseal forearm fractures.

The infection rate after plating of forearm fractures varied between 0.8% (Hertel et al 1996) and 5.5% (Hadden et al 1983).

Moed et al (1986) reported the results of immediate internal fixation of open fractures of the diaphysis of the forearm in 50 patients. Seventy-two of 79 fractures united (91%). As would be expected, the grade 1 compound injuries had a better union rate (96.7%) than the grade 2 (89.6%) or grade 3 injuries (84.2%). The average time to union was 13.2 weeks (12.8 weeks for grade 1 injuries and 13.8 weeks for grade 3 injuries). Excellent or satisfactory results were achieved in 85% of patients, 90% in those with grade 1 injuries as compared with 88% of grade 2 and 70% of grade 3 injuries.

Jones (1991) reported similar functional results following the immediate debridement and plate fixation of grade 3 forearm fractures performed in conjunction with aggressive soft tissue management. He recorded satisfactory results in 66% of his 18 patients.

External fixation

The use of a Hoffmann external fixator for the treatment of acute fractures of the diaphysis of one or both bones of the forearm was reported by Schuind et al (1991). Of the 93 patients reported on, 25 had compound injuries. Non-union occurred in 8.5% of the fractures, the others uniting in a mean of 15 weeks. About 80% had normal forearm rotation.

Smith & Cooney (1990) also recorded the usefulness of external fixation in 32 patients with mainly compound grade 3 injuries. Delayed internal fixation and bone grafting were performed in 16 patients. Using this technique, bony union was achieved in 91% of the fractures. The mean forearm rotation was recorded as 40° of supination and pronation.

Summary

- Undisplaced forearm fractures in adults unite in 6–8 weeks, and displaced fractures heal in 13–20 weeks. 29–59% of patients with displaced fractures treated in above-elbow plaster of paris had a satisfactory result.
- Conservatively treated adult forearm fractures had a non-union rate of 7.2%. Rotation was significantly restricted in 45–60% of patients treated in an above-elbow plaster. Rotation was most restricted in middle third fractures.
- The functional bracing of adult forearm fractures has been reported as achieving excellent results, with a 2% non-union rate and a significant limitation of rotation in 4.5% of patients.
- Union occurred in 91% of adult forearm fractures treated by intramedullary fixation. Union occurred in 10–20 weeks.
- A satisfactory functional end-result was achieved in 84.4% of adult patients after intramedullary fixation of their forearm fractures.
- A union rate of 96.2% occurred following the adequate plating of forearm fractures. The average time to union has been variably reported at 7.4–18.8 weeks. A satisfactory functional result was obtained in 86.7% of patients.
- A 0.8–5.5% infection rate occurred after the plating of forearm fractures.
- There was a 96.7% union rate and a 90% satisfactory functional level achieved after the plating of grade 1 compound fractures.
- An 89.6% union rate and an 88% satisfactory functional level have been reported after the plating of grade 2 compound fractures.
- There was an 84.2% union rate and a 66–70% satisfactory functional level after the plating of grade 3 compound forearm fractures.
- The average time to union after the plating of compound forearm fractures was 13.2 weeks.
- Bony union occurred in 91% of compound fractures treated with external fixators.

Fracture of both bones in children

Fractures of the forearm bones in children respond more readily to conservative treatment than their equivalent fracture in adults: Whipple & St John (1917) reported on the conservative treatment of 95 fractures and reported that 97.9% resulted in a good anatomical result and 96.8% had a good functional result, after an average 18 months' follow-up.

Re-angulation and displacement after closed reduction of pediatric forearm fractures occurred in 7% (Voto et al 1990) to 12.6% (Davis & Green 1976) of patients. The majority of these fractures re-angulate at 1–2 weeks. In the 90 cases reported by Voto et al, all fractures were re-manipulated, all united and all had a functionally satisfactory result.

Thomas et al (1975) found that 65 patients out of 285 (23%) had an unsatisfactory result at 3 months after fracture, but at their 4 year review this number had fallen to eight (3%). All eight patients had incomplete recovery of rotation and none was aware of any functional limitation.

Proximal third fractures

Proximal third fractures account for 7% (Blount et al 1942) to 10% (Cooper 1964) of forearm fractures in children. Fifty percent of Thomas' eight patients with proximal forearm fractures had unsatisfactory results at 3 months, and three patients (37.5%) still had a residual loss of rotation at 4 years, although none was aware of any functional disability. Holdsworth & Sloan (1983) reviewed 51 proximal forearm fractures. Ten patients (19.6%) had lost more than 15° of pronation or supination, but only three were felt to have significant restriction of rotation. Fifteen (29%) had mild symptoms of minor discomfort or aching in cold weather.

Occasionally, these fractures of the proximal forearm in children are unstable with the elbow flexed but stable when the elbow is in extension. Of the 15 patients treated by a cast with the elbow in extension (Walker & Rang 1991), all obtained normal elbow movement at 2 weeks after cast removal and full forearm rotation at follow-up. Only one patient had more than 15° angulation at the time of bony union.

Middle third fractures

Middle third fractures constitute 15 to 18% of forearm fractures in children. Greenstick fractures of the middle third require 4–6 weeks in plaster. Van Herpe (1976) stated that since the diaphysis was the most slowly growing area of bone, virtually no angulation was acceptable at this level. He further stated that there was a great tendency to re-angulation after manipulation unless the intact dorsal bony bridge was broken at the time of reduction. However, Kaya Alpar et al (1981) reported that in his 56 greenstick fractures with angular deformity alone, no subsequent deformity occurred despite leaving the concave cortex intact. Thomas et al (1975) reported that 11 of their 28 middle third fractures (39%) had unsatisfactory results at 3 months, but only two (7%) had a significant restriction of rotation at 4 years. Kaya Alpar et al (1981) found that 10% of their 80 midshaft forearm fractures were angulated by 15° or more, and that all of these had decreased rotation. In those fractures with only one bone displaced in the initial radiograph, conservative treatment was used, but there was a tendency for the fracture to slip, requiring remanipulation. When both bones were displaced the results of conservative treatment were always unsatisfactory, with more than 15° of residual angulation being usual.

Distal third fractures

Distal third forearm fractures account for 75% of forearm fractures in children. Buckle fractures require only 2–3 weeks in a below-elbow plaster. Cooper (1964) stated that 20° of angulation of the distal third of the forearm could be accepted without requiring reduction, while Van Herpe (1976) felt that 30° angulation in children under the age of seven was acceptable. These angulated greenstick fractures and those undisplaced fractures with both cortices broken required a plaster for 6 weeks. Davis & Green (1976) found that 10% of their patients with greenstick fractures re-angulated. They stated that displaced distal third fractures required 6 weeks in plaster after reduction, but 25% of these redisplaced. A similar incidence of re-angulation after manipulation (25.4% of 67 fractures) was noted by Green et al (1998).

Displacement of distal third forearm fractures can occur in a cast even if they were undisplaced or minimally displaced at the time of initial treatment. Schranz & Fagg (1992) reported that the volar (pronation) pattern of greenstick fracture did not seem to progress, while 22.5% of those with a dorsal (supination) pattern of injury showed some radiological progression of the angulation. Of the unicortical fractures, 13.6% showed a progression of the deformity, as compared with 47.6% of the bicortical fractures. Of the unicortical fractures, 7.1% of those showing a dorsal buckle displaced, as compared with 29.4% of those with a cortical breach.

Thomas et al (1975) reported that 45 out of 249 patients (18%) with distal third fractures had unsatisfactory results at 3 months, but only three of 40 patients (7.5%) had an unsatisfactory result at 4 years.

Creasman et al (1984) analysed those factors which might mitigate against a good result (Table 8.7).

Premature closure of the distal ulnar epiphysis has been reported in association with fractures of the distal radius. Ray et al (1996) presented five cases, reviewed the literature, and proposed a classification system and suggested indications for surgical treatment.

Internal fixation

Nielson & Simonsen (1984) reported the results of 29 children with displaced forearm fractures treated with AO plates. All united and there was one case of deep infection. Of 27 patients reviewed, 22 (81.5%) had no loss of rotation and none had lost more than 20° of rotation. They noted a mean total increase in the linear growth of the plated bones of 2.4 mm (range 15 mm lengthening to 6.5 mm shortening), and an average 4.5 mm discrepancy in the lengths of the radius and ulna. This alteration in growth had no obvious effect on function.

Good results have also been reported using intramedullary techniques. The results of the larger reported series are shown in Table 8.8. All the fractures united and the time to union was about 6 weeks (Pugh et al 1999, Lascombe et al 1990). Malunion was not a major complication. Lascombes et al (1990) reported 12 instances of malunion of more than 5° noted immediately postoperatively in their 76 cases. Of these, six had recovered completely 2 years later, while in the other six (8%) some malunion persisted. Three had a deficit of pronation and supination of >20° and one of >30°. Of the 57 forearm fractures reported by Yung et al (1998) five patients (9%) had a residual angulation of 10–15° at a mean follow-up of 20 months.

Van der Reis et al (1998) compared plate and screws fixation with intramedullary nailing for unstable fractures of the radius and ulna in children. A retrospective analysis was made of 23 patients treated with plate-and-screw fixation and 18 who were treated with intramedullary nailing. The functional results, rate of union, and rate of complications were statistically similar for the two groups. Intramedullary fixation allowed a short operative time, excellent cosmesis, minimal soft tissue dissection, ease of hardware removal and early motion after nail removal.

Compound fractures

Haasbeek and Cole (1995) reported their experience of treating 46 children with open forearm fractures. Thirty-five fractures were Gustilo Type I, five Type II and six Type III. Normal union occurred in 36 children (78%),

Table 8.7 Signs suggesting impending problems after children's forearm fractures (after Creasman et al 1984)

Factor	Number of patients with sign	Number (%) unsatisfactory
Angulation 10–30° in any plane	16	5 (31%)
AP bow straightened or reversed	10	6 (60%)
Abnormal bow in lateral plane	8	3 (37.5%)
Displacement >50%	8	2 (25%)
Shortening at distal radioulnar joint	9	3 (33%)
Up to 45° malrotation	9	2 (22%)
Single bone injuries	19	2 (10.5%)
Proximal fractures	6	2 (33%)
Midshaft fractures	31	3 (9.7%)
Distal fractures	20	3 (15%)

Table 8.8 The results of intramedullary fixation of forearm fractures in children

Authors	Number of forearms	Technique	Excellent/ good results	Non-union	Malunions
Lascombes et al (1990)	76	ESIN	70 (92%)	Nil	6 (8%)
Yung et al (1998)	57	K wire	57 (100%)	Nil	5 (9%)
Shoemaker et al (1999)	32	K wire	32 (100%)	Nil	3 (9%)
Pugh et al (1999)	27	SP	32 (100%)	Nil	Nil
Richter et al (1998)	30	ESIN	29 (97%)	Nil	Nil
Total	222		220 (99%)	Nil	14 (6%)

ESIN—Elastic stable intramedullary nailing.

K wire—Kirschner wire.

SP—5/64 inch Steinmann pins.

delayed union was seen in two children (4%), non-union in two (4%), malunion in five (11%) and refracture in four (9%). The long-term results in 38 children were excellent in 21 (55%), good in 12 (32%), fair in four (11%) and poor in one (2%).

Malunion

The remodelling ability of fractures in children is well known, but the degree of residual angulation that can acceptably be left in the knowledge that remodelling will occur is disputed.

Midshaft fractures

Angular deformity resulting from fracture of the midshaft of the forearm will correct poorly, with a resultant reduction in the range of pronation and supination (Gandhi et al 1962). Högström et al (1976) reviewed 25 patients with mainly midshaft fractures, with a minimal angulation at union of 10° (average angulation 20° for the whole group). At final follow-up an average of 10° correction (50% of the original deformity) had occurred. They found that only children under the age of 10 years were able to produce large corrections of growth. They felt that all deformities exceeding 10° in the midshaft should be corrected. Daruwalla (1979) agreed that 10° was the upper limit of angulation that was acceptable in midshaft fractures. Tarr et al (1984) (Table 8.2) confirmed in cadaver studies that a 10° angulation in the midshaft of forearm bones produced less than 20° loss of rotation. Fuller & McCullough (1982) stated that in children aged over 11 years with midshaft fractures spontaneous correction of the malunion could not be anticipated. Roberts (1986) felt that radial deviation of over 15° at the fracture site rather than dorsal angulation was significant in reducing rotation after midshaft fractures.

Price et al (1990) noted a poor correlation between the residual angular deformity and the final range of forearm rotation. Union in malrotation, however, did correlate with restriction of forearm rotation. They noted that complete remodelling occurred in 12 of their 39 patients with malunion, but that remodelling did not correlate with restoration of motion. They concluded that while every effort should be made to obtain anatomic alignment, it was their opinion that 45° of malrotation, 10° of angulation, complete displacement and loss of radial bow could be accepted rather than resorting to open reduction.

Distal third fractures

There would appear to be a better chance of achieving a correction of the malunion of distal third fractures provided that there are enough years left for remodelling to occur before the distal radial epiphysis fuses. This occurs between 15 and 25 years of age (Gandhi 1962). Gandhi found that after 5 years of remodelling there was a 98% correction of the distal third malalignment. Daruwalla (1979) felt that 15° of angulation of the distal third could be expected to remodel, and Friberg (1979) reported that only two of his four patients with 20° of angulation achieved full correction. Fuller & McCullough (1982) reported that a 20° residual angulation produced a 30° loss of rotation, and they felt that limitation of rotation of the forearm was directly related to the angular deformity.

However, Nilsson & Obrant (1977) reported an approximate 20° loss of rotation in 18 fractures that had healed with no angular deformity, implying that factors other than residual deformity were responsible for this dysfunction.

Trousdale & Linscheid (1995) reported the results of 27 consecutive osteotomies for malunited fractures of the forearm. Twenty patients had osteotomy because of functional loss of motion. Those who had their corrective surgery within 12 months of the original injury gained an average of 79° while those whose surgery was delayed beyond 12 months gained an average of only 30°. Six patients had their osteotomy for an unstable and painful distal radio-ulnar joint. Three achieved a painfree stable joint and they lost an average of 7° of forearm rotation. One patient who had a corrective osteotomy for cosmetic reasons lost 10° of rotation. Thirteen patients had some form of complication.

Blackburn et al (1984) reported the results of a drill osteoclasis in 15 children with significant malunion of the forearm. Eleven of these children regained full pronation and supination.

Refracture

In children, refracture of a forearm bone is not uncommon, the reported incidence being between 5% (Schwarz et al 1996) and 6% (Bould et al 1997). Schwarz et al performed a retrospective study of 28 refractures of the forearm in children. The cause for the refractures was incomplete healing of a primary greenstick fracture in 21 cases (84%). In all but one of these there was persistent angulation, usually in a dorsal direction with incomplete consolidation of the original fracture. The gap in the fractured cortex had widened during immobilisation and on this side of the bone there had been no bony bridging before refracture. Conservative treatment of the refracture gave good results in 14 out of 17 patients (82%), the other three patients having a pronounced restriction of forearm rotation. Bould et al (1997) reported that refracture was five times more likely in a mid shaft fracture compared to any other site.

Plastic deformation

Plastic deformation was first described by Barton in 1821 (see King 1984). Borden (1974) described eight patients, but found manipulative reduction of little benefit in six of these. Sanders & Heckman (1984), however, achieved an average correction of 85% of the angulation, but stressed that many minutes of sustained manipulation may be required to reduce the deformity. They described one case in an adult, as did Greene (1982). As discussed above, residual deformity will be related to residual angulation.

Summary

- 97% of children had a satisfactory functional result after the conservative treatment of forearm fractures.
- 20–37.5% of proximal third fractures had more than 15° loss of rotation, although there could still be normal function.
- 7–10% of middle third forearm fractures in children lost more than 15° of rotation.
- 10% of angulated greenstick distal third fractures, and 25% of displaced distal third fractures, will re-angulate in plaster. Significant rotation is lost in 7.5%.
- Children's forearm fractures treated with AO plates achieved full rotation in 81.5% of cases.
- 99% of children's forearm fractures treated by intramedullary techniques had an excellent or good functional result. Malunion occurred in 6% of cases.
- 87% of children with compound forearm fractures had an excellent/good functional result.
- Only 10° of angulation of midshaft forearm fractures in children aged under 10 was acceptable, while in those over the age of 10 even less angulation was acceptable as remodelling was less likely to occur.

- 15° of angulation was acceptable in distal third fractures unless the patient was close to cessation of bone growth.
- Loss of rotation may be related to factors other than residual angulation.
- Osteotomy for malunion may result in an excellent outcome in over 70% of patients.
- Refracture occurs in 5–6% of patients and is most likely to occur in mid shaft fractures.
- An 85% improvement of angulation can be expected in plastic deformation after manipulation.

Isolated fracture of the ulna

Isolated fractures of the shaft of the ulna, without dislocation of the radial head, have a reputation for being slow to heal and of having a high incidence of non-union. This has led some authors to recommend internal fixation as the routine treatment for these fractures.

Smith & Sage (1957) noted a non-union rate of 20% in 79 isolated ulna fractures treated by various intramedullary fixation devices. However, Boriani et al (1991) achieved 100% union in 22 fractures treated by an intramedullary nail. Consolidation occurred at an average of 2.5 months.

The results of the plating of isolated ulna shaft fractures are shown in Table 8.9. Union occurred in 95% of the reported cases, in an average of 8.8–12.7 weeks. Satisfactory functional results were recorded in 83% of cases, although different criteria for assessing function were used in these papers.

Labbe et al (1999) compared 57 patients with isolated ulna shaft fracture treated by open reduction and plate fixation with 56 patients operated on by percutaneous intramedullary nailing. In the group operated on by plate fixation there was a 29.8% complication rate including

Table 8.9 The results of plating of isolated ulnar fractures

Reference	Number of fractures	Number united	Time to union	Satisfactory functional results
Anderson et al (1975)	50	48 (96%)	8.8 weeks	43 of 46 (93.5%)
Corea et al (1981)	47	42 (89%)	12.7 weeks	24 of 35 (69%) (good)
Hooper (1974)	16	16		14 of 16 (87.5%)
Szabo & Skinner (1990)	18	17 (94%)		
Chapman et al (1989)	27	27	12 weeks	22 of 27 (81.5%)
Overall	158	150 (95%)		103 of 124 (83%)

osteomyelitis, non-union, plate breakage, screw loosening and refracture. This compared with a few minor complications in the intramedullary nailing group.

Corea et al (1981) reported that the mean time to union in their 254 cases was 12.7 weeks, with little difference being noticed between conservative treatment or internal fixation.

An above-elbow plaster of paris has been the traditional conservative method of treatment.

The results of plaster immobilisation in the treatment of isolated ulnar fractures is shown in Table 8.10. Union occurred in 98.9% of these fractures between 7 and 10.8 weeks. Satisfactory functional results were seen in 93 and 96.5% of patients. With the use of a forearm brace alone or with elastic support, union was 99% and occurred in 6.7–9.1 weeks, with functional loss being minimal. Most of these cases were undisplaced or minimally displaced (Sarmiento et al 1998).

Brakenbury et al (1981) reported 21 non-unions out of 254 isolated ulnar fractures, the incidence being higher in midshaft fractures. A 20% non-union rate was seen in fractures with more than 50% shaft displacement and open reduction had three times the non-union rate of conservatively treated fractures (4.9% compared with 17.4%).

Summary

■ Conservatively treated isolated ulnar shaft fractures had a low non-union rate (1%) and healed in 7–10.8 weeks. Satisfactory function can be expected in 93–96.5% of patients.

■ Rigid plating of isolated ulnar shaft fractures produced a slower rate to radiological union (8.8–12.7 weeks), satisfactory functional results in 83% and a higher non-union rate (5%). These tend to be higher-energy injuries.

Complications of forearm fractures
Non-union

The incidence of non-union in forearm fractures is discussed under the various sections. Good reports of union

Table 8.10 The results of the conservative treatment of isolated ulnar fractures

Reference	Type of Treatment	Number of cases	Number united	Healing time (weeks)	Function
Altner & Hartman (1972)	AEPOP	151	150 (99%)	7 distal, 10 proximal	94% satisfactory
Du Toit & Gräbe (1979)	AEPOP	63	63	7.6	
Sarmiento et al (1998)	Brace	287	284 (99%)	9.1	(i) Loss 13° rotation Proximal third
					(ii) Loss 12° rotation middle third
					(iii) Loss 12° rotation distal third 89% excellent 7.5% good 3.5% poor
Pollock et al (1983)	(i) AEPOP	12	11 (92%)	10.5	Average loss 8° rotation
	(ii) Brace or nil	42	42	6.7	Average loss 5° rotation
Goel et al (1991)	(i) POP	28	26 (96%)	10.8	92.9% satisfactory
	(ii) Elastic support	32	32	7.8	100% satisfactory

following surgery for non-union of forearm fractures have been provided by various authors. De Buren (1962) reported 34 successes in 36 non-unions (94%) treated with a plate and cancellous bone graft, with 27 uniting in 4 months. Rosen (1979) reported a 95% success rate in 21 non-unions treated with compression plates, applied with and without cancellous bone graft. Union occurred in an average of about 6 months, with hypertrophic non-unions healing in approximately 4 months and atrophic non-unions in 5–8 months.

Scaglietti et al (1965) reported a 92% union rate in 102 non-unions treated with onlay cortical grafts. Christensen (1976) had less success with intramedullary Küntschner nails without grafting. Only 75% of 20 fractures healed primarily and in four of these X-rays were not consolidated at 1 year.

Heppenstall et al (1983) had an 80% union rate in 40 non-unions treated with DC electrical stimulation, but cautioned against its use when large fracture gaps or infections were present. Encouraging results have been reported by Dell & Sheppard (1984) in the use of vascularised fibular grafts in four infected non-unions, converting them to one-bone forearms.

Twenty-four cases of segmental bone loss and associated non-union were treated with an intercalary bone graft and internal fixation with a cortical bone graft fixed opposite to a plate (Moroni et al 1997). The average length of bone defect was 3.6 cms. In 23 cases union was achieved. Sixteen patients had an excellent or satisfactory functional result.

Nerve and tendon lesions

Smith & Sage (1957) reported 53 nerve lesions (31 radial, 10 ulnar, four median, eight mixed) in 338 fractures (15.7%) treated by intramedullary nailing, but one-third of these patients had compound injuries. The true incidence in closed forearm fractures is much lower than this, and lies somewhere between 0.9% (Davis & Green 1976) and 5% (Hadden et al 1983). These lesions are usually transient and all the main nerve trunks have been involved. Altner & Deeney et al (1998) reported seven cases of patients whose flexor digitorum profundus tendons were adherent to the callus of an isolated ulnar fracture, causing impaired function and a pseudo-Volkmann's contracture. Mackay & Simpson (1980) reported the closed rupture of the extensor digitorum communis tendon following a fracture of the lower end of the radius, with anterior displacement.

Six cases of loss of flexor pollicis longus functions after plating of a radius fracture were presented by Keogh et al (1997). The exact aetiology was uncertain but was felt to be a traction neuropraxia of the anterior interosseous nerve branches to the muscle. All six patients had achieved full recovery within 5 months.

Synostosis

Vince and Miller (1987a,b) reported the results of the treatment of 28 patients and 10 children with cross-union as a complication of forearm fractures. They found the overall incidence in adults was 2%. In children the incidence was 5.7% for proximal fractures, while it was very rare in middle and distal third injuries. Bauer et al (1991) found the incidence of synostosis occurring between the radius and ulna was 11 out of 167 forearm fractures (6.6%) treated with plate fixation. They also found that the incidence was increased when a single incision was used to approach both bones, and in fractures of the proximal third of the radius and ulna. Vince & Miller divided cross-union into three types: type 1 occurred in the distal intra-articular part of the radius and ulna; type 2 in the middle, or the non-articular part of the distal third of the radius and ulna; and type 3 cross-union occurred in the proximal third. The type 1 injuries in adults were uncommon (four cases) and none occurred in children. This type occurred after Colles' fractures in each case: all four underwent surgery but only one had a satisfactory result.

Type 2 injuries were most common in adults (14 cases), with only three cases occurring in children. These cases tended to occur after severe trauma and an associated head injury was common. This association with head injury has been noted by others (Hadden et al 1983). Ten type 2 cross-unions in adults were excised; 70% had satisfactory functional results and there were no recurrences. Three were excised in children, with one satisfactory result and one recurrence.

Ten type 3 cross-unions occurred in adults, again associated with severe trauma. Six occurred in children, only two after high-energy injuries, and three of these six children had undergone open reduction. Surgery was performed in three of the adult cases and two synostoses recurred. In three children the radial head was excised in an attempt to improve movement, but a satisfactory result was achieved only in the patient who had a prosthesis inserted to replace the excised radial head.

Failla et al (1989) reported the results of surgical excision of post-traumatic proximal radio-ulnar synostosis in 20 adults. According to their grading system, four patients had an excellent result (at least 50° each of pronation and supination), three a good result (at least 30° each of pronation and supination), four a fair result (a total arc of rotation of more than 30°) and nine poor results. The average total arc of postoperative rotation was 55°. In most of these patients failure was evident within a few months of excision of the area of synostosis. No patient lost more rotation after 6 months, nor did any patient lose motion once motion had remained stable for 3 months postoperatively. None of the patients operated on within 12 months of injury, or more than 3 years after injury, had a good result, suggesting that treatment too soon or too long after injury may be associated with a worse prognosis.

Refracture after plate removal

There is considerable debate concerning the incidence of refracture after plate removal, but it would appear to be a significant rate, especially if the plate is removed less than 1 year from its application. Anderson et al (1975) removed the plates routinely from less than 10% of their 244 patients, and had eight refractures when the plates were removed before 1 year. They now leave the plate for 12–18 months and apply a protective splint for 4–6 weeks after plate removal. However, they do not recommend the routine removal of plates, a view endorsed by Langkamer & Ackroyd (1990), who found that 22 out of 55 patients (40%) who had undergone elective removal of forearm plates had a significant wound infection, five (9%) had a poor scar, 17 (31%) had neurological problems, and two patients (3.6%) refractured. Chia et al (1996) noted two refractures in 82 forearm bones (2.4%) after plate removal, and a similar rate of refracture (4.3%) was reported by Hertel et al (1996) after plate removal in 70 patients. Minor complications ranging from mild superficial wound infection to nerve injury occurred in 20 patients (24.4%) of Chia's series. Nielsen & Simonsen (1984) reported a 3.4% refracture rate after plate removal in 29 children.

Summary

- Non-union of forearm fractures treated with compression plates with and without bone graft healed in 94–95% of cases. Hypertrophic non-unions healed in 4 months and atrophic non-unions in 5–8 months.
- Nerve injuries were associated with 0.9–5% of closed forearm fractures, although these injuries were invariably transient.
- Rarely, flexor or extensor tendons may be compromised by forearm fractures.
- Synostosis occurred in 2–6% of adults and 5.7% of proximal third fractures in children.
- Of cross-unions in adults, 35–52% had satisfactory function after surgery, the most success occurring in the type 2 injuries (70% success rate).
- Of cross-unions in children, 33% had satisfactory function after surgery.

- Refracture after plate removal occurred in up to 4.3% of forearms. Plates should not be removed before 18 months if possible.

Monteggia fracture–dislocation
Incidence and classification

Although uncommon, Monteggia fracture–dislocations of the forearm are by no means rare, occurring in 0.7% of elbow injuries and from 5% (Altner 1981) to 9.9% (May & Mauck 1961) of fractures of the radius and ulna. However, judging from the reported series, a large number are not diagnosed on presentation. Speed & Boyd (1940) reported that 52% of Monteggia fractures were diagnosed 4 weeks or longer after the accident, although the number from the same centre had dropped to 23% by 1969 (Boyd & Boals 1969). However, other articles have quoted the incidence at between 16% (Dormans & Rang 1990) and 21% (Edwards 1952). In a more recent paper, Weisman et al (1999) reported that the diagnosis of dislocation of the radial head, either in isolation or as part of a Monteggia fracture–dislocation, was delayed in 10 of 110 children treated with those injuries. In eight children the dislocation was overlooked on the initial radiographs. However, in two children the radial head was reduced on the initial elbow radiograph but was found to be dislocated 10 days later in one child and 21 days later in the other.

Bado's 1967 classification of Monteggia fractures or lesions is the most widely used:

- type 1—anterior dislocation of the radial head with a fracture of the ulnar diaphysis at any level with anterior angulation
- type 2—posterior or posterolateral dislocation of the radial head with a fracture of the ulnar diaphysis with posterior angulation
- type 3—lateral or anterolateral dislocation of the radial head with a fracture of the ulnar metaphysis
- type 4—anterior dislocation of the radial head with a fracture of the proximal third of the radius and a fracture of the ulna at the same level

He also described some Monteggia equivalent lesions as follows:

- anterior dislocation of the radial head
- a fracture of the ulnar diaphysis with fracture of the neck of the radius
- a fracture of the ulnar diaphysis with fracture of the proximal third of the radius, with the radial fracture always proximal to the ulnar one

- a fracture of the ulnar diaphysis with anterior dislocation of the radial head and fracture of the olecranon
- a posterior dislocation of the elbow and fracture of the ulnar diaphysis, with or without fracture of the proximal radius

Bado pointed out that in the type 2 Monteggia lesion a lesion at the wrist very frequently coexisted.

Monteggia fracture–dislocations in adults

The incidence of the different types of Monteggia fracture–dislocations in adults is shown in Table 8.11. Overall, 50% are type I, and 42% type II, although Ring et al (1998) reported a 78% incidence of the posterior (type II) fracture–dislocation. However, this figure is exceptionally high compared with other reported series.

It is difficult to compare these series because of the differing criteria for functional assessment. Reckling (1982) based his final result on the active range of motion of the wrist, forearm and elbow. A good result was one with less than a 10° loss of motion, a fair result had more than 10° but less than 30° loss of motion, and a poor result had more than 30° loss of motion in either plane. Boyd & Boals' 1969 criteria were as follows:

- excellent—a full range of flexion–extension and pronation–supination

- good—at least 75° motion in flexion–extension and pronation–supination 50% of normal or better
- fair—at least 50° motion in flexion–extension and 50% of pronation–supination
- poor—less than 50° motion in flexion–extension, and less than 50° pronation–supination

Bryan's 1971 criteria, while not exactly the same, were similar, while Ring et al (1998) used a points system.

Table 8.12 is thus constructed using the individual authors' grading for comparison. It can be seen that 63% of patients achieved an excellent or good results, as compared with 37% who achieved a fair or poor result. Although the number of patients reported on is small, no patient achieved a good result by closed methods of treatment of the ulnar fracture. Some form of internal fixation of the ulna gave superior results to closed treatment. Most early series used a variety of non-rigid internal fixations, such as intramedullary rods. Compression plates are the preferred treatment of choice in more modern papers.

An exception to this view, that adult patients with Monteggia fracture–dislocations do not achieve good results if the ulnar fracture is not internally fixed, has come from China. Shang et al (1987) reported the results of the treatment of 259 Monteggia fractures treated by a combination of traditional Chinese and Western medicine,

---

Table 8.11 The incidence of the different types of Monteggia fracture–dislocations in adults

Reference	Number of cases	Type I	Type II	Type III	Type IV
Reckling (1982)	24	19 (79%)	5 (21%)	–	–
Ring et al (1998)	51	8 (16%)	40 (78%)	1 (2%)	2 (4%)
Givon et al (1997)	27	21 (78%)*	1 (4%)	1 (4%)	4 (14%)
Bryan (1971)	23	14 (61%)	6 (26%)	3 (13%)	–
Overall	125	62 (50%)	52 (42%)	5 (4%)	6 (4%)

* Type I and I-equivalent lesions.

Table 8.12 Overall results of the treatment of Monteggia fracture–dislocations in adults

Reference	Number of cases	Excellent/good	Fair/Poor
Reynders et al (1996)	67	36 (54%)	31 (46%)
Boyd & Boals (1969)	74	57 (77%)	17 (23%)
Ring et al (1998)	48	40 (83%)	8 (17%)
Bryan (1971)	27	15 (56%)	12 (44%)
Reckling (1982)	30	6 (20%)	24 (80%)
Overall	246	154 (63%)	92 (37%)

with 159 patients (90%) achieving an excellent or good result (although the criteria for these gradings were not specified).

There is insufficient data in the literature from which to draw any strong conclusions as to the results to be expected from the various types of Monteggia fracture–dislocation. Reynders et al (1996), in their multi-centre review of 67 adult patients with Monteggia lesions, reported excellent results in type I and III lesions and unsatisfactory results in type II and IV lesions. Givon et al (1997) reported significantly worse functional results in their type I equivalent injury. Ring et al (1998) found that the type II lesion was the most difficult to treat; while 83% of patients in their series achieved a satisfactory result, a number of re-operations or reconstructive procedures were necessary in some of these patients. If the result of the index operation alone is taken before re-operation or reconstructions then 16 (33%) of their 48 patients had an unsatisfactory initial outcome as compared with 13 (50%) of the 26 patients with a Bado type II fracture.

Warnock et al (1998) reported the results of the treatment of Bado type I fractures in 21 patients treated by means of open reduction and internal fixation with a compression plate. All fractures united without the need for re-operation. Seventeen (81%) were rated as good or excellent.

Those papers looking exclusively at the posterior (type II) Monteggia fracture are listed in Table 8.13. It can be seen that almost 74% of these fractures have an associated radial head fracture. Approximately 67% of these reported cases had a satisfactory functional result from their treatment.

Barquet & Caresani (1981) reported 14 cases of fracture of the shaft of ulna and radius with associated dislocation of the radial head (type IV). Five of these 14 patients (36%) achieved an excellent/good result by various methods of internal fixation, although they stated a preference for rigid fixation by means of compression plates.

Monteggia fracture–dislocation in children
The incidence of the different types of Monteggia fracture–dislocation in children is shown in Table 8.14.

Table 8.13 The results of the treatment of posterior (type II) Monteggia fractures

Reference	Number of cases	Radial head fractures	Fixation	Results
Ring et al (1998)	38	28	Compression plates	32 satisfactory, 6 unsatisfactory*
Pavel et al (1965)	18	13	Various	7 satisfactory 11 unsatisfactory
Jupiter et al (1991)	13*	10	Compression plates	Function: 6 satisfactory 5 unsatisfactory
Overall	69	51 (74%)		45 (67%) satisfactory 22 (33%) unsatisfactory

* 11 patients assessed for function.

Table 8.14 The incidence of the different types of Monteggia fracture–dislocations in children

Reference	Number of cases	Type I	Type II	Type III	Type IV
Wiley & Galey (1985)	46	22 (48%)	5 (11%)	18 (39%)	1 (2%)
Letts et al (1985)	33	28 (85%)	1 (3%)	4 (12%)	–
Peiró et al (1977)	25	18 (72%)	1 (4%)	6 (24%)	–
Ring & Waters (1996)	36	20 (55.5%)	1 (3%)	11 (30.5%)	4 (11%)
Dormans & Rang (1990)	50	36 (72%)	3 (6%)	9 (18%)	2 (4%)
Overall	190	124 (65%)	11 (6%)	48 (25%)	7 (4%)

Comparison with Table 8.11 shows that the lateral displacement (type III) injury is more common in children, while the posterior displacement (type II) injury is more common in adults.

A comparison of those series reporting the treatment of these fractures in children is given in Table 8.15. While excellent/good results are the rule, poor results do occur, although none was recorded in the larger series that have been shown in Table 8.15. The results appear to be good no matter which type of fracture–dislocation was being reported or which method of treatment was used. Closed reduction of the dislocated radial head and closed manipulation of the fracture with plaster immobilisation would appear to be the treatment of choice. Open reduction of a radial head which remains dislocated despite attempts at closed reduction is occasionally required, as is intramedullary fixation or compression plating for unstable fractures.

Kuksov (1997) preferred open reduction with intramedullary fixation of the ulna with Kirschner wires for unstable type I and type IV fractures. Of the 57 children reviewed, 49 (86%) had an excellent anatomical and functional result with no deformity and a full range of movement. Four patients had radiographic evidence of subluxation of the radial head but full movement. Three patients had a breakage of the transarticular wire and required a further operation. They had a slight restriction of movement. One patient had a radio-ulnar synostosis. It can be seen that these results compare unfavourably with the results of conservative treatment.

Ring & Waters (1996), however, reported good results after operative fixation in 18 cases. The two poor results occurred in patients in whom malalignment and dislocation of the radial head persisted for at least 2 weeks before definitive treatment.

Normal function was usually restored by 2–3 months after injury.

Wiley & Galey (1985) found increased hyperextension of the elbow by 5–10° in 12 patients out of their series of 31 (39%). Similarly, Letts et al (1985) noted that 10 of their 22 patients (45%) had a mild hyperextension of the elbow of 5° more than the uninjured side.

Complications of Monteggia fracture–dislocations
Malunion

Although some patients with persistent subluxation and dislocation of the radial head had almost perfect function of the elbow, the majority had limited movements of flexion–extension and pronation–supination, muscle atrophy, weakness of the extremity, pain on heavy lifting, arthritic changes about the head of the radius and, in children, usually an increase in the carrying angle (Speed & Boyd 1940).

Verboom et al (1999) reviewed 16 patients who had surgery for missed Monteggia fractures. Ten had a proximal ulnar osteotomy, two had resection of the radial head, one an open reduction of the radial head, while three patients had closed treatment. Eight of the 10 patients who had a proximal ulnar osteotomy had a satisfactory result, while the results after radial head resection were poor.

McGuire & Myers (1986) reported the restoration of normal elbow function in seven cases of missed Monteggia fracture treated by simple ulnar osteotomy without a direct operation on the radial head.

Bell Tawse (1965) utilised a strip of fascia from the triceps tendon to refashion the annular ligament. No osteotomy of the ulna was performed. Almost full movement was restored, apart from slight limitation of pronation in some patients.

Nerve lesions

Although the incidence of nerve lesions in Monteggia fracture–dislocations varied from series to series, in those series that have been reviewed the overall incidence was 16%, which correlates well with the 17% occurrence

Table 8.15 The results of treatment of Monteggia fracture–dislocation in children

Reference	Number of patients	Excellent/good	Fair/Poor
Wiley & Galey (1985)	31	31 (100%)	0
Peiró et al (1977)	25	25 (100%)	0
Letts et al (1985)	23	22 (96%)	1 (4%)
Ring & Waters (1996)	36	34 (94%)	2 (6%)
Bado (1967)	18	18 (100%)	0
Overall	133	130 (98%)	3 (2%)

reported by Altner (1981), but it is lower than the 26% incidence of Dormans & Rang (1990). Although the radial nerve or posterior interosseous nerve is usually involved, Wiley & Galey (1985) reported involvement of the anterior interosseous nerve, and Stein et al (1971) reported ulnar nerve involvement. The posterior interosseous nerve is also vulnerable at the time of open reduction of the radial head. In the case reported by Spar (1977), it was actually wrapped round the radial head and was acting as a block to reduction.

Spontaneous recovery of function within 6–8 weeks would appear to be the rule following neuropraxia at time of injury or peroperatively (Dormans & Rang 1990). Although Stein et al (1971) explored six of their seven nerve lesions and recommend surgical decompression of involved nerves, the majority of reported cases have resolved without recourse to decompression.

Tardy palsy of the posterior interosseous nerve has been described following untreated Monteggia lesions. Lichter & Jacobsen (1975) described a case developing 39 years after injury, treated by radial head excision and decompression, with almost full return of function. Austin's 1976 case occurred 65 years after the initial injury. Holst-Nielsen & Jensen (1984) treated their two patients by splitting the ligament of Frohse, with full return of function, 30 and 39 years, respectively, after the intial injury

Summary

- Monteggia fracture–dislocations occurred in 0.7% of elbow injuries and 5–9.9% of fractures of the radius and ulna.
- Wrist lesions have been seen in association with type II injuries and 74% have an associated radial head fracture.
- 50% of Monteggia fracture–dislocations in adults were of type I, 42% were of type II, 4% were of type III, and 4% were of type IV.
- Overall, 63% of adult Monteggia fracture–dislocations achieved an excellent or good result, stable internal fixation with closed or open reduction of the radial head giving the best functional result.
- 65% of Monteggia fracture–dislocations in children were of type 1, 6% were of type II, 25% were of type III, while the 4% type IV lesions.
- An excellent/good result occurred in 98% of children, despite the type of fracture or the method of treatment. The disability time was from 6–12 weeks.
- A mild hyperextension deformity was seen in 39–45% of children after Monteggia fracture–dislocation.

- Persistent dislocation of the radial head limited elbow movement and caused an increase in the carrying angle in some children. Satisfactory improvement in function has been reported following various surgical treatments for persistent malunion.
- Tardy palsy of the posterior interosseous nerve has been reported up to 65 years after initial injury.
- Nerve lesions (usually posterior interosseous) occurred in 16–26% of Monteggia fracture–dislocations. Spontaneous recovery was the rule.

Galeazzi fracture–dislocation
Introduction

The term 'Galeazzi fracture' was originally applied to radial fractures occurring at the junction of the middle and distal thirds of the shaft. It is now more generally used to describe radial fractures at any level associated with disruption of the inferior radio-ulnar joint.

Mikic (1975) reported that 57% of the fractures in his series (of mainly adult patients) occurred at the junction of the middle and distal thirds of the radius and 31% in the middle third of the radial shaft. Only 4% occurred in the distal third of the radius.

Moore et al (1985) reported a 6.8% incidence of Galeazzi fracture (84 cases) out of a series of 1236 forearm fractures in adults. Wong (1967) found the incidence in adults to be slightly higher in Singapore, where 38 cases out of a series of 364 forearm fractures (10.4%) were of the Galeazzi type.

Galeazzi fracture–dislocation in adults

The conservative treatment of this type of fracture in adults has produced poor results, Hughston (1957) reporting only three good ones out of 38 patients (8%) treated by closed reduction and immobilisation. A similar poor result following conservative treatment was reported from Singapore, where Wong (1967) had only three satisfactory results out of 34 patients (9%). Mikic (1975) found that the healing time for these fractures in adults was 2–3 months. On the other hand, Shang et al (1987) reported 81% satisfactory results in 236 cases of Galeazzi fracture treated by a combination of traditional Chinese and Western medicine. However, the criteria for their functional assessment were not stated.

Intramedullary fixation devices and compression plates have been utilised in the operative treatment of this type of fracture. Although Mikic (1975) reported 68% excellent results from 19 Rush intramedullary pins, compared with 50% from 12 cases plated, more recently published papers suggest that rigid fixation for this fracture gives better results.

Reckling (1982) reported good results in all 17 of his patients treated by immediate open reduction. Kraus & Horne (1985) noted 25 satisfactory results in 27 patients (92.5%) treated by plate fixation. Moore et al (1985) reported two non-unions in 36 fractures (5.5%) treated with compression plates, although both united after second plates and bone grafts were applied. Final healing was rated as excellent in 35 of the 36 fractures (97%). Eighty percent of these patients had an excellent range of movement (less than 10° loss of wrist flexion–extension and less than 25° loss of pronation–supination). Similarly, function was rated as excellent in 78% of the patients, while only one patient (3%) had a poor functional result. However, grip strength was normal in only seven patients (20%). The average loss of grip strength was 33% in males and 20% in females. Bhan & Rath (1991) compared the results of the early and late treatment of Galeazzi fractures. Of the 20 patients treated within 2 weeks by plate fixation, 16 (80%) had an excellent functional result. Of the 24 cases treated between 2 and 10 weeks by a plate and bone graft, 19 (79%) had an excellent result. All seven cases treated after 6 months had poor results.

Ulnar and anterior interosseous nerve lesions are occasionally reported in association with Galeazzi fracture–dislocation. Mikic (1975) found only one ulnar nerve injury in his 125 patients with this fracture.

Occasionally, irreducible dislocation of the distal radio-ulnar joint can occur in Galeazzi fractures due to entrapment of extensor tendons. The extensor carpi ulnaris and extensor tendons to the ring and little finger have been implicated (Jenkins et al 1987).

Galeazzi fracture–dislocation in children

The reported results of the treatment of Galeazzi fracture–dislocations in children tend to be better than those for adults, although Wong (1967) reported that all six children in his series had unsatisfactory results after conservative management.

Better results were reported by Walsh et al (1987). In 17 of the 41 patients (41%) in this series, the injury to the distal radio-ulnar joint was not recognised initially. Overall, of 39 fractures treated conservatively, 24 (61.5%) had excellent results and 12 (30.5%) had fair results. Excellent results were more readily achieved when the fracture was at the junction of the middle and distal third (75%), than with fractures of the distal third (47.5%). Below-elbow plasters gave excellent results in seven of 16 cases (43.5%), while above-elbow plasters gave excellent results in 17 of 23 cases (74%). The authors found that the healing time for children with these fractures was 4–6 weeks.

King (1984) stated that 10° of angulation in these radial shaft fractures in children was acceptable, and that no loss of pronation or supination would result.

A variant of the Galeazzi fracture–dislocation in children, in which the fracture of the radius is associated with a Salter–Harris type II epiphyseal fracture of the distal ulnar physis, has been described by Landfried et al (1991). All three cases regained full function after internal fixation.

Summary

- Only 8–9% of adult patients achieved a satisfactory result after the conservative treatment of Galeazzi fracture–dislocations. Satisfactory results have been reported in 68% of patients following intramedullary fixation, and in 80–100% of patients after compression plates.
- Grip strength was impaired by 33% in males and 20% in females after the compression plating of these fractures.
- Nerve palsies were infrequent.
- An excellent result was achieved in 61.5% of conservatively treated Galeazzi fractures in children, while 30.5% achieved a fair result.
- Distal third fractures and treatment in below-elbow plasters resulted in a worse result than fractures at the junction of the middle and distal third and above-elbow immobilisation.
- The healing time in children was 4–6 weeks.
- 10° of angulation can be accepted with no anticipated loss of function.

References

Altner P C 1981 Monteggia fractures. Orthopaedic Review 10: 115–120

Altner P C, Hartman J T 1972 Isolated fractures of the ulnar shaft in the adult. Surgical Clinics of North America 52: 155–170

Anderson L D, Sisk T D, Tooms R E, Park W I 1975 Compression-plate fixation in acute diaphyseal fractures of the radius and ulna. Journal of Bone and Joint Surgery 57A: 287–297

Austin R 1976 Tardy palsy of the radial nerve from a Monteggia fracture. Injury 7: 202–204

Bado J L 1967 The Monteggia lesion. Clinical Orthopaedics 50: 71–86

Barquet A, Caresani J 1981 Fracture of the shaft of the ulna and radius with associated dislocation of the radial head. Injury 12: 471–476

Bauer G, Arand M, Mutschler W 1991 Post-traumatic radioulnar synostosis after forearm fracture osteosynthesis. Archives of Orthopaedics and Traumatic Surgery 110: 142–145

Bell Tawse A J S 1965 The treatment of malunited anterior Monteggia fractures in children. Journal of Bone and Joint Surgery 47B: 718–723

Bhan S, Rath S 1991 Management of the Galeazzi fracture. International Orthopaedics 15: 193–196

Blackburn N, Ziv I, Rang M 1984 Correction of the malunited forearm fracture. Clinical Orthopaedics 188: 54–57

Blount W P, Schaefer A A, Johnson J H 1942 Fractures of the forearm in children. Journal of the American Medical Association 120: 111–117

Bolton H, Quinlan A G 1952 The conservative treatment of fractures of the shaft of the radius and ulna in adults. Lancet 2: 700–705

Borden S 1974 Traumatic bowing of the forearm in children. Journal of Bone and Joint Surgery 56A: 611–616

Boriani S, Lefevre C, Malingue E, Bettelli G 1991 The Lefevre ulnar nail. Chirurgia Degli Organi di Movimento 76: 151–155

Bould M, Bannister G C, Foster R P 1997 Re-fractures of the radius and ulna in children. Journal of Bone and Joint Surgeon 79B: supp II: 187

Boyd H B, Boals J C 1969 The Monteggia lesion. Clinical Orthopaedics 66: 94–100

Bradford E H, Adams R W, Kilfoyle R M 1953 Fractures of both bones of the forearm in adults. Surgery, Gynaecology and Obstetrics 96: 240–244

Brakenbury P H, Corea J R, Blakemore M E 1981 Non-union of the isolated fracture of the ulnar shaft in adults. Injury 12: 371–375

Bryan R S 1971 Monteggia fracture of the forearm. Journal of Trauma 11: 992–998

Burwell H N, Charnley A D 1984 Treatment of forearm fractures in adults with particular reference to plate fixation. Journal of Bone and Joint Surgery 46B: 404–425

Caden J G 1961 Internal fixation of fractures of the forearm. Journal of Bone and Joint Surgery 43A: 1115–1121

Chapman M W, Gordon J E, Zissimos A G 1989 Compression-plate fixation of acute fractures of the diaphyses of the radius and ulna. Journal of Bone and Joint Surgery 71A: 159–170

Chia J, Soh C R, Wong H P, Low Y P 1996 Complications following metal removal: a follow-up of surgically treated forearm fractures. Singapore Medical Journal 37: 268–269

Christensen N O 1976 Küntschner intramedullary reaming and nail fixation for non-union of the forearm. Clinical Orthopaedics 116: 215–221

Cooper R R 1964 Management of common forearm fractures in children. Journal of the Iowa Medical Society 54: 589–598

Corea J R, Brakenbury P H, Blakemore M E 1981 The treatment of isolated fractures of the ulnar shaft in adults. Injury 12: 365–370

Cotler J M, Ingemi B J, Prabhaker M P 1971 Experience with Schneider nailing in forearm fractures. In: Proceedings of the American Academy of Orthopedic Surgeons. Journal of Bone and Joint Surgery 53A: 1228–1229

Creasman C, Zaleske D J, Ehrlich M G 1984 Analyzing forearm fractures in children. Clinical Orthopaedics 188: 40–53

Daruwalla J S 1979 A study of radioulnar movements following fractures of the forearm in children. Clinical Orthopaedics 139: 114–120

Davis D R, Green D P 1976 Forearm fractures in children. Clinical Orthopaedics 120: 172–184

De Buren N 1962 Causes and treatment of non-union in fractures of the radius and ulna. Journal of Bone and Joint Surgery 44B: 614–625

Deeney V F, Kaye J J, Geary S P, Cole W G 1998 Pseudo-Volkmann's contracture due to tethering of flexor digitorum profundus to fractures of the ulna in children. Journal of Pediatric Orthopedics 18: 437–440

Dell P C, Sheppard J E 1984 Vascularized bone grafts in the treatment of infected forearm non-unions. Journal of Hand Surgery 9A: 653–658

Dodge H S, Cady G W 1972 Treatment of fractures of the radius and ulna with compression plates. Journal of Bone and Joint Surgery 54A: 1167–1176

Dormans J P, Rang M 1990 The problem of Monteggia fracture–dislocations in children. Orthopaedic Clinics of North America 21: 251–256

Du Toit F P, Gräbe R P 1979 Isolated fractures of the shaft of the ulna. South African Medical Journal 56: 21–25

Edwards E G 1952 The posterior Monteggia fracture. American Surgeon 18: 323–327

Failla J M, Amadio P C, Morrey B F 1989 Post-traumatic proximal radio-ulnar synostosis. Journal of Bone and Joint Surgery 71A: 1208–1213

Friberg K S I 1979 Remodelling after distal forearm fractures in children. Acta Orthopaedica Scandinavica 50: 731–739

Fuller D S, McCullough C J 1982 Malunited fractures of the forearm in children. Journal of Bone and Joint Surgery 64B: 341–367

Gandhi R K, Wilson P, Mason Brown J J, Macleod W 1962 Spontaneous correction of deformity following fractures of the forearm in children. British Journal of Surgery 50: 5–10

Givon U, Pritsch M, Levy O, Yosepovich A, Amit Y, Horoszowski H 1997 Monteggia and equivalent lesions. A study of 41 cases. Clinical Orthopaedics & Related Research 337: 208–215

Goel S C, Raj K B, Srivastava T P 1991 Isolated fractures of the ulnar shaft. Injury 22: 212–214

Green J S, Williams S C, Finlay D, Harper W M 1998 Distal forearm fractures in children: the role of radiographs during follow up. Injury 29: 309–312

Greene W B 1982 Traumatic bowing of the forearm in an adult. Clinical Orthopaedics 168: 31–34

Haasbeek J F, Cole W G 1995 Open fractures of the arm in children. Journal of Bone and Joint Surgery 77B: 576–581

Hadden W A, Reschauer R, Seggl W 1983 Results of AO plate fixation of forearm shaft fractures in adults. Injury 15: 44–52

Heppenstall R B, Brighton C T, Esterhai J L, Becker C T 1983 Clinical and roentgenographic evaluation of non-union of the forearm in relation to treatment with DC electrical stimulation. Journal of Trauma 23: 740–744

Hertel R, Pisan M, Lambert S, Ballmer F T 1996 Plate osteosynthesis of diaphyseal fractures of the radius and ulna. Injury 27: 545–548

Hicks J H 1961 Fractures of the forearm treated by rigid fixation. Journal of Bone and Joint Surgery 43B: 680–687

Högström H, Nilsson B E, Willner S 1976 Correction with growth following diaphyseal forearm fracture. Acta Orthopaedica Scandinavica 47: 299–303

Holdsworth B J, Sloan J P 1983 Proximal forearm fractures in children: residual disability. Injury 14: 174–179

Holst-Nielson F, Jensen V 1984 Tardy posterior interosseous nerve palsy as a result of an unreduced radial head dislocation in Monteggia fractures: a report of two cases. Journal of Hand Surgery 9A: 572–575

Hooper G 1974 Isolated fractures of the shaft of the ulna. Injury 6: 180–184

Hughston J C 1957 Fractures of the distal radial shaft. Journal of Bone and Joint Surgery 39A: 249–264

Jenkins N H, Mintowt-Czyz W J, Fairclough J A 1987 Irreducible dislocation of the distal radioulnar joint. Injury 18: 40–43

Jones J A 1991 Immediate internal fixation of high-energy open forearm fractures. Journal of Orthopaedic Trauma 5: 272–279

Jupiter J B, Leibovic S J, Ribbans W, Wilk R M 1991 The posterior Monteggia lesion. Journal of Orthopaedic Trauma 5: 395–402

Kaya Alpar E, Thompson K, Owen R, Taylor J F 1981 Midshaft fractures of the forearm bones in children. Injury 13: 153–158

Keogh P, Khan H, Cooke E, McCoy G 1997 Loss of flexor pollicis longus function after plating of the radius: Report of six cases. Journal of Hand Surgery 22B: 375–376

King R E 1984 Fractures of the shafts of the radius and ulna. In: Rockwood C A, Wilkins K E, King R E (eds) Fractures in children. J B Lippincott, Philadelphia, pp 301–362

Knight R A, Purvis G D 1949 Fractures of both bones of the forearm in adults. Journal of Bone and Joint Surgery 31A: 755–764

Kraus B, Horne G 1985 Galeazzi fractures. Journal of Trauma 25: 1093–1095

Kuksov V 1997 Unstable Monteggia fracture dislocations in children. Journal of Bone and Joint Surgery 79B: supp II: 186

Labbe J L, Peres O, Leclair O, Goulon R, Bertrou V, Saint-Lannes 1999 Fixation of isolated ulnar shaft fracture: by open reduction and internal fixation with plate or percutaneous intramedullary nailing. Journal of Bone and Joint Surgery 81B: supp III: 371

Landfried M J, Stenclik M, Susi J G 1991 Variant of Galeazzi fracture–dislocation in children. Journal of Pediatric Orthopaedics 11: 332–335

Langkamer V G, Ackroyd C E 1990 Removal of forearm plates. Journal of Bone and Joint Surgery 72B: 601–604

Langkamer V G, Ackroyd C E 1991 Internal fixation of forearm fractures in the 1980s: lessons to be learnt. Injury 22: 97–102

Lascombes P, Prevot J, Ligier J N, Metaizean J P, Poncelet T 1990 Elastic stable intramedullary nailing in forearm shaft fractures in children. Journal of Pediatric Orthopaedics 10: 167–171

Letts M, Locht R, Wiens J 1985 Monteggia fracture–dislocations in children. Journal of Bone and Joint Surgery 67B: 724–727

Lichter R L, Jacobsen T 1975 Tardy palsy of the posterior interosseous nerve with a Monteggia fracture. Journal of Bone and Joint Surgery 57A: 124–125

Mackay I, Simpson R G 1980 Closed rupture of extensor digitorum communis tendon following fracture of the radius. The Hand 12: 214–216

Matthews W E, Saunders E A 1979 Fractures of the radius and ulna: part II. American Surgeon 45: 321–324

May V R, Mauck W 1961 Dislocation of the radial head with associated fracture of the ulna. Southern Medical Journal 54: 1255–1261

McGuire T P, Myers P 1986 Ulnar osteotomy for missed Monteggia fracture. In: Proceedings of the Australian Orthopaedic Association. Journal of Bone and Joint Surgery 68B: 336

Michels C, Weissman S L 1976 Intramedullary nailing in fractures of the forearm. In: Proceedings of the Association of Surgeons of East Africa. Journal of Bone and Joint Surgery 58B: 380

Mikic Z 1975 Galeazzi fracture–dislocation. Journal of Bone and Joint Surgery 57A: 1071–1080

Moed B R, Kellam J F, Foster R J, Tile M, Hansen S T 1986 Immediate internal fixation of open fractures of the diaphysis of the forearm. Journal of Bone and Joint Surgery 68A: 1008–1017

Moore T M, Klein J P, Patzakis M J, Harvey J P 1985 Results of compression-plating of closed Galeazzi fractures. Journal of Bone and Joint Surgery 67A: 1015–1021

Moerman J, Lenaert A, De Coninck D, Haeck L, Verbeke S, Uyttendaele D, Verdonk R 1996 Intramedullary fixation of forearm fractures in adults. Acta Orthopaedica Belgica 62: 34–40

Moroni A, Rollo G, Guzzardella M, Zinghi G 1997 Surgical treatment of isolated forearm non-union with segmental bone loss. Injury 28: 497–504

Nielsen A B, Simonsen O 1984 Displaced forearm fractures in children treated with AO plates. Injury 15: 393–396

Nilsson B E, Obrant K 1977 The range of motion following fracture of the shaft of the forearm in children. Acta Orthopaedica Scandinavica 48: 600–602

Pavel A, Pitman J M, Larne E M, Wade P A 1965 The posterior Monteggia fracture: a clinical study. Journal of Trauma 5: 185–199

Peiró A, Andres F, Fernandez-Esteve F 1977 Acute Monteggia lesions in children. Journal of Bone and Joint Surgery 59A: 92–97

Pollock F H, Pankovich A M, Prieto J J, Lorenz M 1983 The isolated fracture of the ulnar shaft. Journal of Bone and Joint Surgery 65A: 339–342

Price C T, Scott D S, Kurzner M E, Flynn J C 1990 Malunited forearm fractures in children. Journal of Pediatric Orthopaedics 10: 705–712

Pugh D M W, Galpin R G, Carey T P 1999 Intramedullary Steinmann pin fixation of paediatric forearm fractures—long term results. Journal of Bone and Joint Surgery 81B: supp I: 108–109

Ray T D, Tessler R H, Dell P C 1996 Traumatic ulnar physeal arrest after distal forearm fractures in children. Journal of Pediatric Orthopaedics 16: 195–200

Reckling F W 1982 Unstable fracture–dislocations of the forearm (Monteggia and Galeazzi lesions). Journal of Bone and Joint Surgery 64A: 857–863

Reynders P, De Groote W, Rondia J, Govaerts K, Stoffelen D, Broos P L 1996 Monteggia lesions in adults. A multicenter Bota study. Acta Orthopaedica Belgica 62: supp I: 78–83

Richter D, Ostermann P A, Ekkernkamp A, Muhr G, Hahn M P 1998 Elastic intramedullary nailing: a minimally invasive concept in the treatment of unstable forearm fractures in children. Journal of Pediatric Orthopaedics 18: 457–461

Ring D, Jupiter J B, Simpson N S 1998 Monteggia fractures in adults. Journal of Bone and Joint Surgery 80A: 1733–1744

Ring D, Waters P M 1996 Operative fixation of Monteggia fractures in children. Journal of Bone and Joint Surgery 78B: 734–739

Roberts J A 1986 Angulation of the radius in children's fractures. Journal of Bone and Joint Surgery 68B: 751–754

Rosen H 1979 Compression treatment of long bone pseudarthroses. Clinical Orthopaedics 138: 154–166

Sage F P 1959 Medullary fixation of fractures of the forearm. Journal of Bone and Joint Surgery 41A: 1489–1516

Sanders W E, Heckman J D 1984 Traumatic plastic deformation of the radius and ulna. Clinical Orthopaedics 188: 58–67

Sarmiento A, Cooper J S, Sinclair W F 1975 Forearm fractures: early functional bracing. Journal of Bone and Joint Surgery 57A: 297–304

Sarmiento A, Ebramzadeh E, Brys D, Tarr R 1992 Angular deformities and forearm function. Journal of Orthopaedic Research 10: 121–133

Sarmiento A, Latta L L, Zych G, McKeever P, Zagorski J P 1998 Isolated ulnar shaft fractures treated with functional braces. Journal of Orthopaedic Trauma 12: 420–423

Scaglietti O, Stringa G, Mizzau M 1965 Bone grafting in non-union of the forearm. Clinical Orthopaedics 43: 65–76

Schranz P J, Fagg P S 1992 Greenstick fractures of the distal third of the radius in children. An innocent fracture? Injury 23: 165–167

Schuind F, Andrianne Y, Burny F 1991 Treatment of forearm fractures by Hoffman external fixation. Clinical Orthopaedics 266: 197–204

Schwarz N, Pienaar S, Schwarz A F, Jelen M, Styhler W, Mayr J 1996 Refracture of the forearm in children. Journal of Bone and Joint Surgery 78B: 740–744

Shang T-Y, Gu Y-W, Dong F H 1987 Treatment of forearm bone fractures by an integrated method of traditional Chinese and Western medicine. Clinical Orthopaedics and Related Research 215: 56–64

Shoemaker S D, Comstock C P, Mubarak S J, Wenger D R, Chambers H G 1999 Intramedullary Kirschner wire fixation of open or unstable forearm fractures in children. Journal of Pediatric Orthopaedics 19: 329–337

Smith D K, Cooney W P 1990 External fixation of high-energy upper extremity injuries. Journal of Orthopaedic Trauma 4: 7–18

Smith H, Sage F P 1957 Medullary fixation of forearm fractures. Journal of Bone and Joint Surgery 39A: 91–98

Spar I 1977 A neurologic complication following Monteggia fracture. Clinical Orthopaedics 122: 207–209

Speed J S, Boyd H B 1940 Treatment of fractures of ulna with dislocation of head of radius. Journal of the American Medical Association 115: 1699–1705

Stein F, Grabias S L, Deffer P A 1971 Nerve injuries complicating Monteggia lesions. Journal of Bone and Joint Surgery 53A: 1432–1436

Street D M 1986 Intramedullary forearm nailing. Clinical Orthopaedics 212: 219–230

Szabo R M, Skinner M 1990 Isolated ulnar shaft fractures. Acta Orthopaedica Scandinavica 61: 350–352

Tarr R R, Garfinkel A I, Sarmiento A 1984 The effects of angular and rotational deformities of both bones of the forearm. Journal of Bone and Joint Surgery 66A: 65–70

Thomas E M, Tuson K W R, Browne P S H 1975 Fractures of the radius and ulna in children. Injury 7: 120–124

Trousdale R T, Linscheid R L 1995 Operative treatment of malunited fractures of the forearm. Journal of Bone and Joint Surgery 77A: 894–902

Van der Reis W L, Otsuka N Y, Moroz P, Mah J 1998 Intramedullary nailing versus plate fixation for unstable forearm fractures in children. Journal of Pediatric Orthopaedics 18: 9–13

Van Herpe L B 1976 Fractures of the forearm and wrist. Orthopaedic Clinics of North America 7: 543–556

Verboom W S W, Besselaar P P, Schaap G R, Bollen S M, Van der Zwan A I 1999 Results of treatment of missed Monteggia fractures. Journal of Bone and Joint Surgery 81B: supp II: 191

Vince K G, Miller J E 1987a Cross-union complicating fracture of the forearm, part I: adults. Journal of Bone and Joint Surgery 69A: 640–653

Vince K G, Miller J E 1987b Cross-union complicating fracture of the forearm, part II: children. Journal of Bone and Joint Surgery 69A: 654–661

Voto S J, Weiner D S, Leighley B 1990 Redisplacement after closed reduction of forearm fractures in children. Journal of Pediatric Orthopaedics 10: 79–84

Walker J L, Rang M 1991 Forearm fractures in children. Journal of Bone and Joint Surgery 73B: 299–301

Walsh H P J, McLaren C A N, Owen R 1987 Galeazzi fractures in children. Journal of Bone and Joint Surgery 69B: 730–733

Warnock D, Simpson S, Jupiter J 1998 The adult anterior Monteggia fracture dislocation: long term results of plate fixation. Journal of Bone and Joint Surgery 80B: supp I: 63

Wei S Y, Born C T, Abene A, Ong A, Haydon R, DeLong W G 1999 Diaphyseal forearm fractures treated with and without bone graft. Journal of Trauma-Injury Infection and Critical Care 46: 1045–1048

Weisman D S, Rang M, Cole W G 1999 Tardy displacement of traumatic radial head dislocation in childhood. Journal of Pediatric Orthopedics 19: 523–526

Whipple A O, St John F B 1917 A study of one hundred consecutive fractures of the shafts of both bones of the forearm with the end results in ninety-five. Surgery, Gynaecology and Obstetrics 25: 77–91

Wiley J J, Galey J P 1985 Monteggia injuries in children. Journal of Bone and Joint Surgery 67B: 728–731

Wong P C N 1967 Galeazzi fracture–dislocations in Singapore 1960–64: incidence and results of treatment. Singapore Medical Journal 8: 186–193

Wright R R, Schmeling G J, Schwab J P 1997 The necessity of acute bone grafting in diaphyseal forearm fractures: a retrospective review. Journal of Orthopaedic Trauma 11: 288–294

Yung S H, Lam C Y, Choi K Y, Ng K W, Maffulli N, Cheng J C Y 1998 Percutaneous intramedullary Kirschner wiring for displaced diaphyseal forearm fractures in children. Journal of Bone and Joint Surgery 80B: 91–94

The wrist

Phillip S. Fagg

◼ Fractures of the Distal Radius

It has been estimated that fractures of the distal end of the radius account for 3% of all fractures seen and treated in casualty departments. The mean incidence rate across the whole lifespan is 42 per 10 000 population. The highest age-specific incidence rate is found in the group above 79 years (90 per 10 000), followed by those in the 0–9 years range (80 per 10 000) (Oskam et al 1998). Women significantly outnumber men in the age group of 60 and over.

Fractures of the distal radius may be divided into:

- undisplaced fractures;
- fractures of the distal radius with dorsal displacement (Colles' fracture);
- fractures of the distal radius with palmar displacement (Smith's fracture);
- marginal articular (Barton's) fractures.

The first two groups will be considered together for convenience.

Fractures of the distal radius: undisplaced and with dorsal displacement

In 1814, Colles gave his description of the fracture of the distal radius with dorsal displacement which bears his name. He stated that 'the limb will at some remote period again enjoy perfect freedom in all its motions, and be completely exempt from pain: the deformity, however, will remain undiminished through life' (Dobyns & Linscheid 1984). Since this statement, many articles have appeared on the subject, reporting good and bad overall results, enthusing over a variety of conservative and operative methods of treatment, and reporting factors both radiological and clinical pertaining to good or bad overall results. A full spectrum of opinions can be found with diligent research of the literature. Reports of the overall results are further hampered by the wide variety of classifications of these fractures.

The more recent articles in the literature do appear to challenge the concept held by many surgeons that no specific treatment is needed because the deformity rarely results in a loss of function. This is especially true of the younger patients with complex intra-articular fractures.

Rather than comment on the benefits of each variety of plaster type or functional brace, this chapter will observe the overall results of conservative treatment, and then look more closely at these results as they relate to those factors more widely regarded as important by various authors The results of operative treatment will be reported later.

The overall functional results of conservative treatment

This section looks at the overall results of the conservative treatment of Colles' fractures. The results of the five larger series are shown in Table 9.1. These series had used either the points system of Gartland & Werley (1951), or a modification thereof, or Lidström's 1959 grading to evaluate their functional results. These results show that 78% of patients with Colles' fractures achieved a satisfactory result. Lidström and Frykman (1967) reported that there was no significant deterioration in the overall functional result once recovery had occurred after the injury. Recovery time was reported as being within 6 months of the initial fracture.

Subjective symptoms

A high percentage of patients appear to suffer from subjective symptoms following Colles' fractures despite achieving a reasonable functional result. Bacorn & Kurtzke (1953) retrospectively reviewed 2132 cases from the files of the Workmens Compensation Board of New York State and found that only 62 cases (2.9%) had no subjective symptoms. Flinkkila et al (1998) reported that 72% of 652 patients with Colles' fractures had subjective symptoms. Mild symptoms were reported in 344 cases (52%), moderate symptoms in 84 cases (13%), severe symptoms in 34 cases (5.2%) and very severe symptoms in 8 cases (1.2%). Frykman (1967) reported that 52.3% of 430 patients had symptoms, although just over 28% of the total study group had very mild symptoms. Similarly, Lidström (1959) found 45.8% of 515 patients with subjective symptoms, although 25.8% had very mild symptoms.

Thus subjective symptoms have been reported as occurring in between 46% and 97% of patients with

Table 9.1 The functional results after conservative treatment

Reference	Total fractures	Excellent		Good		Fair		Poor	
		Total	%	Total	%	Total	%	Total	%
Lidström (1959)[†]	515	214	41.5	195	37.9	61	11.9	45	8
Frykman (1967)[†]	430	105	24.4	218	50.7	81	18.8	26	6
Altissimi et al (1986)[‡]	297	113	38.0	145	48.8	35	11.8	4	1
Gupta (1991)[‡]	204	82	40.3	63	30.8	41	20.1	18	8
Giannikas et al	320	93	29	147	46	67	21	13	4
Overall	1766	607	34	768	44	285	16	106	6

78% satisfactory, 22% unsatisfactory

[†] Lidström's categories.

[‡] Gartland & Werley's categories (1951).

Colles' fractures; the overall figure would appear to be 80.5% experiencing some subjective symptoms. This falls to 58% if Bacorn and Kurtzke (1953) are excluded. Their surprisingly high figures may reflect the fact that their cases were involved in Workmens Compensation. Bacorn & Kurtzke felt that there was an average disability of 24% loss of function of the hand after such a fracture, whereas Green & Gay (1956) estimated the average disability to be 17.7% in 75 fractures.

Pain

Pain, from a variety of causes, is a common subjective complaint, and the various types and incidences are shown in Table 9.2. Of the 56 patients in Eelma & McElfresh's 1983 study, 75% had subjective symptoms of pain, compared to only 34% in Smaill's 1965 series.

Fatiguability

A sensation of weakness of the wrist and hand with strenuous activity was noted in 2.3% of Frykman's 430 cases (1967) and 6.6% of the 515 patients in Lidström's series (1959).

Loss of grip strength

Those larger series that specifically reported loss of grip strength in their functional assessment are recorded in Table 9.3. Between 18 and 35% of patients were aware of a feeling of subjective weakness, although objectively the incidence was lower. Eelma & McElfresh (1983) reported a higher subjective incidence of weakness (64.2%), but this was in a younger patient population who tended to be more demanding than older patients. However, only 8.9% of these patients had any evidence of objective weakness.

The average deficit in grip strength following Colles' fracture is from 15.1% (Jenkins & Mintowt-Czyz 1988,

Fernandez 1991) to 31% (Kaukonen et al 1988) of the normal value.

Lagerstrom et al (1999) monitored the recovery of isometric grip strength over a two year period in 33 patients with a displaced Colles' fracture involving the distal radio-ulnar joint. They found that the recovery of grip strength occurred up to 1 year after the fracture.

Algodystrophy and finger stiffness

The incidence and features of algodystrophy (reflex sympathetic dystrophy) following Colles' fracture were reported by Atkins et al (1989). They noted a number of features suggestive of the disorder:

- pain and tenderness in the hand or fingers
- pain in the shoulder of the fractured side
- discolouration of the affected hand
- a history of vasomotor instability of the affected hand occurring since the fracture
- excessive sweating of the affected hand
- swelling of the hand
- thinning of the skin with shininess and dystrophy
- finger stiffness and loss of finger movement
- loss of shoulder movement.

On the basis of a questionnaire they reported that, at 9 weeks post fracture, 27 of 109 patients (25%) showed signs of algodystrophy. No unaffected patients developed the disorder after this time. Of the 19 patients returning for review at 6 months, 12 (62%) still showed some residual abnormalities. Employing more sensitive techniques in a subsequent study, these same authors reported that 24 of 60 patients (37%) had features of algodystrophy at 9 weeks post injury (Atkins et al 1990). A similar incidence of algodystrophy was reported by Laulan et al (1997).

Table 9.2 The incidence and type of painful subjective symptoms following Colles' fractures

Reference	Total sample	Number with symptoms	%
Pain on strenuous use			
Lidström (1959)	515	59	11.5
Vang Hansen et al (1998)	74	17	23
Frykman (1967)	430	58	13.5
Pain on loading			
Lidström (1959)	515	54	10.5
Frykman (1967)	430	61	14.2
Pain with weather change			
Smaill (1965)	41	9	22.0
Frykman (1967)	430	23	5.4
Eelma & McElfresh (1983)	58	23	39.7
Pain from the radio-ulnar joint			
Frykman (1967)	430	59	13.7
Kaukonen et al (1988)	207	46	22
Altissimi et al (1986)	297	108	36.4
Pain on forced dorsiflexion			
Eelma & McElfresh (1983)	58	19	32.8

Table 9.3 The incidence of weakness of grip in Colles' fractures

Reference	Total sample	Number with symptoms	%
Bacorn & Kurtzke (1953) only 3% had severe weakness	2130	737	34.6
Lidström (1959)			
Subjective	515	141	27.4
Objective	481	84	17.5
Frykman (1967)	430	154	35.8
Altissimi et al (1986)	297	53	17.9
Eelma & McElfresh (1983)			
Subjective	56	36	64.2
Objective	56	5	8.9

They performed a prospective study of algodystrophy after fracture of the distal radius in 100 consecutive patients. Algodystrophy was diagnosed in 26% of cases.

Field and Atkins (1997) studied 100 patients with Colles' fractures to see how early the diagnosis of algoneurodystrophy could be made. They had noted that patients developing algodystrophy appeared to get little pain relief when immobilised in a plaster cast. The predictive power of normality of dolorimetry and goniometry 1 week post injury was reported. Normal goniometry at 1 week conveyed only a 4% chance of developing the syndrome, and a normal dolorimetry ratio only a 3% chance.

Zyluk (1998) presented the results of a study into the natural history of post-traumatic algoneurodystrophy of the hand. Thirty patients were observed without treatment; 27 completed the study, three patients requiring treatment before it had finished. A final assessment of these 27 patients was made at an average of 13 months post injury. Only one patient was said to show sufficient features of the condition to warrant the diagnosis of mild algoneurodystrophy, most features having resolved spontaneously in the remaining 26. Pain and swelling disappeared more quickly than other features. But although the signs and symptoms of algoneurodystrophy had largely gone at 13 months, the hands were still functionally impaired because of the weaker grip strength. At the last follow-up 10 patients had a grip strength greater than 50% of the other side, 14 patients between 11 and 50% and 3 patients had grip strength less than 10% of the contralateral side.

Residual finger stiffness alone has been reported to occur in as many as 47.5% of the 2130 patients in Bacorn & Kurtzke's 1953 series, to as low as 0.7% after 430 fractures in Frykman's 1967 series.

Loss of motion

Smaill (1965) reported very little difference in the range of motion of the injured wrist when it was compared with the uninjured one in his 41 patients. The percentage loss of wrist movement after these fractures is recorded in Table 9.4. It can be seen that no clear pattern emerges. In general, palmar flexion, ulnar deviation and supination were more restricted than dorsiflexion, radial deviation and pronation. The degree of the loss of motion varied widely.

Cosmetic appearance

The final cosmetic appearance was found to appear normal in from 36% (Camelot et al 1999) to 60% (Lidström 1959) of patients. The incidence of residual cosmetic

Table 9.4 Loss of motion after Colles' fractures

Reference	Patient sample	Palmar flexion		Dorsiflexion	
		No. decreased	%	No. decreased	%
Bacorn & Kurtzke (1953)	2130		94.5		80
Lidström (1959)	515	210	40.8	73	14.2
More than 20°		92	17.9	43	8.4
Frykman (1967)	430	223	51.9	122	28.4
More than 20°		132	30.7	97	22.6
Eelma & McElfresh (1983)	58	8	13.8	25	43
More than 20°		3	5.2	11	19

Reference	Patient sample	Ulnar deviation		Radial deviation	
		No. decreased	%	No. decreased	%
Lidström (1959)	515	78	15.2	36	7
More than 20°		64	12.4	36	7
Frykman (1967)	430	173	40.2	90	20.9
More than 20°		127	29.5	76	17.7
Eelma & McElfresh (1983)	58	11	19	6	10.4
More than 20°		2	3.5	1	1.7

Reference	Patient sample	Pronation		Supination	
		No. decreased	%	No. decreased	%
Bacorn & Kurtzke (1953)	2130		28.2		36.9
Lidström (1959)	515	38	7.4	47	9.1
More than 20°		26	5.1	26	5.1
Frykman (1967)	430	19	4.4	66	15.4
More than 20°		13	3	49	11.4
Eelma & McElfresh (1983)	58	3	5.2	18	31
More than 20°		2	3.5	6	10.4

deformity varied widely, with a prominent ulna being reported in 7.9% (Frykman 1967) to 46.3% (Smaill 1965) of fractures, radial deviation in 18.3% (Frykman 1967) to 37.9% (Lidström 1959) and dinner fork deformity in 5.6% (Lidström 1959) to 10.9% (Frykman 1967) of cases.

It is sometimes easy to forget the importance to the elderly female patient of a good cosmetic result (Stewart et al 1985a).

Factors affecting functional results
The age of the patient

There appears to be general agreement in the literature that there is a lower incidence of impaired function after extra-articular distal radius fractures in the younger age group than in the older groups. Bacorn & Kurtzke (1953) further stated that the percentage disability in Colles' fractures increased directly with age at a rate of approximately 4% loss of function per decade. Frykman (1967) and Lidström (1959) agreed that the younger age group had better functional results, but they felt that the importance of the age factor on this end result was slight. Stewart et al (1985a) showed that improvement of function between 3 months and 6 months after fracture was statistically more significant in patients aged under 64. As stated previously, Eelma & McElfresh (1983) found a high incidence of subjective symptoms (82%) in their 56 patients aged under 45 years, as compared with the larger series of Frykman (1967) and Lidström (1959), in which the incidence was 52% and 45% respectively. In these young patients they found that 86% of those aged 18–25 years had a good or excellent result, as compared with 62% in those aged 36–45 years.

However, intra-articular fractures of the distal radius in young adults are more difficult to manage and are associated with a high frequency of post-traumatic arthritis (Knirk & Jupiter 1986).

The fracture pattern

Many different classifications have been applied to Colles' fractures (Gartland & Werley 1951, Older et al 1965, Frykman 1967, Lidström 1969). Of these, Frykman's is now the most widely used, but is too complicated to be used as a basis for discussion in this section.

For simplicity, we will examine the results following fissure fractures, extra-articular fractures, intra-articular fractures involving the radiocarpal joint, intra-articular fractures involving the radio-ulnar joint and comminuted fractures.

The original amount of dorsal tilt has been shown to have no appreciable effect on the ultimate end-result (Gartland & Werley 1951, Lidström 1959, Villar et al 1987). However, Stewart et al (1984) felt that the functional result was related to the severity of initial displacement, but that the type of fracture did not influence the final anatomical result.

Table 9.5 shows how the different published classifications fall into the categories that will be assessed in this section. It is obviously difficult to combine classifications and some overlap must occur. The functional results related to the fracture type are given in Table 9.6.

These figures show no great correlation between fracture pattern and final functional outcome. This view was also held by Stewart et al (1984) and Altissimi et al (1986). Certainly, undisplaced fissure fractures gave the best functional results (see Table 9.6A) with 89–100% satisfactory results. Comminuted fractures tended to have the worst functional scores with 25–80.7% satisfactory results. Green & Gay (1956) agreed that the end-results in non-comminuted fractures were generally better, and Cooney et al (1980a) found that comminuted fractures had a higher incidence of complications.

There has been recent interest in the results of intra-articular fractures of the distal radius, especially in young adults, with a view to internal fixation. Melone (1984) classified articular fractures of the distal radius into four types based on displacement of the medial complex which affects the radiocarpal and radio-ulnar joints. Trumble et al (1998), in a review article on intra-articular fractures of the distal radius, describe the various classifications of intra-articular fractures in great detail and the reader should refer to the original article if necessary. The results of intra-articular fractures of the distal radius healing with a step in the articular surface will be discussed later in this chapter.

The other aspects of the fracture pattern do not appear grossly to affect the final functional outcome, although Frykman (1967) felt that involvement of the distal radio-ulnar joint was an important contribution to poor functional results. In his series this group had the lowest percentage of satisfactory results (62.7%), even lower than that for comminuted fractures (69%). The contribution of the involvement of the distal radio-ulnar joint to an inferior functional result has also been commented on by Gartland & Werley (1951), who found that 39% had unsatisfactory results, and Older et al (1965), with 70% poor results from involvement of the distal radio-ulnar joint. Geissler et al (1996) described three types of distal radio-ulnar joint lesions occurring in association with fractures of the distal radius. Type I are stable distal radio-ulnar joint lesions, which could include minimally displaced avulsion of the tip of the ulnar styloid, a stable fracture of the neck of the ulna, an intact or minimally disrupted capsular ligament or triangular fibrocartilage complex. Type II lesions were unstable distal radio-ulnar joints with

Table 9.5 A correlation of previous fracture classifications with the categories used in this section

Reference	Fracture type
A. Fissure fracture	
Frykman (1967)	Fissure fracture
Older et al (1965)	Type I
Lidström (1959)	Type I
B. Extra-articular	
Frykman (1967)	Types I and II
Older et al (1965)	Type II
Lidström (1959)	Types IIA and IIC
Gartland & Werley (1951)	Type I
C. Involving radiocarpal joint	
Frykman (1967)	Types III and IV
Lidström (1959)	Types IIB and IID
Gartland & Werley (1951)	Type II
D. Involving radio-ulnar joint	
Frykman (1967)	Types V and VI
E. Comminuted	
Frykman (1967)	Types VII and VIII
Older et al (1965)	Type IV
Lidström (1959)	Type IIE
Gartland & Werley (1951)	Type III

subluxation or dislocation of the ulnar head due to a massive tear of the triangular fibrocartilage complex and ligaments or an avulsion fracture of the base of the ulnar styloid. Type III lesions were potentially unstable lesions caused by skeletal disruption of the joint surface at the sigmoidnotch. Moharti & Kar (1979) reported that 60 of their 200 patients (30%) had pain and tenderness over the radio ulnar joint after fracture healing. Arthrograms of the inferior radio-ulnar joint were performed and tears of the triangular fibrocartilage complex were found in 27 cases (45%). This abnormality was found even in well-reduced Colles' fractures. Villar et al (1987) reported that involvement of the radio-ulnar joint resulted in an increased loss of grip strength when compared with fractures involving the radiocarpal joint.

Malunion

Unfortunately, not all united and fully reduced Colles' fractures result in an excellent functional end-result. Both Cassebaum (1950) and Frykman (1967) reported poor functional results in association with excellent anatomical results in 2 to 5%. Many authors, however, have reported excellent functional results with poor anatomical healing. Lidström (1959) reported that 52% of his patients with a poor anatomical result had good function, while Frykman (1967) reported a 64% incidence, Stewart et al (1985a) an 81% incidence at 6 months' review, and Cassebaum (1950) satisfactory results in over 85%. However, there is no doubt that the functional end-result deteriorates with increasing deformity. What is disputed in the literature is which radiological parameters are important with regard to ultimate function.

Dorsal angulation   Villar et al (1987) felt that residual dorsal angulation was not significant in producing unsatisfactory results, and Frykman (1967) that it only slightly increased the incidence of unsatisfactory end-results. Lidström (1957) considered that a dorsal angulation of less than 10° was of no consequence, but that any larger angulation caused a rapid decline in the functional results. Hollingsworth & Morris (1976) found that 6% of patients with no dorsal angulation had unsatisfactory results, while with dorsal angulation of 1–10 there were unsatisfactory

Table 9.6 Functional result related to fracture pattern

Reference	Total	Excellent		Good		Fair		Poor	
		No.	%	No.	%	No.	%	No.	%
A. Fissure fracture									
Lidström (1959)	40	40	100						
Older et al (1965)	13	13	100						
Frykman (1967)	19	11	57.9	6	31.5	1	5.3	1	5.3
B. Extra-articular fractures									
Futami & Yamamoto (1989)	126	45	36	72	57	7	5	2	2
Lidström (1959)	339	159	46.9	117	34.5	36	10.6	27	8.0
Stoffelen & Broos (1999)	98	73 satisfactory results (75%)				25 unsatisfactory results (25%)			
Frykman (1967)	156	56	35.9	80	51.2	17	10.9	3	2
Altissimi et al (1986)	90	79 satisfactory results (88%)				11 unsatisfactory results (12%)			
C. Involving radiocarpal joint									
Gartland & Werley (1951)	27	20 satisfactory results (74%)				7 unsatisfactory results (16%)			
Lidström (1959)	107	39	36.5	51	47.7	12	11.2	5	4.6
Frykman (1967)	98	19	19.4	53	54.1	19	19.4	7	7.1
Strange-Vognsen (1991)	28	12	42.9	11	39.3	2	7.1	3	10.7
Altissimi et al (1986)	73	66 satisfactory results (90.4%)				7 unsatisfactory results (9.6%)			
D. Involving radio-ulnar joint									
Frykman (1967)	102	19	18.6	45	44.1	26	25.5	12	11.8
Kaukonen et al (1988)	32	6	18.7	11	34.4	15	46.9	(fair or poor)	
Altissimi et al (1986)	41	38 satisfactory results (92.7%)				3 unsatisfactory results (7.3%)			
E. Comminuted fractures									
Gartland & Werley (1951)	26	15 satisfactory results (58%)				11 unsatisfactory results (42%)			
Lidström (1959)	32	2	6.3	12	37.5	8	25	10	31.2
Older et al (1965)	14	6	42.9	5	35.7			3	24.4
Frykman (1967)	74	11	14.9	40	54.1	19	25.7	4	5.3
Strange-Vognsen (1991)	8	5	62.5	1	12.5	1	12.5	1	12.5
Altissimi et al (1986)	93	75 satisfactory results (80.7%)				18 unsatisfactory results (19.3%)			

results in 19%; with over 10° dorsal angulation this rose to 42%. Altissimi et al (1986) reported 50% unsatisfactory results when dorsal angulation measured more that 15°. Green & Gay (1956) estimated that with up to 10° dorsal angulation there was an average 14% permanent loss of function, and with over 10° angulation this rose to an average of 34% permanent disability. Rubinovich & Rennie (1983) found that a loss of volar tilt adversely affected the functional result by decreasing grip and pinch strength, while Porter & Stockley (1986) found that this occurred only if the dorsal angulation exceeded 20°.

Kelly et al (1997), in their comparison of manipulation under Biers block with plaster immobilisation alone, in 30 elderly patients with moderately displaced Colles' fractures, found no detectable difference between the two groups. They concluded that up to 30° of dorsal angulation could be accepted.

Radial deviation Villar et al (1987) and Gartland & Werley (1951) felt that abnormal radial deviation did not affect the functional end-result. However, Rubinovich & Rennie (1983) concluded that a radial deviation of less than 10° affected the outcome by weakening grip, while Altissimi et al (1986) reported 100% unsatisfactory results when the deviation was less than 5°.

Radial shortening Lidström (1959), Frykman (1967) and Camelot et al (1999) felt that increasing radial shortening caused increasing unsatisfactory results, although Frykman found that this was more so when radial shortening was combined with a degree of dorsal angulation. Camelot et al (1999) reported that radial shortening of more than 3 mm affected the functional outcome, and Villar et al (1987) found that increasing shortening caused decreasing grip strength. Kelly et al (1997) concluded that 5 mm of radial shortening could be accepted in selected elderly patients.

Articular step-off Fernandez (1991) suggested that articular congruity was important. He felt that there was a direct correlation between the subjective and functional findings and the radiographic results, and that there was no evidence of post-traumatic arthrosis when the fractures healed with an anatomic joint congruity or with an articular step-off of up to 1 mm. Knirk & Jupiter (1986) found that 91% of their 24 distal radial fractures in young adults which healed with residual incongruity of the radiocarpal joint had arthritis at a mean follow-up of 6.7 years, as opposed to the 11% incidence in the 19 fractures healing with a congruous joint. Strange-Vognsen (1991), however, reported that residual intra-articular step-off correlated with the development of subsequent arthrosis only, and not with the subjective functional evaluation. Similarly, a strong association was found between the development of osteoarthrosis of the radiocarpal joint and residual displacement of articular fragments at the time of bony union in the 26 patients reported by Catalano et al (1997). However, the functional status did not correlate with the magnitude of the residual articular step at fracture healing.

The value of remanipulation Pool (1973) found that there was no progression of the deformity after 6 weeks from the initial reduction, but Dias et al (1987) reported that it progressed over a 3 month period even after plaster casts had been removed. Lidström (1959) reported that 28% of reduced fractures redisplaced, whilst Porter & Stockley (1986) reported 59%. Redisplacement after remanipulation was reported to occur in 40% (Lidström 1959) and 57.5% (Collert & Isacson 1978) of cases.

Jenkins (1989) studied 121 displaced Colles' fractures, and he felt that the tendency to malunion or chronic instability of the Colles' fracture was determined solely by the initial deformity, and was not related to the intra-articular involvement or the presence of comminution. Roumen et al (1991) believed that the severity of the original soft tissue injury and its complications were the major determinants of functional end-result rather than the severity of initial fracture displacement or final anatomical position. They treated 43 patients whose wrist fracture had displaced within 2 weeks of manipulation; 21 were remanipulated and held by an external fixator, while in the other 22 patients the redisplacement was accepted and conservative treatment continued. The patients treated with external fixation had a good anatomical result, but their function was no better than that of the conservatively treated group.

In a larger study McQueen et al (1996) compared four methods of treatment in 120 patients with redisplaced fractures of the distal radius. The four treatment groups, each containing 30 patients, were remanipulation and plaster, open reduction and bone grafting, and closed external fixation with and without mobilisation of the wrist at 3 weeks. Functional results showed no difference between any of the four groups.

The results of operative treatment

The operative treatment of Colles' fractures falls into five basic groups:

- percutaneous fixation with pins and casts
- external fixation
- internal fixation with plates
- use of bone substitutes
- arthroscopically assisted techniques.

Percutaneous fixation with pins and casts

Many reports have been published concerning the use of percutaneous pins for the treatment of displaced fractures of the distal radius. They may be used to supplement external fixation or bone grafting procedures but are most commonly used with a cast or splint. A number of techniques have been described. Kirschner wires or other intramedullary devices may be passed through the radial styloid or wires are passed through the fracture site to wedge open the distal fragment and prevent redisplacement (Kapandji intrafocal pin).

A further technique is bipolar fixation, in which pins are placed proximal and distal to the fracture, and reduction is obtained and then held by incorporating the pins in the plaster. Subtle differences in the technique used are described, but for simplicity they will be considered together. The functional results obtained by using this technique are shown in Table 9.7, and were satisfactory in 91% of patients. The anatomy was generally better maintained than with pure plaster immobilisation. Between 83% (Fritz et al 1999) and 88% (Raüis et al 1985, Pritchett 1995) had satisfactory anatomical results. The technique is not without its complication rate, however Chapman et al (1982), in a study of 80 cases, reported 21% with loose pins, 20% with pin track infections, 9% with osteomyelitis requiring curettage, and 9% with iatrogenic fracture of the metacarpal or ulna.

External fixation

The functional results of the larger reported series of patients treated by various external fixation devices are shown in Table 9.8. Overall, 88% of patients achieved a satisfactory result, a figure that appears to be slightly inferior to that for bipolar fixation. However, the fractures treated by this method tended to be those with greater disturbance of anatomy. Thus in the study of Kongsholm & Olerud (1989), all of the fractures were comminuted (Frykman type VII and VIII). Final grip strength varied between 54% (Cooney 1983) and 90% (Kongsholm & Olerud 1989) of the uninjured side. Again, there are risks of pin loosening, pin track infection, osteomyelitis and iatrogenic fracture. Cooney et al (1979) reported complications in 27% of their patients.

Internal fixation with plates and screws

Internal fixation is not commonly used for Colles' fractures.

Melone (1984) classified intra-articular fractures of the radius into four types. In 1986 he reported the results of internal fixation in 15 patients with his type 4 injury (the most severe grade, with wide separation or rotation of the intra-articular fragments). These showed that 80% achieved satisfactory functional results and 93% had satisfactory anatomical results. All lost some mobility, being

Table 9.7 The functional results of percutaneous fixation

Reference	Number of fractures	Excellent		Good		Fair		Poor	
		No.	%	No.	%	No.	%	No.	%
Fritz et al (1999)	110	39	35	55	50	11	10	5	5
Pritchett (1995)	50	26	52	22	44	1	2	1	2
Green (1975)	45	10	22.2	29	64.4	2	4.4	4	9
	(objective)								
Rauïs et al (1979)	102	98	96.1	3	2.9			1	1
Suman (1983)	37	8	21.6	22	59.5			7	18.9
Overall	344	181	53	131	38	14	4	18	5

91% satisfactory, 9% unsatisfactory

Table 9.8 The functional results of external fixation

Reference	Number of patients	Excellent		Good		Fair		Poor	
		No.	%	No.	%	No.	%	No.	%
Cooney et al (1979)	60	28	46.7	26	43.3	5	8.3	1	1.7
Kongsholm & Olerud (1989)	68	44	64.7	17	25	6	8.8	1	1.5
Cooney (1983)	100	22	22	64	64	10	10	4	4
D'Anca et al (1984)	81	55	68	21	26	3	4	2	2
Jakim et al (1991)	115	69	60	26	23	14	12	6	5
Overall	424	218	51.4	154	36.3	38	9	14	3.3

87.7% satisfactory, 12.3% unsatisfactory.

intra-articular fractures, while grip strength averaged 84% of that of the uninjured hand.

Axelrod & McMurtry (1990) reported results of 20 patients treated by open reduction after failure of closed means. The overall complication rate was high (50%), but patient satisfaction was also high, with 89% of the 17 patients reviewed returning to their previous occupations. Articular congruency was restored in 88% of cases. Thirteen patients (76.5%) had full satisfaction with the functional outcome, while the other four had mild functional limitations. Grip strength was 83% of the uninjured side, while pinch strength was 90% of normal.

Use of bone substitutes

Early reports have suggested satisfactory results from the use of a calcium-phosphate bone cement that crystallises into an apatite similar to bone mineral. When injected into areas of cancellous comminution after fracture it is supposed to increase stability and improve outcome.

Sanchez-Sotelo and Munvera (1999) reported the results of a prospective randomised trial on 60 patients, comparing 35 patients treated with a bone substitute injected percutaneously after closed reduction and cast immobilisation for 2 or 3 weeks and 34 patients treated with closed reduction and cast immobilisation for 6 weeks. Functional recovery was quicker and loss of reduction less frequent in the bone substitute group.

Kopylov et al (1999) compared the same bone substitute with external fixation in 40 patients with redisplaced distal radial fractures. Whilst there was no difference in function parameters at 3 months' follow-up, the bone substitute group had better grip strength, wrist extension and forearm supination at 7 weeks' follow-up.

Arthroscopically assisted techniques

Recent advances in arthroscopically assisted reduction of intra-articular fractures have made it possible to assess soft tissue injuries associated with distal radial fractures. Geissler et al (1996) reported that 41 (68%) of 60 patients had soft tissue injuries that included the triangular fibrocartilage complex in 26 (43%), the scapholunate interosseous ligament in 19 (32%) and the lunotriquetral interosseous ligament in 9 (15%) (13 patients had two injuries each). Richards et al (1997) reported the findings in 118 acute distal radial fractures assessed arthroscopically. The triangular fibrocartilage complex was torn in 46 of 118 patients (39%) and the scapholunate ligament in 18%. These tears were more common in intra-articular fracture (59% and 22% respectively). A much higher incidence of triangular fibrocartilage complex tears was reported by Lindau et al (1997), 39 out of 50 cases (78%), with a statistical correlation to ulnar styloid fractures. The scapholunate ligament was partially or totally torn in 27 patients (54%), and chondral lesions were found in 16 (32%). It is felt that these chondral and ligament lesions might explain poor outcomes after seemingly well-healed distal fractures of the radius.

Complications of Colles' fractures
Nerve injuries

As a consequence of Colles' fractures, the median and ulnar nerves are at risk from compression within their respective tunnels at the wrist. The incidence of median nerve compression in the larger reported series is recorded in Table 9.9, and varies between 0.2% (Bacorn & Kurtzke 1953) and 17.4% (Stewart et al 1985b). According to the latter authors, this high figure was a reflection of the

Table 9.9 The incidence of median and ulnar nerve compression with Colles' fracture

Reference	Number of patients	Median nerve		Ulnar nerve	
		Number	%	Number	%
Bacorn & Kurtzke (1953)	2130	4	0.2	1	0.05
Jakim et al (1991)	132	11	8.3	1	0.75
Lidström (1959)	515	1	0.5	5	1
Frykman (1967)	430	10	2.3	4	0.9
Altissimi et al (1986)	297	31	10.4	9	3
Aro et al (1988)	166	18	10.8	10	6
Stewart et al (1985b)	213	37	17.4	2	0.9
Overall	3883	112	2.9	32	0.8

patients in their series being reviewed by a hand surgeon. The overall incidence in the largest series was 2.9%.

Although the majority of compressions of the median nerve were noted early on after the fracture, symptoms of compression can be delayed. In nearly 25% of the cases noted by Stewart et al (1985b), the symptoms developed after 3 months. They noted that their cases of median nerve irritability occurred in the older patient and in those who had a greater residual dorsal angulation (average 12.6° in patients with symptoms, compared with 7° in those without). Frykman (1967) found that all 10 cases of median nerve compression in his series were associated with intra-articular fractures. Melone (1984) divided the intra-articular fractures of the distal radius into four types. The type I fracture was stable with minimal comminution and the type II fracture was comminuted and unstable. Ten out of 70 type II fractures (14%) had median nerve compression. His rare type III fracture was comminuted with a ventral spike from the proximal radius, which compressed the median nerve in all three cases of this type until the spike was excised. In the type IV injury, with wide separation of the fragments, 13 of 15 patients (87%) had median nerve compression (Melone 1986).

The majority of median nerve compressions settled down with conservative treatment. A few cases came to carpal tunnel decompression, and the results were usually good, although Lewis (1978) pointed out that the nerve could be compressed by fibrosis as a consequence of haematoma beneath the deep fascia, at the level of the fracture site, well away from the carpal tunnel.

Ulnar nerve compression was less frequent, with an overall incidence of 0.8%.

Tendon injuries

The incidence of rupture of the extensor pollicus longus tendon after Colles' fracture is low; 0.5% (Stewart et al 1985b), 0.7% (Frykman 1967) and 1% (Mason 1953). Engkvist & Lundborg (1979) noted that 39 of the 54 that they presented (72%) occurred in undisplaced fractures, while Hirasawa et al (1990) noted only 11 undisplaced fractures in 14 patients (64%) with EPL rupture. From the Swedish series, 34 of 52 (65%) ruptured within 8 weeks, as did 13 out of 14 (93%) of Hirasawa's series. Rarely, the tendons of extensor communis may rupture as a late consequence of Colles' fracture (Sadr 1984).

Hirasawa et al (1990) performed microvascular studies on five cadavers and showed a poorly vascularised portion of the extensor pollicus longus tendon about 5 mm in length, which may be a cause of spontaneous rupture of the tendon.

Flexor tendons are rarely affected by Colles' fractures. Stuart & Beckenbaugh (1987) reported entrapment of the flexor digitorum profundus tendons to the long and ring fingers in a displaced comminuted Colles' fracture, and Melone (1984, 1986) rupture of flexor pollicus longus and the long flexor to the index finger. Rupture of a flexor tendon occurring 30 years after the original fracture has been reported (Takami et al 1997).

Post-traumatic osteoarthritis

The incidence of post-traumatic arthritis following Colles' fractures is shown in Table 9.10. As can be seen, there is wide variation between an incidence of 3% (Cooney 1983) and 17.8% (Altissimi et al 1986). Certainly, 35 of Lidström's 65 patients included those with only minute osteophytic change. Frykman (1964) described involvement of the radio-ulnar joint in 18.3% of patients. The cases of Altissimi et al (1986) all involved the radiocarpal joint, but there was a longer follow-up of up to 6 years. After a 5–6 year follow-up Smaill (1965) found a 24% incidence of arthritis in 41 patients. However, insufficient data were available to suggest an increasing incidence of

Table 9.10 The incidence of post-traumatic osteoarthritis following Colles' fractures

Reference	Number of patients	Incidence of arthritis	
		Number	**%**
Lidström (1959)	515	65	12.6
Altissimi et al (1986)	297	53	17.8
Mason (1953)	100	4	4
Cooney (1983)	100	3	3
Jakim et al (1991)	115	9	7.2
Overall	1127	134	11.9

degenerative changes with increasing length of follow-up. Only 30% of Smaill's 10 patients with radiological signs of osteoarthrosis were symptomatic, and just 32% of those patients described in Altissimi's 1986 paper had functional results in the fair or poor group.

The comminuted intra-articular fractures had a greater incidence of degenerative changes following fracture. Of 15 patients with type 4 (Melone 1986) intra-articular fractures, 14 had changes. Only one of 339 patients in Lidström's extra-articular groups (IIA and IIC) had changes, as compared with 14 of 32 patients with the comminuted (IIE) fracture.

In young adults with intra-articular fractures of the distal radius, the incidence of late post-traumatic arthritis is very high. Knirk & Jupiter (1986), at a mean follow-up of 6.7 years, noted radiographic evidence of post-traumatic arthritis in 28 (65%) of 43 fractures. Arthritis in the radiocarpal joint developed in 22 (91%) of the 24 wrists that had any degree of articular step-off, but in only two (11%) of the 19 wrists that healed with a congruous joint surface. Similarly, Strange-Vognsen (1991) noted radiographic arthritis in 20 (57%) of 35 cases of young adults with this fracture pattern. Catalano et al (1997) also reported a high incidence of osteoarthrosis after displaced intra-articular fractures in young adults. Seventy-six percent of 16 wrists reviewed at an average of 7.1 years after open reduction and stabilisation had osteoarthritis of the radiocarpal joint. However, all patients had a good or excellent functional outcome irrespective of radiographic evidence of osteoarthrosis of the radiocarpal or the distal radioulnar joint or non-union of the ulnar styloid process.

Dupuytren's contracture and stenosing tenosynovitis

Bacorn & Kurtzke (1953) reported four cases of Dupuytren's contracture (0.2%) in association with 2130 cases of Colles' fracture. Stewart et al (1985b) found that nine (4.2%) of 213 patients had palmar fascia nodules or bands at 3 months' follow-up, increasing to 23 (11%) of 209 patients at 6 months' follow-up. In all cases the Dupuytren's contracture was mild, and presented in older patients.

Stenosing tenosynovitis was noted in 12 of the 101 Colles' fractures in patients over the age of 55 years reported by Roumen et al (1991).

Carpal instability and malunion

Taleisnik (1985) described three types of proximal carpal instability occurring after trauma, these being dorsal carpal and palmar carpal translocation at the radiocarpal joint and midcarpal instability. Stoffelen et al (1998) investigated the incidence and clinical importance of carpal instabilities after distal radial fractures. The overall incidence among the 272 patients studied was 60%. The most frequent deformity was radial translocation, found in 88 patients (32%), followed by scapholunate dissociation and dissociative DISI in 47 (17%) and 32 (12%) patients respectively. Ulnar translocation was noted in just 15 patients (6%) and other instabilities were infrequent. Some patients had more than one instability, however. Only scapholunate dissociation in association with a dissociative DISI and ulnar translocation showed significant clinical differences at 1 year follow-up.

Bickerstaff & Bell (1989) suggested that a dorsiflexion instability pattern is the inevitable response of the carpus to the altered mechanics caused by malunion with dorsal radial tilt. They also reported a strong correlation between final function and dorsal carpal instability. In Rosenthal et al's 1983 series of 190 consecutive fractures of the distal radius, 14 examples (7.4%) of scapholunate dissociation were found, although some of these fractures had palmar displacement. Carpal instability will be discussed more fully in a later section of this chapter.

Cooney et al (1980a) described corrective osteotomy in 14 patients with symptomatic malunion, causing pain, deformity and a decreased range of motion. After surgery, 13 of these had improved grip strength and motion. Fernandez (1982) reported satisfactory results in 15 of 20 corrective osteotomies and, more recently (Fernandez 1988), described a hemiresection arthroplasty in combination with radial osteotomy in 15 patients whose malunion of a fracture of the distal end of the radius was associated with symptoms predominantly in the radioulnar joint with limited rotation of the forearm. Postoperatively, 13 had no pain, while in the other two patients the degree of pain was reduced to a mild level. Grip strength increased by an average of 30%, and 12 had a satisfactory functional result, three a fair result.

Weiland et al (1999) reported the results of osteotomy for 30 patients with an intra-articular malunion. At 41.7 months' follow-up union was achieved in all patients. Sixty-seven percent had no pain, whilst 23% had intermittent pain. Range of motion improved in all patients by an average of 22% in flexion and extension, and grip strength improved by an average of 80% as compared to the contralateral hand.

Non-union

Non-union of a Colles' fracture is very rare, and for this reason the diagnosis may be delayed for some considerable time. Smith & Wright (1999) described five patients treated with internal fixation and iliac bone graft. All were heavy smokers and three had a history of alcohol abuse.

Union was achieved in three patients, one requiring a second operation, but non-union persisted in two and was salvaged with a total wrist fusion.

Ulnar styloid fractures

Fractures of the ulnar styloid in association with fractures of the distal radius are common, often progressing to non-union but not affecting the final outcome (Giannikas et al 1999). Oakarsson et al (1997) reported ulnar styloid fractures occurring in 70 of their 138 patients (53%) with fractures of the distal radius. They found this fracture to be a better predictor of a poor outcome than the intra-articular fracture although the combination of the two carried the worst prognosis.

Ulnar styloid non-unions are frequent, usually show no evidence of bone reaction and are painless. However, Burgess & Watson (1988) reported 11 patients with chronic pain on the ulnar side of the wrist associated with a hypertrophic ulnar styloid non-union. Subperiosteal excision of the non-union fragment relieved the localised pain. Shaw et al (1990) performed biomechanical tests on nine cadavaric forearms, confirming that the triangular fibrocartilage is a major stabiliser of the radio-ulnar joint, and that internal fixation of triangular fibrocartilage–ulnar styloid avulsion fractures restores stability. They advised primary repair of displaced ulnar styloid avulsion fractures as a means of stabilising the radio-ulnar joint and thus preventing the disability associated with chronic instability. In their six patients, all had stability restored after internal fixation. Hauck et al (1996) classified non-union of the ulnar styloid as: Type I, non-union associated with a stable distal radio-ulnar joint; and Type II, non-union associated with subluxation of the distal radio-ulnar joint. Eleven Type I wrists were treated with excision of the fragment, and all patients experienced satisfactory pain relief. Nine Type II wrists had surgery to stabilise the triangular fibrocartilage complex, seven with excellent results, one graded as good and one as fair. Kikuchi and Nakamura (1998) reported two examples of avulsion fractures at the fovea of the ulna, which they felt represented an injury to the triangular fibrocartilage complex. Both responded to conservative treatment.

Fracture of the distal ulna

Distal radial fractures can occur in association with distal ulnar metaphyseal fractures. Biyani et al (1995) reported this association in 19 of 320 (5.9%) patients. They divided them into four types: type 1 was a simple extra-articular fracture with minimal comminution; type 2 was an inverted T- or Y-shaped fracture with an ulnar styloid fragment including a portion of the metaphysis; type 3 was a fracture of the lower end of the ulna with an avulsion fracture of the ulnar styloid; and type 4 was a comminuted fracture of the lower ulnar metaphysis with or without a styloid fracture. Most of the patients were treated conservatively. Fifteen were reviewed after a mean follow-up of 23.8 months; the results were excellent, four (27%), good, five (33%), fair, five (33%) and poor, one (7%). Some loss of forearm rotation occurred in eight patients (53%).

Summary

- 78% of patients with Colles' fractures had a satisfactory end-result.
- Subjective symptoms occurred in 58–80.5% of patients after a Colles' fracture.
- It has been estimated that the average disability following a Colles' fracture is 17.7–24%.
- Up to 75% of patients had reported experiencing some subjective symptoms of pain with various activities after Colles' fracture.
- Fatiguability occurred in 2.3–6.6% of wrists after Colles' fracture.
- 18–35% of patients experienced feelings of subjective weakness after Colles' fracture, although objective weakness occurred in 9–17.5%. The average deficit in grip strength was 15.1–31% of the normal value. Grip strength recovered up to 1 year post fracture.
- Symptoms and signs of algodystrophy have been reported in up to 37% of patients after Colles' fracture. These symptoms do not appear after 9 weeks from injury. Residual finger stiffness occurs in 0.7–47.5% of patients after Colles' fracture.
- Palmar flexion, ulnar deviation and supination were most restricted following Colles' fracture.
- The younger the patient, the better was the overall functional result after extra-articular Colles' fracture, but results were inferior in intra-articular comminuted fractures.
- Undisplaced fissure fractures had 89–100% satisfactory results.
- Comminuted fractures had 25–80% satisfactory results.
- Involvement of the radio-ulnar joint resulted in 30–70% unsatisfactory results.
- 2–5% of patients with an excellent anatomical result had a poor functional result.
- 52–85% of patients with poor anatomical results had satisfactory functional results.
- A dorsal tilt of over 10° may adversely affect the functional end-result.
- A radial deviation of less than 10° and increased radial shortening probably affects the functional end-result, as does a persistent articular step-off.

- 28–59% of manipulated fractures redisplaced, and this displacement occurs up to 3 months after initial reduction.
- 40–57.5% of remanipulated fractures redisplaced.
- Percutaneous fixation resulted in 91% satisfactory functional results and 83–88% satisfactory anatomical results.
- After external fixation, 87.7% of patients achieved a satisfactory result, although these fractures were often more severe.
- Ligamentous injuries are common. Tears of the TFCC occur in 39–78% of patients, and scapholunate ligament injuries in 32–54%. Chondral lesions occur in 16%.
- Median nerve compression has been reported in 0.2–17.4% (average 2.9%) of Colles' fractures, and in 10–25% of these the symptoms developed after 3 months.
- Intra-articular fractures, older patients and residual dorsal angulation are associated with a higher incidence of median nerve compression.
- Ulnar nerve compression occurred in 0.8% of distal radial fractures.
- Rupture of extensor pollicus longus occurred in 0.5–1% of distal radial fractures.
- 44–72% of ruptures of extensor pollicus longus occurred in undisplaced fractures and 65–93% occurred within 8 weeks of fracture.
- 3–18% of fractures of the distal radius resulted in post-traumatic arthritis. In young adults with intra-articular fractures, post-traumatic arthritis occurred in 57–65%.
- 30% of patients with radiological signs of post-traumatic arthritis were symptomatic.
- The incidence of post-traumatic arthritis was higher in comminuted intra-articular fractures. Functional incapacity may be reasonable in the presence of post-traumatic osteoarthrosis.
- There may be an increased incidence of Dupuytren's disease and stenosing tenosynovitis after Colles' fracture.

- Proximal carpal instability may follow malunited fracture of the distal radius and corrective osteotomy was successful in 75–80% of patients.
- 7–17% of distal radial fractures may have associated scapholunate dissociation and DISI.
- Ulnar styloid non-union is often asymptomatic, but hypertrophic ulnar styloid non-union can be painful. Symptomatic non-union is usually successfully treated with surgery.

Fracture of the distal radius with palmar displacement

The description of a fracture of the distal radius with palmar displacement was made by R. W. Smith in 1847. In 1938, J. R. Barton described dorsal marginal fracture of the distal radius and drew attention to the occurrence of the less frequent palmar marginal fracture (Pattee & Thompson 1988). Controversy exists as to whether dorsal marginal fracture alone or dorsal and palmar marginal fractures combined constitute the true Barton's fracture.

Between 3 and 5% of distal radial fractures were of the palmar displacement (Smith's) type (Lidström 1959, Kaukonen et al 1988), and 0.5–1.2% were marginal articular fractures (Kaukonen et al 1988, Pattee & Thompson 1988). These marginal fractures of the distal radius are relatively rare and are said to occur with greater frequency in young men secondary to high-velocity accidents (Pattee & Thompson 1988).

Fractures with palmar displacement are unstable, and Thomas (1957) emphasised the importance of maintaining the forearm in supination. Redisplacement during the course of manipulation and plaster treatment is common, as Table 9.11: illustrates. Although the total numbers are small, the percentage exceeds 60.

The results of conservative treatment in four series are shown in Table 9.12, 75.5% overall being functionally satisfactory. King (1975) reported that all 17 patients with marginal articular fractures in his series had some pain, either weather sensitivity or discomfort with heavy

Table 9.11 Redisplacement after plaster immobilisation in Smith's and Barton's fractures

Reference	Number	Redisplaced
Flandreau et al (1962)	8	5 (62.5%)
Thompson & Grant (1977)	7	5 (71.4%)
Pattee & Thompson (1988)	18	10 (55.6%)
Overall	33	20 (60.6%)

labour, mild weakness and some minor loss of movement. On the other hand, Thomas (1957), who treated his patients with the forearm in full supination, had only one of 11 patients who did not achieve full pronation. Four (36.4%) of the 11 cases of Pattee & Thompson (1988) had mild pain and there was a mean loss of 4° dorsiflexion and 5° palmar flexion. The healing time was 6–8 weeks.

These fractures may be treated by internal fixation with a buttress plate, and the results of surgical treatment are shown in Table 9.13. Overall, 79.8% achieved a satisfactory functional result. Fuller (1973) had satisfactory results in 28 of 31 fractures (90%). The average period of incapacity after internal fixation was 4 months (De Oliveira 1973).

Jupiter et al (1996) reviewed 49 patients who had operative treatment of a volar intra-articular fracture. At an average follow-up of 51 months there were 32 excellent results (65%), nine good (19%), five fair (10%) and three poor (6%). Fifteen patients had a complication, adversely influencing the overall outcome in some form. Nienstedt (1999) also concentrated on intra-articular fractures in his report of 21 fractures treated by operative fixation.

Eighteen patients (86%) had an excellent or good result, two (9%) a fair result and one (5%) a poor result.

Subsequent radiocarpal arthritis was noted in nine (18.4%) of the 49 patients in Jupiter et al's 1996 series, and in three (12.5%) of 24 patients reported by De Oliveira (1973). A much higher incidence was reported by Pattee & Thompson (1988): of their 20 patients, 13 (65%) had some radiographic evidence of post-traumatic arthritis. There were nine patients with mild, two with moderate and two (both with concomitant ipsilateral transscaphoid perilunate fracture–dislocations) with severe changes. They found that the most important correlations between the functional result and post-traumatic arthritis were residual displacement of the articular surface and ipsilateral carpal injuries.

Occasionally, the tendons of extensor pollicus longus and the long extensors to the fingers have been reported as being trapped within these fractures. The median nerve is at risk of irritation as a result of these injuries. van Leeuwen et al (1990) noted this complication in 13 (24.5%) of their 53 cases, mostly due to the initial trauma. All but one recovered completely within 1 year. Three of the 49

Table 9.12 The conservative treatment of distal radial fractures with palmar displacement

Reference	Number of patients	Excellent		Good		Fair		Poor	
		No.	%	No.	%	No.	%	No.	%
Lidström (1959)	13	1	7.7	6	46.2	4	30.8	2	
Flandreau et al (1961)	8	4	50	3	37.5			1	
Frykman (1967)*	17	4	23.5	8	47	4	23.5	1	
Pattee & Thompson (1988)	11	6	54.5	5	45.5				
Overall	49	15	30.6	22	44.9	8	16.3	4	

75.5% satisfactory, 24.5% unsatisfactory
* This series involves four operated cases.

Table 9.13 The results of the surgical treatment of Smith's fractures

Reference	Number	Excellent	Good	Fair	Poor
De Oliveira (1973)	24	9 (37.5%)	11 (45.8%)	3 (12.5%)	1 (4.2%)
van Leeuwen et al (1990)	53	9 (17%)	32 (60.4%)	9 (17%)	3 (5.6%)
Pattee & Thompson (1988)	7	2 (28.6%)	4 (57.1%)	1 (14.3%)	
Overall	84	20 (23.8%)	47 (56%)	13 (15.5%)	4 (4.7%)

79.8% satisfactory, 20.2% unsatisfactory

cases reported in Jupiter et al's 1996 series required a carpal tunnel decompression.

Twenty-five patients had an opening wedge osteotomy for the treatment of a malunited, volarly displaced fracture of the distal end of the radius (Shea et al 1997). Preoperatively, extension of the wrist averaged 25° and grip strength was 42.5% of the contralateral hand. At an average of 61 months after the osteotomy extension of the wrist had improved to an average of 55° and grip strength to 75% of the contralateral hand. The functional result was rated as excellent in 10 patients (40%), good in eight (32%), fair in three (12%) and poor in four (16%).

The association of a Smith's fracture with a scaphoid fracture (van Leeuwen et al 1990) or other carpal injuries (Pattee & Thompson 1988) gave a poor functional result.

Summary

- Anatomical reduction was lost in 60–67% of conservatively treated fractures of the distal radius with palmar displacement.
- A satisfactory result was achieved in 75.5% of distal radial fractures with palmar displacement after conservative treatment. The healing time was 6–8 weeks.
- 80–86% of these fractures had satisfactory results after internal fixation. The average period of incapacity was 4 months.
- Post-traumatic arthritis occurred in 12–65% of these fractures.
- Median nerve irritation was seen in up to 24.5% of patients.

Epiphyseal fractures of the distal radius and ulna

Epiphyseal fractures of the distal radius and ulna are common injuries in childhood. The incidence is variably reported as having occurred in 8.5% (Harbison et al 1978) to 17.9% (Thomas et al 1975) of forearm fractures in children, and in 54.8% of 911 wrist injuries reported by Lee et al (1984). The majority are Salter type II injuries. In the series of 499 epiphyseal injuries presented by Lee et al (1984), 110 (22%) were Salter type I injuries, 288 (57.7%) type II, 13 (2.6%) type III, 10 (2%) type IV, two (0.4%) type V and 76 (15.3%) were unclassified.

Accurate reduction of the fracture was not necessary for a good functional result, only 50% apposition being required, and O'Brien (1984) quoted Aitken as having found no residual deformity in 58 patients reviewed. Plaster immobilisation was required for 3–6 weeks.

Redisplacement can occur, and this happened in four of 53 cases (7.5%) reported by Davis & Green (1976). Premature fusion of the epiphyseal plate after repeated manipulation of these fractures was warned of by O'Brien (1984) and experienced by Lee et al (1984) in six patients out of 22 (27.3%) who underwent two or more attempts at closed reduction.

Open reduction was rarely required but irreducible fractures have been reported, with the block to reduction being the flexor digitorum profundus tendon to the ring and little fingers (Manoli 1982) or the median nerve and flexor pollicis longus tendon (Sumner & Khun 1984).

Guichet et al (1997) described a modification of the Kapandji percutaneous intrafocal pinning in the treatment of unstable Smith's fractures in children. All six patients had a good result.

Although five of 67 patients (7.5%) in Thomas et al's 1975 series were felt to have unsatisfactory results on discharge from review, most patients eventually achieved full function. Harbison et al (1978) reported that their 88 patients with Salter type II epiphyseal injuries all regained full function despite the lack of complete reduction in some.

Premature epiphyseal arrest was the main complication, and its incidence in reported series (4.6% overall) is recorded in Table 9.14. Although this problem usually arose as the result of the compression type V injury, this

Table 9.14 The incidence of premature epiphyseal fusion in fractures of the distal radial epiphysis

Reference	Number of patients	Number with premature fusion	%
Thomas et al (1975)	42	3	7.1
Davis & Green (1976)	53	1	1.9
Harbison et al (1978)	88	2	2.3
Lee et al (1984)	100	7	7
Overall	283	13	4.6

injury was often not diagnosed at initial presentation (O'Brien 1984). It also occurred in type IV and type II injuries (Lee et al 1984), but there is no record of it being found in the rare type III injury. Premature fusion may be partial or complete and produces deformity, weakness of grip and occasional loss of motion. Hove and Engesoeter (1997) performed corrective osteotomies of the distal forearm because of growth disturbance from post-traumatic closure of the distal radial physis in six children. Three patients had a lengthening osteotomy of the radius with bone graft and three had shortening of the ulna. The postoperative pain relief was complete in all patients and the total range of motion was 96% compared with the opposite side. Non-union of a distal radial fracture in a child is extremely uncommon but has been reported (Kwa & Tonkin 1997)

Fractures of the ulnar styloid in children occurred in 45 of the 222 (20.3%) with wrist fracture studied by Stansberry et al (1990). They found that it was seldom an isolated injury, and thus served as a useful signal for the presence of an associated radial fracture.

Fractures of the distal ulnar epiphysis are uncommon, occurring in association with less than 4% of distal radial injuries (Gotz et al 1991); in isolation, too, they are extremely rare (Evans et al 1990). Gotz et al noted that of their 16 patients with fresh injuries, eight had a type I injury, six a type III injury, one a type II and one a type IV. Four patients required open reduction. Premature epiphyseal closure occurred in 10 of the 18 patients (55%) in the whole series. The degree of ulnar minus variance ranged from 2–30 mm. Patients with post-traumatic growth arrest had few symptoms, and indeed most were asymptomatic.

Summary

- Accurate reduction of distal radial epiphyseal fractures was not necessary for a good functional result.
- Redisplacement occurred in 7.5% of patients.
- Repeated manipulation resulted in premature fusion of the epiphysis in 27.3% of patients.
- Premature epiphyseal arrest occurred in 4.6% of patients, and in Salter type II, type IV and type V injuries.
- Premature fusion of the distal ulnar epiphysis occurred in 55% of patients but was usually asymptomatic.

Isolated injury of the distal radio-ulnar joint

Pure dislocation of the distal radio-ulnar joint and tears of the triangular fibrocartilage complex do occur in isolation, but are not common injuries.

Dislocation of the distal radio-ulnar joint

Isolated dorsal or palmar dislocation of the distal ulna can occur. However, this isolated lesion was missed at initial assessment in up to 50% of cases (Alexander 1977). Dorsal dislocation results in a prominent ulna with painful and limited supination. The dislocation is easily reduced when seen in the acute stage and plaster immobilisation is required for 4–6 weeks. A complex dislocation of the distal radio-ulnar joint is characterised by obvious irreducability, recurrent subluxation or dislocation, or a mushy sensation caused by soft tissue interposition when reduction is attempted (Bruckner et al 1995). Manipulative reduction of a dorsal dislocation has been performed successfully 60 days after initial injury (Dameron 1972), although Dobyns & Linscheid (1984) felt that if reduction was delayed beyond 2 weeks then laxity of the distal radio-ulnar joint could occur. This would result in recurrent subluxation in pronation, which might require ligamentous reconstruction or distal excision of the ulna in some cases. Late presentation may require open reduction or excision of the distal ulna. Hanel & Sheid (1988) reported the case of a 12-year-old boy with irreducible dorsal dislocation of the distal radio-ulnar joint due to entrapment of the extensor carpi ulnaris tendon.

Palmar dislocation causes the wrist to appear narrow on the AP X-ray, and pronation is painful or impossible. This type of dislocation tends to be stable when reduced early, although habitual volar subluxation has been reported (Rose-Innes 1960). Late diagnosis may necessitate open reduction or excision of the distal ulna.

Tears of the triangular fibrocartilage complex (TFC)

Tears of the TFC can occur in isolation or in combination with fractures of the distal radius and ulna. Degeneration and perforation of the TFC can also occur with ageing, and 30.6–53% of TFCs in cadavers show perforation (Coleman 1960, Fisk 1984). However, some of these may be congenital perforations. Tan et al (1995) studied the TFC in 120 cadaveric wrists of the foetus and infant and noted 27 perforations in the 120 wrists (22.5%).

Strickner et al (1980) found 53 confirmed lesions of the triangular disc on arthrography in 153 patients (34.6%) with post-traumatic ulnar pain, while Moharti & Kar (1979) reported arthrographically proven tears of the TFC in 27 of 60 patients after a Colles' fracture (45%). Arthroscopic assessment of wrists after fractures of the distal radius has revealed tears of the TFC in 39% (Richards et al 1997) to 43% (Geissler et al 1996).

Dobyns & Linscheid (1984) suggested that if an acute tear of the TFC was suspected then the wrist should be immobilised for 4–6 weeks. They reported that these injuries often improved with time.

Coleman (1960) found that removal of the disc relieved symptoms and did not prejudice function. However, Fisk (1984) suggested that the results of disc excision were disappointing and he felt that instability of the distal radio-ulnar joint was almost inevitable.

Hulsizer et al (1997) arthroscopically debrided 97 patients with central or non-detached ulnar peripheral tears of the TFC. Thirteen patients (13%) had persisting pain. Westkaemper et al (1998) performed arthroscopic debridement on 28 wrists with TFC tears and reported excellent or good results in 21 patients (75%), fair results in two (7%) and poor results in five (18%).

Corso et al (1997) performed an arthroscopic reconstruction of the peripheral attachment of the TFC in 45 wrists. Excellent/good results were reported in 41 patients (91%), whilst one was noted as fair (2%) and three as poor (7%).

Minami and Kato (1998) performed ulnar shortening in 25 patients with TFC tears. Twenty-three (92%) had either complete relief or only occasional mild pain of the wrist.

Summary

- Isolated dislocations of the radio-ulnar joint were frequently missed at initial presentation.
- Early reduction of dorsal dislocation results in good functional recovery, but late presentation may require distal ulnar excision.
- Prompt reduction of volar dislocation tends to be stable, although recurrent subluxation can occur.
- Perforations in the triangular fibrocartilage complex were seen in 30.6–53% of cadavers examined.
- 35–45% of patients with post-traumatic ulnar pain had lesions of the triangular disc.

- Acute tears of the triangular disc may settle with 4–6 weeks in plaster.
- 75–92% of patients may have successful results following surgery on the TFC.

■ Carpal Fractures and Dislocations

Scaphoid fractures

Fractures of the carpal scaphoid are relatively common. Their classification into anatomical thirds (distal, middle and proximal) is adequate to enable consideration of their prognosis, and they can be further divided into undisplaced or displaced fractures. The incidence of scaphoid fractures at the three anatomical sites in some of the larger series is shown in Table 9.15, 22.4% occurring in the distal third overall, 73.3% in the middle third and 4.3% in the proximal third.

The majority of scaphoid fractures are treated by conservative methods, although there is no agreement as to which position of immobilisation is correct. The overall results of conservative treatment will be presented with no consideration to the position of immobilisation. A later section will deal with the results of surgical treatment.

The results of conservative treatment

The overall rate of non-union in conservatively treated scaphoid fractures from seven of the larger reported series is shown in Table 9.16. This gives an overall non-union rate of 7.7%. Herbert & Fisher (1984), writing in support of their compression screw, claimed a non-union rate in the order of 50% after conservative treatment.

Table 9.15 The incidence of scaphoid fractures according to anatomical location

Reference	Number of patients	Distal third		Middle third		Proximal third	
		No.	%	No.	%	No.	%
London (1961)	300	73	24.3	218	72.7	9	3
Stewart (1954)	258	44	17.1	207	80.2	7	2.7
Leslie & Dickson (1981)	222	63	28.4	146	65.8	13	5.8
Clay et al (1991)	285	25	8.8	249	87.4	11	3.8
Langhoff & Andersen (1988)	285	97	34	169	59.3	19	6.7
Overall	1350	302	22.4	989	73.3	59	4.3

The rate at which union occurs at the various anatomical locations will be discussed later in this section. It is perhaps appropriate at this point to stress how unreliable inter-observer agreement is when attempting to assess radiographic criteria for scaphoid fracture or scaphoid union (Dias et al 1988, 1990).

In their review of carpal injuries in Holland, Mink Van Der Molen et al (1999) noted that the average immobilization for 447 scaphoid fractures was 11.1 weeks. The mean time off work was 144 days. Four hundred and thirty-seven patients returned to their original work, four to different work and six patients had a partial or permanent disability.

Although the functional results are generally good, Lindström & Nyström (1990) found that of their study group of 229 patients reviewed with a minimum of a 7 year follow-up, 10.5% noticed weakness of grip and 9.6% noticed pain related to wrist motion. Impaired range of motion was reported in 5.7% and pain at rest occurred in 3.1%. Borgeskov et al (1966) reported three of 71 patients (4%) with complaints severe enough to reduce their working capacity and 30% had slight impairment of function, while Eddeland et al (1975) found that 28% of their 92 patients had a slight decrease in grip strength. Stewart (1954) reported that after removal of plaster following scaphoid fractures, function recovered very quickly, generally in 3.5 weeks.

Amadio et al (1989) found that increasing malunion of scaphoid fracture, eventually resulting in a 'humpback' deformity, was associated with progressively poor clinical and radiological results (Table 9.17). Up to 85% of patients had a good clinical result after healing with normal anatomy, while up to 42% had a poor functional result, healing with severe malunion.

There is an increased frequency of non-union with increased delay in treatment beyond 4 weeks from injury (Langhoff & Andersen 1988). However, in their study of 285 fractures of the scaphoid these authors noted that there was no increase in the time to bony union or in the incidence of non-union if there was a delay of immobilisation of less than 4 weeks. They concluded that it was unnecessary to immobilise the wrist when there was a

Table 9.16 The non-union rate in conservatively treated scaphoid fractures

Reference	Number of patients	Number of non-unions	%
Lindström & Nyström (1990)	412	75	18.2
Stewart (1954)*	306	3	1
London (1961)	227	11	5
Leslie & Dickson (1981)	222	11	5
Russe (1960)	220	6	2.7
Clay et al (1991)	284	26	9.2
Langhoff & Andersen (1988)	251	16	6.4
Overall	1922	148	7.7

* The end-result of some of Stewart's reported fractures was uncertain.

Table 9.17 The relationship of scaphoid malunion to the clinical outcome

Reference	Anatomy	Number	Excellent/good	Fair	Poor
Amadio et al (1989)	Normal	20	17 (85%)	3 (15%)	–
	Malunion	26	16 (61.5%)	7 (26.9%)	3 (11.6%)
Condamine et al (1986) (as quoted by Amadio)	Good position	46	21 (45.7%)	18 (39.1%)	7 (15.2%)
	Moderate malunion	21	2 (9.5%)	13 (61.9%)	6 (28.6%)
	Severe malunion	19	3 (15.8)	8 (42.1%)	8 (42.1%)

clinical suspicion of a fracture which was not demonstrable at X-ray examination. If another X-ray was felt necessary after a clinical examination at 2 weeks and immobilisation was required, the frequency of non-union was not increased. In a further study of the clinical fractured scaphoid, Sjølin & Andersen (1988) compared 108 patients treated with either a supportive bandage or dorsal plaster cast. They found that these injuries always healed irrespective of treatment, and recommended they be treated as a soft tissue injury with a supportive bandage. Only seven patients (6.5%) had a confirmed scaphoid fracture. Duncan & Thurston (1985) found no scaphoid fractures after reviewing 108 patients with a clinical diagnosis of fracture of the scaphoid. Jacobsen et al (1995) reviewed 231 patients with clinical signs of a fractured carpal scaphoid but negative primary radiographs. Only three fractures (1.3%) of the scaphoid were finally diagnosed on subsequent clinical and radiological examination. They also advocated the use of a simple supportive bandage for an observation period.

Munk et al (1995) reported a large multicentre prospective study of 1052 patients with clinical signs of a scaphoid fracture. One hundred and fifty fractures were diagnosed at the first examination. Ten cases of scaphoid fracture (1.1%) were confirmed after a second radiographic examination 10–14 days later. Thus it would seem that plaster immobilisation is not required for a clinical fractured scaphoid but a review appointment should be offered to allow clinical reassessment with radiological examination if indicated. However, with the increasing use of magnetic resonance imaging (MRI) associated wrist injuries in patients with clinical fractured scaphoids are being reported. Kukla et al (1997) performed MRIs on 25 patients with suspect scaphoid injuries. They found eight examples of bony abnormality of the scaphoid, five coincidental bony

lesions and three purely ligamentous lesions. In another study of 59 patients reported by Thorpe et al (1996), four scaphoid fractures, 10 other fractures and three significant ligamentous injuries were noted. Delayed diagnosis and treatment beyond 4 weeks may delay fracture union. Mack et al (1998) retrospectively reviewed 23 subacute scaphoid fractures in which the patients sought medical attention 4 weeks to 6 months after injury. Nine of 10 stable subacute middle third fractures healed at an average of 19 weeks whereas a similar group of stable acute middle third fractures healed in an average of 10 weeks. Five of six unstable subacute middle third fractures healed in an average of 20 weeks. Only one of three subacute proximal third fractures healed after 29 weeks of closed treatment.

Undisplaced fractures of the scaphoid have a significantly higher union rate than displaced fractures. The reported incidences in those series distinguishing the rates of union between these two groups of fractures are shown in Table 9.18. Although these are not large series, it can be seen that the non-union rate in displaced scaphoid fractures averages 27.8%, as compared with 6.8% for undisplaced fractures. Langhoff & Andersen (1988) found that undisplaced fractures healed at an average of 8.5 weeks, while displaced fractures healed at an average of 10.6 weeks from injury.

Leslie & Dickson (1981) felt that non-union was not related to the initial displacement of the fracture but more to those fractures which displaced during treatment. However, Fisk (1984) and Taleisnik (1985) regarded internal fixation of the fractured scaphoid as mandatory when there was displacement of the fracture.

Avascular necrosis was variably reported as occurring in from less than 1% of scaphoid fractures (Borgeskov et al 1966) to up to 40% of proximal scaphoid fractures

Table 9.18 The comparative rates of union between undisplaced and displaced scaphoid fractures

References	Undisplaced fractures			Displaced fractures		
	No. of patients	Non-unions	%	No. of patients	Non-unions	%
Eddeland et al (1975)	82	11	13.4	30	26	83
Clay et al (1991)	126	9	7	74	10	14
Gellman et al (1989)	51	2	4	–	–	–
Langhoff & Andersen (1988)	105	3	3	52	5	9.6
Cooney et al (1980b)	32	2	6	13	6	46
Overall	396	27	6.8	169	47	27.8

(Gellman et al 1989). In their review article Buchler and Nagy (1995) suggest that transient ischaemia is frequent but frank necrosis occurs in probably less than 14% of patients. The incidence of avascular necrosis is increased in fractures that have more than 1 mm of displacement, being reported in up to 50% of patients (Szabo & Manske 1988). It would appear to cause delay in union; in Stewart's 1954 paper, fractures with avascular necrosis healed in an average of 21 weeks, as compared with 10–16 weeks for other fractures. A similar finding was recorded by Gellman et al (1989). In their series, with treatment in either a long or short thumb spica cast, the fractures healed at an average of 9.5 weeks or 12.7 weeks, depending on the type of cast, but this increased to an average duration of immobilisation of 15.3 weeks with the development of avascular necrosis. It is not an impending sign of non-union. Four cases have been reported in which avascular necrosis of the proximal part of the scaphoid developed after apparent healing of the acute fracture (Filan & Herbert 1995).

Results in distal third fractures

Distal third fractures have an overall incidence of 22.4%, and may be further subdivided into those of the scaphoid tubercle and of the intra-articular distal pole, as well as true distal third fractures. Fractures of the tubercle are stable, extra-articular and tend to heal rapidly in 3–6 weeks. Occasionally, delayed union and non-union occur. Langhoff & Andersen (1988) reported two cases of delayed union (3.5%) in the 57 patients with tuberosity fractures that they recorded, while Prosser et al (1988) noted one case of non-union (5%) in 20 patients with this injury.

Ripperger et al (1980) described the intra-articular distal pole fracture. Eight radio-distal cases were diagnosed early and healed in 6–7 weeks with good results. Four ulno-distal cases were diagnosed late and all went on to symptomatic non-union.

Other distal third fractures tend to unite in 4–8 weeks. Borgeskov et al (1966) reported excellent functional results in 11 of 17 patients (64.7%), good results in five (29.4%) and fair results in one (5.9%).

Results in middle third fractures

Fractures of the middle third of the scaphoid account for 73.3% of all scaphoid fractures. The time to union following conservative treatment ranges from 8.5 weeks (Langhoff & Andersen 1988) to 12.7 weeks (Gellman et al 1989). The incidence of delayed union and non-union is shown in Table 9.19. Non-union was reported in 8.2% of middle third scaphoid fractures, while delayed union occurred in 11.7%. Avascular necrosis was noted in five of 40 middle third fractures treated in a cast (12.5%) and two of these cases went on to delayed union (Gellman et al 1989).

In the series reported by Dias et al (1989), of 52 patients with united fractures, nine (17.3%) complained of mild symptoms, 13 (25%) had some local tenderness, and all had an essentially normal range of movement and power of grip. These observations were made at a mean period of 2.1 years after injury. Lindström & Nyström (1990) reported on 229 healed middle third scaphoid fractures with a minimum follow-up of 7 years. A weakness of grip was noted in 10.5%, and pain with wrist motion was seen in 9.6%. An improved range of motion was recorded in 5.7%, and 3.1% had pain at rest. Early radiological signs of radiocarpal arthrosis were seen in 12 cases (5.2%). Of the 84 patients reviewed at 6 months by Hambidge et al (1999), 63 patients (75%) had no pain, 17 (20%) had mild pain, three (4%) had moderate pain and one had severe pain.

Borgeskov et al (1966) found excellent functional results in 32 of 44 patients (72.7%), satisfactory results in 11 patients (25%) and fair results in one (2.3%).

Dias et al (1989) noted a subgroup of patients in their study who appeared to have a healed middle third scaphoid fracture, and yet the site of fracture could be easily identified on radiographs taken more than 1 year after injury. This subgroup tended to be older patients, and predominantly female. Of these 20 patients, 15 (75%) had pain, over half had local tenderness and one-third had appreciable weakness of grip strength, but wrist movement was essentially normal.

Results in proximal third fractures

Proximal third fractures account for 4.3% of all scaphoid fractures. Union after cast immobilisation is noted as occurring in 9–15 weeks. Non-union is reported to occur in from 31% (Clay et al 1991) to 42.1% of cases (Langhoff & Andersen 1988). Avascular necrosis occurred in up to 40% of cases (Gellman et al 1989). The functional results in these fractures were 30% excellent, 60% good and 10% fair, in a 10 patient study (Borgeskov et al 1966).

The results of the operative treatment of fresh scaphoid fractures

Internal fixation of the fractured scaphoid is recommended in displaced fractures, fractures associated with carpal instability and where the fracture is part of a complicated fracture–dislocation.

The largest reported series appears to be that of Wozasek & Moser (1991), reporting on 146 patients treated via a percutaneous screw fixation. Union occurred in 130 patients (89%); 87 patients (60%) had no pain and full

Table 9.19 The incidence of delayed union and non-union in fractures of the middle third of the scaphoid

Reference	Number	Delayed union	Non-union
Langhoff & Andersen (1988)	157	21 (13.4%)	8 (5.1%)
Gellman et al (1989)	40	2 (5%)	1 (2.5%)
Dias et al (1989)*	82	–	10 (12.3%)
Clay et al (1991)*	269	–	22 (8.2%)
Hambidge et al (1999)*	108	–	13 (12%)
Totals			
Non-union	656		54 (8.2%)
Delayed union	197	23 (11.7%)	

* These papers were not concerned with delayed union.

strength, 50 (34%) had occasional pain, seven (5%) had frequent pain and two (1%) had continuous pain. Full function was noted in 107 patients (73%), 30 (20.5%) had 20° or less loss of movement, five (3.5%) lost between 20° and 50°, and four (3%) lost at least 50° range of movement.

Filan & Herbert (1996) achieved good results with the Herbert compression screw, with 87.5% union in 56 cases, and the patients returning to work at a mean of 4.7 weeks. However, they confirmed that the main disadvantage of the screw fixation is that it is technically difficult.

Inoue and Shionoya (1997) described a semi-closed method of Herbert screw fixation for acute fractures of the scaphoid. They used their technique in 40 patients and compared the results with 39 patients treated conservatively. Fracture union was reported for all of the patients treated surgically at an average of 6 weeks as compared with 9.7 weeks in the conservatively treated group. The average return to work time for manual labourers in the conservative group was 10.2 weeks and in the surgical group 5.8 weeks. Three patients in each group had more than 10% loss of movement and/or more than 20% loss of grip strength compared with the uninjured hand.

McLaughlin & Parkes (1969) reported 100% union in a series of 16 fresh scaphoid fractures treated by screw fixation. In 22 fresh fractures treated with a screw, Maudsley & Chen (1972) had 19 unions (86.4%) with all the patients achieving bony union having excellent function, and two of the non-unions nonetheless having good function post-operatively.

Simultaneous fractures of the scaphoid and distal radius

Vukov et al (1988) reported that 26 (4%) of the 650 injuries of the distal radius seen at their clinic in Belgrade had a simultaneous fracture of the scaphoid bone. They found that the fracture of the radius typically had minimal or slight displacement, and the fracture of the scaphoid bone was undisplaced. In eight patients (30.7%) the scaphoid fracture was not recognised at initial presentation. Consolidation of the fractures occurred within 8 weeks. Full movement was obtained in 11 patients, and slightly limited motion was seen in the remaining 15 patients.

Oskam et al (1996) reported that all the scaphoid fractures in their 23 patients were undisplaced and healed without complication. Twelve patients required a primary operative procedure for the distal radius fracture, and in three treated conservatively redisplacement occurred. The final functional result was good in 18 patients (78%), fair in four (17%) and poor in one.

Non-union of the scaphoid

Not every example of scaphoid non-union is necessarily a cause of symptoms. Sometimes, symptoms are provoked by a second injury and may rapidly resolve with conservative measures. This has led some authors (London 1961) to recommend no surgical treatment for established non-union in the absence of significant clinical symptoms. Indeed spontaneous healing of a non-union has been reported (Roolker et al 1998). However, a number of more recent publications have suggested that there is progressive degeneration with an increased period of non-union.

Mack et al (1984) looked at 47 symptomatic scaphoid non-unions. They divided the stages of degeneration into three groups. Group I, with scaphoid changes only, was seen in 23 patients, with an average duration of their non-union of 8.2 years. In group II, 14 patients with radioscaphoid degeneration had had their non-union for

17 years, while in the third group, with generalised arthritis (10 patients), the average was 31.6 years. The authors commented that after 5–10 years of non-union almost all showed cyst formation and resorptive changes within the scaphoid.

Ruby et al (1985) also found an increased incidence and severity of degenerative changes with increasing duration of non-union. Only one (4%) of 23 non-unions of 1–4 years' duration had arthritis, while 92% of 13 patients with non-unions of 5–9 years and all 19 patients with non-union of 10 or more years had degenerative changes.

Vender et al (1987) reported progressive arthritis in 64 patients with scaphoid non-union. When the non-union was over 18 months old, 100% had scaphoid cysts; 75% had radioscaphoid arthritis at 4 years, and only 38% had midcarpal arthritis after this same period of non-union. Inoue and Sakuma (1996) retrospectively reviewed 104 scaphoid non-unions. Osteoarthritis occurred in 22% of those of less than 5 years' duration, 75% of those of 5–9 years' duration and 100% of those of 10 years' duration. Symptomatic non-union of the scaphoid may eventually lead to a type of degenerative arthritis with severe collapse termed 'scaphoid non-union advanced collapse' (SNAC). These and similar findings have led to the conclusion that at least symptomatic and probably asymptomatic scaphoid non-unions should be treated surgically.

Fisk (1970) noted the adverse effects that carpal instability had on scaphoid union. Black et al (1986) reported that 10 of their 64 non-unions had a scapholunate gap, and that the instability was progressive and associated with the earlier onset of arthritis. The presence of displacement at the fracture site and the scapholunate gap did not change in frequency with time, but the incidence of increased scapholunate angle and the dorsal intercalated segmental instability (DISI) pattern increased significantly with a longer duration of non-union. Milliez et al (1987) found that eight of their 32 cases of non-union suffering a single trauma presented with a DISI, which was always accompanied by displacement of the fracture by at least 1 mm.

Inoue and Sakuma (1996) reported an overall incidence of DISI deformity of the wrist in 56% of their cases and they also noted that the frequency of the DISI pattern increased with a longer duration of non-union.

Monsivais et al (1986) performed wrist arthrograms or plain X-rays in 20 consecutive scaphoid non-unions. They found that an intercalated segmental instability was consistently found in wrists with non-union of scaphoid fractures and probably predicted those patients with a greater chance of non-union. Failure to correct this instability and subsequent malunion increased the chances of developing arthritis (Vender et al 1987). Tsuyuguchi et al (1995) emphasised the importance of restoring the scapholunate angulation of the affected wrist when treating the humpback deformity of scaphoid non-union with an anterior wedge-shaped bone graft. They reported the results in 27 patients, all having progressed to bony union, although two patients required a second operation. There was a statistically significant relationship between the wrist score and the postoperative scapho-lunate angulation.

Many techniques have been described for the surgical treatment of scaphoid non-union, and a few of the more commonly used are included below.

Bone graft

Cancellous or corticocancellous bone grafts are inserted using a variety of techniques via dorsal or volar approaches. The results from the larger reported series, which describe slightly differing techniques, are documented in Table 9.20. Overall, the union rate was about 89.3%, union occurring in 15.8–18 weeks.

Table 9.20 The results of bone grafts for scaphoid non-union

Reference	Number of patients	Number united	%
Mulder (1968)	100	97	97
Cooney et al (1980b)	66	58	87.9
Barton (1997)	83*	59	71.1
Green (1985)	45	33	73.3
Stark et al (1988)	151	147	97.4
Brunelli & Brunelli (1991)	52	50	96.2
Overall	497	444	89.3

* 3 different procedures described. Only definite non-unions excluded from total united

Green (1985) described 92% union in patients with good vascularity of the proximal pole of the scaphoid, as compared with no cases of union when the proximal pole was totally avascular.

van Duyvenbode et al (1991) reviewed 100 patients previously reported by Mulder (1968) following the Russe operation for non-union of the scaphoid. Sixty-nine patients at a mean of 27.9 years after operation were functionally assessed; 35 (50.7%) had a good subjective result, 21 (30.4%) a moderate result (slight pain and slight loss of mobility), and 13 (18.9%) had a poor result (moderate to severe pain and loss of mobility). Long-term radiographic findings showed slow progression of osteoarthritis in the pattern described as scapholunate advanced collapse, but as compared to untreated cases the progress of degeneration to severe general osteoarthritis of the carpus was greatly retarded.

Siebel et al (1998) also reported the long-term functional results of 121 patients at an average 11 year follow-up after Matte-Russe bone graft. They found 29% to be excellent, 34% good, 26% fair and 11% poor. Arthrosis was seen in more than 50% of cases, although the subjective result was much better than the radiological result would suggest.

Screw fixation

The results of screw fixation for delayed and non-union of scaphoid fractures are shown in Table 9.21. Union is reported to occur in 86% of cases. Although Enders' 1989 results are excellent, no details of the patients were given in this paper.

Radford et al (1990) noted that 64% of their patients united within 12 weeks. However, 20% required immobil-isation for up to 6 months. Inoue et al (1997) reported a high degree of patient satisfaction following surgery, even in those with persistent non-union. Results were excellent in 80 cases (50%), good in 37 (23%), fair in 33 (21%) and poor in 10 cases (6%). Kvarnes et al (1983) measured the grip strength in their series and noted that in 28 (63.6%) it was equal to or less than 10% reduced compared with the other side; 14 (31.8%) had a grip strength reduced by less than 30%, while only two patients (4.6%) showed a marked loss.

Both Inoue et al (1997) and Shah and Jones (1998) noted that the success rate in their series fell off as the duration of non-union before treatment increased.

Proximal pole fractures of the scaphoid tend to have a worse prognosis due to the risks of avascular necrosis. Herbert and Filan (1999) reported the results of retro-grade screw fixation of 69 patients with symptomatic non-union of the proximal pole. At an average follow-up of 34 months, 59 (85%) were asymptomatic and had regained excellent wrist function, inspite of the fact that sound radiological union was present in only 50% of these. Union was often slow (3–36 months) and appeared to be related to the vascularity of the bone fragments. The 10 patients with unsatisfactory results had all developed late avascular necrosis of the proximal pole. Similarly Inoue et al (1997) reported definite bony union in only 13 of 16 patients after bone graft and retrograde Herbert screw fixation for ununited proximal pole fractures. Clinical results were five excellent, five good, five fair and one poor.

In the presence of an avascular proximal pole, Robbins et al (1995) achieved definite bony union in only nine of 17 patients after Herbert screw and bone graft. The

Table 9.21 The results of screw fixation in delayed union and non-union of scaphoid fractures

Reference	Number	Number united
Ender (1989)*	271	266 (98.2%)
Filan & Herbert (1996)	234	163 (70%)
Radford et al (1990)[†]	50	42 (84%)
Kvarnes & Reikeras (1983)[‡]	44	42 (95.5%)
Shah & Jones (1998)	50	40 (80%)
Inoue et al (1997)	160	144 (90%)
Total	809	697 (86%)

* Bone graft and hook plate.
[†] Herbert screw with or without bone graft.
[‡] Compresson screw with or without bone graft.

functional results were excellent in six patients, good in five, fair in four, and poor in two patients.

Radford et al (1990) confirmed the technical difficulties of the Herbert screw, noting problems in 28% of their cases.

Vascularised bone graft

The subject of avascular necrosis and vascularised bone grafts has been well reviewed by Buchler and Nagy (1995). A number of different techniques have been described.

Mathoulin and Haerle (1998) achieved bony union in all 17 patients using bone graft from the palmar and ulnar aspect of the distal radius and vascularised by the palmar carpal artery. Union occurred at an average of 60 days.

Zaidemberg et al (1991) achieved union in all 11 of their patients at an average of 6.2 weeks using a pedicled vascularised bone graft from the dorsum of the distal radius, and Kawai & Yamanoto (1988) reported that a bone graft on a pronator quadratus pedicle produced early union in all of their eight patients at an average of 8.5 weeks.

Tendon rupture

Occasionally, attritional rupture of flexor pollicus longus and the flexor profundus to the index finger after long-standing non-union of the scaphoid has been reported (McLain & Steyers 1990). This may simulate an anterior interosseous nerve palsy.

Scaphoid fracture in children

Scaphoid fractures in children are not common, although on occasion they have been reported in those under 6 years of age (Larson et al 1987). These occur most commonly in the distal third of the scaphoid. Müssbichler (1961) reported 100 scaphoid fractures in children; 85% occurred in the distal third and 52% were avulsions from the dorso radial surface of the scaphoid. Of Vahranen & Westerlund's (1980) 108 patients, 94 (87%) were distal third and 41 (38%) were avulsion fractures, while in Christodoulou & Colton's 1986 series of 64 patients, 38 (59.4%) were distal third fractures and a further 24 (37.5%) were waist fractures. Proximal third fractures are uncommon in children.

Scaphoid fractures in children generally heal well with conservative measures in 4–7 weeks. Non-union occasionally occurs and was seen in 2% of Müssbichler's 1961 series, 1.6% of Christodoulou & Colton's 1986 series, but in no patients in Vahranen & Westerlund's 1980 series.

Mintzer & Waters (1999) described 13 examples of scaphoid non-union in children, all of which united after cancellous bone grafts alone, or combined with a Herbert screw.

Summary

- The reported incidence of fresh scaphoid fractures was 22.4% in the distal third, 73.3% in the middle third and 4.3% in the proximal third.
- The overall reported incidence of non-union after conservative treatment was 7.7%, although some authorities quoted rates of up to 50%.
- Up to 30% of scaphoid fractures had slight functional impairment and 3–4% had to reduce their working capacity. Up to 28% had some decrease in grip strength. Function recovered about 3.5 weeks after plaster removal. The functional result deteriorated with increasing malunion.
- Patients return to work at an average of 20 weeks after scaphoid fractures.
- Up to 6.5% of patients are subsequently shown to have a scaphoid fracture after a clinical fractured scaphoid.
- There was an increased incidence of non-union with delay in treatment, although union has occurred with conservative treatment.
- Displaced fractures had an increased rate of non-union of 27.8%, as compared with 6.8% in undisplaced fractures.
- Avascular necrosis causes delayed union rather than non-union.
- Fractures of the scaphoid tubercle healed rapidly in 3–6 weeks and non-union was uncommon. Radial distal intra-articular fractures healed well, whereas ulnar distal articular fractures tended to go on to non-union.
- Distal third fractures tended to unite in 4–8 weeks, with 94.1% excellent or good results.
- 92% of middle third fractures united in an average of 8.5–12.7 weeks. Satisfactory functional results were seen in 95–97.7%.
- Proximal third fractures had an increased incidence of non-union of 31–42%, with avascular necrosis in up to 40%. Union in proximal third fractures occurred in 9–15 weeks, with 90% satisfactory results.
- Union rates of 86.4–100% were achieved with screw fixation of fresh fractures, the Herbert screw achieving rates of 87.5–100% in fresh fractures.
- Although scaphoid non-unions may be asymptomatic, degenerative changes slowly develop. After 5–10 years of non-union almost all patients show degenerative changes.
- Carpal instability increases the incidence of non-union and the rate of development of degenerative changes.
- There was an overall union rate of 89.3% after various bone grafting techniques for non-union of the scaphoid. Union occurred in 15.8–18 weeks.

- Avascularity of the proximal pole increased the chances of failure to achieve union.
- Compression screws produced union rates of 86% in scaphoid non-union.
- Flexor tendon rupture after scaphoid non-union has been reported.
- Scaphoid fractures in children are uncommon, and the majority are distal third fractures. Scaphoid fractures in children unite in 4–7 weeks.
- Scaphoid non-union in children occurred in up to 2%, but united well with cancellous bone grafts.

Lunate fractures and Kienböck's disease
Aetiology

The cause of Kienböck's disease and its relation to trauma remain controversial. In 1910, Kienböck maintained that at the moment of injury a transient perilunate dislocation with ligamentous tear occurred, interfering with the vascular supply to the lunate bone. Subsequent reports have suggested the infrequent occurrence of osteonecrosis following perilunate dislocations and fracture–dislocation.

Whether osteonecrosis occurs prior to fracture or whether a single fracture or multiple stress fractures cause the osteonecrosis and secondary avascular changes is disputed.

White & Omer (1984) reviewed 24 fracture–dislocations and found three cases (12.5%) of transient vascular compromise of the lunate, suggested by a relative increase in the radiodensity of this bone. They found that natural resolution of the avascular necrosis was the rule, and none of these cases progressed to the classic avascular necrosis of Kienböck's disease.

Amadio et al (1987) described a patient in whom they showed that suspected osteonecrosis preceded a fracture of the lunate. However, histologic evidence of this osteonecrosis was not obtained. Beckenbaugh et al (1980) also believed that the fracture occurred as a terminal event, rather than as an aetiological one. In Beckenbaugh's paper, 72% of 46 patients had a history of wrist injury and 67% had evidence of fracture or fragmentation of the lunate.

Therkelsen & Anderson (1949) were of the opinion that repetitive trauma played the predominant role in the causation of osteonecrosis. In 109 patients with Kienböck's disease, a history of fairly definite trauma was found in only 42 (38%). Almquist & Burns (1982) also felt that Kienböck's disease was probably caused by microfractures or stress fractures developing within the lunate. That the avascular process is due to repetitive trauma and ischaemia is a view also held by Fisk (1984), while according to Lee (1963) over 30% of lunates are vulnerable to an avascular process due to the pattern of vascularity of the lunate.

Taleisnik (1985) quoted Hulten who, in 1928, described the ulna-minus variant as occurring in 23% of 400 normal wrists and 18 of 23 patients (78%) with Kienböck's disease. A similar association between Kienböck's disease and an ulna-minus variant was noted by Bonzar et al (1998), which they confirmed in 44 patients with Kienböck's and 99 control subjects. Gelberman et al (1975) also showed a statistically significant association between negative ulnar variance and Kienböck's disease. They showed negative ulnar variance in 21% of normal blacks, 29% of normal whites and 13 of 15 (87%) of affected wrists of patients with Kienböck's. The disease is less likely to occur in coloured people. A similar racial difference in Kienböck's disease had previously been noted by Chan & Huang (1971), who commented upon its absence in Chinese patients, despite the same distribution of negative ulnar variance as in Hulten's series.

Negative ulnar variance is believed to subject the lunate to a 'nutcracker' effect between the ulnar border of the radius and the head of the capitate.

Fisk (1984) pointed out that there was no 'step' between the ulnar and radius since the triangular fibrocartilage is thicker with a short ulna and thinner with a long one. However, there may be altered resistance between the cartilaginous end of the radius and this fibrocartilage complex.

Kristensen et al (1986b) suggested that in eight of 47 cases of Kienböck's disease they could demonstrate subchondral bone formation in the distal radius opposite the lunate bone. If these eight wrists were excluded, no statistical difference could be found in the incidence of the ulnar-minus variant in the diseased wrists when compared with normal wrists.

In a recent review article Watson and Guidera (1997) have reviewed the literature on the aetiology of Kienböck's disease and proposed a fault plate hypothesis. They felt that the multiple factors influencing lunate necrosis could be grouped into extrinsic and intrinsic factors. The result of the combination of these factors was the formation of multiple plates or faults within the substance of the lunate. These fault plates interrupt the trabeculae and blood supply to a specific area, resulting in isolation of that area and necrosis. Extrinsic factors were: (a) pile-driver effect of the capitate; (b) abnormal lunate loading; (c) ulnar variance; (d) abnormal loading; and (e) scapholunate dissociation with subsequent destabilisation of the lunate. Intrinsic factors were: (a) the spherical shape of the lunate; (b) cortical strength; (c) type 'V' and 'D' lunates (type V lunates are thinner palmarly and type D lunates are thinner dorsally); (d) trabeculae anatomy; (e) position and type of trabeculae; and (f) vascular anatomy of the lunate. The influence of load on the aetiology of Kienböck's disease may have important medico-legal consequences. A possible association between Kienböck's and the use of vibrating tools has been suggested (Gemme and Saraste 1987, Letz et al 1992). That abnormal loading influences the occurrence of Kienböck's disease is also suggested by its increased incidence in patients with cerebral palsy (Leclercq and Xarchas (1998)

Fresh lunate fractures are rarely reported, but Cetti et al (1982) described three examples, although they could find only three well-documented cases on reviewing the literature. None of their three cases went on to develop Kienböck's disease (one died).

Teisen & Hjarbeck (1988) reported on 17 patients with fresh fractures of the lunate, and proposed a classification according to their radiological appearance (Table 9.22). A long-term radiological follow-up was performed on 11 patients (4–31 years from fracture), and none of these had developed Kienböck's disease. However, Beckenbaugh et al (1980) with two cases, Brolin (1964) with four cases and Stahl (1947) with four cases have all reported fresh lunate fractures as going on to produce the full-blown radiological picture of Kienböck's disease.

Kienböck's disease can be classified into four stages (Lichtman et al 1982):

- Stage I—a normal radiographic appearance of the lunate, although there may be a suggestion of a compression fracture.
- Stage II—the lunate exhibits increased density, but its size and shape are unchanged.
- Stage III—the lunate has collapsed, allowing the capitate to migrate proximally. In stage IIIA the scaphoid maintains its normal position, but in stage IIIB it has moved into a position of fixed rotation.

- Stage IV—secondary degenerative changes are present in the carpus.

The treatment of Kienböck's disease

The treatment of Kienböck's disease remains controversial. Proponents may be found for both conservative and surgical treatment.

The results of conservative treatment

Some authors have reported the failure of conservative treatment to produce significant improvement or to prevent collapse of the lunate. In fact, Lichtman et al (1977) reported that 19 of their 22 patients (86.4%) had unsatisfactory results after non-operative treatment.

Kristensen et al (1986a) reported the 20 year follow-up of 49 patients who had either been treated by plaster immobilisation alone or else had received no treatment. Just under 80% (39 of 49 patients) were pain-free or had pain only on heavy work. Most patients reported that the pain gradually subsided after some years. All had deformed lunates and 67% developed osteoarthritic changes. However, these authors found that there was little correlation between the symptomatic and radiographic status of the patient. This poor correlation between symptoms and radiographic findings has been confirmed by Mirabello et al (1987).

Evans et al (1986) reported on 16 conservatively treated wrists with a 20 year follow-up. 10 patients (62.5%) had a satisfactory result, and two-thirds of this group showed no progression in their radiological changes.

Therkelsen & Anderson (1949) reported that 36 of 48 patients (75%) had satisfactory results. Tajima (1966) found no appreciable difference in the end-results of non-operative versus surgical treatment in 80 wrists seen during a 42 year period, and a similar finding was reported by Delaere et al (1998). In a retrospective study, the latter authors compared 21 cases of Kienböck's disease operated on by various techniques with 22 cases treated

Table 9.22 A classification of lunate fractures (after Teisen & Hjarbeck 1988)

Group	Description	Number of patients
I	Fracture of the volar pole of the lunate	9
II	Chip fracture which does not affect the main blood supply	4
III	Fracture of the dorsal pole of the lunate possibly affecting the dorsal nutrient artery	2
IV	Sagittal fracture through the body of the lunate	1
V	Transverse fracture through the body of the lunate	1

conservatively, with a mean follow-up of 65 months. Those patients treated surgically had similar outcomes to those treated conservatively; moreover, 24% of them lost some mobility and 25% had to change their social activities, while grip strength was only slightly improved.

The results of surgical treatment

Many surgical techniques have been proposed for Kienböck's disease. Only the more commonly used lunate excision and prosthetic replacement, joint levelling operations and arthrodesis will be considered.

Lunate excision and prosthetic replacement Because simple lunate excision is followed by progressive carpal collapse, various lunate implants have been proposed to replace the excised bone. Silicone implants were most commonly used, although recently they have fallen into disfavour because of the reported incidence of silicone synovitis (Palmer 1987).

Stark et al (1981) used a hand-carved silicone rubber spacer in 36 patients and achieved satisfactory relief of pain in 29 of 32 (90.6%) followed up for over 2 years. Progressive loss of carpal height was seen in 77% of these patients.

Lichtman et al (1977) reported 14 satisfactory results out of 20 patients (70%) using the initial Swanson silastic prosthesis, improving to 93.8% satisfactory results (15 of 16 patients) using the newer design (Lichtman et al 1982).

Evans et al (1986) had 43% good, 33% fair and 24% poor results in 21 patients treated by silicone replacement arthroplasty. More than half of these cases had radiological abnormalities, including carpal collapse, scapholunate diastasis and generalised degenerative changes in the carpus. Two patients had changes resembling silicone synovitis.

However, the long-term results of silicone replacement arthroplasty are disappointing. Kaarela et al (1998) reviewed 39 patients at a mean follow-up of 8 years. Sixteen prostheses (41%) had to be removed at a mean of 5.6 years postoperatively, in 15 because of pain and silicone synovitis or cysts.

Replacement of the lunate by fascial interpositional graft has been reported to produce good results at 10 year follow-up in 10 patients, with no carpal collapse (Carroll 1997).

Joint levelling procedures Joint levelling procedures are aimed at neutralising the ulna-minus variant at the wrist by either ulna lengthening or radial shortening operations.

Almquist (1986) quoted the results of radial shortening from seven separate papers and found that 69 of 79 reported cases (87%) had a satisfactory clinical result. Similarly,

Weiss et al (1991) reported that of their 29 patients treated by radial shortening, 25 (86%) had decreased pain, and grip strength improved by an average of 49%.

An even better improvement in the level of pain after radial shortening was noted by Quenzer et al (1997). Pain diminished in 93% of their 68 patients, and 13% were completely pain free. Grip strength improved in 74% of patients, and 74% continued in their original occupations including heavy labour. One-third of patients demonstrated lunate healing after joint leveling.

Good results have also been reported following ulna lengthening procedures. This operation is technically easier, but the rate of non-union of the osteotomy is higher.

Armistead et al (1982) reported 90% satisfactory pain relief in 20 patients, with some increase in the range of movement and a 17% improvement in grip strength. Although 13 patients showed no change in the degree of sclerosis of their lunates, six exhibited decreased sclerosis and only one showed increased sclerosis.

Sundberg & Linscheid (1984) had 18 of 19 patients (95%) with satisfactory pain relief and a 20% improvement in grip strength. Eight showed less sclerosis of the lunate at follow-up, while three showed increased sclerosis.

Arthrodesis Radiocarpal arthrodesis for severe disease and various intercarpal arthrodeses have been suggested as means of treating Kienböck's disease (Taleisnik 1985, Almquist 1986).

Voche et al (1992) reported the results of 16 triscaphe arthrodeses performed for Kienböck's. In three patients the pain disappeared completely, nine had mild pain, two were unchanged and two patients were worse. Grip strength improved by an average of 32%. However, the range of motion was quite markedly restricted.

Watson et al (1996) reported the long-term results of 28 cases of Kienböck's disease treated by scaphotrapezio-trapezoid arthrodesis at an average follow-up of 51 months. Nine required late lunate excision for pain and limited movement. Overall the patients rated their pain relief as excellent in 12 cases (44%), good in nine (33%), fair in four (15%) and poor in two (7%) cases (one case was omitted because of co-existing disease).

Summary

■ Kienböck's disease is unlikely to be the result of a transient perilunar dislocation. Transient vascular compromise without progression to osteonecrosis occurred in only 12.5% of patients.

■ Repetitive trauma may be a cause of Kienböck's disease. An ulna-minus variant may predispose to this repetitive trauma. It occurred in 78–87% of patients with Kienböck's disease, but it may be an apparent abnormality secondary to degeneration rather than a primary abnormality.

- It is suggested by some authors that a primary fracture causes Kienböck's disease.
- There may be an association between Kienböck's disease and the use of vibrating tools.
- The failure rate after the conservative treatment of Kienböck's disease has been reported to be as high as 86.4%, although other authors have reported 62.5–80% satisfactory symptomatic results after the long-term follow-up of such treatment.
- Silicone replacement arthroplasty has produced satisfactory results in 90–100% of patients. However, progressive radiological abnormalities and silicone synovitis are causing silicone replacement arthroplasty to fall into disfavour.
- Joint levelling procedures have produced satisfactory results in 86–95% of patients.

Isolated injury to other carpal bones

Although uncommon when compared to the frequency with which the scaphoid is fractured, every carpal bone is capable of being fractured or dislocated in isolation, as shown in the following sections.

Triquetrum

After the scaphoid, fractures of the triquetrum are said to be the next most common carpal fractures. The reported incidence varies from 3.5% (Bonnin & Greening 1943) to 20.2% (Borgeskov et al 1966).

The importance of triquetral fractures is not so much the problems that occur when the fracture is in isolation, but the fact that dorsal chip fractures or fractures through the body of the triquetrum may be the only sign of a spontaneously reduced complex carpal dislocation (Taleisnik 1985).

Triquetral fractures fall into three main types. Dorsal chip fractures are common. In Bonnin & Greening's 1943 series of 60 triquetral fractures, 49 (82%) were of this kind, as were 28 of the 29 triquetral fractures (97%) in Borgeskov et al's 1966 series. Bartone & Grieco (1956) reported on 46 triquetral fractures, 70% were isolated chip fractures, 2% were isolated body fractures and the other 28% were combined body and dorsal chip fractures.

Dorsal chip fractures require immobilisation for 2–4 weeks. There is a relatively high incidence of non-union, but complete functional recovery is the rule despite this. However, Bartone & Grieco (1956) suggested that if these fractures are misdiagnosed and not immobilised then chronic residual pain may persist for several months, although this does not interfere with ordinary use of the wrist.

Volar chip fractures have only recently been reported (Smith & Murray 1996). The authors described five examples of volar triquetral avulsion fractures occurring in young men as a result of falls suffered while playing sports. All five patients had persistent pain and carpal instability of variable severity 1year after injury. Patients with this fracture require careful evaluation for associated ligament injury and carpal instability.

Fractures of the body tend to be undisplaced and unite after immobilisation in a plaster cast for 4–6 weeks. Herbert (1986) has reported the use of his compression screw in the treatment of these fractures. Complete functional recovery is the rule.

Avascular necrosis has not been reported. Non-union is rare after fractures of the body but has been noted (Durbin 1950), although in this patient it caused only a slight decrease in the range of motion and no pain.

Isolated dislocation of the triquetrum is rare but can occur volarly (Soucascos & Hartefilakidis-Garofalidis 1981) or dorsally (Goldberg & Heller 1987), and fracture–dislocation can occur (Porter & Seehra 1991). The diagnosis tends to be overlooked in the initial stage. Excision of the triquetrum has been used to treat these dislocations with no obvious functional impairment, although reduction either closed or open is to be preferred (Taleisnik 1985).

Summary

- Triquetral injuries comprised 3.5–20.2% of carpal fractures, and they may be the only radiological sign of a complex carpal dislocation.
- Dorsal chip fractures are common, heal in 2–4 weeks and rarely cause any functional disturbance even though non-union is common.
- Volar chip fractures are rare and may be a subtle sign of carpal instability.
- Triquetral body fractures are uncommon, but heal in 6 weeks and cause little functional disturbance.
- Non-union in body fractures is rare but causes little disability.
- Dislocation, either dorsal or volar, is rare and causes little long-term disability.

Pisiform

Injuries to the pisiform are rare, and occur in 0.7% (Borgeskov et al 1966) to 3% (Dobyns & Linscheid 1984) of reported series. Fracture patterns include avulsions of the distal portion, vertical fractures or osteochondral fractures of the articular surface (Dobyns & Linscheid, 1984). Immobilisation for 3–4 weeks is all that is required for the fracture to become asymptomatic. Post-traumatic degenerative changes in the piso-triquetral joint have been reported following intra-articular fracture (Jenkins 1951). Should pain persist, or degeneration develop following a pisiform fracture, excision of the whole bone produces excellent results (Palmieri 1982).

Occasionally, a dislocation of the pisiform bone occurs. Minami et al (1984) reported a case which, despite open reduction and Kirschner wire fixation, went on to redislocate, requiring excision of the bone. They reviewed the six previously reported cases, three of which were excised, and recommended that the pisiform be removed in cases of isolated dislocation.

A rare case of dislocated pisiform in a child, associated with a Salter-Harris type II fracture of the distal radius and ulna, was reported by Ashkan et al (1998). Closed reduction followed by immobilisation achieved a good clinical result.

Ulnar nerve palsy has been reported to occur in association with a fracture of the pisiform (Howard 1964).

Summary

- Pisiform fractures and dislocations occur in 0.7–3% of carpal injuries.
- Immobilisation for 3–4 weeks is generally sufficient.
- Symptomatic fractures, degeneration of the piso-triquetral joint and isolated dislocation of the pisiform are treated by excision of the pisiform, with excellent results.

Trapezium

Fractures of the trapezium are reported as occurring in 1% (Dobyns & Linscheid 1984) to 5% (Cordrey & Ferrer-Torrels 1960) of carpal fractures. They may affect the body of the trapezium or may be trapezial ridge fractures.

Cordrey & Ferrer-Torrels (1960) reviewed the world literature and found 75 reported cases; 60% of these had persistent pain and swelling, with diminished movement of the wrist and thumb at the end of treatment. In none was open reduction and internal fixation advocated.

Walker et al (1988) proposed a classification of fractures of the body of the trapezium based on their 10 cases. Type I is a horizontal fracture not involving either the carpometacarpal or scaphotrapezial joints. Type II fractures involve the radial tuberosity, and type III the ulnar tuberosity. Type IV are vertical fractures running through

the articular surface of the first carpometacarpal joint, often accompanied by subluxation of the first metacarpal. Type V are comminuted. Five of their fractures were of type IV. The two treated conservatively were not problematic; nor were two of the three treated by open reduction and internal fixation. The fifth patient with a poor result had a grade III compound injury.

Jones & Ghorbal (1985) reported three vertical fractures, two being treated with plaster cast immobilisation and one having percutaneous Kirschner wire fixation without accurate reduction of the fracture. All three patients had residual symptoms with approximately 50% loss of movement and strength of power, pinch and key grip. They all experienced aching with prolonged writing and repetitive work.

In contrast to the generally poor results after conservative treatment, those of open reduction and internal fixation have been good. Cordrey & Ferrer-Torrels (1960) reported excellent results in five vertical fractures treated with open reduction and Kirschner wire fixation, the fractures healing in 8 weeks. Griffin et al (1988) described four cases of fracture of the dorso-ulnar tubercle of the trapezium (type III). In three of the four patients the fracture was not initially recognised. Of the three with follow-up, all healed well, but two required immobilisation for 6 months.

Trapezial ridge fractures were described as the 'missed fracture' by McClain & Boyes (1966), as all four of their cases (plus two of the three reported by Palmer in 1981) were diagnosed late. Palmer (1981) described two types. The type I trapezial ridge fracture occurs at the base of the ridge of the trapezium, and his one case healed with immobilisation. The more common type II (an avulsion fracture from the tip of the volar ridge) tends to progress to non-union. In the four cases reported by McClain & Boyes (1966) and in one of the two cases of non-union reported by Palmer (1981), excision of the avulsed fragment was performed. However, late surgical treatment did not result in immediate relief of symptoms, and a relatively long delay in returning to normal work was the rule (McClain & Boyes 1966). In over half of the cases reported in these two papers, there were signs and symptoms of irritability of the median nerve within the carpal tunnel.

Dislocation of the trapezium may occur in an ulnar-volar or dorsal-radial direction and seemingly with equal frequency in both directions. Siegal & Hertzberg (1969) reviewed the literature and found only two cases of true dislocation, previously reported by Peterson, and these had been treated by excision of the trapezium. Goldberg et al (1981) excised the trapezium in their case of an ulnar–volar dislocation but found some shortening of the thumb, with reasonable preservation of pinch grip but poor opposition. If possible, closed reduction is the ideal treatment but this is rarely achieved, and even when achieved is often unstable. Open reduction and Kirschner wire fixation has produced good results (Sherlock 1987) but two cases of ulnar–volar dislocation treated in this way resulted in fusion of the first carpometacarpal joint, with some loss of movement and poor opposition (Siegel & Hertzberg 1969, Seimon 1972).

Summary

- The incidence of fractures of the trapezium was 1–5%.
- Conservative treatment of displaced vertical fractures produced over 60% residual symptoms.
- The results of the operative fixation of vertical fractures were good.
- Trapezial ridge fractures were often overlooked and frequently went on to non-union, and recovery—even after surgical excision of the non-union—was slow.
- Over 50% of trapezial ridge fractures were associated with median nerve irritability.
- Dislocations of the trapezium generally did well with open reduction and Kirschner wire fixation, although premature fusion of the first carpometacarpal joint has been reported to occur.

Trapezoid

Less than 0.7% of carpal fractures occur at the trapezoid (Borgeskov et al 1966) and they are rarely reported. Isolated fractures may be treated in a plaster cast for 3–6 weeks, but secondary degenerative changes may occur between the trapezoid and second metacarpal, necessitating a later arthrodesis (Bryan & Dobyns 1980). In a case reported by Watanabe et al (1997) there was dorsal displacement of a fractured trapezoid. This was initially untreated and the patient complained of pain and poor grip. Despite open reduction and Kirschner wire fixation being delayed for 2 months the final outcome was said to be satisfactory.

Dislocation of the trapezoid, while uncommon, would appear to be more frequent than fracture, and may occur in a dorsal or volar direction. Treatment consists of closed manipulation and plaster immobilisation (Meyn & Roth 1980), open reduction and Kirschner wire fixation (Stein 1971), or open reduction and primary limited arthrodesis (Goodman & Shankman 1984). The shape of the trapezoid prevents closed reduction in palmar dislocations.

Avascular necrosis of the trapezoid may occur after open reduction (Meyn & Roth 1980).

If further surgery is required due to secondary degenerative changes, limited arthrodesis is to be preferred to simple excision of the trapezoid, because the second metacarpal and trapezium will migrate into the defect and produce symptomatic disability (Meyn & Roth 1980, Taleisnik 1985).

Summary

- Trapezoid fractures occurred in less than 0.7% of carpal fractures.
- Trapezoid fractures heal with plaster immobilisation in 3–6 weeks, although secondary arthritis may occur.
- Dislocation may occur in a dorsal or volar direction. Avascular necrosis may follow open reduction.
- If secondary symptoms require surgery, limited arthrodesis is to be preferred to excision of the trapezoid.

Capitate

The incidence of capitate fractures is 0.4–1.4% of all carpal fractures (Borgeskov et al 1966, Dobyns & Linscheid 1984). Fractures of the capitate may occur as isolated injuries, as part of the scaphocapitate (naviculo-capitate) syndrome, or in association with other carpal or metacarpal fractures.

Although Adlar & Shafton (1962) found 79 reported cases in the world literature, of which 48 were isolated capitate fractures, there have been few reports of the isolated fracture since then. They added five cases, with follow-up in three of them. These five healed after plaster immobilisation for 3–6 weeks and the two without previous arthritis had full function. Rand et al (1982) noted three isolated capitate fractures, two of which went on to non-union. In a previous article from the same centre, Bryan & Dobyns (1980) had reported that non-union of the capitate was common, and Freeman & Hay (1985) noted that it healed well with bone grafting.

Rand et al (1982) found that five of their seven patients without a perilunar dislocation had a mean range of motion of 73% and a grip strength of 78% of the contralateral normal hand. Four of six patients with follow-up radiographs revealed post-traumatic arthritis. The two patients without arthritis had a shorter follow-up period (less than 3 years), as compared with a mean follow-up of 10 years 5 months for the four patients with arthritis.

The scaphocapitate syndrome has been well described (Stein & Siegel 1969). It involves a fracture of the scaphoid, with a fracture of the proximal pole of the capitate rotated 90° or 180° to its long axis, with or without an associated-perilunar dislocation.

Plaster immobilisation in the rotated position has resulted in union with no pain and 25% loss of full motion (Jones 1955). However, non-union and avascular necrosis of the proximal pole are more likely to occur (Marsh & Lampros 1959). Fenton (1956) recommended excision of the proximal pole with reasonable preservation of function but some loss of movement, while Meyers et al (1971) performed an open reduction with wire fixation and reported the return of full function.

Vance et al (1980) resorted to open reduction and pin fixation in four cases after the failure of attempts at closed reduction. Rand et al (1982) reported that four of five patients with trans-scaphoid, transcapitate perilunar fracture–dislocations had a mean range of 65% and grip strength of 68% of the contralateral hand. Three of the four patients with adequate follow-up had degenerative arthritis (mean follow-up 3 years 9 months) and only the patient followed up for 1 year was free of this.

A case of volar dislocation of the capitate in a complex wrist injury has been reported (Lowray et al 1984).

Summary

- Capitate fractures occurred in 0.4–1.4% of carpal injuries.
- Fractures of the body of the capitate resulted in a range of motion of 73% of the contralateral wrist, while grip strength was 78% of that of the opposite wrist.
- Non-union is not uncommon, and degenerative change was the rule after a 10-year follow-up.
- Open reduction of the scaphocapitate syndrome was the treatment of choice.
- Perilunar scaphocapitate fracture–dislocations resulted in 65% motion and 68% grip strength of the contralateral wrist at follow-up. Degenerative changes were common after a 4 year follow-up.

The hamate

Fractures of the hamate occurred in from 0.5% (Dobyns & Linscheid 1984) to 4.6% (Taleisnik 1985) of carpal fractures.

They manifest through either the body or the hook of the hamate. Fractures of the body are uncommon, although Bowen (1973) reviewed the literature and discovered 44 recorded cases, 29 of the body, five of the hook and 10 the site of which was unrecorded. Although he found only five fractures of the hook of the hamate, they would now appear to occur more frequently than body fractures. This is probably due to increased recognition of this type of fracture, as well as their increasing frequency from racquet and club sports.

Fractures of the body may be dorsal oblique (coronal) in association with subluxation of the base of the ulnar metacarpals. Ebraheim et al (1995) reported on 11 patients with coronal fractures of the hamate bone, all involving dislocation of the hamate metacarpal bone. They classified them into: Type A—a fracture that passes through the centre of the body in the coronal plate; Type B—extending in a more oblique direction and involving a significant portion of the distal articular surface; and Type C—a true carpometacarpal joint fracture-dislocation with the hamate coronal fracture representing an avulsion fracture that was found to be highly unstable. They identified one Type A, three Type B, and seven Type C fractures. In all cases the fracture was found to be unstable. Ten patients underwent surgical stabilisation, four being treated with open reduction and internal fixation with Kirschner wires or screws, whilst six had closed reduction and percutaneous pinning. All patients treated surgically maintained reduction of their joints. The one patient treated with closed reduction and plaster cast alone developed residual subluxation of the hamate-metacarpal joint. At an average 20 months' follow-up one patient complained of moderate pain due to the development of arthritis at the hamate-metacarpal joint, and four of occasional pain in the ulnar aspect of the hand. The patient who had persistent subluxation complained of pain with daily activities and a loss of grip strength.

True body fractures may pass to the ulnar side or, more commonly, radial to the hook of the hamate. These fractures are usually stable and require 4–6 weeks in plaster cast to become asymptomatic, even if fibrous union alone is achieved (Taleisnik 1985). Open reduction and internal fixation is required if the fracture is displaced.

Terrono et al (1989) reported a case of non-union of the body of the hamate, the patient complaining of intermittent pain on activity and weakness. He became asymptomatic after internal fixation with a cortical mini lag screw. Moller & Lybecker (1987) described a simultaneous fracture of the body of the hamate and capitate bones in a child, which healed completely after 6 weeks in a plaster cast.

Proximal pole osteochondral fractures may occur (Dobyns & Linscheid 1984). Howard (1964) described two patients with fractures of the body of the hamate who had associated ulnar nerve palsies.

Fractures of the hook of the hamate are more common and there is an almost 100% progression to non-union. This is not only due to the fact that they are often diagnosed late, as even after immediate treatment non-union is not uncommon (Stark et al 1989). No record could be found of primary bone union of hook of hamate fractures until the recent reports of Bishop & Beckenbaugh (1988), in which two examples are recorded, and Jensen & Christensen (1990), who described one patient.

Non-union of the hook of the hamate tends to result in local tenderness and pain on gripping, grip strength averaging 20% less than that of the uninjured hand (Stark et al 1989). However, cast immobilisation can sometimes resolve these symptoms, presumably due to fibrous union (Egawa & Asai 1983). In 59 of the 62 patients (95%) in Stark et al's 1989 series, surgery was required. Occasionally, bone graft and screw fixation has been performed (Bishop & Beckenbaugh 1988, Watson & Rogers 1989), although one of the three patients in the 1988 series went on to non-union. Excision of the ununited fragment gives universally good results (Egawa & Asai 1983, Foucher et al 1985, Bishop & Beckenbaugh 1988, Stark et al 1989). In the 1988 series all 18 employed patients returned to work and sport. Eight (42%) had no symptoms, six (32%) had mild symptoms and five (26%) had moderate or multiple symptoms. In the series of Stark et al (1989), 57 of the 59 patients (97%) who were followed up had relief of all their pre-operative complaints and resumed all of their usual activities. They had normal grip strength by 6 months after the operation. The athletes resumed their former athletic pursuits at an average of 8 weeks after operation. The two patients who had had a crush injury continued to complain of occasional pain in the wrist, and both had a 50% loss of grip strength. One patient developed tingling and numbness of the little finger 8 years after the operation, due to new bone formation where the fractured hook had been removed.

Flexor tendon tendonitis or rupture has been reported in association with non-united hook of hamate fractures (Foucher et al 1985, Milek & Boulas 1990). Foucher et al noted that five of their six patients with non-union had fraying or rupture of flexor tendons, whereas Stark et al (1989) reported only two cases of flexor tendon involvement in 62 patients. Bishop & Beckenbaugh (1988) have estimated that 15–20% of hook of hamate non-unions are associated with flexor tendon involvement. In the present review, 24 reported cases of flexor tendon injury have been found in 141 reported cases of fracture of the hook of the hamate, an incidence of 17%.

Involvement of the ulnar nerve with hook of hamate fractures was reported by Howard (1964), while Egawa & Asai (1983) reported that four of their six cases of hook of hamate fracture had hypoaesthesia in an ulnar nerve distribution. Bishop & Beckenbaugh (1988) noted ulnar nerve involvement in 5 of 21 cases (23.8%). Occasionally, median nerve irritability has been found (Bishop & Beckenbaugh 1988). Tardy ulnar nerve palsy has been reported due to perineural fibrosis (Baird & Friedenberg 1968).

No case of avascular necrosis has been reported.

Dislocation of the hamate can occur in a volar or dorsal direction. It can sometimes be reduced closed (Duke 1963), but open reduction is usually required (Gunn 1985). The functional result after reduction is generally good.

Summary

- The incidence of hamate fractures was 0.5–4.6%.
- Dorsal oblique (coronal) fractures heal with good functional results if reduced well.
- True body fractures tend to be stable and heal with 4–6 weeks in a plaster cast.
- Fractures of the hook of the hamate have an almost 100% non-union rate. Excision of the ununited fragment is the procedure of choice. 42–97% will be asymptomatic, although 32% have been reported to have mild symptoms.
- Ulnar nerve neuropathy may occur with body and hook fractures. Tardy ulnar palsy can occur, as can median nerve neuropathy.
- Flexor tendonitis or rupture was reported in 15–20% of hook of hamate non-unions.
- Dislocation of the hamate occasionally occurs.

Dislocations and fracture–dislocations of the carpus

Dislocations and fracture dislocations of the carpus comprised 1–2% of all fractures (Morawa et al 1976) and 4.8–13.8% of all carpal injuries (Dobyns & Linscheid 1984), and many varieties and combinations can occur.

Most carpal dislocations and fractures are confined to an area contained within a 'lesser arc' that closely hugs the lunate and a 'greater arc' that crosses the middle third of the scaphoid and runs distal to the midcarpal joint in an ulnar direction to cross the triquetrum (Taleisnik 1985). Based on these two arcs, carpal dislocations and fracture dislocations can be classified into four main groups:

- I—lunate and perilunate dislocations.
- II—trans-scaphoid perilunate fracture–dislocation (with or without other carpal bones) in the 'greater arc'.
- III—variants of the above pattern including scaphocapitate syndrome and isolated dislocation of other carpal bones.
- IV—radiocarpal dislocations.

Lunate and perilunate dislocations

Mayfield et al (1980) investigated the pathomechanics of carpal instability in perilunate and lunate dislocations in

32 cadaver wrists. They described four stages in a progressive perilunar instability, ranging from stage I, scapholunate diastasis, the least significant degree of perilunar instability, through stage II, an additional dorsal dislocation of the capitate, and stage III, with additional triquetrolunate diastasis, and finally to stage IV, dislocation of the lunate. This study supported previous clinical assumptions that perilunate dislocation precedes lunate dislocation and that both are manifestations of the same injury. Thus, both injuries will be reviewed together.

Dorsal perilunar and volar lunate dislocation

This injury is often missed on initial presentation. Rawlings (1981) found that only 17 of 30 such patients (57%) were diagnosed on the day of admission. Campbell et al (1964) reported that 66% of their patients (22 of 33) were treated within 2 weeks of diagnosis, and Green & O'Brien (1978) found that 15 of their 22 patients (68.2%) were treated soon after injury.

Acute perilunate and lunate dislocations are usually relatively easy to reduce. If, after closed reduction, carpal alignment is anatomical, plaster immobilisation is maintained, with radiological checks on alignment, for 8–10 weeks (Taleisnik 1985). Adkison & Chapman (1982) found that anatomical alignment was maintained in only 40% of their 10 patients treated by closed reduction alone. Many authors recommend percutaneous Kirschner wire fixation after closed reduction to maintain this alignment. If rotary subluxation of the scaphoid or instability of the lunate persisted, then this was reduced by further closed manipulation or open reduction with Kirschner wire fixation. Inoue and Kuwahata (1997) retrospectively reviewed 14 cases of acute perilunate dislocation. Four patients had closed reduction followed by percutaneous Kirschner wire fixation, eight had open reduction with repair of the torn scapholunate ligaments and Kirschner wire fixation, and two had open reduction with cast immobilisation alone. In the patients who had ligamentous repair the scapholunate relationship was maintained more consistently. They concluded that open reduction, direct repair of the scapholunate ligament and Kirschner wire fixation of the carpus was the treatment of choice.

Morawa et al (1974) stated that the presence of a scaphoid subluxation did not mitigate against an excellent prognosis. However, Rawlings (1981) found that nine out of his 12 patients with a poor result had an increase in the scapholunate gap suggestive of scapholunate dissociation, as compared with only two of the 12 patients who had a satisfactory result—and in these two patients, the increase in the scapholunate gap was only borderline. Panting et al (1984) reported that five of their 12 patients (41.6%) with carpal instability had unsatisfactory results, while Green & O'Brien (1979), Mayfield et al (1980) and Minami et al (1986) all suggested that the existence of a scapholunate gap after reduction of the dislocation gave an increased chance of a poor result.

The results of the treatment of lunate and perilunate dislocation are recorded in Table 9.23. Satisfactory results were seen in between 43 and 91% of patients (70% overall). In Rawling's 1981 series with a 43% satisfactory result overall, 85% (11 of 13 patients) achieved their results after early diagnosis and treatment as compared with 35% (six of 17 patients) diagnosed and treated after some delay. Inoue and Kuwahata (1997) found that the average postoperative flexion-extension arc of the wrist was 106°, or 80% of the uninjured wrist. Grip strength averaged 85% of

Table 9.23 The results of the treatment of lunate and perilunate dislocations

Reference	Number of patients	Satisfactory		Unsatisfactory	
		No.	%	No.	%
Campbell et al (1964)	15	12	80	3	20
Morawa et al (1974)	24	22	91	2	9
Green & O'Brien (1978)	16	9	56	7	44
Rawlings (1981)	30	13	43	17	57
Panting et al (1984)	29	24	83	5	17
Inoue & Kuwahata (1997)	14	10	71	4	29
Overall	128	90	70	38	30

the uninjuored wrist. Nine patients (64%) were totally pain-free.

Green & O'Brien (1978) stressed the fact that virtually all of these patients had some permanent limitation of motion, and it took several months before the maximum benefit of rehabilitation was obtained. They found that rarely had their patients been able to return to an occupation requiring the heavy use of the hands before 6 months.

Campbell et al (1964) reported good results following-proximal row carpectomy for some cases of chronic dislocation. Excision of the lunate was seldom felt to be indicated and reduction of the chronically displaced lunate, if possible, was also considered to give a satisfactory wrist. Siegart et al (1988) reported on 16 cases of chronic dislocation and concluded that open reduction should be the treatment of choice. All six of their patients so treated had a satisfactory result. In these chronic cases proximal row carpectomy and wrist fusion was preferred to isolated lunate excision.

Of the five cases of late open reduction of lunate or perilunate dislocation reported by Weir (1992), the radiological results were generally poor and there was a considerable restriction of wrist movement, on average to 42% of that of the other wrist. However, the functional recovery was surprisingly good, with all patients returning to normal activities, including heavy manual work. Vegter (1987) reported the successful late reduction of two dislocated lunates using an external fixator.

Avascular necrosis of the lunate with collapse is extremely uncommon. White & Omer (1984) recorded only three cases of transient ischaemia in 24 fracture–dislocations (12.5%). The clinical course of these cases was for resolution to occur and none progressed to collapse. Avascular necrosis with collapse of the lunate occurred in one of the cases reported by Weir (1992).

The incidence of symptoms related to median nerve compression within the carpal tunnel is reported as occurring in between 16% (Adkison & Chapman 1982) and 56.6% (Rawlings 1981) of all perilunate dislocations and fracture–dislocations. These symptoms are usually transient, but the longer they persist the worse the final outcome is.

Chen (1995) reported on 10 patients who had median nerve neuropathy in association with chronic volar dislocation of the lunate. The average time from injury to evaluation was 21 months. All 10 patients had pain as well as sensory and motor dysfunction in the distribution of the median nerve. Carpal tunnel release was performed with a proximal row carpectomy in four and excision of the lunate alone in six. Three distinct sites of nerve compression were identified: the volar and dorsal edges of the lunate and the proximal edge of the transverse carpal ligament. All patients except one were satisfied with the outcome.

A transient ulnar nerve palsy associated with a volar dislocation of the lunate has also been described (Yamada et al 1995).

Stern (1981) reported the rupture of the flexor pollicus longus and flexor digitorum superficialis and profundus tendons to the index and long fingers in a case of chronic volar dislocation of the lunate, while Minami et al (1989) described rupture of the extensor tendons in association with a palmar perilunar dislocation.

Volar perilunar and dorsal lunate dislocation

Dorsal dislocation of the lunate is extremely rare and only isolated case reports are recorded (Bilos & Hui 1981). Volar perilunar dislocation is only slightly more common (Niazi 1996). Treatment of these injuries is along the lines of the more common dorsal perilunar and volar lunar dislocations. Closed reduction of the volar perilunar dislocation is said to be more difficult and it is more unstable once reduced (Taleisnik 1985).

The case of an old dorsal lunate dislocation with associated multiple extensor tendon ruptures was reported by Schwartz et al (1990).

Dislocations and fracture–dislocations of the greater arc

Trans-scaphoid perilunar fracture dislocation of the carpus is the common injury in this group. In many ways, with regard to treatment, it may be looked upon as a variety of perilunate dislocation, but the displacement occurs through the body of the scaphoid rather than the scapholunate ligament.

Closed treatment may be considered if anatomical reduction of the scaphoid can be achieved and maintained. Healing of the scaphoid fracture may be delayed and avascular necrosis of the proximal scaphoid fragment is common. However, avascular necrosis does not imply non-union. In Adkison & Chapman's 1982 series, 13 of 19 patients (68%) lost the anatomical position with conservative treatment. If an anatomical position of the scaphoid-cannot be maintained, then the incidence of non-union of the scaphoid is increased, in Adkison & Chapman's series to 75%.

Wagner (1956) recommended primary wrist arthrodesis for the displaced trans-scaphoid perilunate fracture–dislocation. However, most authors recommend open reduction, with the scaphoid being held reduced with wires or screws, with or without bone graft (Morawa et al 1974, Green & O'Brien 1978, Cooney et al 1987).

The incidence of median nerve irritation after trans-scaphoid perilunate fracture–dislocations varies between 14% (Inoue and Imaeda 1997) and 30% (Cooney et al 1987). These injuries were usually transient.

The results of the treatment of trans-scaphoid perilunate fracture–dislocations are recorded in Table 9.24. Overall, 73% of these patients achieved a satisfactory result. This table includes patients treated both surgically and conservatively. Morawa et al (1974), Adkison & Chapman (1982) and Cooney et al (1987) all emphasised the improved results obtained by operative, as compared to conservative, treatment.

Loss of wrist motion is a problem after these injuries. Cooney et al (1987) found the average wrist flexion to be 40° and the average extension 36° in 22 patients treated operatively. Only nine of the 22 patients (41%) had no pain, nine (41%) had mild but tolerable pain and four (18%) had severe pain; 13 (59%) of the patients in this group had no weakness, six (27%) had mild to moderate weakness and three (14%) had severe weakness. Of cases seen at an average of 4.3 years following treatment, 56% had radiographic evidence of intercarpal arthritis and 54% evidence of radiocarpal arthritis. In the series of 29 wrist injuries reported by Inoue & Imaeda (1997) the average postoperative flexion-extension arc of the wrist was 114° in those immobilised for 4 weeks after surgical reduction, as compared to 96° in those immobilised for longer than 5 weeks. The average grip strength was 81% of the normal wrist. Green (1982) pointed out that return to heavy work occurred 6 months to 1 year after these injuries.

Occasionally, these fracture–dislocations have proved to be irreducible by closed means, due either to the prox-imal pole of the scaphoid dislocating volar to the lunate (Weiss et al 1970) or to interposition of the dorsal capsule (Jasmine et al 1988).

The late treatment of unreduced perilunate fracture dislocations was reported by Inoue and Shionoya (1999). In their series of 28 patients, 18 were fracture dislocations and 10 were pure ligamentous injuries. Open reduction and temporary Kirschner wire fixation at an average of 16 weeks after injury led to three good results, one fair and two poor. Proximal row carpectomy performed at an average interval of 14 months after injury resulted in 10 fair and six poor results. Three of the four patients treated by lunate excision had a poor result, with the fourth patient reporting a fair result. The two cases of carpal tunnel release and partial excision of the lunate had a fair result.

Sousa et al (1995) used pre-operative progressive distraction in three patients. Subsequent surgical reduction and scaphoid osteosynthesis was said to be easily performed.

Lowdon et al (1984) described a case of recurrent dorsal trans-scaphoid perilunate dislocation through a scaphoid non-union.

Occasionally, a palmar trans-scaphoid lunate fracture–dislocation occurs. Green & O'Brien (1978) and Viegas et al (1987) reported poor results in a total of four cases treated by surgery. However, Stern (1984) noted good results following surgery in two cases.

Palmar trans-scaphoid perilunate fracture–dislocation is also occasionally reported. Green & O'Brien (1978) and Fernandes et al (1983) achieved good results in patients treated by screw fixation, while Aitken & Nalebuff (1960) had a good functional result in a patient

Table 9.24 The results of the treatment of trans-scaphoid perilunate fracture–dislocations

Reference	Number of patients	Satisfactory		Unsatisfactory	
		No.	%	No.	%
Morawa et al (1974)	21	18	86	3	14
Green & O'Brien (1978)	18	12	67	6	33
Inoue & Imaeda (1997)*	29	19	66	10	34
Panting et al (1984)	19	13	68	6	32
Cooney et al (1987)†	26	20	77	6	23
Overall	113	82	73	31	27

* Includes some group III variants.

† This series includes patients treated by open reduction only.

despite a scaphoid non-union after closed treatment. Cooney et al (1987) had a poor result with their one patient.

Variants

Many of these have been discussed in the section on fracture and dislocation of the individual carpal bone. Isolated dislocation of the scaphoid or scaphoid and lunate will be discussed in this section.

Isolated dislocations of the scaphoid are rare injuries. The dislocation may be radial, dorsal or palmar (Leung et al 1998). Reduction is generally achieved closed—in 16 of 20 reported cases (Amamilo et al 1985)—and the functional end-result was usually good, with only occasional discomfort. Szabo et al (1995) reported three examples, describing the spectrum of ligamentous damage that occurs, which ranges from rupture of the radio-scapho-capitate ligament to complete rupture of ligaments about the scaphoid. They suggest that the initial treatment should be closed reduction with percutaneous pinning if an anatomical reduction was obtained. They used arthroscopy to assist percutaneous pinning in one patient. Open reduction, ligament repair and internal fixation are required if initial attempts at closed reduction fail to reduce the proximal pole. Avascular necrosis of the scaphoid occurred in one of their patients.

Dislocation of the scaphoid and lunate may occur as a unit (Sarrafian & Breihan 1990), as a trans-scapholunate dislocation (Barros et al 1997), or with both bones in isolation from each other (Baulot et al 1999). In all earlier case reports open reduction was required, avascular necrosis of the lunate was common and the functional results were poor. More recent reports are more optimistic. In their case of divergent dislocation Baulot et al (1999) noted an almost full range of motion, no residual pain and grip strength of 75% of the opposite side at 3.5 year follow-up. Barros et al (1997) performed immediate open reduction and internal fixation in their patient with bilateral trans-scapholunate dislocations. The patient was asymptomatic 18 months after injury.

Radiocarpal dislocation

Isolated radiocarpal dislocations are rare. Varodompun et al (1985) reported the fourth example of isolated dorsal dislocation. Closed reduction was usually easy and full function was restored (Freund & Ovesen 1977).

Isolated volar dislocation is also rare. Moore & McMahon (1988) reported the fifth example. Closed reduction was usually easy and function was invariably fully restored (Fehring & Milek 1984), although Moore & McMahon's patient described a feeling of occasional weakness, and early degenerative changes were noted.

With increasing severity of injury there is an increasingly complex fracture–dislocation. Dislocations are classified as Type I without intercarpal injuries and Type II with them. Mudgal et al (1999) reported on 12 patients, 10 Type I injuries and two Type II injuries. In 11 patients the carpus was displaced dorsally and in one there was palmar displacement. Open reduction and internal fixation was performed in each case. At mean follow-up of 36 months, eight patients had returned to their original jobs. Four patients complained of mild pain with heavy labour, six patients noted wrist stiffness in the morning and four complained of weak grip. Three patients had a poor functional outcome, three had slight narrowing of the joint space when assessed radiographically, and seven had a pre-operative sensory impairment, mainly affecting the median nerve. In six of these the deficit resolved very shortly after correction of the deformity. Moniem et al (1985) described four patients with isolated radiocarpal dislocation with marginal fractures of the radius and ulna. Closed reduction was successful in three patients and the functional end-results were generally good. Three patients had associated intercarpal injuries, open reduction was required and the results were inferior with two unsatisfactory results.

Axial dislocation

Axial dislocations of the carpus are rare injuries usually resulting from severe trauma. As a result, the carpus is separated longitudinally and is usually displaced with the respective metacarpals. Garcia-Elias et al (1989) reviewed 40 patients reported in the literature and suggested a classification according to the direction of the instability: axial–ulnar, axial–radial or combined axial–radial–ulnar disruption. Axial–ulnar injuries had a three times greater incidence of ulnar nerve injuries, and these injuries influenced the final results. Indeed, the prognosis was determined more by the associated soft tissue injury than by the carpal derangement.

Summary

- Lunate and perilunate dislocation were missed on initial presentation in 32–43% of patients.
- Anatomical alignment was maintained in only 40% of cases of lunate and perilunate dislocation treated by closed reduction and plaster immobilisation.
- An increased scapholunate gap or scapholunate angle gave a poor result in 42–75% of cases of lunate and perilunate dislocation.
- A satisfactory result was seen in 70% of cases of lunate and perilunate dislocation, but delay in treatment increased the risk of a poor result. An 80% flexion-

extension arc of wrist movement and 85% grip strength compared with the uninjured wrist are to be expected.

- Median nerve symptoms were seen in 16–57% of cases of lunate and perilunate dislocation but were usually transient.
- Flexor tendon rupture has been reported in an old unreduced case of volar dislocation.
- 68% of conservatively treated trans-scaphoid perilunate fracture–dislocations lost their anatomical position. The incidence of non-union of the scaphoid with non-anatomical reduction was at least 75%.
- Median nerve irritation occurred in 14–30% of cases of trans-scaphoid perilunate fracture–dislocation, although these symptoms were usually transient.
- 73% of trans-scaphoid perilunate fracture–dislocations achieved a satisfactory result. Better results were achieved by surgical treatment. These patients tended to have an arc of flexion-extension of 114°. Pain was absent in 41% and grip strength was normal in 59% after treatment, averaging 81% of normal. Return to heavy work occurred in 6 months to 1 year.
- Degenerative changes were seen in over 50% of wrists after trans-scaphoid perilunate fracture–dislocation at an average of 4.3 years after the injury.
- Isolated scaphoid dislocations were usually easily reduced by closed manipulation and the functional results were generally good.
- Isolated scaphoid–lunate dislocation usually required open reduction and the functional results were variable.
- Isolated radiocarpal dislocations had a good prognosis, whereas comminuted or compound fracture–dislocations had a poor (25%) outcome.
- Axial dislocations are rare, and the prognosis is related to the soft tissue injury.

Traumatic carpal instability
Classification

Post-traumatic carpal instability was first referred to by Gilford and associates in 1943 (see Linscheid et al 1972), Fisk (1970) used the term 'carpal instability' when referring to the concertina deformity seen in some wrists after scaphoid fractures. Put simply, however, carpal instability is the inability to bear physiological loads with an associated loss of the normal carpal alignment. Linscheid et al (1972) classified carpal instabilities into dorsiflexed intercalated segment instability (DISI) and volar (palmar) flexed intercalated segment instability (VISI). Since this paper, much has been written about these classifications, which may be further divided into static forms of carpal instab-

ility, when the malalignment is permanent regardless of the load being applied, and where the collapse patterns may be recognised on routine radiographs; and dynamic forms which occur sporadically under certain loading conditions and in which routine radiographs may be normal. But the concept of carpal instability continues to evolve with subsequent changes in the classification (Ruby 1995, Garcia-Elias 1997), in the case of the latter author as follows:

- Dissociative carpal instability (CID)
  — proximal dissociative carpal instability (proximal CID)
  — distal dissociative carpal instability (distal CID)
- Non-dissociative carpal instability (CIND)
  — non-dissociative radiocarpal instability (radiocarpal CIND)
  — midcarpal non-dissociative instability (midcarpal CIND)
  — combined radiocarpal and midcarpal CIND
- Complex carpal instability (CIC)

Whilst trauma is the commonest cause, many different condition such as inflammation, infection, tumour and congenital disease may result in an unstable wrist.

Dissociative carpal instability (CID)
Proximal dissociative carpal instability (proximal CID)

This pattern of instability is most commonly seen in:

- unstable scaphoid non-unions
- scapholunate dissociation
- triquetrolunate dissociations

Scaphoid non-union has been discussed earlier in this chapter.

Scapholunate dissociation is the most common form of carpal instability. It may be primary, secondary to more extensive injury or disease, or associated with extracarpal injuries. It usually occurs following trauma, but is also seen in association with rheumatoid arthritis, infection, spastic paralysis and congenital ligament laxity.

Persistence of intercarpal collapse would seem to result in significant degenerative changes. The rate of progression of this degeneration is uncertain, although it has been reported to occur as early as within 3 months of injury (Linscheid et al 1972, Taleisnik 1985). This untreated chronic scapholunate dissociation commonly results in a pattern of osteoarthritis and subluxation that has been called scapholunate advanced collapse (SLAC) (Watson & Ballet 1984). The progression of these degenerative changes in the SLAC wrist occurs in three stages. In the first stage degenerative changes are limited to the tip of the styloid. In the second stage the arthritis has spread to the entire radioscaphoid joint, and in the third stage there is additional involvement of the capitolunate joint. Hudson et al (1976) found evidence of articular cartilage narrowing and osteophyte formation in 11 of 19 cases (58%).

Treatment of scapholunate dissociation is more successful if initiated early, and its aim is to re-establish the anatomical alignment of the carpus. This can be achieved by closed reduction alone or by arthroscopically assisted reduction supplemented by percutaneous Kirschner wires. Open reduction may be required, and again percutaneous Kirschner wires may be used to provide stability. Palmer et al (1978) reported on 17 patients treated within 1 month of injury by closed reduction, open reduction alone or combined with direct suture of torn ligaments or ligament reconstruction. Of these 17 patients, nine (53%) had no pain, while six (35%) had only slight pain. Grip strength was 53–80% of normal and the average range of movement was decreased from normal by almost 50%. Patient satisfaction was good in nine patients (53%), fair in five patients (29%) and poor in three (18%).

Chronic scapholunate dissociation without radiocarpal arthritis may be treated either by soft tissue reconstruction or by intercarpal arthrodes if surgical treatment is required.

The results of ligament reconstruction were also reported by Palmer et al (1978). In the 30 patients with chronic scapholunate dissociation without arthritis, 20 (66%) had no pain, nine (30%) had slight pain and only one patient had moderate pain. The range of wrist movement was decreased to approximately 45° of palmar flexion and dorsiflexion. Grip strength was improved in 19 patients (63%) and averaged 76% of normal. The scapholunate gap and scapholunate angle were restored to normal in 24% of the patients.

Glickel & Millender (1982) reported the results of ligament reconstruction in 21 patients. Only two patients were pain-free, although 18 (86%) noticed a decrease in their pain. They found that grip strength was generally only slightly increased and the range of motion was reduced to an average of 41° of palmar flexion and 53° of dorsiflexion. They also discovered that while the scapholunate angle was initially improved, as follow-up continued the scapholunate gap and scapholunate angle increased, suggesting that the repairs 'stretch out' with time and use.

Almquist et al (1991) wrote enthusiastically of their four-bone ligament reconstruction for chronic complete scapholunate separation. Of their 36 patients (average follow-up 4.8 years), 35% reported no pain, 35% reported pain with heavy labour, and 24% reported pain with light labour. The average postoperative range of wrist extension was 52° and 37° flexion. Grip strength averaged 73% of the uninvolved side. Eighty-six percent of patients returned to their pre-injury activities, including heavy labour. No patient showed radiological evidence of advancing arthritic changes. However, other authors have found the technique of soft tissue reconstruction unreliable and/or demanding (Taleisnik 1988, Deshmukh et al 1999).

Deshmukh et al (1999) reviewed 44 cases of chronic scapholunate dissociation treated by dorsal capsulodesis. Only 21 patients (48%) had good or excellent pain relief. There was a significant postoperative reduction of wrist movement with the loss averaging 22° in extension, 31° in flexion, 13° in radial and 13° in ulnar deviation. Grip strength was only 65% of the unaffected side. The presence of a compensation claim was a statistically significant factor in a poor result.

Limited intercarpal fusion produced satisfactory results in 80% of patients (Kleinman 1989). Union of the arthrodesis was sometimes difficult to achieve and in Hastings & Silver's 1984 series of six patients, three had a non-union. However, Kleinman (1989) achieved a 90% bony union rate in 41 patients. Range of motion was decreased but averaged approximately 65–80% of the pre-operative range (Hastings and Silver 1984, Kleinman 1989). Grip strength was also improved as compared with the pre-operative strength, and Eckenrode et al (1986) reported that grip strength was 74% of normal, while pinch grip was 86% of normal.

When chronic scapholunate instability is associated with extensive degenerative changes at the radioscaphoid or lunocapitate joints then treatment is either by midcarpal fusion with resection of the scaphoid or by proximal row carpectomy. Wyrick et al 1995 compared 17 patients treated with scaphoid excision and four corner arthrodesis with 11 treated with proximal row carpectomy for scapholunate advanced collapse wrists. The total arc of motion averaged 95° in the arthrodesis patients and 115° in the proximal row carpectomy patients. Grip strength averaged 74% of the opposite wrist in the arthrodesis group and 94% in the proximal row carpectomy group. They recommended proximal row carpectomy as the motion-preserving procedure of choice.

Triquetrolunate dissociation occurs with complete disruption of the triquetrolunate ligament, resulting in a dissociative VISI pattern. A patient with an acute triquetrolunate dissociation often has a history of a rotational injury of the wrist, commonly as the result of holding a power drill when the drill bit has jammed (Ruby 1995). Triquetrolunate dissociation often exhibits minimal disability after acute injury and the need for surgical correction is infrequent (Taleisnik 1985). Should surgery be required then ligament reconstruction or intercarpal fusion produces good results in the majority of patients (Reagan et al 1984). In acute cases anatomic reduction, with percutaneous pinning or open repair of the triquetrolunate ligament combined with dorsal capsulodesis, is recommended. In chronic cases triquetrolunate arthrodesis or ulnar recession osteotomy is indicated. Koppel et al (1997) reported the results of 47 ulnar shortening osteotomies carried out for ulnar carpal impaction and/or ulnar carpal instability. The overall result was excellent in 22, good in 15, fair in six and poor in four patients.

Trumble et al (1988) described seven patients with static or dynamic VISI. They felt that the instability occurred between the proximal lunate and triquetrum, and distal hamate and capitate. Arthrodesis of the proximal and distal rows of the ulnar carpus provided relief of wrist pain in five of six patients. Flexion–extension was 63% of normal, radial and ulnar deviation 57%, and grip strength 74%.

Distal dissociative carpal instability

This is an uncommon problem usually caused by a crush or blast injury. The transverse intercarpal ligament binding the bones of the distal row rupture, so that the distal row divides into two columns which separate, giving rise to the so-called axial fracture dislocation (Garcia-Elias et al 1989).

Non-dissociative carpal instability (CIND)
Non-dissociative radiocarpal instability

Radiocarpal CIND follows major disruption of the radiocarpal ligament support or changes in the alignment of the distal articular surface of the radius, while dorsal radiocarpal CIND occurs secondary to intra-articular or extra-articular mal-united fractures of the distal radius. Extra-articular malunions are treated by a dorsal open wedge osteotomy to correct the dorsal angulation of the distal articular surface. Intra-articular fractures without degenerative changes require an osteotomy along the plane of the fracture. In the presence of degeneration a radiolunate or radioscapholunate fusion may be required.

Saffar (1996) reported the results of 11 cases of symptomatic distal radial intra-articular malunion treated by radiolunate arthrodesis. Union was achieved in 10 of the 11 patients in 45–90 days. Pain was absent or moderate after 4 months. The arc of flexion-extension was 72° and of radial and ulnar deviation 46°. The average postoperative grip strength was 57% of the opposite side. All were male manual workers. Eight returned to their previous work while two returned to lighter work.

Palmar radiocarpal CIND also occurs in association with intra-articular mal-united fractures of the distal radius. Smith's fractures do not appear to result in this type of instability. Bellinghausen et al (1983) have described two patients with a pure post-traumatic palmar carpal subluxation, both with an associated ulnar translocation. They were treated by plaster immobilisation. Although recurrent subluxation occurred in both patients, there was discomfort in the wrist only after heavy work.

Ulnar translocation

Ulnar translocation usually follows inflammatory arthritis but can occur as a post-traumatic event. According to Taleisnik (1985) there are two types: type I involves an ulnar shift of the whole carpus, while in type II the scaphoid remains in its normal relationship to the radius. This produces a scapholunate gap which must not be confused with the gap seen in scapholunate dissociation. Ulnar translocation is frequently accompanied by volar flexion instability of the proximal part of the carpus (Taleisnik 1988).

Taleisnik (1985) describes the acute injury as being associated with marked swelling and an extreme loss of the range of movement and grip strength. There is often a cosmetic deformity. He feels that surgical correction is invariably required and should involve either radiolunate or radioscapholunate fusion.

Rayhack et al (1987) described traumatic ulnar translocation in eight patients. The initial diagnosis was delayed by an average of 7.3 months. Seven patients underwent ligament repair with or without tendon augmentation. Three achieved a good result, two a fair result and two required conversion to a wrist arthrodesis at an average follow-up of 32 months.

Midcarpal non dissociative instability

If the midcarpal ligament is torn, absent or lax, when placed under load the lunate is forced by the scaphoid into palmar flexion. This places the distal carpal row palmar to the flexion-extension axis of the wrist, resulting in a non-dissociative VISI deformity of the proximal carpal row.

Johnson & Carrera (1986) noted a chronic capitolunate instability in 12 patients, all with a remote dorsiflexion injury to the symptomatic wrist. They described a dorsal-displacement stress test to show dorsal subluxation of the capitate out of the cup of the lunate. Eleven patients had surgery which involved shortening of the radial capitate ligament, with satisfactory results in nine of the patients. However, the significance of the stress test is uncertain, as some of the asymptomatic contralateral wrists that were tested had more displacement than the symptomatic wrists.

Ono et al (1996) described five patients with dorsal wrist pain who had a positive dorsal capitate-displacement test. They were all felt to have capitolunate instability. Conservative treatment did not produce long-term pain relief.

Apergis (1996) reported a retrospective study of 12 young women (14 wrists) complaining of chronic wrist pain, obscure numbness and a reduction of grip strength. All wrists were in VISI alignment. The dorsal-displacement stress test showed subluxation of the capitolunate joint (in nine cases), or both the capitolunate and the radiolunate joint, accompanied by a marked feeling of apprehension. All patients had ligamentous reefing of the whole palmar aspect of the midcarpal joint, and the radiolunate joint when needed, with an additional neurectomy of the terminal branch of the anterior interosseous nerve in four cases. The result was excellent in eight cases, good in five and fair in one.

Summary

- Scapholunate dissociation resulted in significant degenerative changes in up to 58% of patients.
- Early treatment of scapholunate dissociation involves closed or open reduction with or without percutaneous wire fixation, and resulted in minimal or no pain in 88% of patients, almost a 50% reduction in wrist movement, and a 53–80% reduction in grip strength.
- Soft tissue reconstructions for chronic scapholunate dissociation produced early relief of symptoms with no or little pain in 70–96% of patients, almost a 50% loss of motion and 73–76% of normal grip strength. These soft tissue repairs may not produce good long-term results, however.
- Intercarpal arthrodesis for chronic scapholunate dissociation produced satisfactory results in up to 80% of patients. Union occurred in up to 90% of cases. The range of motion averaged 65–80% of normal. Grip strength improved to 74% of normal and pinch grip to 86%. Proximal row carpectomy may produce an acceptable result.
- Triquetrolunate dissociation produces a dynamic or static VISI deformity. Triquetrolunate instability may result in few symptoms. If surgery is required, ligament reconstruction, limited arthrodesis or ulnar shortening osteotomy produces satisfactory results.

- Dorsal radiocarpal CIND requires distal radial osteotomy or fusion.
- Palmar radiocarpal CIND tends to be unstable.
- Ulnar translocation is a rare injury, which results in reasonable early results after ligament repair and tendon augmentation. Arthrodesis may be used primarily or to treat failed ligament repairs.
- Chronic capitolunate instability may be a post-traumatic instability, and appears to produce a reasonable result from shortening of the radial capitate ligament.

References

Adkison J W, Chapman M W 1982 Treatment of acute lunate and perilunate dislocations. Clinical Orthopaedics 164: 199–207

Adler J B, Shafton G W 1982 Fractures of the capitate. Journal of Bone and Joint Surgery 44A: 1537–1547

Aitken A P, Nalebuff E A 1960 Volar transnavicular perilunar dislocation of the carpus. Journal of Bone and Joint Surgery 42A: 1051–1057

Alexander A H 1977 Bilateral traumatic dislocation of the distal radioulnar joint, ulna dorsal. Clinical Orthopaedics 129: 238–244

Almquist E E 1986 Kienböck's disease. Clinical Orthopaedics 202: 68–78

Almquist E E, Burns J F 1982 Radial shortening for the treatment of Kienbock's disease—a 5 to 10 year follow-up. Journal of Hand Surgery 7: 348–352

Altissimi M, Anterucci R, Fiacca C, Mancini G B 1986 Long-term results of conservative treatment of fractures of the distal radius. Clinical Orthopaedics 206: 202–210

Amadio P C, Berquist T H, Smith D K, Ilstrup D M, Cooney W P, Linscheid R L 1989 Scaphoid malunion. Journal of Hand Surgery 14A: 679–687

Amadio P C, Hanssen A D, Berquist T H 1987 The genesis of Kienbock's disease: evaluation of a case by magnetic resonance imaging. Journal of Hand Surgery 12A: 1044–1049

Amamilo S C, Uppal R, Samuel A W 1985 Isolated dislocation of carpal scaphoid. Journal of Hand Surgery 10B: 385–388

Apergis E P 1996 The unstable capitolunate and radiolunate joints as a source of wrist pain in young women. Journal of Hand Surgery 21B: 501–506

Armistead R B, Linscheid R L, Dobyns J H, Beckenbaugh R D 1982 Ulnar lengthening in the treatment of Kienböck's disease. Journal of Bone and Joint Surgery 64A: 170–178

Aro H, Koivunen T, Katevuo K, Nieminen S, Aho H J 1988 Late compression neuropathies after Colles' fractures. Clinical Orthopaedics 233: 217–225

Ashkar K, O'Connor D, Lambert S 1998 Dislocation of the pisiform in a 9 year old child. Journal of Hand Surgery 23B: 269–270

Atkins R M, Duckworth T, Kanis J A 1989 Algodystrophy following Colles' fracture. Journal of Hand Surgery 14B: 161–164

Atkins R M, Duckworth T, Kanis J A 1990 Features of algodystrophy after Colles' fracture. Journal of Bone and Joint Surgery 72B: 105–110

Axelrod T S, McMurtry R Y 1990 Open reduction and internal fixation of comminuted intraarticular fractures of the distal radius. Journal of Hand Surgery 15A: 1–11

Bacorn R W, Kurtzke J F 1953 Colles' fracture. Journal of Bone and Joint Surgery 35A: 643–658

Baird D B, Friedenberg Z B 1968 Delayed ulnar-nerve palsy following a fracture of the hamate. Journal of Bone and Joint Surgery 50A: 570–572

Barros J W, Oliveira D J, Fernandes C D 1997 Bilateral transscapholunate dislocations. Journal of Hand Surgery 22B: 169–172

Barton N J 1997 Experience with scaphoid grafting. Journal of Hand Surgery 22B: 153–160.

Bartone N F, Grieco R V 1956 Fractures of the triquetrum. Journal of Bone and Joint Surgery 38A: 353–356

Baulot E, Perez A, Hallonet D, Grammont P M 1997 Scaphoid and lunate palmar divergent dislocation. A case report. Journal of Bone and Joint Surgery 81B: supp III: 349

Beckenbaugh R D, Shives T C, Dobyns J H, Linscheid R L 1980 Kienböck's disease: the natural history of Kienböck's disease and consideration of lunate fractures. Clinical Orthopaedics 149: 98–106

Bellinghausen H W, Gilula L A, Young L V, Weeks P M 1983 Post-traumatic palmar carpal subluxation. Journal of Bone and Joint Surgery 65A: 998–1006

Bickerstaff D R, Bell M J 1989 Carpal malalignment in Colles' fractures. Journal of Hand Surgery 14B: 155–160

Bilos Z J, Hui P W T 1981 Dorsal dislocation of the lunate with carpal collapse. Journal of Bone and Joint Surgery 63A: 1484–1486

Bishop A T, Beckenbaugh R D 1988 Fracture of the hamate hook. Journal of Hand Surgery 13A: 135–139

Biyani A, Simison A J M, Klenerman L 1995 Fractures of the distal radius and ulna. Journal of Hand Surgery 20B: 357–364

Black D M, Watson H K, Vender M I 1986 Scapholunate gap with scaphoid non-union. Clinical Orthopaedics 224: 205–209

Bonnin J G, Greening W P 1943 Fractures of the triquetrum. British Journal of Surgery 31: 278–283

Bonzar M, Firrell J C, Hainer M, Mah E T, McCabe S J 1998 Kienbock disease and negative ulnar variance. Journal of Bone and Joint Surgery 80A: 1154–1157

Borgeskov S, Christiansen B, Kjaer A, Balslev I 1966 Fractures of the carpal bones. Acta Orthopaedica Scandinavica 37: 276–287

Bowen T L 1973 Injuries of the hamate bone. The Hand 5: 235–237

Brolin I 1964 Post-traumatic lesions of the lunate bone. Acta Orthopaedica Scandinavica 34: 167–182

Bruckner J D, Alexander A H, Lichman D M 1995 Acute dislocations of the distal radio-ulnar joint. Journal of Bone and Joint Surgery 77A: 958–968

Brunelli G A, Brunelli G R 1991 A personal technique for treatment of scaphoid non-union. Journal of Hand Surgery 16B: 148–152

Bryan R S, Dobyns J H 1980 Fractures of the carpal bones other than lunate and navicular. Clinical Orthopaedics 149: 107–111

Buchler U, Nagy L 1995 The issue of vascularity in fractures and non union of the scaphoid. Journal of Hand Surgery 20B: 726–735

Burgess R C, Watson H K 1988 Hypertrophic ulnar styloid non-union. Clinical Orthopaedics 228: 215–217

Camelot C, Ramaré S, Lemoine J, Saillant G 1999 Conservative treatment for displaced fractures of the distal end of the radius according to Judet: Anatomical and functional results of 280 cases. Journal of Bone and Joint Surgery 81B: supp III: 363

Campbell R D, Lance E M, Yeoh C B 1964 Lunate and perilunar dislocations. Journal of Bone and Joint Surgery 46B: 55–72

Carroll R E 1997 Long-term review of fascial replacement after excision of the carpal lunate bone. Clinical Orthopaedics and Related Research 342: 59–63

Cassebaum W H 1950 Colles' fracture. Journal of the American Medical Association 143: 963–965

Catalano L W, Cole R J, Gelberman R H, Evanoff B A, Gilula L A, Borelli J 1997 Displaced intra-articular fractures of the distal aspect of the radius. Journal of Bone and Joint Surgery 79A: 1290–1302

Cetti R, Christensen S-E, Reuther K 1982 Fracture of the lunate bone. The Hand 14: 80–84

Chan K P, Huang P 1971 Anatomic variations in radial and ulnar lengths in the wrists of Chinese. Clinical Orthopaedics 80: 17–20

Chen W S 1995 Median nerve neuropathy associated with chronic anterior dislocation of the lunate. Journal of Bone and Joint Surgery 77A: 1853–1857

Christodoulou A G, Colton C L 1986 Scaphoid fractures in children. Journal of Pediatric Orthopaedics 6: 37–39

Clay N R, Dias J J, Costigan P S, Grigg P J, Barton N J 1991 Need the thumb be immobilised in scaphoid fractures? Journal of Bone and Joint Surgery 73B: 828–832

Coleman H M 1960 Injuries of the articular disc at the wrist. Journal of Bone and Joint Surgery 42B: 522–529

Collert S, Isacson J 1978 Management of redislocated Colles' fractures. Clinical Orthopaedics 135: 183–186

Cooney W P 1983 External fixation of distal radial fractures. Clinical Orthopaedics 180: 44–49

Cooney W P, Bussey R, Dobyns J H, Linscheid R L 1987 Difficult wrist fractures: perilunate fracture–dislocations of the wrist. Clinical Orthopaedics 214: 136–147

Cooney W P, Dobyns J H, Linscheid R L 1980a Complications of Colles' fractures. Journal of Bone and Joint Surgery 62A: 613–619

Cooney W P, Dobyns J H, Linscheid R L 1980b Fractures of the scaphoid: a rational approach to management. Clinical Orthopaedics 149: 90–97

Cooney W P, Linscheid R L, Dobyns J H 1979 External pin fixation for unstable Colles' fractures. Journal of Bone and Joint Surgery 61A: 840–845

Cordrey L J, Ferrer-Torels M 1960 Management of fractures of the greater multangular. Journal of Bone and Joint Surgery 42A: 1111–1118

Corso S J, Savoie F H, Geissler W B, Whipple T L, Jiminez W, Jenkins N 1997 Arthroscopic repair of peripheral avulsions of the triangular fibrocartilage complex of the wrist: a multicenter study. Arthroscopy 13: 78–84

D'Anca A F, Sternlieb S B, Byron T W, Feinstein P A 1984 External fixator management of unstable Colles' fractures. Orthopaedics 7: 853–859

Dameron T B 1972 Traumatic dislocation of the distal radio-ulnar joint. Clinical Orthopaedics 83: 55–63

Davis D R, Green D P 1976 Forearm fractures in children. Clinical Orthopaedics 120: 172–184

Delaere O, Dury M, Molderez A, Foucher G 1998 Conservative versus operative treatment for Kienbock's disease. Journal of Hand Surgery 23B: 33–36

De Oliveira J C 1973 Barton's fractures. Journal of Bone and Joint Surgery 55A: 586–594

Deshmukh S C, Givissis P, Belloso D, Stanley J K, Trail I A 1999 Blatt's capsulodesis for chronic scapholunate dissociation. Journal of Hand Surgery 24B: 215–220

Dias J J, Brenkel I J, Irvine G B 1989 Patterns of union in fractures of the waist of the scaphoid. Journal of Bone and Joint Surgery 71B: 307–310

Dias J J, Taylor M, Thompson J, Brenkel I J, Gregg P J 1988 Radiographic signs of union of scaphoid fractures. Journal of Bone and Joint Surgery 70B: 299–301

Dias J J, Thompson J, Barton N J, Gregg P J 1990 Suspected scaphoid fractures. Journal of Bone and Joint Surgery 72B: 98–101

Dias J J, Wray C C, Jones J M, Gregg P J 1987 The value of early mobilisation in the treatment of Colles' fractures. Journal of Bone and Joint Surgery 69B: 463–467

Dobyns J H, Linscheid R L 1984 Fractures and dislocations of the wrist. In: Rockwood C A, Green D P (eds) Fractures in adults. J B Lippincott, Philadelphia, pp 411–510

Duke R 1963 Dislocation of the hamate bone. Journal of Bone and Joint Surgery 45B: 744

Duncan D S, Thurston A J 1985 Clinical fracture of the carpal scaphoid—an illusionary diagnosis. Journal of Hand Surgery 10B: 375–376

Durbin F C 1950 Non-union of the triquetrum. Journal of Bone and Joint Surgery 32B: 388

Ebraheim N A, Skie M C, Savolaine E R, Jackson W T 1995 Coronal fracture of the body of the hamate. Journal of Trauma-Injury Infection and Critical Care 38: 169–174

Eckenrode J F, Louis D S, Greene T L 1986 Scaphoid–trapezium–trapezoid fusion in the treatment of chronic scapholunate instability. Journal of Hand Surgery 11A: 497–502

Eddeland A, Eiken O, Hellgren E, Ohlsson N-M 1975 Fractures of the scaphoid. Scandinavian Journal of Plastic and Reconstructive Surgery 9: 234–239

Eelma J, McElfresh E C 1983 Colles' fractures in young adults. Minnesota Medicine 66: 487–490

Egawa M, Asai T 1983 Fracture of the hook of the hamate. Journal of Hand Surgery 8: 393–398

Ender H G, Herbert T J 1989 Treatment of problem fractures and non-unions of the scaphoid. Orthopaedics 12: 195–202

Engkvist O, Lundborg G 1979 Rupture of the extensor pollicis longus tendon after fracture of the lower end of the radius—a clinical and microangiographic study. The Hand 11: 76–85

Evans D L, Stauber M, Frykman G K 1990 Irreducible epiphyseal plate fracture of the distal ulna due to interposition of the extensor carpi ulnaris tendon. Clinical Orthopaedics 251: 162–165

Evans G, Burke F D, Barton N J 1986 A comparison of conservative treatment and silicone replacement arthroplasty in Kienböck's disease. Journal of Hand Surgery 11B: 98–102

Fehring T K, Milek M A 1984 Isolated volar dislocation of the radiocarpal joint. Journal of Bone and Joint Surgery 66A: 464–466

Fenton R L 1956 The naviculo-capitate fracture syndrome. Journal of Bone and Joint Surgery 38A: 681–684

Fernandes H J A, Köberle G, Ferreira G H S, Camargo J N 1983 Volar transscaphoid perilunar dislocation. The Hand 15: 276–280

Fernandez D L 1982 Correction of post-traumatic wrist deformity in adults by osteotomy, bone grafting, and internal fixation. Journal of Bone and Joint Surgery 64A: 1164–1178

Fernandez D L 1988 Radial osteotomy and Bowers arthroplasty for malunited fractures of the distal end of the radius. Journal of Bone and Joint Surgery 70A: 1538–1551

Fernandez D L 1991 Treatment of displaced articular fractures of the radius. Journal of Hand Surgery 16A: 375–384

Field J, Atkins R M 1997 Algodystrophy is an early complication of Colles' fracture. Journal of Hand Surgery 22B: 178–182

Filan S L, Herbert T J 1995 Avascular necrosis of the proximal scaphoid after fracture union. Journal of Hand Surgery 20B: 551–556

Filan S L, Herbert T J 1996 Herbert screw fixation of scaphoid fractures. Journal of Bone and Joint Surgery 78B: 519–529

Fisk G R 1970 Carpal instability and the fractured scaphoid. Annals of the Royal College of Surgeons of England 46: 63–76

Fisk G R 1984 The wrist. Journal of Bone and Joint Surgery 66B: 396–407

Flandreau R H, Sweeney R M, O'Sullivan W D 1962 Clinical experience with a series of Smith's fractures. Archives of Surgery 84: 36–39

Flinkkila T, Raatikainen T, Hamalainen M 1998 AO and Frykman's classifications of Colles' fracture. No prognostic value in 652 patients evaluated after 5 years. Acta Orthopaedica Scandinavica 69: 77–81

Foucher G, Schuind F, Merle M, Brunelli F 1985 Fractures of the hook of the hamate. Journal of Hand Surgery 10B: 205–210

Freeman B H, Hay E L 1985 Non-union of the capitate. Journal of Hand Surgery 10A: 187–190

Freund L G, Ovesen J 1977 Isolated dorsal dislocation of the radiocarpal joint. Journal of Bone and Joint Surgery 59A: 277

Fritz T, Wersching D, Klavora R, Kreiglstein C, Friedl W 1999 Combined Kirschner wire fixation in the treatment of Colles' fracture. A prospective controlled trial. Archives of Orthopaedic & Trauma Surgery 119: 171–178

Frykman G 1967 Fracture of the distal radius including sequelae. Acta Orthopaedica Scandinavica (suppl) 108

Futami T, Yamanoto M 1989 Chinese external fixation treatment for fractures of the distal end of the radius. Journal of Hand Surgery 14A: 1028–1032

Garcia-Elias M 1997 The treatment of wrist instability. Journal of Bone and Joint Surgery 79B: 684–690

Garcia-Elias M, Dobyns J H, Cooney W P, Linscheid R L 1989 Traumatic axial dislocations of the carpus. Journal of Hand Surgery 14A: 446–457

Gartland J J, Werley C W 1951 Evaluation of healed Colles' fractures. Journal of Bone and Joint Surgery 33A: 895–907

Geissler W S B, Fernandez D L, Lamey D M 1996 Distal radioulnar joint injuries associated with fractures of the distal radius. Clinical Orthopaedics and Related Research 327: 135–146

Geissler W B, Freeland A E, Savoie F H, McIntyre L W, Whipple T L 1996 Intracarpal soft-tissue lesions associated with an intra-articular fracture of the distal end of the radius. Journal of Bone and Joint Surgery 78A: 357–365

Gelberman R H, Salamon P B, Jurist J M, Posch J L 1975 Ulnar variance in Kienböck's disease. Journal of Bone and Joint Surgery 37A: 674–676

Gellman H, Caputo R J, Carter V, Aboulafia A, McKay M 1989 Comparison of short and long thumb spica casts for non-displaced fractures of the carpal scaphoid. Journal of Bone and Joint Surgery 71A: 354–357

Gemme G, Saraste H 1987 Bone and joint pathology in workers using hand held vibrating tools. An overview. Scandinavian Journal of Work Environment and Health 13: 290–300

Giannikas D, Tylliankis M, Lambiris E 1999 Long term results of conservative treatment of intra articular fractures of the distal radius. Journal of Bone and Joint Surgery 81B: supp II: 166–167

Goldberg B, Heller A P 1987 Dorsal dislocation of the triquetrum with rotary subluxation of the scaphoid. Journal of Hand Surgery 12A: 119–122

Goldberg I, Amit S, Bahar A, Seelenfreund M 1981 Complete dislocation of the trapezium. Journal of Hand Surgery 6: 193–195

Goodman M L, Shankman G B 1984 Palmar dislocation of the trapezoid. Journal of Hand Surgery 9A: 127–131

Gotz R J, Grogan D P, Greene T L, Belsole R J, Ogden J A 1991 Distal ulnar physeal injury. Journal of Pediatric Orthopaedics 11: 318–326

Green D P 1975 Pins and plaster treatment of comminuted fractures of the distal end of the radius. Journal of Bone and Joint Surgery 57A: 304–310

Green D P 1982 Operative hand surgery, vol 1. Churchill Livingstone, Edinburgh

Green D P 1985 The effect of avascular necrosis on Russe bone grafting for scaphoid non-union. Journal of Hand Surgery 10A: 597–605

Green D P, O'Brien E T 1978 Open reduction of carpal dislocations: indications and operative techniques. Journal of Hand Surgery 3: 250–265

Green D P, O'Brien E T 1979 Classification and management of carpal dislocations. Clinical Orthopaedics 149: 55–72

Green J T, Gay F H 1956 Colles' fracture—residual disability. American Journal of Surgery 91: 636–642

Griffin A C, Gilula L A, Young V L, Strecker W B, Weeks P M 1988 Fracture of the dorsoulnar tubercle of the trapezium. Journal of Hand Surgery 13A: 622–626

Guichet J M, Moller C C, Dautel G, Lascombes P 1997 A modified Kapandji procedure for Smith's fracture in children. Journal of Bone and Joint Surgery 79B: 734–737

Gunn R S 1985 Dislocation of the hamate bone. Journal of Hand Surgery 10B: 107–108

Gupta A 1991 The treatment of Colles' fracture. Journal of Bone and Joint Surgery 73B: 312–315

Hambidge J E, Desai V V, Schranz P J, Compson J P, David T R C, Barton N J 1999 Treatment by cast immobilisation with the wrist in flexion or extension. Journal of Bone and Joint Surgery 81B: 91–92

Hanel D P, Scheid D K 1988 Irreducible fracture–dislocation of the distal radioulnar joint secondary to entrapment of the extensor carpi ulnaris tendon. Clinical Orthopaedics 234: 56–60

Harbison J S, Stevenson T M, Lipert J R 1978 Forearm fractures in children. Australia and New Zealand Journal of Surgery 48: 84–88

Hastings D E, Silver R L 1984 Intercarpal arthrodesis in the management of chronic carpal instability after trauma. Journal of Hand Surgery 9A: 834–840

Hauck R M, Skahen J, Palmer A K 1996 Classification and treatment of ulnar styloid non union. Journal of Hand Surgery 21A: 418–422

Herbert T J 1986 Use of the Herbert bone screw in surgery of the wrist. Clinical Orthopaedics 202: 79–92

Herbert T J, Filan S L 1999 Proximal scaphoid non union—osteosynthesis Hardchirurgie, Mikzrochirurgie, Plastische Chirurgie 31: 169–173

Herbert T J, Fisher W E 1984 Management of the fractured scaphoid using a new bone screw. Journal of Bone and Joint Surgery 66B: 114–123

Hirasawa Y, Katsumi Y, Akiyoshi T, Tamai K, Tokioka T 1990 Clinical and microangiographic studies on rupture of the EPL tendon after distal radial fractures. Journal of Hand Surgery 15B: 51–57

Hollingsworth R, Morris J 1976 The importance of the ulnar side of the wrist in fractures of the distal end of the radius. Injury 7: 263–266

Hove L M, Engesaeter L B 1997 Corrective osteotomies after injuries of the distal radial physis in children. Journal of Hand Surgery 22B: 699–704

Howard F M 1964 Ulnar-nerve palsy in wrist fractures. Journal of Bone and Joint Surgery 43A: 1197–1201

Hudson T M, Caragol W J, Kaye J J 1976 Isolated rotatory subluxation of the carpal navicular. American Journal of Roentgenology 126: 601–611

Hulsizer D, Weiss A P, Akelman E 1997 Ulna shortening osteotomy after failed arthroscopic debridement of the triangular fibrocartilage complex. Journal of Hand Surgery 22A: 694–698

Inoue G, Imaeda T 1997 Management of trans-scaphoid perilunate dislocations. Herbert screw fixation, ligamentous repair and early wrist mobilization. Archives of Orthopaedics & Trauma Surgery 116: 338–340

Inoue G, Kuwahata Y 1997 Management of acute perilunate dislocations without fracture of the scaphoid. Journal of Hand Surgery 22B: 647–652

Inoue G, Sakuma M 1996 The natural history of scaphoid non union. Radiographical and clinical analysis in 102 cases. Archives of Orthopaedic & Trauma Surgery 115: 1–4

Inoue G, Shionoya K 1997 Herbert screw fixation by limited access for acute fractures of the scaphoid. Journal of Bone and Joint Surgery 79B: 418–421

Inoue G, Shionoya K 1999 Late treatment of unreduced perilunate dislocations. Journal of Hand Surgery 24B: 221–225

Inoue G, Shionoya K, Kuwahata Y 1997a Herbert screw fixation for scaphoid non unions. An analysis of factors influencing outcome. Clinical Orthopaedics & Related Research 343: 99–106

Inoue G, Shionoya K, Kuwahata Y 1997b Ununited proximal pole scaphoid fractures. Treatment with a Herbert screw in 16 cases followed for 0.5 to 8 years. Acta Orthopaedica Scandinavica 68: 124–127

Jacobsen S, Hassani G, Hansen D, Christensen O 1995 Suspected scaphoid fractures. Can we avoid overkill? Acta Orthopaedica Belgica 61: 74–78

Jakim I, Pieterse H S, Sweet M B E 1991 External fixation for intra-articular fractures of the distal radius. Journal of Bone and Joint Surgery 73B: 302–306

Jasmine M S, Packer J W, Edwards G S 1988 Irreducible trans-scaphoid perilunate dislocation. Journal of Hand Surgery 13A: 212–215

Jenkins N H 1989 The unstable Colles' fractures. Journal of Hand Surgery 14B: 149–154

Jenkins N H, Mintowt-Czyz W J 1988 Malunion and dysfunction in Colles' fractures. Journal of Hand Surgery 13B: 291–293

Jenkins S A 1951 Osteoarthritis of the pisiform-triquetral joint. Journal of Bone and Joint Surgery 33B: 532

Jensen B V, Christensen C 1990 An unusual combination of simultaneous fracture of the tuberosity of the trapezium and the hook of the hamate. Journal of Hand Surgery 15A: 285–287

Johnson R P, Carrera G F 1986 Chronic capitolunate instability. Journal of Bone and Joint Surgery 68A: 1164–1176

Jones G B 1955 An unusual fracture–dislocation of the carpus. Journal of Bone and Joint Surgery 37B: 146–147

Jones W A, Ghorbal M S 1985 Fractures of the trapezium: a report of three cases. Journal of Hand Surgery 10B: 227–230

Jupiter J B, Fernandez D L, Toh C L, Fellman T, Ring D 1996 Operative treatment of volar intra-articular fractures of the distal end of the radius. Journal of Bone and Joint Surgery 78A: 1817–1828

Kaarela O I, Raatikainen T K, Torniainen P J 1998 Silicone replacement arthroplasty for Kienbock's disease. Journal of Hand Surgery 23B: 735–740

Kaukonen J-P, Karaharju E O, Porras M, Lüthje P, Jakobsson A 1988a Functional recovery after fractures of the distal forearm. Annales Chirurgiae et Gynaecologiae 77: 27–31

Kaukonen J-P, Porras M, Karaharju E 1988b Anatomical results after distal forearm fractures. Annales Chirurgiae et Gynaecologiae 77: 21–26

Kawai H, Yamamoto K 1988 Pronator quadratus pedicled bone graft for old scaphoid fractures. Journal of Bone and Joint Surgery 70B: 829–831

Kelly A J, Warwick D, Crichlow T P, Bannister G C 1997 Is manipulation of moderately displaced Colles' fracture worthwhile? A prospective randomized trial. Injury 28: 283–287

Kienböck R 1980 Concerning traumatic malacia of the lunate and its consequences: degeneration and compression fractures: the classic. Clinical Orthopaedics 149: 4–8

Kikuchi Y, Nakamura T 1998 Avulsion fracture at the fovea of the ulna. Journal of Hand Surgery 23B: 176–178

King R E 1975 Barton's fracture–dislocation of the wrist. Current Practice in Orthopaedic Surgery 6: 133–144

Kleinman W B 1989 Long term study of chronic scapho-lunate instability treated by scapho-trapezio-trapezoid arthrodesis. Journal of Hand Surgery 14A: 429–445

Knirk J L, Jupiter J B 1986 Intra-articular fractures of the distal end of the radius in young adults. Journal of Bone and Joint Surgery 68A: 647–659

Kongsholm J, Olerud C 1989 Plaster cast versus external fixation for unstable intraarticular Colles' fractures. Clinical Orthopaedics 241: 57–65

Koppel M, Hargreaves I C, Herbert T J 1997 Ulnar shortening osteotomy for ulnar carpal instability and ulnar carpal impaction. Journal of Hand Surgery 22B: 451–456

Kopylov P, Runnqvist K, Jonsson K, Aspenberg P 1999 Norian SRS versus external fixation in redisplaced distal radial fractures. Acta Orthopaedica Scandinavica 70: 1–5

Kristensen S S, Thomassen E, Christensen F 1986a Kienböck's disease—late results by nonsurgical treatment. Journal of Hand Surgery 11B: 422–425

Kristensen S S, Thomassen E, Christensen F 1986b Ulnar variance in Kienböck's disease. Journal of Hand Surgery 11B: 258–260

Kukla C, Gaebler C, Breitenseher M J, Tratting S, Vecsei V 1997 Occult fractures of the scaphoid. The diagnostic usefulness and indirect economic repercussions of radiography versus magnetic resonance scanning. Journal of Hand Surgery 22B: 810–813

Kvarnes L, Reikeras O 1983 Non-union of the carpal navicular. The Hand 15: 252–257

Kwa S, Tonkin M A 1997 Nonunion of a distal radial fracture in a healthy child. Journal of Hand Surgery 22B: 175–177

Lagerstrom C, Nordgren B, Rahme H 1999 Recovery of isometric grip strength after Colles' fracture: a prospective two-year study. Scandinavian Journal of Rehabilitation Medicine 31: 55–62

Langhoff O, Andersen J L 1988 Consequences of late immobilisation of scaphoid fractures. Journal of Hand Surgery 13B: 77–79

Larson B, Light T R, Ogden J A 1987 Fracture and ischemic necrosis of the immature scaphoid. Journal of Hand Surgery 12A: 122–127

Laulan J, Bismuth J P, Sicre G, Garaud P 1997 The different types of algodystrophy after fracture of the distal radius. Journal of Hand Surgery 22B: 441–447

Leclercq C, Xarchas C 1998 Kienbock's disease in cerebral palsy. Journal of Hand Surgery 23B: 746–748

Lee B S, Esterhai J L, Das M 1984 Fracture of the distal radial epiphysis. Clinical Orthopaedics 185: 90–96

Lee M L H 1963 The intraosseous arterial pattern of the carpal lunate bone and its relationship to avascular necrosis. Acta Orthopaedica Scandinavica 33: 43–55

Leslie I J, Dickson R A 1981 The fractured carpal scaphoid. Journal of Bone and Joint Surgery 63B: 225–230

Letz R, Cherniack M G, Gerr F, Herschman D, Pace P 1992 A cross sectional epidemiological survey of shipyard workers exposed to hand-arm vibration. British Journal of Industrial Medicine 49: 53–62

Leung Y F, Wai Y L, Kam W L, Ip P S 1998 Solitary dislocation of the scaphoid. Journal of Hand Surgery 23B: 88–92

Lewis M H 1978 Median nerve decompression after Colles' fracture. Journal of Bone and Joint Surgery 60B: 195–196

Lichtman D M, Alexander H, Mack G R, Gunther S F 1982 Kienböck's disease—update on silicone replacement arthroplasty. Journal of Hand Surgery 7: 343–347

Lichtman D M, Mack G R, Macdonald R I, Gunther S F, Wilson J N 1977 Kienböck's disease: the role of silicone replacement arthroplasty. Journal of Bone and Joint Surgery 59A: 899–908

Lidström A 1959 Fractures of the distal end of the radius. Acta Orthopaedica Scandinavica (suppl) 41

Lindau T, Arner M, Hagberg L 1997 Intra-articular lesions in distal fractures of the radius in young adults. Journal of Hand Surgery 22B: 638–643

Lindström G, Nyström A 1990 Incidence of post-traumatic arthrosis after primary healing of scaphoid fractures: a clinical and radiological study. Journal of Hand Surgery 15B: 11–13

Linscheid R L, Dobyns J H, Beabout J W, Bryan R S 1972 Traumatic instability of the wrist. Journal of Bone and Joint Surgery 54A: 1612–1632

London P S 1961 The broken scaphoid bone. Journal of Bone and Joint Surgery 43B: 237–244

Lowdon I M R, Simpson A H R W, Burge P 1984 Recurrent dorsal trans-scaphoid perilunate dislocation. Journal of Hand Surgery 9B: 307–310

Lowrey D G, Moss S H, Wolff T W 1984 Volar dislocation of the capitate. Journal of Bone and Joint Surgery 66A: 611–613

Mack G R, Bosse M J, Gelberman R H, Yu E 1984 The natural history of scaphoid non-union. Journal of Bone and Joint Surgery 66A: 504–509

Mack G R, Wilkens J H, McPherson S A 1998 Subacute scaphoid fractures. A closer look at closed treatment. American Journal of Sports Medicine 26: 56–58

Manoli A 1982 Irreducible fracture-separation of the distal radial epiphysis. Journal of Bone and Joint Surgery 64A: 1095–1096

Marsh A P, Lampros P J 1959 The naviculo-capitate fracture syndrome. American Journal of Roentgenology 82: 255–256

Mason M L 1953 Colles' fracture. British Journal of Surgery 40: 340–346

Mathoulin C, Haerle M 1998 Vascularized bone graft from the palmar carpal artery for treatment of scaphoid nonunion. Journal of Hand Surgery 23B: 318–323

Maudsley R H, Chen S C 1972 Screw fixation in the management of the fractured carpal scaphoid. Journal of Bone and Joint Surgery 54B: 432–441

Mayfield J K, Johnson R P, Kilcoyne R K 1980 Carpal dislocations: pathomechanics and progressive perilunar instability. Journal of Hand Surgery 5: 226–241

McClain E J, Boyes J H 1966 Missed fractures of the greater multangular. Journal of Bone and Joint Surgery 48A: 1525–1528

McLain R F, Steyers C M 1990 Tendon ruptures with scaphoid nonunion. Clinical Orthopaedics 255: 117–120

McLaughlin H L, Parkes J C 1969 Fracture of the carpal navicular bone: gradations in therapy based upon pathology. Journal of Trauma 9: 311–319

McQueen M M, Hajducka C, Court-Brown C M 1996 Redisplaced unstable fractures of the distal radius. Journal of Bone and Joint Surgery 78B: 404–409

Melone C P 1984 Articular fractures of the distal radius. Orthopaedic of Clinics North America 15 (2): 217–236

Melone C P 1986 Open treatment for displaced articular fractures of the distal radius. Clinical Orthopaedics 202: 103–111

Meyers M H, Wells R, Harvey J P 1971 Naviculo-capitate fracture syndrome. Journal of Bone and Joint Surgery 53A: 1383–1386

Meyn M A, Roth A M 1980 Isolated dislocation of the trapezoid bone. Journal of Hand Surgery 5: 602–604

Milek M A, Boulas H J 1990 Flexor tendon ruptures secondary to hamate hook fractures. Journal of Hand Surgery 15A: 740–744

Milliez P Y, Courandier J M, Thomine J M, Biga N 1987 The natural history of scaphoid non-union. Annales de Chirurgie de la Main 6: 195–202

Minami A, Kato H 1998 Ulnar shortening for triangular fibrocartilage complex tears associated with ulnar positive variance. Journal of Hand Surgery 23A: 904–908

Minami A, Ogino T, Hamada M 1989 Rupture of extensor tendons associated with a palmar perilunar dislocation. Journal of Hand Surgery 14A: 843–847

Minami A, Ogino T, Ohshio I, Minami M 1986 Correlation between clinical results and carpal instabilities in patients after reduction of lunate and perilunar dislocation. Journal of Hand Surgery 11B: 213–220

Minami M, Yamazaki J, Ishii S 1984 Isolated dislocation of the pisiform. Journal of Hand Surgery 9A: 125–127

Mink Van Der Molen A B, Groothoff J W, Visser G J P, Robinson P H, Eisnia W H 1999 Time off work due to scaphoid fractures and other carpal injuries in the Netherlands in the period 1990 to 1993. Journal of Hand Surgery 24B: 193–198

Mintzer C M, Waters P M 1999 Surgical treatment of pediatric scaphoid fracture non unions. Journal of Pediatric Orthopaedics 19: 236–239

Mirabello S C, Rosenthal D I, Smith R J 1987 Correlation of clinical and radiographic findings in Kienböck's disease. Journal of Hand Surgery 12A: 1049–1054

Moharti R C, Kar N 1979 Study of the triangular fibrocartilage of the wrist joint in Colles' fracture. Injury 11: 321–324

Moller J T, Lybecker H 1987 Simultaneous fracture of the hamate and the capitate bones. Archives of Orthopaedic & Trauma Surgery 106: 331–332

Monsivais J J, Nitz P A, Scully T J 1986 The role of carpal instability in scaphoid non-union: casual or causal? Journal of Hand Surgery 11B: 201–206

Moore D P, McMahon B A 1988 Anterior radio-carpal dislocation: an isolated injury. Journal of Hand Surgery 13B: 215–217

Morawa L G, Ross P M, Schock C C 1976 Fractures and dislocations involving the navicular-lunate axis. Clinical Orthopaedics 118: 48–53

Mudgal C S, Psenica J, Jupiter J B 1999 Radiocarpal fracture-dislocation. Journal of Hand Surgery 24B: 92–98

Mulder J D 1968 The results of 100 cases of pseudarthrosis in the scaphoid bone treated by the Matti–Russe operation. Journal of Bone and Joint Surgery 50B: 110–115

Munk B, Frokjaer J, Larsen C F, Johannsen H G, Rasmussen L L, Edal A, Rasmussen L D 1995 Diagnosis of scaphoid fractures. A prospective multicenter study of 1052 patients with 160 fractures. Acta Orthopaedica Scandinavica 66: 359–360

Müssbichler H 1961 Injuries of the carpal scaphoid in children. Acta Radiologica 56: 361–368

Niazi T B 1996 Volar perilunate dislocation of the carpus: a case report and elucidation of its mechanism of occurrence. Injury 27: 209–211

Nienstedt F 1999 The operative treatment of intra-articular Smith fractures. Journal of Hand Surgery 24B: 99–103

O'Brien E T 1984 Fractures of the hand and wrist region. In: Rockwood C A, Wilkins K E, King R E (eds) Fractures in children. J B Lippincott, Philadelphia, pp 229–300

Older T M, Stabler E V, Cassebaum W H 1965 Colles' fracture: evaluation and selection of therapy. Journal of Trauma 5: 469–476

Ona H, Gilula L A, Evanoff B A, Graid D 1996 Midcarpal instability: is capitolunate instability pattern a clinical condition? Journal of Hand Surgery 21B: 197–201

Oskam J, De Graaf J S, Klasen H J 1996 Fractures of the distal radius and scaphoid. Journal of Hand Surgery 21B: 772–774

Oskam J, Kingma J, Klasen H J 1998 Fracture of the distal forearm: epidemiological developments in the period 1971–1995 Injury 29: 353–355

Oskarsson G V, Aaser P, Hjall A 1997 Do we underestimate the predictive value of the ulnar styloid affection in Colles' fractures? Archives of Orthopaedic & Trauma Surgery 116: 341–344

Palmer A K 1981 Trapezial ridge fractures. Journal of Hand Surgery 6: 561–564

Palmer A K 1987 Kienböck's disease (editorial). Journal of Hand Surgery 12B: 291–293

Palmer A K, Dobyns J H, Linscheid R L 1978 Management of posttraumatic instability of the wrist secondary to ligament rupture. Journal of Hand Surgery 3: 507–532

Palmieri T J 1982 The excision of painful pisiform bone fractures. Orthopaedic Review 11: 99

Panting A L, Lamb D W, Noble J, Haw C S 1984 Dislocations of the lunate with and without fracture of the scaphoid. Journal of Bone and Joint Surgery 66B: 391–395

Pattee G A, Thompson G H 1988 Anterior and posterior marginal fracture–dislocations of the distal radius. Clinical Orthopaedics 231: 183–195

Pool C 1973 Colles' fracture. Journal of Bone and Joint Surgery 55B: 540–544

Porter M L, Seehra K 1991 Fracture–dislocation of the triquetrum treated with a Herbert screw. Journal of Bone and Joint Surgery 73B: 347–348

Porter M L, Stockley I 1986 Fracture of the distal radius: intermediate and end results in relation to radiological parameters. In: Proceedings of the British Orthopaedic Association. Journal of Bone and Joint Surgery 68B: 666

Pritchett J W 1995 External fixation or closed medullary pinning for unstable Colles' fractures? Journal of Bone and Joint Surgery 77B: 267–269

Prosser A J, Brenkel I J, Irvine G B 1988 Articular fractures of the distal scaphoid. Journal of Hand Surgery 13B: 87–91

Quenzer D E, Dobyns J H, Linscheid R L, Trail I A, Vidal M A 1997 Radial recession osteotomy for Kienböck's disease. Journal of Hand Surgery 22A: 386–395

Radford P J, Matthewson M H, Meggitt B F 1990 The Herbert screw for delayed and non-union of scaphoid fractures: a review of fifty cases. Journal of Hand Surgery 15B: 455–459

Rand J A, Linscheid R L, Dobyns J H 1982 Capitate fractures: a long term follow-up. Clinical Orthopaedics 165: 209–216

Rauïs A, Ledoux A, Thiebaut A, van der Ghinst M 1979 Bipolar fixation of fractures of the distal end of the radius. International Orthopaedics 3: 89–96

Rawlings D 1981 The management of dislocations of the carpal lunate. Injury 12: 319–330

Rayhack J M, Linscheid R L, Dobyns J H, Smith J H 1987 Post traumatic ulnar translation of the carpus. Journal of Hand Surgery 12A: 180–189

Reagan D S, Linscheid R L, Dobyns J H 1984 Lunotriquetral sprains. Journal of Hand Surgery 9A: 502–514

Richards R S, Bennett J D, Roth J H, Milne K 1997 Arthroscopic diagnosis of intra-articular soft tissue injuries associated with distal radial fractures. Journal of Hand Surgery 22A: 772–776

Ripperger R R, Cooney W P, Linscheid R L 1980 Distal pole scaphoid fractures. Orthopaedic Transactions 4: 18

Robbins R R, Carter P R 1995 Iliac crest bone grafting and Herbert screw fixation of non unions of the scaphoid with avascular proximal poles. Journal of Hand Surgery 20A: 818–831

Roolker W, Ritt M J P F, Bos K E 1998 Spontaneous healing of a nonunion of the scaphoid. Journal of Hand Surgery 23B: 86–87

Rose-Innes A P 1960 Anterior dislocation of the ulna at the inferior radio-ulnar joint. Journal of Bone and Joint Surgery 42B: 515–521

Rosenthal D I, Schwartz M, Phillips W C, Jupiter J 1983 Fracture of the radius with instability of the wrist. American Journal of Roentgenology 141: 113–116

Roumen R M H, Hesp W L E M, Bruggink E D M 1991 Unstable Colles' fractures in elderly patients. Journal of Bone and Joint Surgery 73B: 307–311

Rubinovich R M, Rennie W R 1983 Colles' fracture: end results in relation to radiologic parameters. Canadian Journal of Surgery 26: 361–363

Ruby L K 1995 Carpal instability. Journal of Bone and Joint Surgery 77A: 476–487

Ruby L K, Stinson J, Belsky M R 1985 The natural history of scaphoid non-union. Journal of Bone and Joint Surgery 67A: 428–433

Russe O 1960 Fracture of the carpal navicular. Journal of Bone and Joint Surgery 42A: 759–768

Sadr B 1984 Sequential rupture of extensor tendons after a Colles' fracture. Journal of Hand Surgery 9A: 144–145

Saffer P 1996 Radio-lunate arthrodesis for distal radial intra-articular malunion. Journal of Hand Surgery 21B: 14–20

Sanchez-Sotela J, Munuera L 1999 Norian SRS for the treatment of distal radius fractures: A prospective randomized study. Journal of Bone and Joint Surgery 81B: supp II: 166

Schwartz M G, Green S M, Couille F A 1990 Dorsal dislocation of the lunate with multiple extensor tendon ruptures. Journal of Hand Surgery 15A: 132–133

Seimon L P 1972 Compound dislocation of the trapezium. Journal of Bone and Joint Surgery 54A: 1297–1300

Shah J, Jones W A 1998 Factors affecting the outcome in 50 cases of scaphoid nonunion treated with Herbert screw fixation. Journal of Hand Surgery 23B: 680–685

Shea K, Fernandez D L, Jupiter J B, Martin C 1997 Corrective osteotomy for malunited, volarly displaced fractures of the distal end of the radius. Journal of Bone and Joint Surgery 79A: 1816–1826

Sherlock D A 1987 Traumatic dorsoradial dislocation of the trapezium. Journal of Hand Surgery 12A: 262–265

Siebel T, Kleber R, Russel C, Schmitt E, Kaefer W 1998 Long-term outcome of Matti–Russe plasty after scaphoid non-union. Journal of Bone and Joint Surgery 80B: supp I: 6

Siegel M W, Hertzberg H 1969 Complete dislocation of the greater multangular (trapezium). Journal of Bone and Joint Surgery 51A: 769–772

Siegert J J, Frassica F J, Amadio P C 1988 Treatment of chronic per-ilunate dislocations. Journal of Hand Surgery 13A: 206–212

Sjølin S U, Andersen J C 1988 Clinical fracture of the carpal scaphoid—supportive bandage or plaster cast immobilisation? Journal of Hand Surgery 13B: 75–76

Smaill G B 1965 Long term follow up of Colles' fracture. Journal of Bone and Joint Surgery 47B: 80–85

Smith D K, Murray R M 1996 Avulsion fractures of the volar aspect of triquetral bone of the wrist: a subtle sign of carpal ligament injury. American Journal of Roentgenology 166: 609–614

Smith V A, Wright T W 1999 Nonunion of the distal radius. Journal of Hand Surgery 24B: 601–603

Soucacos P N, Hartefilakidis-Garofalidis G C 1981 Dislocation of the triangular bone. Journal of Bone and Joint Surgery 63A: 1012–1013

Sousa H P, Fernandes H, Botelheiro J C 1995 Preoperative progres-sive distraction in old transcapho-peri-lunate dislocations. Journal of Hand Surgery 20B: 603–605

Stahl F 1947 On lunatomalacia. Acta Chirurgica Scandinavica 95 (suppl) 126

Stansberry S D, Swischuk L E, Swischuk J L, Midgett T A 1990 Significance of ulnar styloid fractures in childhood. Pediatric Emergency Care 6: 99–103

Stark H H, Chao E-K, Zemel N P, Rickard T A, Ashworth C R 1989 Fracture of the hook of the hamate. Journal of Bone and Joint Surgery 71A: 1202–1207

Stark H H, Rickard T A, Zemel N P, Ashworth C R 1988 Treatment of ununited fractures of the scaphoid by iliac bone grafts and Kirschner-wire fixation. Journal of Bone and Joint Surgery 70A: 982–991

Stark H H, Zemel N P, Ashworth C R 1981 Use of a hand-carved sil-icone rubber spacer for advanced Kienböck's disease. Journal of Bone Joint Surgery 63A: 1359–1370

Stein A H 1971 Dorsal dislocation of the lesser multangular bone. Journal of Bone and Joint Surgery 53A: 377–379

Stein F, Siegel M W 1969 Naviculocapitate fracture syndrome. Journal of Bone and Joint Surgery 51A: 391–395

Stern P J 1981 Multiple flexor tendon ruptures following an old anterior dislocation of the lunate. Journal of Bone and Joint Surgery 63A: 489–490

Stern P J 1984 Transscaphoid–lunate dislocation; a report of two cases. Journal of Hand Surgery 9A: 370–373

Stewart H D, Innes A R, Burke F D 1984 Functional cast-bracing for Colles' fractures. Journal of Bone and Joint Surgery 66B: 749–753

Stewart H D, Innes A R, Burke F D 1985a Factors affecting the out-come of Colles' fracture: an anatomical and functional study. Injury 16: 289–295

Stewart H D, Innes A R, Burke F D 1985b The hand complications of Colles' fractures. Journal of Hand Surgery 10B: 103–106

Stewart M J 1954 Fractures of the carpal navicular (scaphoid). Journal of Bone and Joint Surgery 36A: 998–1006

Stoffelen D, De Mulder K, Broos P 1998 The clinical importance of carpal instabilities following distal radial fractures. Journal of Hand Surgery 23B: 512–516

Stoffelen D V C, Broos P L 1999 Closed reduction versus Kapandji-pinning for extra-articular distal radial fractures. Journal of Hand Surgery 24B: 89–91

Strange-Vognsen H H 1991 Intraarticular fractures of the distal end of the radius in young adults. Acta Orthopaedica Scandinavica 62: 527–530

Strickner M, Martinek H, Spängler H 1980 Post-traumatic pain in the ulnar part of the wrist joint. In: Proceedings of the South African Orthopaedic Association. Journal of Bone and Joint Surgery 62B: 507

Stuart M J, Beckenbaugh R D 1987 Flexor digitorum profundus entrapment after closed treatment of a displaced Colles' fracture. Journal of Hand Surgery 12A: 413–415

Suman R K 1983 Unstable fractures of the distal end of the radius (transfixion pins and a cast). Injury 15: 206–211

Sumner J M, Khun S M 1984 Entrapment of the median nerve and flexor pollicis longus tendon in an epiphyseal fracture–disloca-tion of the distal radioulnar joint: a case report. Journal of Hand Surgery 9A: 711–714

Sundberg S B, Linscheid R L 1984 Kienböck's disease: results of treatment with ulnar lengthening. Clinical Orthopaedics 187: 43–51

Szabo R M, Manske D 1988 Displaced fractures of the scaphoid. Clinical Orthopaedics 230: 30–38

Szabo R M, Newland C C, Johnson P G, Steinberg D R, Tortosa R 1995 Spectrum of injury and treatment options for isolated dislo-cation of the scaphoid. Journal of Bone and Joint Surgery 77A: 608–615

Tajima T 1966 An investigation of the treatment of Kienböck's dis-ease. In: Proceedings of the Australian Orthopaedic Association. Journal of Bone and Joint Surgery 48A: 1649

Takami H, Takahashi S, Ando M 1997 Attritional flexor tendon rup-tures after a malunited intra-articular fracture of the distal radius. Archives of Orthopaedic & Trauma Surgery 116: 507–509

Taleisnik J 1985 The wrist. Churchill Livingstone, Edinburgh

Taleisnik J 1988 Carpal instability. Journal of Bone and Joint Surgery 70A: 1262–1268

Tan A B H, Tan S K, Yung S W, Wong M K, Kalinga M 1995 Congenital perforations of the triangular fibrocartilage of the wrist. Journal of Hand Surgery 20B: 342–345

Teisen H, Hjarbeck J 1988 Classification of fresh fractures of the lunate. Journal of Hand Surgery 13B: 458–462

Terrono A, Ferenz C C, Nalebuff E A 1989 Delayed diagnosis in non-union of the body of the hamate: a case report. Journal of Hand Surgery 14B: 329–331

Therkelsen F, Andersen K 1949 Lunatomalacia. Acta Chirurgica Scandinavica 97: 503–526

Thomas F M, Tusan K W R, Browne P S H 1975 Fractures of the radius and ulna in children. Injury 7: 120–124

Thomas F B 1957 Reduction of Smith's fracture. Journal of Bone and Joint Surgery 39B: 463–470

Thompson G H, Grant T T 1977 Barton's fractures—reverse Barton's fractures. Clinical Orthopaedics 122: 210–221

Thorpe A P, Murray A D, Smith F W, Ferguson J 1996 Clinically sus-pected scaphoid fracture: a comparison of magnetic resonance imaging and bone scintigraphy. British Journal of Radiology 69: 109–113

Trumble T, Bour C J, Smith R J, Edwards G S 1988 Intercarpal arthrodesis for static and dynamic volar intercalated segment instability. Journal of Hand Surgery 13A: 396–402

Trumble T E, Culp R, Hanel D P, Geissler W B, Berger R A 1998 Intra-articular fractures of the distal aspect of the radius. Journal of Bone and Joint Surgery 80A: 582–600

Tsuyuguchi Y, Murase T, Hidaka N, Ohno H, Kawai H 1995 Anterior wedge-shaped bone grafts for old scaphoid fractures or non-unions. Journal of Hand Surgery 20B: 194–200

Vahranen V, Westerland M 1980 Fracture of the carpal scaphoid in children. Acta Orthopaedica Scandinavica 51: 909–913

van Duyvenbode J F F H, Keijser L C M, Hauet E J, Obermann W R, Rozing P M 1991 Pseudarthrosis of the scaphoid treated by the Matti–Russe operation. Journal of Bone and Joint Surgery 73B: 603–606

van Leeuwen P A M, Reynders P A, Rommers P M, Broos P L O 1990 Operative treatment of Smith–Goyrand fractures. Injury 21: 358–360

Vance R M, Gelberman R H, Evans E F 1980 Scaphocapitate frac-tures. Journal of Bone and Joint Surgery 62A: 271–276

Vang Hansen F, Staunstrup H, Mikkelsen S 1998 A comparison of 3 and 5 weeks' immobilization for older Type 1 and 2 Colles' frac-tures. Journal of Hand Surgery 23B: 400–401

Varodompun N, Limpivest P, Prinyaroj P 1985 Isolated dorsal radio-carpal dislocation: case report and literature review. Journal of Hand Surgery 10A: 708–710

Vegter J 1987 Late reduction of the dislocated lunate. Journal of Bone and Joint Surgery 69B: 734–736

Vender M I, Watson H K, Wiener B D, Black D M 1987 Degenerative change in symptomatic scaphoid non-union. Journal of Hand Surgery 12A: 514–519

Viegas S F, Bean J W, Schram R A 1987 Trans-scaphoid fracture dis-locations treated with open reduction and Herbert screw internal fixation. Journal of Hand Surgery 12A: 992–999

Villar R N, Marsh D, Rushton N, Greatorex R A 1987 Three years after Colles' fracture. Journal of Bone and Joint Surgery 69B: 635–638

Voche P, Bour C, Merle M 1992 Scapho-trapezio-trapezoid arthrode-sis in the treatment of Kienböck's disease. Journal of Hand Surgery 17B: 5–11

Vukov V, Ristic K, Stevanovic M, Bumbasirevic 1988 Simultaneous fractures of the distal end of the radius and the scaphoid bone. Journal of Orthopaedic Trauma 2: 120–123

Wagner C J 1956 Perilunar dislocations. Journal of Bone and Joint Surgery 38A: 1198–1207

Walker J L, Greene T L, Lunseth P A 1988 Fractures of the body of the trapezium. Journal of Orthopaedic Trauma 2: 22–28

Watanabe H, Hamada Y, Yamamoto Y 1999 A case of old trapezoid fracture. Archives of Orthopaedic & Trauma Surgery 119: 356–357

Watson H K, Ballet F L 1984 The SLAC wrist: ScaphoLunate Advanced Collapse pattern of degenerative arthritis. Journal of Hand Surgery 9A: 358–365

Watson H K, Guidera P M 1997 Aetiology of Kienböck's disease. Journal of Hand Surgery 22B: 5–7

Watson H K, Monacelli D M, Milford R S, Ashmead D 1996 Treatment of Kienböck's disease with scapho-trapezio-trapezoid arthrodesis. Journal of Hand Surgery 21A: 9–15

Watson H K, Rogers W D 1989 Nonunion of the hook of the hamate: an argument for bone grafting the nonunion. Journal of Hand Surgery 14A: 486–490

Weiland A J, Saffar P, Raskin K, Mezara K 1999 Treatment of distal radial intra-articular malunions with osteotomy: Review of 30 patients. Journal of Bone and Joint Surgery 81B: supp I: 6

Weir I G C 1992 The late reduction of carpal dislocations. Journal of Hand Surgery 17B: 137–139

Weiss A-P, Weiland A J, Moore J R, Wilgis E F S 1991 Radial short-ening for Kienböck's disease. Journal of Bone and Joint Surgery 73A: 384–391

Weiss C, Laskin R S, Spinner M 1970 Irreducible trans-scaphoid perilunate dislocation. Journal of Bone and Joint Surgery 52A: 565–568

Westkaemper J G, Mitsionis G, Giannakopoulos P N, Sotereanos D G 1998 Wrist arthroscopy for the treatment of ligament and trian-gular fibrocartilage complex injuries. Arthroscopy 14: 479–483

White R E, Omer G E 1984 Transient vascular compromise of the lunate after fracture–dislocation or dislocation of the carpus. Journal of Hand Surgery 9A: 181–184

Wozasek G E, Moser K-D 1991 Percutaneous screw fixation for frac-tures of the scaphoid. Journal of Bone and Joint Surgery 73B: 138–142

Wyrick J D, Stern P J, Kiefhaber T R 1995 Motion-preserving proced-ures in the treatment of scapholunate advanced collapse wrist: proximal row carpectomy versus four-corner arthrodesis. Journal of Hand Surgery 20A: 965–970

Yamada K, Sekiya S, Oka S, Norimatsu H 1995 Lunate disloca-tion with ulnar nerve paresis. Journal of Hand Surgery 20B: 206–209

Zaidemberg C, Siebert J W, Angrigiani C 1991 A new vascularized bone graft for scaphoid nonunion. Journal of Hand Surgery 16A: 474–478

Zyluk A 1998 The natural history of post-traumatic reflex sympa-thetic dystrophy. Journal of Hand Surgery 23B: 20–23

Hand injuries

Peter Lunn and Satouro Chamberlain

▓ Introduction

In primitive times, man had to use his hands to ensure his survival and development. Manual dexterity was required in different ways to obtain food, for defence, in creative functions such as the manufacture of utensils, and in expressive functions to assist in communication with other humans. In our present, largely industrial society, our hands still serve the same functions and are still as important to us despite the engineering and technological advances that have been made. It might even be argued that, as the 'machine' has appeared to become an increasingly important member of our society, man feels even more strongly the need to be able to control his personal contact with his environment in order to retain his own sense of value to the community. A hand injury, or debilitating hand disorder, with resulting loss of manual dexterity, is therefore a distressing event in anyone's life; it raises the question—am I able still to fulfil a useful function in society, or am I like the wounded animal that trails at the back of the herd and may eventually be left behind?

Hand injuries are a common cause of time off work and, for different reasons, cause great concern to employers as well as employees. In the Derby audit in 1990 (Burke 1990) the incidence of hand injuries was noted to be 475/100 000 population, and of these 22% occurred at work. If this figure is converted to apply to the country as a whole it amounts to an incidence of 9500 hand injuries at work in the UK per year. In addition, there will be others who develop work-related conditions in the hand such as tenosynovitis, triggering of the flexor tendons and other similar conditions.

The Health and Safety Executive (HSE) statistics show that there are 18 million working days lost per year in the UK because of industrial accidents (HSE 1994). Upper limb injuries are easily the largest category of injuries responsible for time off work for 3 days or more in the manufacturing industries; more than twice as much as back and neck injuries. The cost involved amounts to the equivalent of approximately 10% of all the UK companies' trading profits. It is estimated that 70% of industrial accidents are preventable.

These work injuries will therefore have a number of far-reaching effects which extend beyond the medical aspects of the treatment and rehabilitation. There will be financial consequences directly affecting the patient in terms of possible lost wages and these could also have secondary effects on the family and dependents. The employer will also be affected financially by the initial injury and also by any subsequent insurance claim or litigation; a secondary effect of this may be to change the relationship between the employer and the employee, depending on the circumstances of the accident. This inevitably results in effects on workforce morale generally and is very much influenced by the culture in which we live. In Hong Kong, there is still a tradition of preserving harmony in personal relationships ('kuan hsi') which, in many instances, has the result of influencing the worker away from litigation in order to avoid harming relationships with the employer (Cheng YH 1997). In the USA, conversely, litigation is considered to be very much a normal part of life, and indeed possibly a measure of 'human rights'. It is helpful to have an overview of our own social situation in the UK so that we can see the true context of the litigation system and, in particular, the function of the Medical Report within that.

The medical report has an important role in the compensation process and the subsequent rehabilitation. The mechanism of injury, the level of disability, and the relationship of the two are important aspects of the medical report of any hand injury. In clinical work we aim to make sure that the treatment is appropriate to the disease or injury; in medical reports we need to ensure that there is a logical relationship between the mechanism of injury, the resulting disability and the claims by the plaintiff and defendant.

Formulation of the medical report

The Woolf Report (1995) has resulted in changes in the structure of medical reports generally, but there are a number of specific points which are worth emphasising in relation to the way in which medicolegal reporting of a hand injury is carried out.

1. *Patient's details*. These should include occupation and hand dominance.
2. *History*. It is important to know the mechanism of injury. For example, if the hand was 'injured in a machine' it is necessary to know whether it was a sharp, blunt or crush injury, and whether or not there was any heat or other

component to the injury. The details of treatment need to be outlined, including any physiotherapy or occupational therapy. Time off work should be recorded, and whether the patient returned to normal or light duties.

3. *The present situation*. This should include present symptoms and how they affect activity at work and at home.

4. *Clinical examination*. Concise findings of the examination of the injured part must be expressed in such a way that both solicitors and other medical experts can understand. Normal findings, where relevant, are also useful. Specific measurements can be helpful, but some measurements such as grip strength can be positively misleading if a standard 'grip meter' is used. This measurement will record only what the patient wishes to convey as his grip strength; it is much more effective for the examiner to make his own assessment of strength on clinical grounds. (New devices are being developed with a view to obtaining objective measurements of grip strength, but are not generally available yet.) Diagrams and photographs are an effective means of demonstrating many of the physical findings.

5. *Investigations*. X-rays are frequently of value and may be used to describe the nature of the bony injury and any soft tissue swelling. They can also often demonstrate some pre-existing changes which may be relevant in relation to both the present state of the patient and the possibility of future deterioration.

6. *Opinion and prognosis*. This is one of the main reasons why the solicitor requests the report, so it is important to commit oneself and give positive views, with percentages to indicate the degree of disability. It may also be necessary to give an opinion on the mechanism of injury (there is sometimes inconsistency between the type of injury and the level of the resulting disability), the response to treatment, and the length of time off work. It is reasonable in some instances to comment on the patient's level of motivation, bearing in mind the words of Seneca (4 BC—65 AD): 'It is part of the cure to wish to be cured.' Sometimes this desire for a cure is tempered by a desire for recompense which can significantly alter the natural history of the healing process. Long-term disability and any anticipated future complication should be included in this section.

■ Soft Tissue Injuries

Skin

The skin on both the palmar and dorsal aspects of the hand is very specialised. Palmar skin is thick, has attachments to the underlying fascia and has a very intricate nerve supply; the dorsal skin is thin, very elastic and freely mobile in relation to the underlying soft tissues. Wounds on the palm heal well but may result in loss of normal skin texture, which is vital for accurate sensation and gripping ability; palmar skin loss is difficult to replace as any form of skin graft or even a skin flap will not reproduce the normal combination of skin stability and flexibility. Scarring on the back of the hand frequently causes adhesions and restriction of gliding of the extensor tendons. Skin grafting (if the fascia and epitenon are intact) is effective, or skin flap cover for deeper soft tissue loss can result in better functional recovery than on the palmar surface of the hand.

Injuries to the skin may be either clean or contaminated, and either sharp or crushing in nature. A contaminated wound will not only require more intensive and prolonged treatment and therefore more time off work, but it is also more likely to result in a greater degree of scarring and fibrosis. There is therefore a higher risk of the development of an unsatisfactory result after such an injury, and this can be reflected in a greater functional deficit. Similarly, a crushing injury carries a greater risk of complications than a sharp injury. It is important therefore to include these factors in both the history and the prognosis of a hand injury.

The cosmetic appearance of the hand is also an important consideration in that scarring or deformity does constitute a significant disability which may sometimes be overlooked. The hand is certainly important cosmetically because it is used in a tactile manner when shaking hands and greeting someone, but it is also used expressively when speaking and any deformity is often noticeable and may cause embarrassment.

Prognosis

The two main problems that may occur after skin injuries are as follows:

- *Scar contracture*. This is likely to develop if a longitudinal scar extends across a flexor crease, and is especially a problem in burns and crush injuries. In severe cases the contracture will appear early (in a few weeks or months) but in less severe cases it may be several years before a contracture develops.

- *Cosmetic disability*. The 'immature' scar tissue is frequently discoloured and therefore may be much more unsightly than at a year or so after the injury. On the other hand, 'mature' scars (9–12 months after injury) on extensor surfaces of joints (especially the elbow) can stretch and become unsightly.

Finger-tip injuries

The skin of the finger-tip is very specialised in many ways and an injury will inevitably result in some impairment of these specialised functions.

Impairment of sensation

The finger-tip is a very precise sensory organ allowing precise, detailed appreciation of light touch, proprioception, temperature, two-point discrimination and deep pain. Because of the many nerve endings in the finger pulp an injury may result in a variety of different impairments. Most commonly there is some reduction of the normal detailed localisation of sensation giving, at the worst, an area of numbness or, at the best, an area of vague, indistinct sensation or tingling.

A more difficult problem occurs if there is an injury to one of the larger branches or nerve trunks causing a neuroma. This will result in an acutely sensitive area directly over the neuroma with impaired sensation more distally. Sometimes the effect of a neuroma is to cause extreme pain which prevents any useful function in the whole finger or even marked impairment throughout the hand because of the fear of anything touching the sensitive area of the neuroma. This functional inhibition can often be modified and reduced considerably if treated early by desensitisation therapy. These techniques are practised by hand therapists who are specially trained to recognise and treat patients who may be prone to develop pain syndromes following hand injuries.

Cold sensitivity

Any injury to the finger-tip, but especially crushing injuries, can result in some degree of cold intolerance due to effects on the control of the blood-flow in the small vessels at the periphery, normally involved in temperature control. The fingers affected will be prone to become numb and go white or blue in cold conditions, often accompanied by some discomfort; they will then take a long time to warm up when the patient returns to warm conditions and may again have painful tingling as the circulation returns the temperature of the finger-tip to normal.

The effects of cold intolerance are worst soon after the injury but tend to improve and diminish for a period of about 3 years, and, although it used to be thought they would resolve completely, it seems that in more serious crushing injuries cold intolerance continues, to some extent, permanently.

Pulp scarring

The skin of the finger-tip has subcutaneous fat which provides 'padding' from the underlying bone. There are also fine fascial strands which limit the mobility of the skin so that it allows precise positioning and grasping of small objects. (The skin on the back of the hand, conversely, is very mobile on the subcutaneous tissues.) The slight mobility of the skin on the pulp and the underlying padding together allow the soft tissues to conform to the shape of objects that are being held and therefore allow very precise manipulation. (This can be seen by observing the indentations that occur in the pulps of the thumb and index fingers after holding a pen.)

Injury and scarring of the pulp of the finger-tip may therefore result in some loss of the normal fatty padding, which will cause some discomfort when gripping objects. There will also be some loss of manual dexterity for manipulation of small objects due to the loss of the normal texture of the skin and its attachments to the underlying tissues.

Finger-nail injuries

The finger-nail serves a number of useful functions quite apart from its cosmetic effect on the general appearance of the hand. The two main functions of the nail are, first, to form an external support for the pulp of the finger beyond the end of the distal phalanx, and, secondly, to allow 'nail-to-nail' grasping of very small objects as when picking up a needle.

Injuries to the nail can cause scarring of the nail-bed with resulting ridging, splitting or other deformity of the nail. Sometimes these can cause considerable discomfort if the free edge of the nail is curled over the finger-tip and gets caught in objects which are being handled, or if the distal nail-bed is exposed it can be very sensitive when gripping or grasping objects.

Nerve injury

Any injury to a nerve, other than a mild neuropraxia, will lead to some permanent impairment in an adult. The most common injury is a crush of the cutaneous nerves at the fingertip, which may cause some degree of hypersensitivity to light touch, and may cause the patient to neglect this finger and transfer normal functions to an adjacent finger. This problem can often be alleviated by appropriate 'desensitisation' therapy which, although not curing the underlying hypersensitivity, may well enable the patient to retain the function of the affected finger for most tasks.

A partial or complete laceration of a nerve trunk will usually be explored and repaired surgically. The recovery of nerve function will depend mainly on the type of nerve injured; a 'pure' nerve such as a digital nerve, which contains only sensory fibres, will have the best result; while a 'mixed' nerve, such as the median or ulnar nerve, will have a significantly poorer result. The type of injury will also affect the outcome, so that a clean, sharp laceration will favour a good result, whereas a contaminated crush injury is likely to result in poor recovery of the nerve.

Results

As a rough guide, it is reasonable to advise that the *best* possible outcome from a nerve injury (such as a sharp laceration to a digital nerve which is repaired under magnification as a primary procedure) can be expected to give only about 80% return of nerve function. In the case of a digital nerve this will mean that a very small area of the fingertip will have diminished sensation, and because of 'overlap' from the adjacent digital nerve the overall disability will be slight. However, the ulnar side of the thumbtip and the radial side of the index finger and middle finger are the areas which will be associated with significant disability if there is impairment of sensation, because these are the most important sensory areas of the hand.

A study of 108 digital nerve injuries (Chow & Ng 1993a) showed that if no repair was carried out there would be some improvement in sensation for a period of 3–6 months only, and the end-result would be inferior to repaired nerves. Sensibility in repaired nerves would continue to improve for up to 2 years; using the MRC grading (Medical Research Council 1954; see Table 10.1), 90% of the study group achieved a recovery of S3+ or S4 (SO is no sensation, S4 is normal sensation). In the group of patients in whom the nerves were not repaired, only 6% achieved this level of recovery.

Division of the median nerve is more disabling than of the ulnar nerve because it is the major sensory nerve to the hand. The level of disability can be assessed in various ways. It can be calculated roughly by assessing it as half the disability of the amputation of that part of the hand (Fig. 10.1), or it can be assessed more accurately using the chart devised by the American Academy of Orthopedic Surgeons and modified by Rank et al (1973) (Fig. 10.2).

The actual percentage disability rating will depend on the opinion of the examining doctor, who may well adjust the figure slightly in order to take into account the requirements of the individual patient. For example, a bricklayer who has cold intolerance following a crush injury of the fingers will be considerably more disabled by this problem than a managing director or solicitor.

It is important to have some idea of what is involved in a patient's occupation or hobbies, because this will obvious-

Table 10.1 The MRC grading of nerve injuries (after Medical Research Centre 1954)

Motor Recovery

M0	No constraction
M1	Return of perceptible contraction in the proximal muscles
M2	Return of perceptible contraction in both proximal and distal muscles
M3	Return of function in both proximal and distal muscles of such degree that all *important* muscles are sufficiently powerful to act against resistance
M4	Return of function as in stage 3, with the addition that all synergistic and independent movements are possible
M5	Complete recovery

Sensory recovery

S0	Absence of sensibility in the autonomous area
S1	Recovery of deep cutaneous pain sensibility within the *autonomous* area of the nerve
S2	Return of some degree of superficial cutaneous pain and tactile sensibility within the autonomous area of the nerve
S3	Return of superficial cutaneous pain and tactile sensibility throughout the autonomous area, with disappearance of any previous over-reaction
S3+	Return of sensibility as in stage 3, with the additional that there is some recovery of two-point discrimination within the autonomous area
S4	Complete recovery

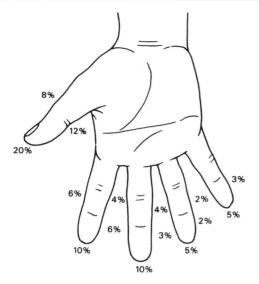

Fig. 10.1 Sensory impairment: relative value to the whole hand for total sensory loss of digit and comparative loss of radial and ulnar sides. Sensory loss is calculated at 50% that of amputation (from Swanson et al 1987, with permission).

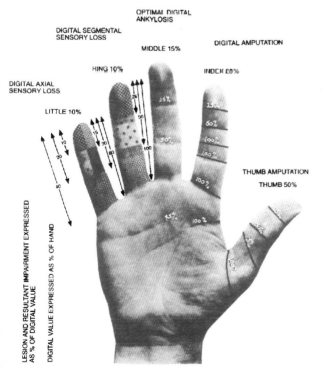

Fig. 10.2 A schematic illustration of working basis for estimating the order of residual disability after hand injuries (from Rank et al 1973, with permission).

ly affect his level of disability. For example, a right-handed violinist will be more disabled by injury to his *left* hand, because this is the one that requires a greater degree of dexterity and accurate sensation when playing the violin.

Assessment of the outcome following nerve injury should involve functional evaluation as well as the normal tests of sensory and motor function. It has been demonstrated that, despite the importance of sensation in the hand, the tests of sensibility do not predict accurately the patients' ability to use their hands in everyday activities (Jerosch-Herold 1993); measurement of performance in selected activities of daily living (ADI) is a better indication of function than assessment of two-point discrimination (Marsh 1990).

Prognosis

The following factors need to be taken into account when assessing the long-term results of nerve injuries:

- *Age.* In patients under 10 years of age nerve recovery is good, but the results become progressively worse with increasing age and the results after 50 are poor.
- *Time.* Full recovery may take 6–9 months in a digital nerve and twice as long in the median or ulnar nerves at the wrist.
- *Neuroma.* Most nerve repairs are tender locally when knocked or palpated. However, the clinical diagnosis of a neuroma is made only when there are the following symptoms and signs: swelling, pain (often constant but made worse by local pressure on the neuroma), distal paraesthesiae on percussion over the neuroma and loss of function (sometimes the function of the whole hand is impaired by a small fingertip neuroma).
- *Cold intolerance.* This can occur after any peripheral nerve injury, but is most marked after a crush injury. The symptoms are worst in the first year and tend to improve for about 3 years but are unlikely to disappear completely. The condition will not worsen and no serious long-term complications have been reported.

Marsh has also shown that a delay between the time of injury and the time of nerve repair is associated with a poor result (Marsh 1990). He does not specify what length of delay is acceptable, but it appears that primary repair can be carried out successfully up to about 10–14 days from the time of injury.

Nerve compression syndromes

Carpal tunnel syndrome is the most common compression neuropathy in the hand, although entrapment of the ulnar nerve in Guyon's canal is also seen and can be associated with an occupational cause. From the medicolegal point of view, the main difficulty arises when dealing with the possible cause of a nerve compression syndrome, particularly in carpal tunnel syndrome. It is well known that this condition occurs very frequently in the general population, often without any known cause; it is also recognised that the following are aetiological factors which may be associated with carpal tunnel syndrome (Leach & Udom 1968; Bleecker 1987):

- Decreased cross-sectional area of carpal tunnel, e.g. rheumatoid arthritis, trauma (wrist fracture), constitutional etc. The MRI scan allows such measurements to be made (Cobb et al 1992).
- Increased volume of the contents of the carpal canal, e.g. flexor tenosynovitis, fluid retention (especially associated with hormonal abnormalities such as pregnancy, menopause, diabetes, thyroid disorders, acromegaly etc.).
- Enlargement of the median nerve (rare cause).

The medical expert has to decide whether the carpal tunnel syndrome has developed as a direct result of the patient's occupation or whether other aetiological factors are involved. The overall incidence of carpal tunnel syndrome is highest in females (a ratio of more than 2:1 female:male) between the ages of 40 and 60 years, and if a patient is in this category, or has one of the predisposing causes listed above, it will be necessary to make a judgement of the relative importance of these factors and the type of work with regard to the development of the nerve compression.

The relationship between manual work and the development of carpal tunnel syndrome has still not been clearly established. Some authors feel that there is a link, and this is related to the repetitive nature of the work rather than to the force applied through the hand (Silverstein 1985); other authors have carried out large studies which do *not* show a direct link between work and carpal tunnel syndrome (Nathan et al 1992). This is never easy. However, it may at least be helpful to give an assessment of the likelihood of the patient developing carpal tunnel syndrome, even if he had not been involved in this work: is it greater or less than 50%, for instance? This will be a useful basis for discussions to take place with regard to the level of 'blame' that can be attributed to an employer insofar as he is responsible for the nature of the work in which his employees are involved.

Compression of the ulnar nerve in Guyon's canal is much less common and is a much less contentious issue; it more commonly has a direct relationship to local trauma on the ulnar side of the hand ('hypothenar hammer syndrome' etc.).

Results

Surgical decompression of the carpal tunnel gives good relief of symptoms when the compression has been present for only 6 months or less (Semple & Cargill 1969). Where is a longer history, and where there is an 'occupational' aetiology, the results are not so predictable. In 'occupational' carpal tunnel syndrome some authorities therefore advocate alteration of the working conditions and a trial of conservative measures such as splintage and steroid injection as a first line of management (Eversmann 1988).

Similarly, the results of ulnar nerve decompression are good if there is only a short history, but are less satisfactory if the compression has been present for over 6–12 months.

Prognosis

The factors associated with *poor* recovery following nerve compression are as follows:

- A long history.
- Age—the older the patient is, the longer the recovery period will be, and the lower the chance will be of full recovery.
- Systemic abnormalities, e.g. diabetes.

Carpal tunnel syndrome

This is a common condition characterised by compression of the Median nerve at the wrist. It occurs more commonly in women than in men, but there is considerable variation in the range of frequency in studies in the medical literature, which quotes rates of 1.4 times (Atroshi 1999) to 5 times (de Krom 1990). It occurs most commonly in the fourth and fifth decades of life, particularly in times of major hormonal changes during pregnancy and at the menopause. The history and clinical features of carpal tunnel syndrome are very characteristic of this condition and it is acknowledged that in the majority of patients symptoms can be temporarily relieved or eased by night splints and cortisone injections, but that surgical decompression of the carpal tunnel usually gives not only quite rapid but also lasting relief.

Carpal tunnel syndrome occurs commonly in the adult population with an incidence varying from 51 to 346 per 100 000 population per year in hospital studies (Burke 2000), whereas a study of a random sample of 3000 adults in Sweden (Atroshi 1999) showed that approximately 3% were suffering from carpal tunnel syndrome diagnosed by both clinical examination and electrophysiological testing. This study also revealed that 14% of the population had experienced some transient symptoms in the median nerve distribution at least twice weekly during the preceding 4 weeks, although the majority of these did not fulfil the clinical and neurophysiological criteria for carpal tunnel syndrome.

The relationship between carpal tunnel syndrome and work-related activities is still indistinct and needs clarification. It seems there are three main theories about the possible mechanism of the causation of carpal tunnel syndrome as a result of work.

Flexor tenosynovitis

It is suggested that frequent, repetitive, forceful movements of the flexor tendons may cause the development of inflammatory changes in the surrounding synovium and the resulting swelling leads to secondary compression of the median nerve in the carpal tunnel. This seems reasonable as a theory but is not borne out in clinical practice. Patients in this situation rarely have the typical clinical signs of flexor synovitis, nor do the symptoms seem to improve when they are rested; sometimes the symptoms actually progress when the patient stops work.

Changes in the carpal ligament

Repeated movement of the flexor tendons causes changes in the carpal ligament with resulting compression of the median nerve. It would be expected that if this were the case, surgical release of the carpal ligament (carpal tunnel decompression) should result in resolution of the symptoms but it is acknowledged that the results of surgery are less successful in work-related carpal tunnel syndrome (Terrono 1996). It has been shown that there is an increased risk of carpal tunnel syndrome in patients with vibration white finger and it may be that this is due to a combination of the physical effects of vibration both on the carpal ligament and on the median nerve itself (Boyle 1988).

Changes in the median nerve

There have been interesting observations made on the mobility of various nerves and especially the median nerve in the carpal tunnel as this is a site of particular mobility, the nerve gliding approximately 1.5 cm during wrist movements. It is reasonable to hypothesise that there may be an element of 'friction' neuritis as a result of these movements, while others have postulated tethering of the nerve and 'adverse neural tension'.

It has to be accepted that carpal tunnel syndrome does develop in people of working age (but so does baldness in men and fibroids in women), and although there may be instances when the work activities are responsible for causing the condition, frequently the onset is related primarily to constitutional factors—or sometimes the work may simply accelerate the onset of the condition. There are several conditions which have been implicated as possibly having an association with carpal tunnel syndrome and a number of studies have been carried out to look at objective evidence for this (de Krom 1990; Nathan et al 1994; Szabo 1998; Szabo & King 2000). The factors which studies have shown to increase the risk of carpal tunnel syndrome are:

- Obesity
- Rheumatoid arthritis
- Pregnancy
- Menopause

Possible associations (yet to be proven) with carpal tunnel syndrome are:

- Activities with extremes of wrist motion
- High repetition, high force activities

Other factors thought to be associated with an increased risk are:

- Hysterectomy
- Thyroid disease
- Diabetes
- Varicose veins (in men)

One of the main problems with the 'overuse' concept as a cause of many hand and upper limb conditions, including carpal tunnel syndrome, is that there is, as yet, no effective definition of 'normal' use, let alone a definition of *over*use. The concept, therefore, remains very much in the field of hypothesis at present.

In order to make a case for an occupational cause the following criteria need to be established:

- Patients involved in a particular working practice develop carpal tunnel syndrome with a greater frequency than would be expected in the general population.
- The work has characteristics which are likely to cause pressure on the median nerve by either direct or indirect means. Direct would be pressure over the carpal tunnel, indirect would be secondary to conditions that might cause swelling or increased pressure in the carpal tunnel such as flexor tenosynovitis.
- Removal of the provocative stimulus results in an improvement in the symptoms.
- The patients respond to the normal treatment measures.

Tendons

Flexor tendon injuries are a well-recognised source of problems in both the short and the long term. In the acute stage, the tendon injury may be missed, but if it is treated it should give a satisfactory result; the exception to this is an injury in zone 2, which has a universally poor outlook (Fig. 10.3, showing zones of tendon injury in the hand).

Extensor tendon injuries are generally easier to treat, heal quicker and have fewer complications than injuries involving flexor tendons. However, the main functional problem which can result is a loss of flexion due to tenodesis of the extensor tendon, which hinders gliding. If there is a loss of full extension of a finger this is unlikely to cause much functional deficit unless the extension loss is more than about 45°.

It is important to ascertain the mechanism of injury (i.e. sharp, crush, associated injuries etc.), as this will have a significant bearing on the ultimate result.

Mallet finger

This is a relatively common injury, usually caused by axial loading of the finger with forced flexion of the distal interphalangeal joint. The majority are closed injuries which can be treated with splintage for 6 weeks; open injuries are likely to require surgical repair of the extensor tendon.

There is a significant incidence of minor complications with splintage, mainly due to skin problems, but there is also often some loss of movement (Stern & Kastrup 1988). This series of 123 patients, who were treated by either splintage or surgery, showed that there is commonly an extension lag, which may be anything up to 40°, and that flexion can also be limited following treatment with a splint. There was a higher incidence of complications and greater restriction of flexion after surgical treatment.

Results

With regard to **flexor tendons**, as with any specialised surgery, the results depend on a number of factors, including the type of injury, the timing of repair (primary repair within 1 week of injury appears to give better results), associated injuries and, in particular, the site of injury; the rehabilitation technique may well also influence the end-result significantly (Duran & Houser 1975). The results of flexor tendon repair in zone 2 are predictably worse than at other sites (Amadio & Hunter 1987). Strickland's review of the results of flexor tendon repairs is probably the best analysis of this subject (Strickland & Glogovac 1987) and shows that the best results achieved in zone 2 in the published series are excellent or good in 65 to 80%. These results are from highly specialised units, and therefore it is not unreasonable to suggest that the best results

expected in zone 2 repairs from an 'average' treatment centre such as a district general hospital may well be nearer 50% satisfactory results.

A flexor tendon injury can result in several weeks or months of treatment involving time off work and, in the worst cases (especially zone 2 injuries), there may be significant long-term disability mainly in terms of loss of active movement of the digits involved. This can result in some loss of manual dexterity and also reduced grip strength; approximately a loss of 25% of grip strength according to Gault in a study of 67 patients with 176 repaired flexor tendons (Gault 1987).

Rehabilitation following a flexor tendon repair is always a delicate balancing-act aiming to recover as much active motion and gliding of the tendon without sustaining a rupture or dehiscence of the tendon repair. Insufficient mobilisation will result in adhesions forming, thereby preventing gliding of the tendon, whereas early active motion may result in tendon rupture. Following flexor tendon repairs, especially in zone 2, there are recorded rupture rates of approximately 5 to 10% in the finger flexors, and a higher rate up to 16% in the flexor pollicis longus tendon of the thumb (Small et al 1989; Elliot et al 1994).

If the rehabilitation is complicated by tendon adhesions and loss of active 'pull-through', tenolysis may be indicated; this is most effective once the soft tissues have stabilised, ideally at least 3–6 months after the primary surgery. Any other complicating factors such as joint stiffness or infection are contraindications to tenolysis and

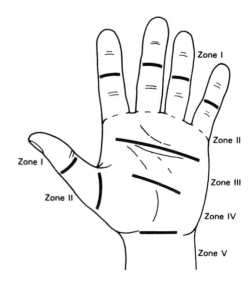

Fig. 10.3 Zone classification of flexor injuries (from Leddy 1988, with permission).

would need to be resolved before surgery of this type can be embarked upon.

With regard to **extensor tendons**, their repair results in a satisfactory outcome in the majority of cases. It is important to test flexion as well as extension in order to ensure that there is no tenodesis which is limiting flexion.

Prognosis

Following primary tendon repair, the long-term result can usually be assessed at 9–12 months post injury. If tenolysis is indicated it is normally carried out between 3 and 9 months after the primary repair (Strickland 1987). If the repair fails and the tendon ruptures this can be treated either by direct secondary repair or by tendon grafting. There is unlikely to be any significant alteration in the clinical situation in the long term once a 'steady state' has been reached.

Tenosynovitis

This diagnosis is made very commonly by doctors for almost any hand or wrist pain even though the main symptoms and physical signs are not present. It is frequently included by the general practitioner in the patient's medical records, and there is often also some comment about the condition being related to work. Unfortunately, this frequently causes significant problems later on because medical experts and lawyers have to argue about the basis for these observations and whether in fact there is any evidence to support either the diagnosis or the relationship of the symptoms to working practices and activities.

The term, 'tenosynovitis', is itself misleading because the condition does not, as was first thought, develop due to inflammation, although some of the secondary effects are associated with the presence of some inflammatory cells. However, the clinical features are quite specific and are as follows:

- Pain over the affected tendon(s), particularly when the tendon is stressed against resistance
- Swelling over the affected tendon(s)
- Inflammation of the skin and overlying soft tissues
- Crepitus with movement of the affected tendon(s).

Natural history

The symptoms of tenosynovitis are exacerbated by any activity which causes the affected tendon(s) to work against resistance, or, in the worst cases, the pain can occur with movement of the tendon alone, regardless of whether or not there is any resistance. Similarly, rest is one of the mainstays of treatment and, in the majority of cases, will allow the symptoms and signs to settle. The condition may recur on returning to manual activities but the risk of this can be reduced by the following:

- ensuring adequate rest (usually a period of approximately 2 weeks is sufficient to allow the changes to settle)
- sometimes, using a splint in the short term, which may be helpful in ensuring that the affected tendon is adequately rested and protected
- modifying activities
- taking anti-inflammatory medication
- steroid injections, which are helpful both diagnostically and therapeutically.

Outcome

In general clinical practice it is unusual to see long-term effects of tenosynovitis unless there is a systemic inflammatory cause such as rheumatoid arthritis; certainly, serious disability or long-term complications are *not* typical features of this condition. In medicolegal reporting it is not uncommon to see patients who are supposedly suffering from tenosynovitis but give a completely different clinical picture. In particular, patients often complain that the symptoms persist or even deteriorate when they stop work; this would seem, by definition, to exclude a diagnosis of tenosynovitis and would suggest that an alternative diagnosis should be made.

Amputations

Although a generalisation, the hand can be regarded from the functional point of view as being made up of two main parts: the 'sensory' side, which consists of the thumb, index and middle fingers (the radial side); and the 'power' side, which consists of the ring and little fingers (the ulnar side).

An amputation on the radial side of the hand will therefore result mainly in impairment of sensation and fine, delicate activities. An amputation on the ulnar side of the hand has its main effect in causing impairment of power grip.

Values of the functional loss following amputation, as a percentage of the function of the hand as a whole, are given in Fig. 10.2. Loss of length of the digit is not directly related to the functional deficit, so that amputation at the level of the distal interphalangeal joint (a loss of about one-quarter of the length of the finger) results in about 50% loss of function of that digit. Similarly, amputation at the proximal interphalangeal joint level results in a 90 to 100% loss of function in that digit.

Results

The level of disability following an amputation of part or all of a digit must not be based solely on the level of amputation, but should also take into account other factors which may warrant an increase in the percentage of disability.

Sensory changes, such as numbness or hypersensitivity, will impair function, and cold intolerance is almost invariable—this is particularly disabling in people who work out of doors in all weathers.

A deformity of the fingernail can affect the function of a finger, either because the nail 'curls over' a shortened finger pulp or because a small spicule of nail remains following incomplete excision of the nail bed. This can be a painful situation, as the nail remnant gets caught on objects and can be torn or develop secondary infection.

Prognosis

The amputation stump of a finger has usually healed fully and reached a stable state by about 3–6 months post injury. If revision of the stump is required, this is normally carried out during this time. The other surgical measures which may be required in the long term are excision of nail remnant and nail bed, excision or burying of a neuroma or, in some patients, complete revision by 'ray' amputation. This is indicated in patients who have the 'gap hand' with complete amputation of the middle or ring fingers, leaving a gap which is not only cosmetically unsatisfactory but which can also cause functional difficulties due to small objects falling out of the hand through the gap left by the amputated finger. The narrowing of the hand from ray amputation is associated with some decrease in the grip strength and is therefore less likely to be of benefit in a manual labourer than in someone involved in a sedentary occupation.

Other long-term complications are uncommon, but the basic disability will obviously be permanent.

Less Common Conditions

Burns

Sykes (1991) has written a comprehensive review article on severe burns of the hand, including descriptions of the different types of burn which are commonly sustained, the treatment measures which are appropriate and possible complications which may develop.

The history is of great importance, as the results and prognosis will vary considerably depending on whether the injury was caused by a simple scald from boiling water, for instance, or an electrical burn—the latter injury having a very much worse prognosis. 'Combination' injuries such as the crush and burn from heated presses or rollers also have a poor prognosis.

Results

The cosmetic and functional aspects of the injury should both be assessed. Cosmetic disability will depend on the site and extent of scarring as well as any secondary deformities such as joint contractures. The functional deficit will be related to the skin texture and sensitivity, as well as joint and tendon mobility with any resulting loss of motion.

Prognosis

A skin graft may take a year or more to 'mature'. The following complications may occur in the long term:

- Contracture, which can cause secondary joint deformities and may require further surgery in the form of further skin cover or Z-plasty
- Splitting or fissuring of the grafted area, particularly in cold conditions. This mainly affects those involved in heavy manual work out of doors, and may necessitate the use of protective gloves or, in severe cases, surgical revision of the graft by using a skin flap.

Injection injuries

High-pressure guns are used widely in industry and can cause severe injury due to penetration of the hand by fluids under pressure. Lubricants, paints, hydraulic solutions, animal vaccines and other fluids may be accidentally injected subcutaneously, causing widespread toxic effects to the surrounding tissues.

Results

Intense pain is the main presenting symptom, often without much to see on clinical examination except a very small puncture wound at the entry site: therefore, the seriousness of the condition is often not recognised initially by inexperienced medical staff. Progressive damage occurs due to a combination of the compartment syndrome caused by the high pressure in the finger and the toxic effects of the chemical on the soft tissues.

Stiffness is the main problem after these injuries because of the widespread fibrosis. However, this should be minimised by early surgical exploration, thorough lavage and debridement. Infection is often an early complication which can additionally increase the fibrotic response and will also delay mobilisation of the hand. Frequently, it is necessary to use an 'open wound' technique, with either delayed primary closure or healing by secondary intention.

Most patients will require an intensive course of rehabilitation therapy before returning to work.

Amputation of the affected digit is reported in 16 to 48% of cases in the literature (Ramos et al 1970; Schoo et al 1980).

Prognosis

Lewis (1985) indicates that the outcome after a high-pressure injection injury is dependent on the following factors:

- The type of material injected: oil-based solvents have a particularly poor prognosis, as do some of the vaccines used by animal workers
- The amount of material injected
- Infection
- The time interval between injury and definitive surgery.

If the condition has been recognised and treated early, the patient may gradually regain full function in a matter of some weeks depending on the severity of the injury. Pinto et al (1993) have reported the results of 25 patients treated by an aggressive open-wound technique. Their results are some of the best in the literature: they have a 16% amputation rate and 64% of patients regained virtually normal hand function at an average follow-up of 10 months. All of the patients had a flexion lag (loss of full active flexion) and in nine cases this amounted to a lag of more than 2.5 cm; nevertheless, 92% returned to their previous jobs. Those cases in which the treatment has been delayed are likely to develop marked stiffness of the affected finger(s) and, in some cases, if only one finger is involved and the disability is severe, amputation may be necessary to improve the function of the hand.

The clinical state of the hand has usually stabilised within 6–9 months of the injury and further deterioration would not be expected after that time.

Vibration white finger

This condition was recognised as an occupational disease by the Department of Health and Social Security in the UK in 1985. It was originally described in forestry workers who had used chain saws for many years, but it has also subsequently been described in other workers, including rock-drill operators and foundry workers. In the foundries it is the fettlers who are particularly at risk, as they are constantly exposed to vibration through the use of powered grinding wheels to smooth down rough iron castings.

Results

The Taylor & Pelmear classification is at present accepted as the best means of recording the severity or staging of this condition (Taylor & Pelmear 1975). The assessment is based on the patient's symptoms, as there are as yet no reliable objective criteria which can be used for staging, although a number of investigations have been studied with this in mind. These include finger plethysmography, finger systolic pressure measurement, cold provocation tests and infra-red thermography, but none of these has as yet been found to be suitable for routine grading of this condition.

Prognosis

The natural history of this syndrome is not yet clearly known, but it certainly appears that continued exposure to vibration results in progressive vasospastic symptoms over many years. What is uncertain is whether there is an early stage at which the symptoms are reversible, nor whether—in the worst cases—the condition can progress despite avoidance of the use of vibrating tools.

Cold conditions provoke symptoms, so that affected patients may have to avoid working outside in winter or else wear gloves to try and minimise the effects.

There have been no reports of serious vascular complications, such as tissue necrosis or gangrenous changes, occurring in affected digits, but compression of the median nerve at the wrist has been described in 30 to 60% of the reported series (Boyle et al 1988). Cystic changes in the carpal bones have been noted on X-rays of patients in some series, but there is some contention as to whether these are directly associated with the vibration or whether they are simply related to the age of the patients and the heavy manual work in which they are involved.

Dupuytren's disease

This condition is so common, particularly in men, that it is not surprising that many workers feel that it must, in some way, be related to the nature of their work; this applies both to manual and sedentary workers who may associate the development of the condition either to the way in which they have to use their hands for their normal work, or else to an injury which they have sustained during their work.

It is well known that there are genetic factors in Dupuytren's disease (Ling 1963). Racial and geographical factors, associations with other diseases (such as diabetes, epilepsy and alcoholism) and also structural changes in the collagen in these patients. McFarlane (1991), who is an acknowledged researcher and an expert in this field, has studied all the different factors involved and concludes that 'there is not sufficient evidence from epidemiologic studies to state that manual work either hastens the onset of Dupuytren's disease or the progression of existing disease'. He does also conclude, however, that an injury may precipitate the onset of the disease in someone who is 'genetically susceptible'. It is unusual for the disease to develop in a man before the age of 40 or in a woman before the age of 50 unless they have a strong predisposition to the condition, and this can usually be determined if they have a family history of Dupuytren's disease, bilateral hand involvement or other manifestations (such as knuckle pads, plantar nodules or Peyronie's disease). Onset before these ages without this evidence of the Dupuytren's diathesis would suggest that the condition has possibly been precipitated (but not necessarily caused) by some other factor, such as an injury.

Disability Rating

Disability is a relative term depending on the nature of the injury, but more importantly the nature of the patient, the level of motivation and other factors which determine why some patients have more disability than others following a similar type of injury.

There seems to be no doubt from the American experience that patients who are involved in litigation ('worker's compensation' cases) do not have such a good result as those for whom there is no litigation involved. Conversely, in other countries there may be social factors which lead patients to cope with their disability in a different way. In Hong Kong, there is still a tradition of preserving harmony in personal relationships ('kuan hsi') which, in many instances, mitigates against the likelihood of a worker suing an employer for negligence (Cheng 1997).

Occupational Arm Pain (Symptoms without signs)

There are a significant number of patients who present for medical reports with upper limb symptoms allegedly caused by the nature of the work in which they are involved. In many patients it is possible to make a definite diagnosis of a common upper limb condition such as carpal tunnel syndrome or tenosynovitis and the main problem is then to decide whether this has developed directly as a result of the work activities, is it partially attributable, or is it completely unrelated?

A more complex situation arises when a patient has upper limb symptoms but no signs. Is it reasonable to

make a decision about the diagnosis, possible treatment measures and prognosis based purely on the history alone? It could be argued that in normal clinical practice a diagnosis of a condition such as carpal tunnel syndrome is frequently made on the history and there may not be any significant neurological signs at all at the time of presentation. Yet many surgeons would make a diagnosis and treat the patient on the basis of these findings alone. It has to be accepted, however, that in medicolegal practice it is important to make a diagnosis that can be supported by more than just the word of the patient and *without reasonable doubt*. In practice, this would seem to mean that a clinician must be able to support his or her diagnosis with some other proof of the condition.

An example of this would be a patient who complains of symptoms suggestive of carpal tunnel syndrome. If such a patient were not to have any relief from the use of a night splint nor to have any benefit from a carpal tunnel decompression operation there seems very little grounds for supporting the original diagnosis. Similarly, a patient who is diagnosed as suffering from tenosynovitis which is related to a particular form of work activity should notice a significant improvement once the provoking activity is ceased or modified. Patients who continue to experience symptoms after stopping this work, or find the condition progressively worsens, do not have tenosynovitis because it is well recognised that these are not the typical features of this condition.

It seems reasonable, therefore, to have some guidelines by which a diagnosis can be made or sustained in the absence of any typical physical signs:

1. The history, as given by the patient must include the typical symptoms of the condition.
2. The condition must behave in the way that is described in the standard medical literature.
3. Standard investigations for this condition, if carried out, should be positive.
4. The condition must respond to the normal treatment methods.

If the patient without any physical signs meets these criteria then it would be reasonable to sustain the diagnosis. If, on the other hand, the patient fails to meet these criteria a diagnosis of 'Occupational Arm Pain' has to be made until a definitive diagnosis is reached.

Summary

Ambrose Bierce (1842–1914), in his 'Devil's Dictionary', defined the hand as: 'A singular instrument worn at the end of the human arm and commonly thrust into somebody's pocket'. In compiling a medicolegal report, the medical expert's opinion will often help determine whose pocket is going to supply the requisite compensation and how much compensation there will be.

The patient with a hand injury deserves every sympathy and also every encouragement to regain as much useful function as possible. It is regrettable that the system of litigation and compensation in this country gives very little encouragement or motivation to patients to assist in the rehabilitation following an injury; more commonly, the process of the law acts as a disincentive to return to normal activities as soon as possible. Nevertheless, it is to be hoped that objective medical evidence can at least go some way to help providing a just outcome and allow the patient to feel that the system has functioned fairly.

■ References

Amadio P C, Hunter J M 1987 Prognostic factors in flexor tendon surgery in zone 2. In: Hunter J M, Schneider L H, Mackin E J (eds) Tendon surgery in the hand. C V Mosby, St Louis, 138–147

Atroshi I, Gummesson C, Johnsson R, Ornstein E, Ranstam J, Rosen I 1999 Prevalence of Carpal Tunnel syndrome in a general population. Journal Of American Medical Association 282(2): 153–158

Barton N J 1979 Fractures of the shafts of the phalanges of the hand. The Hand 11 (2): 119–133

Bertelsen A, Capener N 1960 Fingers, compensation and King Canute. Journal of Bone and Joint Surgery 42: 390–392

Bleecker M I 1987 Medical surveillance for carpal tunnel syndrome in workers. Journal of Hand Surgery 12A: 845–848

Boyle J C, Smith N J, Burke F D 1988 Vibration white finger. Journal of Hand Surgery 13B: 171–176

Burke F D 2000 Leading article: Carpal tunnel syndrome: Reconciling 'demand management' with clinical need. Journal of Hand Surgery 25B: 2: 121–127

Burke F D, Dias J J, Lunn P G, Bradley M 1991 Providing care for hand disorders: trauma and elective. Journal of Hand Surgery 16B: 13–18

Cheng Y H 1997 Explaining disablement in modern times: hand-injured workers' accounts of their injuries in Hong Kong. Soc Sci Med Sept 45(5): 739–950

Chow S P, Ng C 1993a Can a divided digital nerve on one side of the finger be left unrepaired? Journal of Hand Surgery 18B: 629–630

Chow S P, Ng C 1993b Hand function after digital amputation. Journal of Hand Surgery 18B: 125–128

Chow S P, Pon W K, Su Y C et al 1991 A prospective study of 245 open digital fractures of the hand. Journal of Hand Surgery 16B: 137–140

Cobb T K, Dalley B K, Posterard R H, Lewis R C 1992 Establishment of carpal contents/canal ratio by means of magnetic resonance imaging. Journal of Hand Surgery 17A: 843–849

De Krom M C, Kester A D, Knipschild P G, Spaans F 1990 Risk factors for carpal tunnel syndrome. American Journal of Epidemiology 132(6): 1102–1110

Derkash R S, Matyas J R, Weaver J K 1987 Acute surgical repair of the Skier's Thumb. Clinical Orthopedics and Related Research 216: 29–33

Duran R J, Houser R S 1975 Controlled passive motion following flexor tendon repair in zones 2 and 3. In: AAOS symposium on tendon surgery in the hand. C V Mosby, St Louis, pp 105–114

Elliot D, Moiemen N S, Flemming A F, Harris S B, Foster A J 1994 The rupture rate of acute flexor tendon repairs mobilized by the controlled active motion regimen. Journal of Hand Surgery 19B (5): 607–612

Eversmann W W Jr 1988 Entrapment and compression neuropathies. In: Green D P (ed) Operative hand surgery, vol 2, 2nd edn. Churchill Livingstone, Edinburgh, pp 1423–1478

Gault D T 1987 Reduction of grip strength, finger flexion pressure, finger pinch pressure and key pinch following flexor tendon repair. Journal of Hand Surgery (British and European) Jun 12(2): 182–184

Health and Safety Executive 1992 Health and safety statistics 1990–1991. Employment Gazette, Suppl 3 vol 100, no 9, September

Jerosch-Herold C 1993 Measuring outcome in median nerve injuries. Journal of Hand Surgery 18B: 624–628

Johns A M 1981 Time off work after hand injury. Injury 12(5): 417–424

Kelsey J L, Pastides H, Kreiger N, Harris C, Chernow R A 1980 Upper extremity disorders: a survey of their frequency and cost in the United States. C V Mosby, St Louis

Leach R E, Odom J A 1968 Systemic causes of the carpal tunnel syndrome. Postgraduate Medicine 44: 127–131

Leddy J P 1988 Flexor tendons—acute injuries. In: Green D P (ed) Operative hand surgery. Churchill Livingstone, Edinburgh

Lewis R C Jr 1985 High-compression injection injuries to the hand. Emergency Medical Clinics of North America 3: 373–381

Ling R S M 1963 The genetic factors in Dupuytren's disease. Journal of Bone and Joint Surgery 45B: 709–718

Marsh D 1990 The validation of measures of outcome following suture of divided peripheral nerves supplying the hand. Journal of Hand Surgery 15B: 25–34

McFarlane R M 1991 Dupuytren's disease: relation to work and injury. Journal of Hand Surgery 16A: 775–779

Medical Research Council 1951 Peripheral nerve injuries. Special Report Series no 282. HMSO, London

Nathan P A, Keniston R C, Myers L D, Meadows K D 1992 Longitudinal study of median nerve sensory conduction in industry. Journal of Hand Surgery 17A: 850–861

Nathan P A, Takigawa K, Keniston R C, Meadows K D, Lockwood R S 1994 Slowing of sensory conduction of the median nerve and carpal tunnel syndrome in Japanese and American industrial workers. Journal of Hand Surgery 19(B): 30–34

Pinto M R, Cooney W P, Wood M B, Dobyns J H 1993 High pressure injection injuries of the hand: review of 25 patients managed by open wound technique. Journal of Hand Surgery 18A: 125–130

Ramos H, Posch J L, Lie K K 1970 High-pressure injection injuries of the hand. Plastic and Reconstructive Surgery 45: 221–226

Rank B K, Wakefield A R, Hueston J T 1973 Surgery of repair as applied to hand injuries, 4th edn. Churchill Livingstone, Edinburgh, p 376

Saetta J P, Phair I C, Quinton D N 1992 Ulnar collateral ligament repair of the metacarpophalangeal joint of the thumb: a study comparing two methods of repair. Journal of Hand Surgery 17B: 160–163

Schoo M J, Scott R A, Boswick J A Jr 1980 High pressure injection injuries of the hand. Journal of Trauma 20: 229–238

Semple J C, Cargill A O 1969 Carpal tunnel syndrome: results of surgical decompression. Lancet i: 918

Silverstein B 1985 The prevalence of upper limb cumulative trauma disorders in industry. PhD dissertation, University of Michigan, Ann Arbor, Michigan

Small J O, Brennen M D, Colville J 1989 Early active mobilization following flexor tendon repair in zone 2. Journal of Hand Surgery 14B (4): 383–391

Smith R J 1977 Post-traumatic instability of the metacarpophalangeal joint of the thumb. Journal of Bone and Joint Surgery 59A (1): 14–21

Stener B 1962 Displacement of the ruptured ulnar collateral ligament of the metacarpophalangeal joint of the thumb: a clinical and anatomical study. Journal of Bone and Joint Surgery 44B (4): 869–879

Stern P J, Kastrup J J 1988 Complications and prognosis of treatment of mallet finger. Journal of Hand Surgery 13A: 341–346

Strickland J W 1987 Flexor tendon injuries, part 5: flexor tenolysis, rehabilitation and results. Orthopaedic Review XVI: 33–49

Strickland J W, Glogovac S V 1980 Digital function following flexor tendon repair in zone 2. Journal of Hand Surgery 5(6): 537

Swanson A B, Gorgan-Hagert C, Swanson G de G 1987 Evaluation of impairment in the upper extremity. Journal of Hand Surgery 12A: 896–926

Sykes P J 1991 Severe burns of the hand: a practical guide to their management. Journal of Hand Surgery 16B: 6–12

Szabo R M 1998 Carpal tunnel syndrome as a repetitive motion disorder. Clinical Orthopaedics 351: 78–89

Szabo R M, King K J 2000 Repetitive strain injury: Diagnosis or self-fulfilling prophecy? Journal of Bone and Joint Surgery 82A(9): 1314–1328

Taylor W, Pelmear P L (eds) 1975 Vibration white finger in industry. Academic Press, London, pp XVII–XXII

Terrono A L, Millender L H 1996 Management of work-related upper-extremity nerve entrapments. Orthopaedic Clinics of North America 27(4): 783–793

Tubiana R 1985 Incidence and cost of injuries to the hand (including the Kelsey Report). In: The hand, vol II. W B Saunders, Philadelphia, pp 159–164

Wilppola E, Nummi J 1979 Surgical treatment of ruptured ulnar collateral ligament of the metacarpo-phalangeal joint of the thumb. Injury 2(1): 69–72

Hand Fractures

The hand is arguably the most frequently injured portion of the human body, owing to its simultaneous use as a sensory organ and also as our most important manipulator of the environment. This scenario frequently leads us to endanger our hands with consequent fracture of the bony skeleton and concomitant soft tissue damage. Furthermore, as we all use our hands in our work, it is not surprising that hand fractures are a common work-related injury.

We now have clearly established guidelines for the assessment of the degree of disability related to loss of function in the hand (Swanson et al 1987). It would therefore seem to be a simple matter to classify the fracture type and then assess the functional capacity at the end of healing. However, with the introduction of very sophisticated internal fixation devices, eager and aggressive hand therapists and a philosophy of early stable fixation and aggressive early motion, we have improved our functional results dramatically.

Classification of Fractures

Paramount to any discussion of fractures or fracture management is an understanding of the exact character of the traumatic lesion. This understanding will give the treating surgeon an idea of the likely outcomes of all forms of treatment pertaining to that injury. Furthermore, an exact description will allow us to compare the results of various forms of treatment. It seems that all fractures in the distal limb have a distinct 'personality' dependent upon the anatomy and physiology of the traumatised part, the mechanism and force of the injury, and particularly on the ability and motivation of the patient to use and rehabilitate the injured hand.

There have been many classification systems published in the scientific literature over the last 70 years (London 1971; McElfresh & Dobyns 1983; Hastings 1987 and more recently Schenck 1994). It may seem cynical to imply that with this many classification systems, each must be fundamentally flawed. In general, each indicates the mind set of its author.

It is the author's belief, however, that these classification systems do not offer a panacea for the treating surgeon and he prefers to rely on basic orthopaedic tenets.

Regarding the fracture itself:

1. Open or closed fracture configuration (potentially contaminated)
2. Fracture location (will determine the rehabilitative possibilities) and configuration (will determine the treatment options including splintage, implant size and form, and surgical approach)
3. Associated injuries (determining the rehabilitative possibilities).

Clearly, once the goals of fracture toilet, debridement and stabilisation have been achieved, then it is the associated injuries that will determine the outcomes of management. It should not be left unsaid that patient motivation heavily influences the timing and success of rehabilitative goals.

The hand is the primary prehensile instrument of man. Outcomes after injury are determined mainly by four factors:

1. Sensibility in the injured part, being determined by the associated injury
2. Pain, being a combination of both soft tissue and bony rehabilitation
3. Mobility, being determined by intact and competent motors
4. Stability of the intercalated bony segments and restoration of joint motion.

The following discussion will be arranged by anatomical region, discussing both the periarticular regions and diaphyseal fractures concurrently.

Distal segment fractures

Distal phalangeal fractures are classically divided into three categories:

1. Tuft fractures
2. Diaphyseal fractures
3. Basal fractures.

Among hand fractures these distal segment injuries are frequent and often disabling (Barton 1984). Butt (1962) described these fractures as being the most common hand injury occurring predominately in the medius and thumb. A more recent review by Packer (1993) found that the so–called Boxer's fracture has usurped the distal fracture in rate of occurrence. Fractured fifth metacarpal neck fractures accounted for 30% of all hand fractures. Distal segment fractures were found most commonly in the ring finger in this study. This difference may reflect the changing nature of 'leisure' time activities from 1962 to 1993.

Tuft fractures

These fractures are commonly occurring industrial accidents being caused or cut/crushing trauma in machinery presses or pinion mechanisms. They present as bursting contaminated injuries of the pulp, bone and nail bed. DaCruz (1998) has shown that these are not the simple injuries that they at first appear. He found that symptoms often persist for between 3–6 months and that there are frequently long–lasting if not permanent sequelae with cold intolerance, numbness, stiffness and nail deformity. There is often delayed/non-union of the fracture elements, however, these fragments rarely have any functional sequelae (Green & Rowland 1991). The fracture fragments themselves rarely require any direct treatment; rather, it is the stabilisation and rehabilitation of the specialised pulp tissues and nail bed structure that determine the functional and cosmetic outcome. There have been many writers on the subject of nail bed injuries (Seymour 1966; Herndon 1976; Fingbar & Clancy 1978; Simon 1981; Zook 1984; Browne 1994). The debate has ranged around removal of the nail and stabilisation of the fractured phalanx. It seems that stabilisation of the fracture is not enough (Fingbar & Clancy 1978). Even more, the risk of infection is high with internal fixation, and the consequences of bone infection are severe, not infrequently resulting in amputation (Browne 1994). It would seem that the optimal treatment is surgically to lavage and toilet the wound and then stabilise the fingertip with nail bed repair and replacement of the nail plate or a splint within the nail fold. Supplemental stabilisation by external splintage should augment the primary repair. Immobilisation for 2–3 weeks is usually all that is required.

Diaphyseal fractures

These fractures are subdivided into longitudinal and transverse fractures. It would seem that only the unstable transverse fractures would benefit from internal fixation (Green & Rowland 1991), usually in the form of K-wire or even Herbert screw (Richards 1988; Schneider 1988). Complications from these fractures are rare and there are only occasional reports in the literature of interventions for symptomatic non-union or malunion. Once again these fractures may be compounded through the nail plate and appropriate surgical lavage and nail bed reconstruction would seem prudent following the results of distal tuft fractures.

Basal fractures

The mechanism in these fractures is either a shearing/avulsion force manifest through the pull of the FDP or EDC tendons or a pilon injury with commensurate cartilage damage to both the distal phalangeal base and also the condyles of the middle phalanx. Here the literature is ambiguous as there is rarely a distinction made between these pilon injuries and the less violent shearing/avulsion fractures. Most of the literature deals with these fractures as mallet fractures. Clearly the outcomes will depend not only upon the configuration of the fracture (i.e. is there a mallet fragment) but also upon the mechanism of the injury and the amount of comminution and associated articular cartilage damage. Wehbe & Schneider (1984) concluded that the literature did not support either internal fixation or external splintage and that the only advantage of surgery was to be found in those fractures with a large dorsal fragment and subluxation of the joint. Seemingly, these fractures are more of the shearing configuration and have not suffered significant cartilage damage. In these cases internal fixation is indicated. By analogy it would seem that the very comminuted basal pilon fractures did not benefit from any of the various modes of internal fixation.

FDP avulsions

These injuries can be classified into three groups after Leddy (1977, 1985) and a fourth group after Smith (1981):

- Type I   Soft tissue avulsion to the palm destroying the viniculum
- Type II   Small bony fragment avulsion caught at the FDS decussation with intact vinicula
- Type III   Large bony fragment often caught at the A4 pulley

- Type IIIa   As for above but the tendon pulls away from the fragment (Robins & Dobyns 1975)
- Type IV   Associated with an intra–articular fracture component.

Originally described by Von Zander in 1891 this is a relatively common injury in young athletes. It is said to be most common in the ring finger because of anatomical variations in the flexor tendon origin and extensor tendon interconnections. This lesion can occur in any finger that is forcibly extended against active resistance. Because the enthesis is the weakest portion of the musculo-tendinous unit, the avulsion occurs at the distal phalanx (McMaster 1933). Clearly the nutritional supply to the tendon is jeopardised and early repair will restore the best chance of healing. It is said that in the Type II injury the tendon is nourished by the intact vinicula and the synovial fluid so that a delayed repair is acceptable. The early reconstitution of tendon gliding and release of the tension on the vascular viniculae must give the best chance for tendon rehabilitation. It would seem prudent to undertake repair at the earliest opportunity.

Repair will consist of operative internal fixation of the fractured distal phalanx and strong reattachment of the profundus tendon to its insertion.

Management of late cases is problematic, with the literature presenting all cases. Fusion of the DIP joint stabilises that joint and maintains good PIP joint function at the expense of DIP mobility. It will not modify grip strength as compared to the pretreatment group. Tenodesis is technically difficult in the setting of an avulsion and has the propensity to stretch. Tendon grafting is fraught with difficulties. It may jeopardise the existing FDS function and thereby worsen the hand function. There are enthusiasts for all the treatment groups and the options must be clearly thought through with the patient's requirements in mind.

Mallet fractures

These fractures are relatively uncommon and are usually considered in the spectrum of mallet finger deformities:

a) Closed injuries: attrition ruptures of the common extensor tendon at the DIP joint level (Warren et al 1988)
b) Open injuries: either laceration or with skin or tendon loss
c) Associated with fracture:
   (i) Trans-epiphyseal
   (ii) Articular fracture <30%
   (iii) Articular fracture with subluxation.

Much has been written about the various internal fixation options and the outcomes of these various treatments (Stark & Boyes 1962; Wehbe & Scheider 1984; Lange & Engber 1987; Stark et al 1987). The debate now revolves only around those fractures with volar subluxation and extensive capsular disruption. These are uncommon fractures: Stark (1987) had five in a series of 168 mallet fractures, Abouna & Brown (1986) found eight in 148 cases of mallet finger. Other mallet fractures not associated with joint incongruity seem best managed non-operatively with extension splinting for a period of 4–6 weeks.

For those fractures with large articular components and joint subluxations, Lange & Engber (1987) advocated accurate reduction and internal fixation with wires. Wehbe & Scheider (1984) advocated extension splinting even in the cases of subluxation, commenting that the fracture healing was good and that healing even in malunion allowed stability and good range of motion with a lower morbidity from the management itself. Crawford (1984) has even claimed good results with the ubiquitous polythene stack splint.

Distal segment fractures in children

Finger fractures in children are common and may be the most common childhood fracture. Clearly there is a close race between distal forearm fractures and collective fractures of the hand (Barton 1979; Hastings & Simmons 1984; Worlock & Stower 1986). Barton (1979) found that 20% of his fractures involved the distal phalanx in his prospective study. The other studies indicate an incidence in the order of 8 to 10%. There is significant difficulty in interpreting these papers as they are usually retrospective and their populations are not well defined. Worlock & Stower (1986) admit that there is bias in their paper as many of the distal segment injuries were not treated in their unit. Suffice it to say that distal segment fractures are common but rarely require tertiary specialist care. The exception to this rule is the juxta-epiphyseal injury of the distal phalnx which is often compound through the proximal one-third of the nail plate and fold. Here there is often debate as to whether the nail should be discarded; Seymour (1966) advocates thorough debridement and replacing the nail under the nail fold. Supplemental internal fixation is rarely required and not infrequently accompanied by infection with dire consequences.

Tuft and shaft fractures are best managed with nail bed repair, re-insertion of the nail plate and external splintage.

Middle and proximal phalangeal fractures

It is convenient and practical to divide the discussion of phalangeal fractures into periarticular fractures around the proximal interphalangeal and metacapophalangeal joints and those of the phalangeal diaphyses. Our initial discussion will focus on the diaphyseal fractures and then subsequently upon the peri-articular group.

Diaphyseal fractures of the middle and proximal phalanx

Fractures of the proximal phalanx are characteristically more common (especially in children where they are often Salter-Harris type II injuries) and usually oblique or spiral with volar angulation. Those in the middle phalanx are more likely transverse and have a variable angulation dependent upon many factors such as the trauma force, pull of the FDS insertion or extensor insertion and rehabilitation regimen. Anatomically, these sections of the phalanges are cloaked by both the extensor hood mechanism with its associated intrinsic tendons and also the complex flexor tendon arrangements within the essential flexor sheath. Fracture healing with external callus and or surgical approaches to these segments will interfere with free tendon gliding and adversely affect the outcome in terms of functional range of movement.

In the following discussion the various management options will be discussed and the relative merits of each investigated. Most of the literature is anachronistic now and predominately deals with a conglomerate of both phalangeal and metacarpal fractures. Clearly the significant associated tissues are quite different between the metacarpals and the middle phalanx. However, if one keeps the notion to the front of one's mind that each fracture has its own character and that the associated injuries must be evaluated on their own merits, then some good information can be gained by an investigation of these combined studies.

Many factors come into play to determine the outcome from phalangeal factors. Strickland (1982) has written the landmark paper on this topic. He divides the issues into the three major groupings described below.

(i) Patient factors

Elderly patients, those with associated medical conditions, those from lower socio-economic classes and those patients with a poor understanding of '. . . the full ramifications of the injury. . . ' were all shown by Strickland (1982) to have a poor total range of motion at the end of the rehabilitation programme.

(ii) Fracture factors

Anatomical location, fracture configuration, displacement and comminution, stability and associated injuries were all factors that influenced the final outcome in management of these fractures. Flatt (1966) has emphasised the significance of soft tissue injury and has put forward the concept of 'injury at depth': clearly the force is transmitted from external to internal and all of the intervening structures have been damaged prior to the bone fracture. Their

rehabilitation will determine the distal function in the damaged part.

It can be interpreted from the studies of Strickland (1982) and many similar investigations that it is the associated injuries and in particular the tendon excursions that determine the ultimate combined outcomes in these fractures. Woods (1988) and other investigators (James 1962; Huffaker & Wray 1979) have shown that the final range of motion is clearly dependent upon restoration of flexor and extensor tendon excursion. Even more, in Woods' opinion, the flexor tendon gliding has the stronger influence on total range of motion. In contrast, it is Strickland's and James' deduction that the extensor tendon plays a more significant role in the total range of motion following a phalangeal fracture. Irrespective of the management technique clearly prolonged immobilisation of phalangeal fractures has a detrimental effect on functional outcome.

(iii) Management factors

Factors such as recognition of the injury, soft tissue management, fracture reduction and maintenance, mobilisation and intervention for complications were all shown to be significant in attaining the final range of motion.

Strickland (1982) has shown that the outcomes from these fractures as a group is strongly correlated with the total immobilisation time (< 4 wks = 80% TAM; > 4 wks = 60% TAM). He did not find any real benefit in mobilisation earlier than 4 weeks; in fact, in the case of markedly displaced fractures he found that mobilisation during the first and second weeks adversely affected the final total range of motion. However, these opinions are in conflict with previous reports which range in opinion from no movement (Flatt 1966) to the immediate active mobilisation favoured by the AO group.

These management factors are the only factors clearly modifiable by the surgeon so it would seem worthwhile investigating the outcome results from the various forms of treatment.

Manipulation and splinting This is surely the traditional and most popular technique for managing phalangeal fractures. Barton (1984) has shown that only one in four fractures required any form of manipulation and that approximately 5% required internal fixation to maintain the reduction. Jahss (1936) is traditionally thought of as the first to describe a method for reduction and stable immobilisation. He advocated taping of the interphalangeal joints in flexion and leaving the MP joint free to mobilise. Since Jahss's time, however, complications with skin necrosis and IP joint stiffness have dissuaded present day surgeons from using this form of immobilisation. However, his reduction technique is still widely used. James (1962) investigated and discussed the concept of the 'safe position' of the hand. He advocated immobilisation in 70° MCP joint flexion and IP joint extension to resist the contracture of collateral ligaments. Many authors since that time have proposed varying methods of reduction and positions of immobilisation. However, most of these dissertations have become anachronistic in the present light of efficient anaesthesia and new improved techniques for internal fixation and early mobilisation. Reyes, in 1987, has made a convincing argument that these techniques of manipulation and immobilisation in plaster of paris can be effective with a very acceptable complication rate, even in those difficult unstable proximal phalangeal shaft fractures. In his study of 158 proximal phalangeal fractures Reyes reported 91% successful results in basal fractures and 80% functionally successful results in the diaphyseal fractures. In both these groups of fractures he found that the results at 6 weeks can be extrapolated to the final outcome: 'the chances of improving the final results are much better than the chances of worsening after 6 weeks'.

Traction   Closed reduction and traction devices have had a prominent position in orthopaedic history. It seems that the experiences from the closed treatment of large bone fractures were at first popularly adapted to small bone fractures. However, due to the difficulty with proximal stabilisation of the splints and distal attachment of the traction devices, this form of treatment has fallen from popularity. Fitzgerald & Kahn (1984) had outstanding results with a complex management protocol of reduction and traction, reporting full movement in 16 of 18 patients within 3 months. Moberg (1950) has made the important point that transgression of the vital gliding surfaces of the extensor tendon will inhibit the results and he favoured a traction device placed through the pulp. Schenck (1994) has been a recent advocate of this form of treatment in intra-articular fractures. However, in the setting of diaphyseal fractures there has been little to encourage the operator in this technique lately.

External fixation   Once again, following on from the successes of external fixation in long bone fractures along with the recent miniaturisation of existing frame systems, it has become popular to adapt the concepts of ligamentotaxis and 'anatomical form' alignment to the small bones of the hand. Freeland (1987) has presented 12 patients with severe injuries to the hand treated with external fixation. He has outlined the spectrum of care possible with this form of treatment. However, the results are not comparable to those cases of simple isolated phalangeal fractures. When the issues are soft tissue coverage and stabilisation of the grossly unstable, multiply injured part,

external fixation seems a very acceptable modality. Nagy (1993) has presented a review of the application of external fixation to the hand. He presents the philosophical differences that have modified the usage of these fixators within Europe and the rest of the world. Union rates and complication rates for both simple and complex fractures are documented to be in the same order as those from other forms of operative intervention. Notably, the infection rate attendant with these miniature fixators is much lower than the documented rates for long bone fixateurs (5% to 20% as compared with 2% to 6%).

Percutaneous pinning   Has the advantages of being relatively simple to use, low in cost, an easy inventory, limited soft tissue dissection and versatility. Belsky & Eaton (1988) claim that the main advantages are simplicity and major reduction in costs. Using a variety of techniques in 100 patients they claim a 90% success rate with good or excellent results. The majority of papers presenting these techniques require the K-wire to be driven across the adjacent joint and secondary protection with plaster casting. Longitudinal wires are removed at 3 weeks with transverse wires remaining until the fourth week. Splinting and intensive therapy are continued for a subsequent 3 weeks. There is no mention of pin site infection nor secondary septic arthritis. Caspi (1984) illustrates that new bone may form at the site of transarticular wires. However, it remains that percutaneous wires are acceptable treatment and low in cost.

Open reduction and internal fixation   As previously stated, most of the phalangeal fractures are stable and well managed by immobilisation during the acute phase (usually not lasting longer than 3 weeks) and then rehabilitation with active mobilisation. Those fractures that are simple and yet unstable or unreduced are usually managed with closed reduction and percutaneous pinning, predominately because of the simplicity of this treatment. However, there are a significant number of fractures that are not suitable for these simple managements. Pun (1989) reported that those fractures that were unstable and treated with smooth pin fixation had a poor or fair result in 70% of cases. Open fractures, comminuted fractures and significant associated soft tissue injuries were all found to be poor prognostic indicators.

Many authors (Crawford 1976; Segmuller 1977; Belsole 1980; Heime et al 1982; Hastings 1987) have recorded excellent results with AO techniques in phalangeal fractures. However, it is clear that the technique is demanding and not directly transferable from those in major long bone trauma. Steel (1978) set down some of the criteria for internal fixation. He stated clearly that lag screw fixation would be successful only if the fracture line was oblique and two times the diameter of the bone at the fracture site. Steel would admonish us to use precise fixation in order that we may obtain favourable results. Similarly, there have been many attempts to describe the most favourable surgical approach to minimise the stripping of periosteum and damage to the complex gliding structures in the finger (Pratt 1959; Posner 1977; Heime et al 1982).

Wallace Jones (1987) has written a very good paper on the biomechanics of small bone fixation. In this paper he discusses the relative merits of various forms of fixation and also describes the difficulty in trying to compare various fixation techniques. These factors are:

- the quality and type of bone (and from which animal)
- fracture configuration and energy dissipated in fracture formation
- testing mode (repetitive, cycling, 4-pt, 3-pt, bending, cantilever forces)
- the constructs are not comparable.

He highlights the fallacies in previous reports and illuminates the process of choosing the best fixation from an armamentarium of various techniques. His inference is that we must be very proficient in many techniques and apply them judiciously to each individual fracture. He outlines the goals of internal fixation to be:

- anatomical reduction and maintenance of the fracture
- early soft tissue rehabilitation
- union of the fracture.

Further, he states that when used correctly, plates and screws most closely approximate natural bone strength and will allow early bone and soft tissue rehabilitation.

As opposed to other techniques such as tension band wire, interosseous wiring, K-wiring, intramedullary wiring and other intramedullary devices, plates and screws can perform a variety of tasks:

- Compression (tension band principle of Pauwels)
- Neutralisation
- Buttress
- Bridging

Concomitant to any discussion of open reduction and internal fixation is the discussion of implant removal. There are many issues to be considered such as:

1. Patient request
2. Implant failure and impingement
3. Shielding and bone erosion
4. Implant erosion
5. Ion release (allergy and oncogenesis).

A discussion of all the issues would encompass a text in itself. However, it would seem on balance that there is no good evidence that the implants are a biological liability over time, but that they are not infrequently a physical impediment to native usage. However, these physical liabilities are not confined to plate and screw fixation (Burstein 1972; Mathew 1972, 1984; Namba 1987).

Periarticular and articular fractures of the interphalangeal and metacarpophalaneal joints

Fractures of the distal interphalangeal joint

These are rare injuries and occur most commonly in the medius and ring fingers in sporting accidents.

Steel (1988) discusses the incidence of these fractures and deems them to be about 20% of all hand fractures, most being predominately mallet type avulsion injuries. Condylar fractures of the middle phalanx are rarities and therefore large series outlining their treatment are lacking from the literature.

The anatomy of the DIP joint and its ligament restraints has been investigated in prior reports (Shrewsbury & Johnson 1980; Gigis & Kucynski 1982). Recently, there has been some debate as to the likelihood of post-traumatic arthritis in these articular fractures. Schneider (1994), quoting the work of O'Rourke et al (1989), considers that the inevitable onset of arthritis following these fractures is not supported. Schneider therefore stands as a devotee of nonoperative treatment and thereby highlights the complications attendent upon operating on this distal joint.

Those fractures of the DIP joint involving only the distal phalanx have already been addressed in the discussion of distal phalangeal fractures.

Condylar fractures

These are generally classified after the system by London (1971):

1. unicondylar undisplaced
2. unicondylar displaced
3. bicondylar or comminuted (at the DIP joint Type 3 fractures are more frequent, illustrating the higher incidence of crushing injuries at this joint)

Type 1 fractures, if maintaining their position, are responsive to simple immobilisation and early rehabilitation. Unfortunately, these fractures have a tendency to be converted to the unstable Type 2.

Type 3 fractures are difficult to manage due to the poor soft tissue coverage, the tiny fracture fragments, their precarious blood supply and the complicated ligament attachments. In general terms, it seems that K-wire fixation is the only practical technique in this setting. If they cannot be reconstructed then a salvage procedure must be undertaken. Schneider (1994) comments that amputation or primary arthrodesis may be necessary. Zimmerman (1989) has shown favourable results with silicone interpositional arthroplasty as a salavage.

Type 2 fractures are unstable and cannot be maintained by external splintage. Malunion or non-union will result in angular and rotatory deformity with loss of joint function. Most authors agree that operative reduction through a dorsal approach or percutaneously under X-ray control and fixation (usually with wires) is the most appropriate.

Much of these same discussions hold true for condylar fractures of the PIP joint. However, in the setting of the PIP joint there are larger fragments and better soft tissue coverage which would allow the introduction of lag screw principles to maintain compression and allow early active mobilisation.

Proximal interphalangeal joint fractures

Articular fractures of the hand are difficult to manage due to their intricate anatomy and interrelated function. Wolfe & Dick (1991) have written a good overview of the approach to small joint injury in the hand. They emphasise the 'essential triad' of Stability: Mobility: Congruency. Congruency is further defined as joint topography and alignment. These features are important in the decision-making process in management of injuries to the complex PIP joint of the finger.

Classification of PIP joint fractures:

Schenck (1994) has most recently elaborated a comprehensive categorisation of PIP joint fractures. He divides them into proximal phalanx and middle phalanx fractures. Of the middle phalangeal fractures (being the most common) he divides them into groups depending upon both fracture fragment size and degree of dislocation. Of those in the proximal phalanx he uses the usual Uni- and Bi-condylar fracture classification, as outlined in the section on distal interphalangeal joint fractures. In this article Schenk discusses the other prominent classifications from past authors and makes the sound argument that it will continue to be difficult to interpret outcome data as long as the fracture continues to be rare and the descriptions of treatments are varied and idiosyncratic.

Anatomy of PIP joint

Fibonacci (Leonardo of Pisa 1170–1230) positions the PIP joint at the centre of the intercalated segments, between the tip of the finger and the MCP joint. In terms of leaver arms this demonstrates the importance of the PIP joint in grasping.

Several authors have discussed the intricate anatomy of the PIP joints. These discussions demonstrate why the PIP joint has such a bad reputation for stiffness following fractures (Kuczynski 1968; Minamikawa 1993; Leibovic & Bowers 1994). The condylar cross-section of the head is trapezoidal, the radius of curvature of each condyle is different, and there is a condylar tilt towards the middle finger. These factors all contribute to both rotation and tilt as the PIP joint flexes. They determine the notable convergence of the fingers during grasp, leading to the popular test for rotatory malalignment.

The collateral ligament arises at a pit on the dorsolateral region of the proximal phalanx. The origin of the collateral ligament then descends on to the adjacent flat lateral surface which also doubles for the running surface of the collateral ligament as the finger moves into flexion. This anatomical feature is the foundation for many of the problems associated with shortening and adherence of the collateral ligaments and thereby loss of function of the PIP joint.

Unlike the knee joint and the MCP joint, the PIP joint does not appreciably change its pivot centre of rotation during flexion (Kuczynski 1968); however, the accessory collateral ligament and the volar plate are lax in flexion and are liable to contracture and loss of extension. This is in direct conflict with the cam effect of the MCP joints, where the collateral ligament is lax in extension and can lead to a loss of MCP joint flexion.

Management

The management of these difficult fractures is wide and varied, ranging from simple buddy strapping and closed reduction and pinning, through continuous active traction and distraction, to those who advocate early joint arthroplasty both by replacement and by interposition characterised by Eaton's volar plate arthroplasty (Eaton & Malerish 1980; Malerish & Eaton 1994). The results in the literature are mixed, with a wide range of results. There are several series from each of the major devotees with excellent results (although with relatively few cases and relatively short follow-up). However, it is clear from the literature that there is not one excellent management protocol for PIP joint fractures and that there are devotees of disparate types of treatment. It may be most prudent for this author to outline some of these treatments and reference them for further investigation.

Extension block splinting

Pioneered and formalised by J H Dobyns and E C McElfresh from the Mayo Clinic, this technique elaborates the universal orthopaedic concepts of:

Early active mobilization and

Stable arc splinting

Active mobilisation is understood as progressively increasing motion from limited to maximum as determined by the stable arc of motion. Stable arc of motion is that range of motion through which the joint is protected from either increasing deformity or chronic instability.

There is a very long history of results going back to Dobyns' original unpublished work during the 1950s. The splint is modified for each patient, being arm based or hand based. It is adjusted weekly until full range is gained somewhere between the third to eighth week following fracture.

Results are divided into three main groups:

1. Ideal group: Simple dorsal dislocations or fracture dislocations with less than 40% articular fracture and a stable arc to within less than 45° of full extension. At 12 months the results should be approximately: (1) 10–90° R.O.M. at the PIP joint; (2) 230° flexion; (3) 85% grip strength and 75% endurance; (4) PIP joint swelling slight, pain minimal or absent. With continued improvement up to 3–5 years.
2. Marginal group: These are complicated fractures with associated ligament injuries, intra-articular impingement, stable arc in excess of 60% flexion, and those from the ideal group who have been allowed to fall into joint incongruity. At 12 months the results are said to be less than those from the ideal group and they will not continue to improve over time.
3. Questionable group: These are salvageable joints with greater that 50% joint incongruity or a dislocation period greater than 6 weeks. These patients have a 20% worse result at 12 months and the results tend to deteriorate with time.

Dobyns & McElfresh (1994) comment that the technique is safe, salvageable and cheap, but accept that the results in selected cases may well be improved by more exacting and eleborate techniques such as traction, vector apparatus or open reduction and bone grafting.

Dynamic traction and external fixation

This technique was popularised by R R Schenck from Chicago USA. It was first described in 1986 then revisited in 1994 (Schenck 1994). Schenck has shown his results to persist or improve over time. He states that he has had 100% compliance and no major pin tract complications. He quotes comparative studies demonstrating results comparable to those of Dobyns in his Ideal group. However, in his original series of 10 patients the average joint involvement was 63%. In this group Schenck has

shown no deterioration over a 9 year interval. Schenck also compares his results to those of Hastings & Ernst (1993). Hastings has developed and modified a complex system of dynamic external fixation, which he has applied in both closed management and also as an adjuvant to open reduction and bone grafting. His results were similar to those of Schenck, although there was the added complication from the pivot pin placement.

Open reduction and internal fixation

As previously quoted, Barton (1984) has shown that only somewhere between 5 to 10% of all hand fractures will benefit from open reduction and internal fixation. The advantage of internal fixation is that in the unstable and displaced fractures, accurate reduction with interfragmentary compression can be expected to improve the final outcome (Freeland & Benoist 1994). It has been stated (Heim & Pfeiffer 1989) that this anatomical reduction reduces the pain and swelling of the fracture and allows a good basis for early active mobilisation. Fractures about the PIP joint have a tendency to stiffness, extension lag and fixed flexion contracture. This tendency is worsened by age and associated injuries, and complicated by multiple fractures and the poorly compliant patient. In selected cases it would seem that well planned fixation would benefit these patients in both the short and long term.

It should be noted that the fracture configuration and fragment size will determine the implant form. This precept indicates that a wide range of techniques and implant alternatives must be available to deal with these varied fracture situations. In general terms, it seems that internal fixation techniques are more applicable to the proximal phalanx than the middle phalanx, except in the setting of a large single fragment usually larger than 3 mm. This is a relatively rare finding in the pilon injury of the base of the middle phalanx.

Arthroplasty

Extensive results have been gathered from the work of Swanson with implant arthroplasty for degenerative disease of the MCP joints (Swanson & De Groot-Swanson 1994). These results have led to the expansion of this technique to the PIP joint with favourable results. Several authors have expanded the technique even further to the usage in immediate arthroplasty in the unsalavable PIP & MCP joint injury (Nagle et al 1989).

Malerish & Eaton have presented their technique and results of volar plate arthroplasty in several publications over the last 29 years (Eaton & Malerish 1980; Malerish & Eaton 1994). In the acute case the overall results are comparable to those quoted by Dobyns for his Ideal group with an average range of motion of 95° if performed within the first 6 weeks and 87° in the late cases even if performed up to 2 years after injury. Durham-Smith has reproduced Eaton's results with 87% of patients achieving 95° of motion within 2 months. They quote an overall satisfaction rate of 94% (Durham-Smith & McCarten 1992).

Comminuted fractures

These fractures are differentiated from their lesser cousins by the forces involved, the multiplicity of injured parts and the associated soft tissue damage and loss. High dissipated forces, periosteal stripping and contamination, unstable soft tissue constraints and an unstable skeleton all lead to a higher incidence of complications, and therefore a more aggressive mode of management is required. It should be said that it is a requirement of internal fixation devices that there are good soft tissue restraints and coverage so that early mobilisation is possible. In these injuries often the soft tissues will not tolerate early motion nor are there sufficient motors to mobilise an unstable part effectively. In these cases the advantage of elaborate internal fixation devises are already lost and it may be imprudent to introduce further soft tissue damage and foreign material as well as prolongation of ischaemia time. It is often prudent to rely on external splint, simple K-wiring techniques or formal external fixation devices. Unfortunately, the grading of these injuries is difficult so that the comparision of outcomes is similarly difficult. Often the result is idiosyncratic and a success in one man's eyes may be moderate in another's.

Metacarpal head fractures

These fractures are rare and are often difficult to image on X-ray examinations. McElfresh & Dobyns in 1983 reported on 103 such fractures and there is very good outline in 'Fractures of the Hand and Wrist' (McElfresh 1988). They divide these fractures into complicated groupings dependent upon the mechanism of injury and configuration of the fracture. Unfortunately the individual groups are small and the management protocols are pragmatic so it is difficult to compare different management options. In general terms, being an articular surface it seems prudent to engage in open reduction and internal fixation. However, the fracture fragment size will determine the form of the implant so once again a wide variety of operative techniques are required for these fractures.

Metacarpal fractures

Much of the information regarding diaphyseal fractures has already been presented in the sections on diaphyseal fractures of the phalanges. But unlike the phalanges, the metacarpals are relatively well covered by soft tissue, supported by distal and proximal ligaments binding them to the adjacent metacarpal and splinted by their adjacent partner. However, in the case of multiple metacarpal fractures, border digit injuries or high energy shearing/rotation injuries with disruption of the intermetacarpal ligaments, these fractures present an unstable configuration that will lead to loss of distal function as well as function in the palm.

Metacarpal neck fractures

These are arguably the most common fracture in the hand (if not the whole upper limb). They are usually sustained with an inefficient punching technique with flexed MCP joint. They are commonly called a Boxer's fracture (more aptly: Brawler's fracture), especially when involving the little finger metacarpal. Here the differentiation between being injured by a blow and being injured while inflicting a blow can be clearly made. The issues in the past have been angulation and rotational deformity along with prominence of the metacarpal head in the palm and loss of extension.

In general terms, these neck fractures heal well with simple immobilisation and there is little evidence to support complicated methods of fracture manipulation and fixation (Loudon 1986; McKerrel 1987). However, in the case of the index or middle finger metacarpal there is little compensatory movement of the CMC joint and it would seem prudent to correct the deformity at an early stage.

Metacarpal shaft fractures

These fractures usually result from direct trauma to the hand or as the sequelae of high torque injuries. They can be topograpically divided into transverse, oblique or comminuted types. Border digit fractures tend to be less well tolerated and generally require operative stabilisation. Spiral and oblique fractures are potentially unstable with a propensity to shortening and malrotation. Opgrande & Westphal (1983) stated that 1° of malrotation will result in amplification of the deformity and crossing of the fingers. In terms of management options, they are very similar to those already outlined for the diaphyseal fractures of the phalanges.

Carpometacapal joint fractures

This is a relatively uncommon injury, and is said to occur as 1% of all hand and wrist fractures (Mueller 1986; Dobyns et al 1988). With the increase in road traffic there has been a changing spectrum of injury. These injuries can be classified topographically to:

(i) CMC joint of thumb (to be discussed in the section on thumbs)

(ii) CMC joint index and middle

(iii) CMC joint ring and little

(iv) Multiple CMC joint injuries (Gunther 1984; Dobyns 1988).

Most of these injuries are fracture dislocations with true isolated dislocations rare but occasionally found in the index or middle finger. There is a progressive specialisation in the joints as one moves across the wrist from the index to the little finger with a very stable index joint and specialised supple saddle joints in the ring and little finger rays. Nearby structures may be occasionally involved in the injury (Peterson & Sacks 1986).

Early closed reduction is usually easily accomplished; however, the reductions are often unstable, requiring some sort of fixation, usually with K-wires, to hold the reduction. Occasionally, open reduction will be required in the case of marked swelling, delayed treatment or interposition of tendon (usually the ERCL tendon). Dobyns (1988) states that persistent subluxation of the CMC joint does interfere with muscular balance and will lead to a type of secondary clawing.

High speed multiple fracture dislocations are an indication of the widespread forces dissipated on the hand. These injuries may well require fasciotomy and or exploration of the palmar vascular arches or the ulnar nerve to repair acute insufficiency. In these cases stabilisation of the skeleton is an important adjuvant to soft tissue rehabilitation.

Thumb fractures

The vast majority of thumb fracture are extra-articular metacarpal fractures occurring as 80% of all thumb fractures. The three-dimensional mobility of the thumb allows a greater leeway for angular deformity to be accepted.

Phalangeal fractures of the thumb

These are managed with the same protocols as for finger fractures. Intra-articular extensions of diaphyseal fractures or pure condylar fractures/impaction fractures are rare. However, accurate reduction will be necessary to maintain joint mobility and to protect against late development of painful arthrosis (Stern 1993).

Avulsion fractures at the base of the proximal phalanx are often a manifestation of avulsion of the ulnar collateral ligament. In the case of significant instability, the fracture fragment should be either reattached or excised and the ligament attached to the fossa with pull out sutures or bone anchors.

Metacarpal shaft fractures

These usually occur adjacent to the base due to the mobility of the ray and the dissipation of the forces from the cort-

ical bone onto the metaphyseal region. These fractures are well managed with closed reduction and cast immobilisation. Up to 30° angulation is easily compensated for by the great mobility of the CMC joint.

Occasionally, dosal angulation may be severe enough to cause compensatory hyperextension at the IP joint and will require corrective osteotomy (Peterson & Sacks 1986).

Bennett's and Rolando fractures

(From Bennett 1882, Bennett 1886 and Rolando 1910). The basilar joint of the thumb is complex due to the high forces generated during power pinch and its requirement for both stability under load and mobility for dexterity (Cooney & Chao 1977; Breen et al 1988). The anatomic considerations for these fractures have been well described by several previous authors (Gedda 1954; Pellegrini 1988). It is often difficult to get a true radiographic account of the fracture position and this is especially true for intraoperative films, especially those taken on the image intensifiers. These difficulties have complicated long-term outcome studies and studies comparing different forms of operative treatment. Billing & Gedda (1952) have described the proper technique for visualising the small avulsion fragment in basal thumb fractures.

Many different techniques for management have been advocated. However, the debate revolves around accurate reduction and stable immobilisation. In terms of outcome following various forms of treatment it would seem that the clinical effects of post-traumatic arthritis of the thumb do not manifest themselves before the tenth post-injury year. Livesley (1990) found that a large percentage of his conservatively treated fractures manifested limited range of motion and degenerative arthritis. However, in Cannon's group (1986) at 10 years, there were very few patients with degenerative arthritis and among those with arthritis only about 2% had suffered a Bennett's fracture. These patients had been treated in the same era; however, they have been reviewed at a time separated by a decade and it would appear that this extra 10 years has made all the difference.

Following on from the studies on Bennett's fractures, it is understood that the outcome of Rolando fractures is poor if treated consevatively. There have been many advocates of open reduction and internal fixation with either pins or plates and screws. More recently, the application of external fixation either as the definative treatment or as an adjuvant to internal fixation and grafting has become popular (Buchler et al 1991).

Children's fractures

Children's fractures are rarely a complicated dilemma in the hand. They will heal quickly with little loss of adjacent joint function. Ireland & Taleisnik (1986) presented their findings of two cases of non-union as the largest series in the literature.

Fractures are most commonly seen as a complex injury of the distal phalanx with associated nail bed injury. Here again the issue does not lie with the bone union, which is almost universally adequate, but with the deformity from the nail bed injury itself.

Most commonly seen in the pre-adolescent child is the growth plate fracture of the proximal phalanx. This is usually a minimally angulated Salter–Harris II type fracture.

Much has been written about growth deformity with fractures in the immature hand. Light & Ogden (1987) found that growth arrest can occur even in the setting of an undisplaced peri-physeal injury. Mintzer et al (1994) more recently have investigated the remodelling of phalangeal neck fractures, indicating that there is a good capacity for correction of deformity with growth. Remodelling in the plain of motion of the joint can be expected to decrease the deformity over time while that portion of the deformity not in the plain of motion will be only slightly modified by the effects of growth in length and apposition growth.

Rarely is operative intervention required and it is usual that K-wire fixation supported by external splintage will be adequate due to the rapid rate of healing in these fractures. However, articular and periarticular fractures carry a poorer prognosis and will benefit from open reduction and internal fixation (Hastings & Simmons 1984; O'Brien 1991).

■ References

Abouna JM, Brown H 1968 The treatment of Mallet finger, the results in a series of 148 consecutive cases and a review of the literature. British Journal of Surgery 55: 653–667

Barton NJ 1979 Fractures of the phalanges of the hand in children. The Hand 11:2: 134–143

Barton NJ 1984 Fractures of the hand. J B S 66B: 159–167

Belsky MR, Eaton RG 1988 Fractures of the shafts of the phalanges: percutaneous wire fixation in fractures of the hand and wrist. E Barton NJ Churchill Livingstone, London

Belsole R 1980 Physiological fixation of displaced and unstable fractures of the hand. Orthopaedic Clinics of North America 11: 393–404

Bennett EH 1882 Fractures of the metacarpal bones. Dublin Journal of Medical Science 73: 72–75

Bennett EH 1886 On fractures of the metacarpal bone of the thumb. British Medical Journal 2: 12–13 {68} {70}

Billing L, Gedda KO 1952 Roentgen examination of Bennett's fracture. Acta Radiologica 38: 471

Breen T, Gelbermen R, Jupiter J 1988 Intra-articular fractures of the basilar joint of the thumb. Hand Clinics 4: 491–501

Brown JR 1959 Epiphyseal growth arrest in fractured metacarpals. Journal of Bane and Joint Surgery 41A: 494–496

Browne E 1994 Complications of fingertip injuries. Hand Clinics 10(1): 125–137 {72}

Buchler U 1991 Comminuted basilar fracture of the thumb. Journal of Hand Surgery 16a: 556–560

Burstein 1972 Bone strength: the effect of screw holes. Journal of Bane and Joint Surgery 54a: 1143

Butt WD 1962 Fractures of the hand. Canadian Medical Association 86: 731–735 {18} {34}

Cannon SR 1986 A long term follow up of Bennett's fracture. 10 years follow up. Journal of Hand Surgery 11b: 426–431

Caspi I 1984 Intra-articular bone formation in the hand following wire fixation. Orthopaedic Review 13: 91–92

Cooney W, Chao E 1977 Biomechanical analysis of the static forces in the thumb during hand function. Journal of Bone and Joint Surgery 59a: 27–36

Crawford GP 1976 Screw fixation for certain fractures of the phalanges and metacarpals. Journal of Bone and Joint Surgery 58a: 487–492

Crawford GP 1984 The moulded polythene splint for mallet finger deformities. Journal of Hand Surgery 9a: 231–237

DaCruz DJ 1988 Fractures of the distal phalanges. Journal of Hand Surgery 13B: 350–352

Dobyns J 1988 In: Barton NJ Fractures of the wrist and hand. Churchill Livingstone

Dobyns J, McElfresh E 1994 Extension block splinting. Hand Clinics 10(2) 229

Dobyns J, Linscheid R, Cooney W 1988 Fractures of the hand and wrist, then and now. Journal of Hand Surgery: 687–690

Durham-Smith G, McCarten G 1992 Volar plate arthroplasty for closed proximal interphalangeal joint injuries. Journal of Hand Surgery 17b: 422–428

Eaton RG, Malerish M 1980 Volar plate arthroplasty for the proximal interphalangeal joint: A ten year review. Journal of Hand Surgery 5: 260–268

Fingbar MD, Clancy WG 1978 Traumatic avulsion of the finger nail. Journal of Bone and Joint Surgery 60a: 713–714

Fitzgerald JW, Kahn MA 1984 The conservative management of fractures of the shafts of the phalanges of the fingers by combined traction–splintage. Journal of Hand Surgery 9B: 303–306

Flatt AE 1966 Closed and open fractures of the hand: fundamentals of management. Journal of Postgraduate Medicine 39: 17–26

Freeland AE 1987 External fixation for skeletal stabilization of severe open fractures of the hand. Clinical Orthopaedics and Related Research 214: 93–100

Freeland A, Benoist L 1994 Open reduction and internal fixation method for fractures at the proximal interphalangeal joint. Hand Clinics 10(2)

Gedda KO 1954 Studies on Bennett's fracture: Anatomy, roentgenology and therapy. Acta Chirurgica Scandinavica Supplement: 193

Gigis P, Kucynski K 1982 The distal interphalangeal joint of human fingers. Journal of Hand Surgery 7: 176–182

Green DP, Rowland SA 1991 In: Rockwood and Green's Fractures in adults, 3rd edn. Lippincott

Gunther S 1984 The carpometacarpal joints. Orthopaedic Clinics of North America 15: 259–277

Hastings H 1987 Unstable metacarpal and phalangeal fracture treatment with screws and plates. Clinical Orthopaedics and Related Research 214: 37–52

Hastings H, Ernst JM 1993 Dynamic external fixation for fractures of the proximal interphalangeal joint. Hand Clinics 9: 659

Hastings H, Simmons MD 1984 Hand fractures in children: a statistical analysis. Clinical Orthopaedics and Related Research 188: 120–130

Heim U, Pfeiffer KM 1989 Internal fixation of small fractures. Springer-Verlag, Berlin

Heime U, Pfeiffer KM, Meuli HD 1982 Small fragment set manual. Springer-Verlag, New York

Herndon JH 1976 Management of painful neuroma's in the hand. Journal of Bone and Joint Surgery 58a: 367–373

Huffaker WH Wray RC 1979 Factors influencing final range of motion in the fingers after fracture of the hand. Journal of Plastic and Reconstructive Surgery 63: 82–87

Ireland MD, Taleisnik J 1986 Non union of metacarpal extra aticular fractures in children. Journal of Pediatric Orthopaedics 6: 352–355

Jahss SA 1936 Fractures of the proximal phalanges: Alignment and immobilization. Journal of Bone and Joint Surgery 18: 726–731

James JP 1962 Fractures of the proximal and middle phalanges of the fingers. Acta Orthopaedica Scandinavica 32: 401–412

Jones WW 1987 Biomechanics of small bone fixation. Clinical Orthopaedics and Related Research 214: 11–18

Kuczynski K 1968 The proximal interphalangeal joint: Anatomy and causes of stiffness in the fingers. Journal of Bone and Joint Surgery 50B: 656

Lange RH, Engber WD 1987 Hyperextension mallet finger. Orthopaedics 6: 1426–1431

Leddy JP 1977 Avulsion of the profundus tendon insertion in athletes. Journal of Hand Surgery 2: 66–69

Leddy JP 1985 Avulsion of the flexor digitorum profunds. Hand Clinics 1: 77–83

Leibovic S Bowers W 1994 Anatomy of the proximal interphalangeal joint. Hand Clinics 10(2): 169

Light TR Ogden JA 1987 Metacarpal epiphyseal fracture. Journal of Hand Surgery 12A: 460–464

Livesley PJ 1990 The conservative management of Bennett's fracture dislocation. A 26 year follow up. Journal of Hand Surgery 15B: 291

London P 1971 Sprains and fractures involving the interphalangeal joints. The Hand 3: 155–158

Loudon IMR 1986 Fractures of the metacarpal neck of the little finger. Injury 17: 189–192

Malerish M, Eaton RG 1994 The volar plate reconstruction for fracture dislocation of the proximal interphalangeal joint. Hand Clinics 10(2): 251

Mathew LS 1972 Temperatures in drilling. Journal of Bone and Joint Surgery 54A: 297

Mathew LS 1984 Temperatures in drilling. Journal of Bone and Joint Surgery 66A: 1077

McElfresh E 1988 Fractures of the hand and wrist (Chapter 9). Ed Barton NJ. Churchill Livingstone

McElfresh E, Dobyns J 1983 Intra-articular metacarpal head fractures. Journal of Hand Surgery 8: 383–393

McKerrel J 1987 Boxer's fracture: Conservative or operative management? Journal of Trauma 27: 486–490

McMaster PE 1933 Tendon and muscle ruptures: Clinical and experimental studies on the cause and location of subcutaneous ruptures. Journal of Bone and Joint Surgery 15: 705

Minamikawa Y 1993 Stability and restraint of the proximal interphalangeal joint. Journal of Hand Surgery 18A: 198

Mintzer CM, Waters PM, Brown DJ 1994 Remodelling of a displaced phalangeal neck fracture

Moberg E 1950 The use of traction treatment for fractures of the phalanges and metacarpals. Acta Chirurgica Scandinavica 99: 341–352

Mueller J 1986 Carpometacarpal dislocations: a report of five cases and a review of the literature. Journal of Hand Surgery 11A: 184–188

Nagle DJ, Ekenstam F, Lister G 1989 Immediate silastic arthroplasty for non-salvagable intra-articular phalangeal fractures. Scandanavian Journal of Plastic and Reconstructive Surgery 23: 47–50

Nagy L 1993 Static external fixation of finger fractures. Hand Clinics 9(4): 651–657

Namba R 1987 Biomechanical effects of point configuration in kirschner wire fixation. Clinical Orthopaedics and Related Research 214: 19–22

O'Brien ET 1991 Fractures of the hand and wrist region. Rockwood, Williams & King, Fractures in children, Lippincote

Opgrande J, Westphal S 1983 Fractures of the hand. Orthopaedic Clinics of North America 14: 779–792

O'Rourke S, Gaur S, Barton NJ 1989 Long term outcome of articular fractures of the phalanges. Journal of Hand Surgery 14B: 183–193

Packer GJ, Saahern MA 1993 Patterns of hand fractures and dislocations in a district general hospital. Journal of Hand Surgery 18B: 511–514

Pellegrini VD 1988 Fractures at the base of the thumb. Hand Clinics 4: 87–101

Peterson P Sacks S 1986 Fracture dislocation of the base of the fifth metacarpal associated with injury to the deep motor branch of the ulnar nerve. Journal of Hand Surgery 11A: 525–528

Posner MA 1977 Injuries to the hand and wrist in athletes. Orthopaedic Clinics of North America 8: 593–618

Pratt DR 1959 Exposing fractures of the proximal phalanx of the finger longitudinally through the dorsal extensor apparatus. Clinical Orthopaedics and Related Research 15: 22–26

Pun WK 1989 A prospective study on 284 digital fractures of the hand. Journal of Hand Surgery 14A: 474–481

Reyes FA, Latta LL 1987 Conservative management of difficult phalangeal fractures. Clinical Orthopaedics and Related Research 214: 23–30

Richards RR 1988 Internal fixation of an open fracture of the distal phalanx with a Herbert screw. Journal of Hand Surgery 13A: 428–432

Robins PR, Dobyns JH 1975 Avulsion of the insertion of the flexor digitorum profundus tendon associated with fracture of the distal phalanx. AAOS symposium on tendon surgery in the hand. CV Mosby

Rolando S 1910 Fracture de la base du premier metacarpien, et principalement sur une variete non encore decrite. Presse Medicale 33: 303

Schenck R 1994 The dynamic traction method. Hand Clinics 10(2): 187

Schenck R 1994 Classification of fractures and dislocations of the proximal interphalangeal joint. Hand Clinics 10(2): 179

Schneider LH 1988 Fractures of the distal phalanx. Hand Clinics 4: 537–547

Schneider LH 1994 Fractures of the distal interphalangeal joint. Hand Clinics 10(4): 277

Schrewsbury M, Johnson R 1980 Ligaments of the distal interphalangeal joint and the mallet position. Journal of Hand Surgery 5: 214–216

Segmuller G 1977 Surgical stabilization of the skeleton of the hand. Williams and Wilkins, Baltimore

Seymour N 1966 Juxta-epiphyseal fractures of the terminal phalanx of the finger. Journal of Bone and Joint Surgery 48B: 347–349

Smith R 1981 Avulsion of profoundus tendon with simultaneous intraarticular fracture of the distal phalanx. Journal of Hand Surgery 6: 600–601

Stark HH 1987 Operative treatment of intra-articular fractures of the dorsal aspect of the distal phalanx of the digits. Journal of Bone and Joint Surgery 69A: 892–896

Stark HH, Boyes JH 1962 Mallet finger. Journal of Bone and Joint Surgery 44A: 1061–1068

Steel WM 1978 The A. O. small fragment set in hand fractures. Hand 10: 246–253

Steel WM 1988 Articular fractures. In: Barton NJ (ed) Fractures of the hand and wrist. Churchill Livingstone

Stern P 1993 Fractures of the metacarpals and phalanges. In Green D (ed) Operative Hand surgery. Churchill Livingstone

Strickland JW 1982 In difficult problems in hand surgery. C V Mosby, St Louis

Strickland JW, Steichen JB 1982 Phalangeal fractures: Factors influencing digital performance. Orthopaedic Review 11: 39–50

Swanson A, De Groot-Swanson G 1994 Flexible implant resection arthroplasty of the proximal interphalangeal joint. Hand Clinics 10(2)

Von Zander 1891 Trommlerlahmung Inaug Dissertation. Berlin

Warren RA, Kay NRM, Norris SH 1988 The microvascular anatomy of the distal digital extensor tendon. Journal of Hand Surgery 13B: 151–153

Wehbe MA, Scheider LH 1984 Mallet fractures. Journal of Bone and Joint Surgery 66A: 658–669

Wolfe S, Dick H 1991 Articular fractures of the hand. Orthopaedic Review 20(1): 27

Woods GL 1988 Troublesome shaft fractures of the proximal phalanx. Hand Clinics 4: 75–85

Worlock PH, Stower MJ 1986 The incidence and pattern of hand fractures in children. Journal of Hand Surgery 14B(2): 198–200

Zimmerman N, Suhey P, Clark G Silicone interpositional arthroplasty of the distal interphalangeal joint. Journal of Hand Surgery 14A: 882–887

Zook E 1984 A study of nail bed injuries: Causes, treatments and prognosis. Journal of Hand Surgery 9A: 247–252

Section 3

Results following lower limb fractures

Chapter 11

The hip

John P. Ivory, Mike Rigby, Michael A. Foy

Introduction

Fractures and dislocations about the hip are common injuries. Their patterns vary with the mechanism and velocity of the trauma, and with the age and general health of the patient. The injuries themselves are so diverse that their classifications will be discussed within the individual sections rather than in this introduction.

Acetabular fractures

The long-term results of acetabular fractures can become obscured within complex classifications of fracture patterns, as outlined by Judet et al (1964) and modified by Tile (1984). These classifications are vital to an understanding of the pathological anatomy, and to the planning of fracture management, but they do not provide clear guidelines for the prognosis. Within this section Judet's classification will be used. In assessing the prognosis of posterior wall fractures, the common association with hip dislocation is important. An apparently good result from the acetabular fracture may be prejudiced by injury to or subsequent avascular necrosis of the femoral head.

Tile has pointed out that spurious conclusions may be reached when results of methods of treatment of dissimilar fractures are compared. It is obviously quite unscientific to compare the results of conservative treatment of undisplaced acetabular fractures with those of operative treatment of displaced fractures. Tile pointed out that the literature is full of such comparisons.

Prognostic factors

From the reports in the orthopaedic literature on the conservative and surgical management of acetabular fractures, it is possible to identify certain factors which directly affect the prognosis.

Residual fracture displacement at the conclusion of treatment

This is the most critical factor in determining long-term results and is relevant to both conservative and operative treatment. If at the conclusion of treatment the acetabulum has been satisfactorily reduced then a good clinical result can be anticipated. Pennal et al (1980) reported a series of 103 patients with a mean follow-up of 7 years. Residual displacement was found in 66 patients, with a mean Toronto hip score of 14 (indicating a fair clinical result), of which 72% of these developed degenerative changes. The 37 patients with no residual displacement did significantly better with a mean Toronto hip score of 16.5 (indicating a good or excellent clinical result) and only 30% developed degenerative changes.

It is not always possible to achieve a perfect anatomical reduction. Matta et al (1985) graded the reduction as anatomical (0–1 mm of displacement), imperfect (residual 2–3 mm displacement) and poor (more than 3 mm). His initial results suggested that there was no significant difference between the anatomical and the imperfect group. A later report (Matta 1996) with 225 cases, following up at a mean of 6 years, showed that this was no longer true, with good or excellent clinical results seen in 83% of the 185 anatomical, 68% of the 52 imperfect and 50% of the 18 poor reductions. Anatomical reduction was easier to achieve in simpler fracture configurations, patients younger than 40 years of age and reductions carried out less than 2 weeks from injury. Matta now stresses that the goal of treatment should be anatomical reduction.

The largest series of patients with surgically treated acetabular fractures was presented by Letournel and Judet (1993); 569 fractures were treated by operation within 3 weeks of the injury of which 492 were available for follow-up at a minimum of 2 years. Of 336 patients with acetabular fractures treated by operation where a perfect reduction was obtained, 301 (82%) achieved a very good or good clinical result. Despite a perfect reduction and good clinical result, 18 (5%) of the patients in their series still developed osteoarthritis. Of the 126 patients with less than perfect reduction, 81 (65%) still had a very good to excellent result.

Comminution of the acetabular dome

Tile (1984) reported that the degree of comminution of the weight-bearing acetabular dome was important in determining the outcome of acetabular fractures. Pennal et al (1980) found that comminution of the acetabular dome resulted in post-traumatic arthritis in 84% of patients, compared to a 46% incidence of post-traumatic arthritis in those without comminution.

Fracture type

The fracture type is less important than residual acetabular displacement in determining the long-term results. Pennal et al (1980) pointed out that single-column fractures carried a better overall prognosis than two-column fractures, and that the T-fracture carried the worst prognosis of the two-column fractures. Matta (1996) found no significant association between fracture type and outcome with the exception of a cluster of poor results in the T-shaped posterior wall type (five of 14 cases). Letournel & Judet (1993) reported excellent and good clinical results in over 80% of cases, whatever the fracture type, following operative treatment.

Age of the patient

Pennal et al (1980) reported that patients over the age of 40 had significantly worse results following acetabular fractures. Letournel & Judet (1993) reported an 82% incidence of very good or excellent results in 259 patients aged under 40, but only a 64% incidence in 233 patients over 40, while Matta (1996) found 81% of 134 patients aged less than 40 years had good or excellent results compared to 68% of 96 patients aged over 40.

Delay to treatment

Johnson et al (1994) reported a multicentre review of patients treated after 21 days from injury. They showed that the results were poorer than studies of early treatment, with good or excellent results seen in only 65% of cases.

Associated injuries to the pelvic ring or femoral head

Pennal et al (1980) also identified certain other pelvic ring injuries associated with a poor result when combined with an acetabular fracture. They found that disruption of the pubic symphysis, a double vertical fracture (of the Malgaigne type) and an associated fracture, extending from the weight-bearing aspect of the acetabulum to the iliac crest, were all associated with a poorer result than would be expected from the acetabular injury alone. Similarly, Austin (1971), Rowe & Lowell (1961) and Tile (1984) pointed out that acetabular injuries with associated femoral head fractures have an increased risk of developing post-traumatic arthritis. Matta (1996) found 60% good or excellent results in the 50 hips with femoral head damage compared to 80% in the 212 hips with no such damage.

Incidence of osteoarthritis and avascular necrosis

The development of osteoarthritis depends mainly upon the degree of residual acetabular displacement and the damage to the femoral head. Letournel & Judet (1993) reported osteoarthritis in 116 (24%) of 492 patients treated operatively and subsequently reviewed. This is difficult to compare with Pennal et al's 1980 report of 56% degenerative change (58 out of 103 acetabular fractures). However, this brings us back to Tile's 1984 point regarding the comparison of dissimilar cases. The different incidence may well be explained by the fact that all of Letournel & Judet's patients were treated operatively, compared with only 33% of Pennal et al's. Matta (1996) found osteoarthritic change in 46%, of which 23% was mild, 11% moderate and 12% severe. There was a strong association between the radiographic and clinical results. Poor results were seen in wear of the femoral head (12 of 13 hips) and osteonecrosis (six of eight hips). Ruesch et al (1994) found osteoathritis in 40% of 89 hips (mild 20%, moderate 10% and severe 10%). Letournel and Judet (1993) reported osteonecrosis in 3% of 492 fractures.

Timing of medico-legal reports

From the medico-legal point of view, the time when these injuries stabilise is important. Rowe & Lowell (1961), Austin (1971) and Pennal et al (1980) all reported that the functional level 1 year after injury provided an accurate measure of the final outcome. This was well summarised by Lowell (1979), who suggested that a 1 year rule can be devised that allows considerable accuracy in predicting prognosis. Ninety-four percent of patients rated excellent or good 1 year after injury will remain so. Ninety-one percent of patients ultimately developing significant osteoarthritis or avascular necrosis will show at least early changes at the end of this same period, or will have failed to achieve good or excellent function.

However, the long-term follow-up results presented in Letournel & Judet's book (1993) are interesting. Of 110 patients operated on between 1966 and 1971, 89 were classified as very good or excellent in 1971. When reviewed in 1978, three had deteriorated and in 1990 a further four. Of the 87 patients operated on between 1971 and 1978, 57 were rated as excellent in 1978 but seven had deteriorated by 1990. However, of the 18 very good results in this group in 1978, 11 deteriorated. Similarly, Matta (1996) found that with longer follow-up, patients with imperfect reductions were more likely to have a poorer outcome. Lovell's 1 year rule could be qualified such that patients with an anatomical reduction and an excellent clinical result at 1 year are likely to remain so in the longer term. Prognosis in other groups should be more guarded.

Timing of return to work and leisure activities

Pennal et al (1980) found that 71% of their 103 patients returned to their original occupations. The average time lost from work was 11 months. Within this group, 34 patients were treated surgically, and 67% of these were able to return to their original occupations after an average time off work of 12 months (with a range of 3.5–26 months). The slight delay in return to work in the surgically treated group probably reflects the increased severity of the surgically treated injuries, together with the complications inherent in the surgery itself.

Austin (1971) followed up 25 patients for 4–20 years after their injury. Of these, 17 were treated conservatively and in none of these was an anatomical position obtained. Of the eight who underwent open reduction, only two had an anatomical reduction, while six reductions were unsuccessful or incomplete. In this group 20 patients were able to follow their normal or equivalent occupations. Five (20%) had to change their jobs. Of the 19 who were involved in active pastimes, eight (42%) had to modify their leisure activities.

Complications of surgical treatment

Tile (1984) pointed out that some of the late complications of acetabular fractures are inherent in the fracture (i.e. due to type, degree of displacement and degree of comminution), whereas others are a consequence of the treatment. The majority of the results quoted in this section originate from centres with a special interest and expertise in acetabular fractures. Most orthopaedic surgeons will not treat enough acetabular fractures to develop such expertise. Indeed, Tile et al (1985) pointed out that the results of surgical treatment of acetabular fractures varied markedly with the skill of the surgical team.

Certain complications, such as venous thrombosis or infection, may occur after any operation. Other complications are specific to this type of surgery, such as sciatic nerve palsy and heterotopic ossification.

Sciatic nerve palsy

Fassler et al (1993) pointed out that sciatic nerve injury associated with an acetabular fracture occurs most commonly when the femoral head is dislocated posteriorly.

Letournel & Judet (1993) reported 36 postoperative sciatic nerve palsies in 569 patients (6.3%). Thirty-four of these occurred early, whereas two developed later. Of the 34 patients with immediate postoperative palsies, 19 had not been examined adequately pre-operatively. Therefore, some of these palsies may have been present before operation. As this happened in a centre of excellence, it is important to stress the early assessment of sciatic nerve function because of the obvious medico-legal implications.

The incidence of sciatic nerve palsy was 9% in 377 posterior approaches but only 2% in 179 ilioinguinal approaches in this series. Letournel & Judet reviewed the 34 immediate postoperative palsies and found that nine (26%) had totally recovered, 12 (35%) made a good recovery and one did not recover at all. They concluded that 'While serious, the prognosis of post-operative sciatic nerve palsy is not especially gloomy'. Recovery takes place up to 3 years after operation.

Tile et al (1985) reported six postoperative sciatic nerve palsies in 102 displaced acetabular fractures, of which five (83%) recovered fully. They also reported 16 cases of post-traumatic sciatic nerve palsy in their 102 cases, i.e. an incidence of 15%. Only four of these made a complete recovery, i.e. in this group of patients there is a 12% incidence of permanent nerve deficit as a result of injury. The degree of disability is not clear. This figure is similar to that quoted by Wilson (1982), who found a 10% incidence of permanent sciatic nerve paralysis in 40 patients.

Fassler et al (1993) gave a detailed assessment of the functional outcome in 14 patients who had an injury of the sciatic nerve associated with an acetabular fracture. In three of the patients the injury was iatrogenic. They found that all but one of the patients had a satisfactory (fair or better) outcome, but 11 had residual neurological sequelae ranging from minor paraesthesiae to foot drop.

Matta (1996) found 32 (12%) injury-related nerve palsies out of 262 hips. Nine further palsies (3%) occurred during surgery. The clinical results did not appear to be significantly different to those without palsy.

Heterotopic ossification

Letournel & Judet (1993) reported heterotopic ossification in 139 of 569 patients (24%), while Tile et al (1985) found that it occurred in 18 of 102 cases (17.5%). It appeared early on the postoperative X-rays and matured 6–12 months after the operation. In the cases reported by Letournel & Judet (1993), 78% had no or minimal restriction of movement and only 14 came to excision of the bone. Matta (1996) found heterotopic ossification in 18% of their series, of which half had a 20% loss of motion. The incidence was approach related, occurring in 8% of the 112 Kocher-Langebeck, 20% of the 59 extended iliofemoral approaches but only 2% of the 87 ilioinguinal approaches.

The incidence of heterotopic ossification is considerably lower in the cases treated conservatively, Rowe & Lowell (1961) and Pennal et al (1980) reported a figure of only 5% in their series.

Total hip arthroplasty after acetabular fractures

The reported incidence of osteoarthritis after fractures of the acetabulum ranges from 24 to 56% (Pennal et al 1980, Letournel & Judet 1993 and Matta 1996). Factors that predispose to degenerative arthritis include comminution, involvement of the weight-bearing surface and malunion. Avascular necrosis of the femoral head occurs in 3% of cases.

The early Wrightington experience was that many technical difficulties were encountered at operation in a series of 66 cemented arthroplasties (Boardman & Charnley 1978). Difficulty in dislocation of the hip was found in over 50%. There were defects in the acetabular rim in 21% and in the floor in 9%. The acetabulum was enlarged in 13% requiring more cement than usual. The mean age at fracture was 40 years and at arthroplasty 55 years. Pain, function and movement were improved from 3.1, 2.9 and 2.8 (out of a maximum of 6) to 5.9, 5.6 and 5.5 respectively.

The largest series (66 arthroplasties) with the longest follow-up (mean 9.6 years) is from the Mayo Clinic (Weber et al 1998), in patients who had had operative treatment of their acetabular fracture. The prostheses used were a mixture of cemented and uncemented components. The mean age at fracture was 43 years and at arthroplasty 52 years. Three patients had died by the time of review and three were lost to follow-up. The mean rise in the Harris Hip Score was from 49 pre-operatively to 93 (out of a maximum of 100) at latest review in those patients who were not revised. Seventeen arthroplasties were revised of which 16 were for aseptic loosening (nine acetabular and 11 femoral components) and one for recurrent dislocation. Of the unrevised cases, radiographic loosening was observed in a further nine (14%) of the hips, six acetabular and four femoral components.

Survivorship analysis with revision as failure at 10 years was 76%, dropping to 67% at 15 years. If mechanical failure (revision or loosening) is used as the endpoint then the survivorship figures at 10 and 15 years are 73% and 60% respectively. Patients with combined cavitatory and segmental bone loss in the acetabulum pre-operatively were associated with poor survival of the acetabular component at 10 years (27% versus 93% for the rest of the group). Failure was higher in younger males.

Heterotopic ossification is a significant problem in these patients with extensive new bone seen in 22% of the Wrightington series. A leg length discrepancy was noted before operation in 73% of patients which is improved by surgery to 13%. Sciatic nerve palsy was not reported to be more common than usual with hip arthroplasty.

Summary

- Following acetabular fractures, accurate prognosis may be given approximately 1 year after the injury in those patients who have a good result with an anatomical reduction. The functional level at that time is an accurate reflection of the final outcome. In those patients where the reduction is less than perfect (more than 1 mm displacement) prognosis needs to be more guarded.

- Comminution of the superior weight-bearing surface of the acetabulum is a poor prognostic sign.

- The type of acetabular fracture has some bearing on the end-result, T-fractures faring worst. In posterior fractures, where there is also hip dislocation, subsequent avascular necrosis of the femoral head may give rise to a poor result despite a good anatomical reduction.

- Additional damage to the pelvic ring (through the pubic symphysis, iliac wing or sacroiliac joint) worsens the prognosis, as does associated femoral head fracture.

- Patients over the age of 40 fare worse than those under 40.

- The most significant indicator of long-term prognosis is the amount of residual displacement of the articular surface at the conclusion of treatment. Residual displacement of greater than 1 mm is associated with a less satisfactory result.

- There is a 5–12% incidence of permanent sciatic nerve deficit after acetabular fractures. The incidence of sciatic nerve deficit increases after operative treatment, particularly when a posterior approach is used. The prognosis of postoperative sciatic nerve palsy is good.

- There is a small (5% or less) incidence of heterotopic ossification in conservatively treated patients. This increases to 20–30% following operation. Over 75% of these cases are either not functionally impaired or have only minimal limitation of motion.

- Total hip arthroplasty performed for late problems after fracture dislocations about the hip provides good relief of pain and improvement in function and movement.

- The average age at arthroplasty is in the middle of the sixth decade, 5–15 years after the fracture.

- The long-term outlook for the arthroplasty is worse than would be expected for a similar young male with osteoarthritis that was not traumatic in nature, mainly due to acetabular component failure. The expected revision rate at 10 years is 24%. Technical difficulties at operation may explain some of these poor results.

- Significant heterotopic ossification occurs in 22% of arthroplasties in this situation.

Hip dislocations and femoral head fractures

Anterior dislocations

The two largest series of anterior dislocation of the hip were reported by Epstein (1980) and Brav (1962). There were 54 cases with a mean follow-up of 70 months in Epstein's series and 34 cases with a mean follow-up of 80 months in Brav's—88 cases in all. More recently, Dreinhofer et al (1994) have reported on a further 12 patients with a mean follow-up of 8 years. The results were classified after Thompson & Epstein (1951), as shown in Table 11.1. The clinical results are shown in Table 11.2.

There was an overall incidence of excellent/good results of 76% and fair/poor results of 24%. There were five cases of avascular necrosis reported in the three series (5%). Epstein quoted an incidence of post-traumatic arthritis of 17% and of myositis ossificans of 4%. These occurred in patients with fair or poor results. Despite the relatively high incidence of satisfactory (excellent/good) results in Brav's series, only 10 (29%) had no trouble at all with the hip and only 19 (56%) felt that they could engage in all ordinary activities.

Posterior dislocations

Evaluation of the results following posterior dislocation of the hip is difficult because of the differing classifications used in reports of this condition. As the Thompson & Epstein (1951) classification is the most widely used and because Epstein (1980) has reported, in his monograph, the largest series of cases on record, this classification will be used here.

The five types of posterior dislocation according to Thompson & Epstein (1951) are as follows:

- type I—posterior dislocation without fracture
- type II—posterior dislocation with a large posterior acetabular rim fragment
- type III—posterior dislocation with comminution of the posterior acetabular rim
- type IV—posterior dislocation with a fracture of the acetabular rim and floor
- type V—posterior dislocation with fracture of the femoral head

The series of Hunter (1969) and Upadhyay & Moulton (1981) will also be incorporated in the aggregated results. The latter report is particularly useful as it gives

Table 11.1 Classification of results (Thompson & Epstein 1951)

Excellent
1. No pain
2. Full range of movements
3. No limp
4. No X-ray evidence of progressive changes

Good
1. No pain
2. A 75% range of hip movements
3. Slight limp
4. Minimal X-ray changes

Fair
Any one or more of the following:
1. Pain, but not disabling
2. Limited range of hip movements but no adduction deformity
3. Moderate limp
4. Moderate to severe X-ray changes

Poor
Any one or more of the following:
1. Disabling pain
2. Marked limitation of movement or adduction deformity
3. Redislocation
4. Progressive X-ray changes

a much longer mean follow-up (12.5 years) than any other series.

Epstein (1980) assessed his results according to whether closed reduction, closed reduction followed by later open reduction or primary open reduction was employed. However, the results will be presented irrespective of the particular treatment as the numbers within these groups are small.

Type I posterior dislocation (posterior dislocation without fracture or with minimal chip fracture of posterior acetabular rim)

Epstein (1980), Upadhyay & Moulton (1981) and more recently Dreinhofer et al (1994) broke down the results into the categories shown in Table 11.1. The clinical results in 217 patients from these three series are shown in Table 11.3.

As might be expected, there is a much higher chance of a poor clinical result if avascular necrosis of the femoral head occurs. The incidence of avascular necrosis varies from series to series, but overall, as shown in Table 11.4, is approximately 16%.

Dreinhofer et al (1994) found that reduction of the dislocation within 3 hours made no difference to the incidence of avascular necrosis or the clinical result.

Brav (1962) analysed the effect of avascular necrosis on the clinical result. A total of 85 patients had an excellent or good clinical result, only five of these (6%) having avascular necrosis. However, of the 25 patients with a fair or poor clinical result, 19 (76%) had avascular necrosis. Dreinhofer et al (1994) supported these findings.

Upadhyay & Moulton (1981) suggested that 26% of type I dislocations will ultimately develop osteoarthritis. They also commented that there was an impression in the literature that type I injuries had few complications and always gave an excellent result. This does not appear to be the case, particularly when dislocation is complicated by avascular necrosis.

Type II posterior dislocations (where a large posterior acetabular fragment is present)

Brav (1962) found that the incidence of avascular necrosis in type II and III dislocations was 25% (23 of 91 cases). As with the type I dislocations, there was a much greater

Table 11.2 Clinical results following anterior dislocation of the hip

	Epstein (1980)	Dreinhofer et al (1994)	Brav (1962)	Combined series
Excellent	17	9	29	76 (76%)
Good	21			
Fair	11	3	5	24 (24%)
Poor	5			
Total	54	12	34	100

Table 11.3 Clinical results following type I posterior dislocation of the hip (from Epstein 1980, Upadhyay & Moulton 1981, Dreinhofer et al 1994)

Result	Number	%
Excellent/good	141	65
Fair/poor	76	35
Total	217	

Table 11.4 The incidence of avascular necrosis following type I posterior dislocation of the hip

Reference	Number of cases	Number with avascular necrosis
Epstein (1980)	134	20
Brav (1962)	110	24
Upadhyay & Moulton (1981)	53	3
Dreinhofer et al (1994)	30	6
Total	327	53 (16%)

chance of a fair or poor clinical result if avascular necrosis developed. Of 65 excellent or good results, only five (7.7%) had avascular necrosis, but of 26 with fair or poor results, 18 (69%) had avascular necrosis. The results of Epstein (1980) and Upadhyay & Moulton (1981) are summarised in Table 11.5. It can be seen from these figures that Brav reports a higher incidence of excellent/good results in types II and III dislocations than either Epstein or Upadhyay & Moulton. The reason for this is not clear, as the three reports used similar criteria for classifying their results. It is possible that Brav's methods were not quite so stringent as those of Epstein (listed in Table 11.1).

Type III posterior dislocations (posterior dislocations with comminution of the posterior acetabular rim)

The clinical results following type III posterior dislocations are shown in Table 11.6.

The incidence of avascular necrosis in types II and III dislocations is 25% according to Brav's figures. The presence of comminution of the posterior rim appears to worsen the outcome, with a lower incidence of excellent, good and fair results and a higher incidence of poor results.

Type IV posterior dislocation (posterior dislocation with fracture of the acetabular rim and floor)

Epstein (1980) reported 69 patients with this injury, and the clinical results are shown in Table 11.7. The prognosis is significantly worse, with over half of the patients having a poor clinical result. Epstein reported 20 cases (29%) of avascular necrosis in this group.

Type V posterior dislocations (posterior dislocation with fracture of the femoral head)

This injury was reviewed and subclassified by Pipkin (1957) into four types:

Table 11.5 Results following type II posterior dislocation of the hip (from Epstein 1980, Upadhyay & Moulton 1981)

Result	Number	%	
Excellent	5	8	47% excellent/good
Good	24	39	
Fair	16	26	53% fair/poor
Poor	17	27	
Total	62		

Table 11.6 Results following type III posterior dislocation of the hip (from Epstein 1980, Upadhyay & Moulton 1981)

Results	Number	%	
Excellent	0	0	37% excellent/good
Good	53	37	
Fair	30	21	63% fair/poor
Poor	60	42	
Total	143		

Table 11.7 Results following type IV posterior dislocation of the hip (from Epstein 1980)

Results	Number	%	
Excellent	0	0	23% excellent/good
Good	16	23	
Fair	18	26	77% fair/poor
Poor	35	51	
Total	69		

1. Hip dislocation with fracture of the head caudad to fovea centralis
2. Hip dislocation with fracture cephalad to fovea
3. Type 1 or 2 injury combined with fracture of femoral neck
4. Type 1 or 2 injury combined with acetabular rim fracture

Epstein et al (1985) reported 46 cases treated by closed reduction, or by closed followed by open reduction or by primary open reduction. The overall results are shown in Table 11.8.

Marchetti et al (1996) has shown that the results seem to be better in Pipkin types 1 (n=8, 75% good, 25% fair) and 2 (n=9, 78% good, 22% fair). There were only two patients in category 3, one of whom had a good result and one a fair result. In the Pipkin 4 group (n=14) 57% had a good result, 7% fair and 36% poor. There were no excellent results.

These results show that this is an injury with a relatively poor prognosis. The figures also suggested that long-term results were better after primary open reduction than after conservative or delayed open reduction. Epstein (1980) noted only 11 cases (24%) of avascular necrosis in this group, Marchetti et al (1996) an incidence of 10% in 30 cases. Arthritic changes were seen at a mean of 49 months in 75%, but 92% of these were mild and only 8% severe. Dreinhofer et al (1996) found avascular necrosis in five of 26 cases (19%), mild arthritis in four (15%) and moderate in two (8%). The outcome was fair to poor in 15 of 26 cases (58%). Brav (1962) reported an incidence of 70% avascular necrosis in types IV and V dislocations. The reason for this high rate is not clear.

Time from injury to reduction of dislocation

Hougaard & Thomsen (1987) showed that reduction of posterior dislocations more than 6 hours after injury was associated with a significant increase in the incidence of avascular necrosis and osteoarthritis (Table 11.9). This suggests that reduction should be carried out within 6 hours unless contraindicated on other grounds.

The irreducible dislocation

McKee et al (1998) have reported a series of 25 patients who had high energy injuries with dislocations that could not be reduced closed. These were frequently associated with other injuries including sciatic nerve palsies (28%) and femoral head or neck fractures (36%). Only six patients had a good or excellent outcome. Poor results were associated with a delay to reduction or associated femoral head or neck fracture.

Timing of medico-legal reports

It is difficult to forecast accurately a time at which the results following these diverse injuries reach a plateau. Brav (1962) looked at 189 patients with dislocations that were symptomatic at the time of his study. In all, 81 (43%) stated that their hip complaints had been present since the time of injury. Of the remaining 108, 19 (10%) had onset of complaints 2–5 months after injury, 24 (13%) had onset of

Table 11.8 Results following type V posterior dislocation of the hip (from Epstein et al 1985)

Results	Number	%	
Excellent	0	0 ⎫	28% excellent/good
Good	13	28 ⎭	
Fair	11	24 ⎫	7% fair/poor
Poor	22	48 ⎭	
Total	46		

Table 11.9 The development of osteoarthritis and avascular necrosis after posterior dislocation of the hip in relation to time of reduction (adapted from Hougaard & Thomsen 1987)

Time from injury to reduction	Number of patients	Osteoarthritis developed	Avascular necrosis developed
Less than 6 hours	83	25 (30%)	4 (5%)
More than 6 hours	17	13 (76%)	10 (58%)

complaints 6–11 months after injury and 65 (34%) did not develop symptoms until 1 year or more after their injury. In four patients (2%) no symptoms were experienced until 5 years after injury.

Brav (1962) also pointed out that it may take up to 2 years to detect the radiographic changes of avascular necrosis. This should be borne in mind in the timing of medico-legal reports. Modern isotope and magnetic resonance imaging techniques make it possible to assess the vascularity of the femoral head and consequent prognosis for the hip much earlier. After hip dislocation, final medical reports should probably be delayed for 18–24 months from the time of the injury.

Summary

- After anterior dislocation of the hip there is a 76% chance of achieving an excellent or good clinical result.
- Following type I posterior dislocation there is an excellent or good clinical result in 68% of patients. There is a 16% incidence of avascular necrosis, and the clinical result is likely to be worse if avascular necrosis develops.
- Following type II posterior dislocations there is an excellent or good clinical result in 47% of patients. There is a 25% incidence of avascular necrosis, and the clinical result is significantly worse if it does develop.
- Following type III posterior dislocations there were no excellent results; good results were reported in 37% of patients.
- Following type IV posterior dislocations there were no excellent results; good results were reported in only 23% of patients. The incidence of avascular necrosis was 29%.
- Following type V posterior dislocations there were no excellent results; good results were reported in only 28% of patients. Epstein (1980) reported the incidence of avascular necrosis as 24%, and Brav (1962) as 70% in a combined series of types IV and V dislocations. Pipkin types 1 and 2 do better than types 3 and 4.
- Final medico-legal reports may need to be delayed until 18–24 months after the injury.
- The quoted results cannot be related to operative or non-operative management because the subgroups are too small.
- The incidence of avascular necrosis and osteoarthritis is higher in posterior dislocations reduced more than 6 hours after the injury.

Fractures of the neck of the femur

Classification

Both intracapsular and extracapsular fractures of the proximal femur will be considered in this section. The Garden (1961) system will be used to classify the intracapsular fractures, as follows:

- stage I—the abduction or impaction injury, where the inferior cortex has not been completely breached
- stage II—complete fracture without displacement
- stage III—complete fracture with partial displacement
- stage IV—complete fracture with full displacement

It can be difficult to distinguish stage I from stage II, and stage III from stage IV and, as will be shown, both stage I and stage II can often be considered together from a prognostic viewpoint, as can stages III and IV.

Extracapsular or trochanteric fractures tend to be classified according to their stability rather than the situation of the fracture line. Stable fractures consist of two main fragments. Unstable fractures were defined by Dimon & Hughston (1967) as fractures where there is 'lack of continuity of bone cortex on the opposing surfaces of the proximal and distal fragments'. A lesser trochanteric fragment (including the calcar) or a separate posterior fragment will reduce stability, and in the more unstable injuries there may be four or more fragments. On this basis trochanteric fractures will be classified as stable or unstable.

Intracapsular fractures

There is a vast bibliography on the long-term results of intracapsular fractures of the femoral neck. The majority of patients are elderly and have very osteoporotic bone which fractures with relatively minor trauma. In patients under the age of 50 (unless there is osteoporosis secondary to conditions such as renal disease, steroid therapy or alcoholism), fractures of the neck of the femur are usually associated with severe trauma.

It is not the brief of this volume to examine the subtle differences in the results of many different treatment methods for intracapsular fractures of the femur in elderly patients. Nevertheless, the common complications and sequelae of these fractures in elderly patients will be reviewed, as the results do give clues to the outlook in younger patients. The differences in the nature of the trauma and the quality of the bone in those aged under 50 warrant their consideration as a separate group, and they will be reviewed later in this chapter.

There is still much controversy regarding the place of hemiarthroplasty versus reduction and internal fixation in displaced intracapsular fractures. Sikorski & Barrington (1981) showed no difference in mortality between hemiarthroplasty and internal fixation, with Bray & Smith-Hoefer (1988) and Skinner & Riley (1989) agreeing. Revision rates, however, are much lower with hemiarthroplasty (11%) than with internal fixation (42%) in elderly patients with intracapsular fractures. The merits of various types of internal fixation techniques are also disputed. These issues will be addressed, but the two principal complications of avascular necrosis and non-union will be considered in more detail.

The most thorough appraisal of the results, and the factors influencing the results, following subcapital fractures was provided by Barnes et al (1976) in a prospective multicentre study prepared for the British Medical Research Council. Drennan Lowell (1980), in a comprehensive review of the results and complications of femoral neck fractures, observed that reports varied on the incidence of non-union and avascular necrosis rates. Union rates in the literature vary from 66 to 100%, while rates of avascular necrosis and late segmental collapse vary from 7 to 84%. These data require more detailed analysis and, as Barnes et al (1976) indicated, there are many factors which contribute to the end-result. There are those over which the surgeon has no control, such as old age, female sex, osteoporosis and Garden type III or IV fracture, and those over which the surgeon has a measure of control, i.e. acceptance of valgus or varus reduction, extreme retroversion or anteversion in reduction,

positioning of the fixation device and timing of ambulation. These factors are considered in detail in the reports by Barnes et al (1976) and Chua et al (1998). Many recent papers unfortunately group results of displaced and undisplaced fractures, which is unhelpful in predicting outcome in specific fractures. Nevertheless they can give us a good overview of union rates and incidence of avascular necrosis.

The clinical results and complications in Garden stage I/II fractures and Garden stage III/IV fractures will be considered below.

Reduction and internal fixation
Garden stage I/II fractures

Barnes et al (1976) reported on 295 stage I fractures (they classified 19 as stage II and did not report them as a separate group). The results are broken down according to sex and are summarised in Table 11.10. There was little difference between the rates of union in the two sexes; at 6 months it is 153/248 (62%), at 12 months 220/237 (93%) and at 24 months 233/236 (99%). In the same paper the incidence of late segmental collapse was reported as 16% after 3 years follow-up in Garden stage I fractures.

Banks (1962) provided another comprehensive review of intracapsular fractures, albeit with significantly fewer numbers (189 for whom the end-result was definable; 66 of these were Garden stage I or II). There was only a 1 year minimum follow-up. Banks found that 53 of 59 (90%) Garden stage I/II fractures healed with a good clinical result and the rate of avascular necrosis was 4/59 (7%).

Table 11.10 The rate of union related to time after injury in Garden I fractures (adapted from Barnes et al 1976)

Time after injury (months)	Union	
	Female (*n* = 250)	Male (*n* = 45)
6	135/216 (62.5%)	18/32 (56%)
12	192/205 (93.5%)	28/32 (88%)
24	203/204 (99.5%)	30/32 (94%)

Table 11.11 Rates of avascular necrosis after Garden stage I/II fractures

Time after injury (years)	Author	Rate
1	Banks (1962)	7% (4/59)
1	Parker (1994)	5% (9/185)
1	Heyse-Moore (1996)	3% (1/37)
3	Barnes (1976)	16% (38/236)
4	Asnis (1998)	19.5% (8/41)

These results are very similar to those reported by Barnes et al (1976) at 12 months.

Asnis (1994) reported results of 141 patients treated with cannulated hip screws. Of 41 patients with Garden stage I/II fractures, the incidence of avascular necrosis was 19.5% at 4 years. Heyse-Moore (1996) and Parker (1994) both reviewed patients at 1 year following stage I/II fractures. They agree union rates are high (100% and 92% respectively) and avascular necrosis rates are low (3% and 5% respectively). It is clear rates of avascular necrosis rise after 1 year, influencing the timing of any medical report. Rates of avascular necrosis are summarised in Table 11.11.

Garden stage III/IV fractures

When the rate of union is considered following reduction and internal fixation in these fractures, there is little difference between stage III and IV. The union rates are broken down by Barnes et al according to sex and are summarised in Table 11.12.

The incidence of symptomatic avascular necrosis in these patients is important. Swiontkowski (1994) observed that the higher the functional demands on the hip, the more significant the symptoms. Meyers (1985) noted that although avascular necrosis occurs frequently in ununited fractures, progress to late segmental collapse does not occur in these patients. Late segmental collapse occurs only when there is avascular necrosis in association with union of the fracture. Again, there is little difference between stage III and IV fractures in the Barnes series, and the incidence of late segmental collapse is summarised in Table 11.13. It can be seen that there is a significantly higher incidence of late segmental collapse in females. Asnis et al (1994) have shown similar figures with an incidence of avascular necrosis of 25% in stage III/IV fractures and Sikorski & Barrington (1981) showed an incidence of 20%. Lu-Yao et al (1994) performed a meta-analysis of 106 published reports, and noted that stage III/IV fractures had a 16% chance of avascular necrosis and a 33% chance of non-union in the reviewed articles. Rates of avascular necrosis are summarised in Table 11.14.

Table 11.12 The rate of union related to time after injury in Garden III and IV fractures (adapted from Barnes et al 1976)

Time after injury (months)	Union	
	Female (n = 988)	Male (n = 195)
6	117/811 (14%)	16/143 (11%)
12	360/747 (48%)	65/136 (48%)
24	458/728 (63%)	88/131 (67%)
36	474/722 (66%)	93/129 (72%)

Table 11.13 The incidence of late segmental collapse in united Garden III/IV fractures (adapted from Barnes et al 1976)

Time after injury (months)	Females	Males
12	38/360 (10.5%)	2/65 (3%)
24	105/458 (23%)	9/88 (10%)
36	131/474 (28%)	17/83 (18%)

Table 11.14 Rates of avascular necrosis in Garden stage III/IV fractures

Time after injury (years)	Author	Avascular necrosis rate
1	Heyse-Moore (1996)	31% (5/16)
2	Sikorski (1981)	20% (9/44)
3	Barnes (1976)	26% (148/557)
4	Asnis (1994)	25% (18/70)

Residual disability in patients with late segmental collapse is of profound importance in medico-legal reporting. Barnes et al (1976) referred to this in their report, and their findings are reproduced in Table 11.15. Overall, late segmental collapse was disabling in only 53 of 181 patients (29%), and in only 32 of these patients (18% of the total) was a salvage operation performed. In the remaining 128 patients with segmental collapse, the disability was functionally acceptable in 84 (46%) and asymptomatic in 44 (24%).

Holmberg et al (1987) analysed results of 2418 patients admitted for treatment of intracapsular femoral neck fractures. Garden stage is unfortunately not documented, but of 268 patients with late segmental collapse after internal fixation only 160 had symptoms which required arthroplasty.

Stromquist (1983) has documented the risk of developing avascular necrosis and/or non-union based on digitised bone scans obtained in the first 2–3 weeks after injury. A femoral head uptake ratio of 90% or less of the opposite (normal) side translates to an 84% risk of avascular necrosis or non-union.

Endoprosthesis

Patients with endoprostheses were specifically excluded from the Barnes series. Johnson & Crothers (1975) pointed out that the reported incidence of poor results after prosthetic replacement ranged from 12 to 33%. They followed up their patients with Austin Moore hemiarthroplasties for an average of 32 years. Similar reports were provided by Hinchey & Day (1964), Whittaker et al (1972) and Skinner & Riley (1989). The criteria for judging the subjective results in these series vary slightly in their complexity, but can be broadly classified into three groups, as follows:

- Good: no pain or minimal pain; can walk unsupported or with one stick.
- Fair: mild to moderate pain; may require two sticks or a walking frame.
- Poor: pain interfering with normal activities or severe pain; confined to bed or house; secondary operation may be required.

The results are summarised in Table 11.16. In the present context, there is little merit in comparing the detailed results of different endoprostheses following displaced fractures of the femoral neck. No single design is demonstrably superior. Wetherell & Hinves (1990) described the use of a bipolar hemiarthroplasty for displaced subcapital fractures. A group of 91 patients had been followed for a mean of 4 years 10 months and of these 95% had no pain or slight pain. They found that the ratio of acetabular erosion was halved when compared with an earlier group treated with a cemented

Table 11.15 The effect of late segmental collapse on residual disability in intracapsular fractures (from Barnes et al 1976 ©, Journal of Bone and Joint Surgery)

	Females	Males
Salvage operation performed	30 (18%)	2 (11%)
Disabling, but no operation performed	19 (21%)	2 (11%)
Functionally acceptable	77 (47%)	7 (39%)
Asymptomatic	37 (23%)	7 (39%)
Total	163	18

Table 11.16 Clinical results following insertion of endoprostheses for displaced (Garden III/IV) fractures of the femoral neck

Reference	Prosthesis used	Good	Fair	Poor
Johnson et al (1975)	Moore	24	12	8
Anderson et al (1964)	Moore/Thompson	28	4	1
Hinchey & Day (1964)	Moore	67	8	8
Whittaker et al (1972)	Moore/Thompson	65	36	12
Skinner & Riley (1989)	Moore	66	22	15
	Total	250 (66%)	82 (22%)	44 (12%)

Thompson prosthesis at the same institution. They reviewed the literature and found an incidence of good or excellent results in 47 to 82% of patients treated with single compartment hemiarthroplasty (Austin Moore/Thompson) compared to 70 to 94% with biarticular prostheses. Bray et al (1987) and Skinner & Riley (1989) agree that the mortality associated with hemiarthroplasty is not statistically different from that of internal fixation. Sikorski & Barrington (1981) showed a dislocation rate of 4% after hemiarthroplasty and Koval et al (1996) a dislocation rate of <2%.

Total hip replacement as a primary treatment for intracapsular femoral neck fracture

Total hip replacement as a primary treatment of intracapsular hip fractures has been advocated in those patients with pre-existing disease of the hip, i.e. osteoarthritis or rheumatoid arthritis. It has also been recommended as the primary treatment of displaced fractures to avoid some of the complications of hemiarthroplasty, e.g. loosening and acetabular erosion.

The follow-up studies are limited by the relatively high mortality figures within the first year after operation pre-venting acquisition of long-term data. Results of representative studies showing postoperative pain relief and function are shown in Table 11.17.

There is good relief of pain following hip replacement. However, there is not such a predictable effect on mobility because of pre-existing medical and mobility problems. A recent paper by Squires and Bannister (1999) compared the outcome of patients who had either a primary total hip replacement or a hemiarthroplasty for displaced intracapsular femoral neck fractures and who were mobile and socially independent prior to their injury. At a mean follow-up of 3.8 years, 86% of 32 patients who had a total hip replacement had a good or excellent result as measured by the Harris Hip Score compared to only 12% of 42 patients who had a hemiarthroplasty.

Several authors have drawn attention to the high complication rate when this is performed as a primary procedure (Table 11.18). It is generally felt that the high dislocation rate is attributable to the good pre-operative range of movement not usually seen with hip replacements for osteoarthritis. The low incidence of dislocation in Delamarter's 1987 series may be influenced by a high

Table 11.17 Clinical results of total hip replacement as primary treatment of intracapsular hip fracture

Author	No	Mean FU (mths)	Pain		Function	
			None/Mild	Mod/Sev	Good/Exc	Satis/Poor
Coates 1980	54	17	89%	11%	87%	13%
Sim 1980	85	12	99%	1%	61%	39%
Taine 1985	57	42	98%	2%	61%	39%
Delamarter 1987	27	45	85%	15%	70%	30%
Chiu 1995	40	74	100%	0%	85%	15%
Total	249	38	94%	6%	73%	27%

Table 11.18 Complications following THR as primary treatment of displaced hip fracture

Author	No	FU mths	Dislocation	Infection	Loose	Revisions
Coates 1980	54	17	8%	7%	N/A	2%
Sim 1980	85	12	11%	1%	0%	1%
Taine 1985	57	42	12%	3%	6%	11%
Delamarter 1987	27	45	0%	4%	0%	0%
Greenough 1988	37	56	8%	3%	54%	32%
Chiu 1995	40	74	10%	0%	5%	2.5%
Squires 1999	32	41	6%	0%	N/A	0%
Total	332	41	8%	3%	13%	8%

percentage of patients already showing signs of arthritis in their fractured hips which is likely to reduce dislocation rate. The overall high incidence of loosening may be due to a combination of imperfect technique and poor bone quality. Although the operative procedure for total hip replacement involves more extensive surgery than either hemiarthroplasty or internal fixation there is no significant increase in mortality. The good results in the series reported by Chiu et al (1995) may be partly because of a relatively young group of patients aged 52–72 years at operation. The results of Squires and Bannister (1999) suggest that in the mobile and socially independent patient total hip replacement is better than hemiarthoplasty in the short term. Young patients with displaced intracapsular fractures should have reduction and internal fixation of the fracture, total hip replacement being reserved for a failure of fixation should that ensue (Parker & Pryor 1993).

The outcome of total hip arthroplasty done as a salvage procedure following failure of initial treatment of a femoral neck fracture

The incidence of non-union after reduction of displaced femoral neck fractures (Garden III/IV) and fixation using a variety of methods averages 21% on meta-analysis (Parker & Pryor 1993). The majority of the 21% will have further surgery for disabling symptoms. The incidence of radiological evidence of late segmental collapse due to avascular necrosis following reduction and internal fixation of these fractures averages 12% on meta-analysis (Parker & Pryor 1993). However, only one-third to one-half of these with radiological changes of avascular necrosis have symptoms of sufficient severity to merit further surgery (Christie et al 1988, Stromqvist et al 1984). Younger and more active patients more frequently require further surgery. Total hip arthroplasty is the most common re-operation performed for non-union and late segmental collapse. In a large consecutive series of 640 cases of displaced hip fractures treated initially by reduction and fixation, 18% subsequently went on to have a secondary hip arthroplasty because of failure of the primary treatment (Nilsson 1989). Parker & Pryor (1993) suggested that the overall estimated re-operation rate for failure of internal fixation requiring conversion to total hip replacement is approximately 24%.

Similarly, there is a conversion rate of failed hemiarthroplasty to hip replacement. The usual indications are loosening (10% of endoprostheses performed), acetabular erosion (19%) and fracture of the femur around the prosthesis (6%)

Table 11.19 The early clinical results following conversion of failed endoprosthesis or internal fixation to total hip replacement

	No	FU	Pain		Mobility	
			Good/Exc	Fair/Poor	Good/Exc	Fair/Poor
Sarmiento 1978	90	33 mth	98%	2%	93%	7%
Amstutz 1979	41	3 yr	70%	30%	70%	30%*
Turner 1984	205	2.8 yr	89%	11%	75%	25%
Stambough 1.986	59	6.2 yr	95%	5%**		
Total	395	3.7 yr	88%	12%	79%	21%

* figures for pain and mobility in this paper were combined
** figures based on survival data

Table 11.20 Complications of conversion operations to total hip replacement after failed endo prosthesis or internal fixation

	No	FU	Dislocation	Infection	Loosening
Sarmiento 1978	90	33 mth	3 (3.3%)	2 (2.2%)	5 (5.5%)
Amstutz 1979	41	3 yr	2 (4.9%)	6 (14.6%)	17 (41.5%)
Turner 1984	205	2.8 yr	9 (4.4%)	8 (3.9%)	7 (3.4%)
Franzen 1990	84	5–12 yr	5 (6%)	2 (2.4%)	8 (8.9%)
Total	420	3.4 yr	4.5%	4.3%	8.8%

(Parker & Pryor 1993). Not all come to re-operation, the number varying between 2% (Obrant & Carlson 1987) and 24% (Kofoed & Kofod 1983). The use of an uncemented hemiarthroplasty prosthesis appears to be associated with an increased likelihood of revision (Kofoed & Kofod 1983). The meta-analysis suggests the re-operation rate for failed hemiarthroplasty and conversion to total hip replacement is approximately 9% (Parker & Pryor 1993).

The early results of surgery for these indications show a predictable relief of pain and return of function after the total hip replacement (Table 11.19). The early clinical results of conversions to hip replacement have been found by some authors (Amstutz & Smith 1979 and Stambough et al 1986) to be similar to primary total hip replacements. The complications associated with these conversions to hip arthroplasty are similar to those seen after primary total hip replacement performed for osteoarthritis but some deserve special mention (Table 11.20). Poor clinical results appear to be related to sepsis, dislocation and pre-existing co-morbidity that prevents mobilisation.

There are two longer-term follow-up studies which look at survival of the implant. Franzen et al (1990) compared the results of secondary total hip replacement for failure of primary internal fixation of femoral neck fractures with a similar group of patients who had hip replacements for osteoarthritis at the same institution. Overall, the prosthetic failure rate was 2.5 times higher after failure of fixation of femoral neck fracture. This was age specific, however, the increased risk applicable only to those aged over 70 years. Loosening was always of the femoral component, no acetabular loosenings being seen. The overall risk of revision was 15% at 5 years.

Llinas et al (1991) compared survival analyses of converted hemiarthroplasties to standard primary total hip replacements performed for arthritis. Total hip replacements done as conversions from hemiarthroplasties showed no greater incidence of loosening of the acetabular component but the risk of femoral loosening was significantly higher (30% at 10 years). This is probably related to previous violation of the medullary canal of the femur by the hemiarthroplasty. The risk of re-operation after the conversion to total hip replacement was 6% at a mean of 7 years. The lower revision rate of hip replacements done in this study may be due to the age group being younger than that in Franzen's study (1990).

Extracapsular (trochanteric) fractures

The problems of non-union and avascular necrosis are infrequent in trochanteric fractures. An excellent review of the results following internal fixation of trochanteric frac-

tures was provided in two separate papers by Steen Jensen et al (1980a,b), one dealing with stable fractures, and one with unstable fractures (375 and 1071 fractures respectively). Stable fractures treated with a variety of methods healed well, with 93% healing in the postoperative position. Four percent of patients required re-operation due to fixation failure. Of the 1071 unstable fractures, 346 were treated with a dynamic hip screw (DHS). There were 21 failures (6%). Failure rates with other forms of treatment were much higher (McLaughlin and Jewett nail plates and Enders nails). The authors concluded that sliding screw-plate fixation was the only suitable method of fixation for unstable intertrochanteric fractures because of its low failure rate and its low re-operation rate.

These findings were supported by Regazzoni & Reudi (1985) in a paper on the AO dynamic hip screw which reported an incidence of 0.5% of cases (three of 530) of avascular necrosis of the femoral head following trochanteric fractures. Further work by Koval et al (1996) has again shown the sliding screw-plate to result in low rates of failure, with only 2.2% (three of 138) failure of fixation in stable fractures and 4.3% (three of 70) failure in unstable fractures. Five of these six failures could be attributed to poor surgical technique.

Poor surgical technique has been shown to cause a high rate of failure of hip screws. Davis et al (1990) showed an overall DHS cut out rate of 12.6% when they performed a prospective study on 230 intertrochanteric fractures. Posterior placed screws had a cut out rate of 28% (13 of 46) whereas central screws had a cut out rate of only 7% (nine of 121).

There have been several good prospective randomised trials comparing treatment of extra capsular femoral neck fractures with either DHS, intra-medullary hip screw or gamma nails. Bridle and Patel et al (1991) looked at 100 fractures and were unable to demonstrate a clinical difference in outcome between groups (DHS v. gamma nail). There were no differences in operating time, blood loss, wound complications, hospital stay or patient mobility. Cut out rates were equal (6% v. 4%). They did, however, have an 8% (four of 50) femoral shaft fracture at the tip of the gamma nail postoperatively, which obviously necessitated further major surgery. O'Brien and Meek et al (1995) also failed to demonstrate a difference between DHS fixation and the gamma nail. In their series of 102 patients they did notice that there was a higher incidence of local complications during insertion of the gamma nail. They therefore concluded that the DHS should be the implant of choice for intertrochanteric fractures. Madsen et al (1998) did show the DHS to be superior to the Gamma nail. Overall in the 175 patients they treated with unstable trochanteric fractures there was a 5.9% re-operation rate with the DHS and an 8% re-operation rate with the gamma nail. This group of patients included two (4%) with fractures of the femoral shaft at the tip of the nail.

Fractures of the femoral neck in adults under the age of 50

This group is singled out because there is more likelihood of litigation following femoral neck fractures in those aged under 50 due to the nature of the trauma involved. Klenerman (1985) thought that fractures in patients under 50 were rare because their bone was dense and therefore considerable violence was required to break it. However, in young adults with osteoporosis from an underlying condition such as steroid therapy, chronic renal failure or alcoholism, only slight trauma may be required to fracture the neck of the femur, and these cases behave like those in elderly patients. Interestingly, while alcoholism can result in osteonecrosis of the femoral head, alcoholic patients do not appear to be at increased risk after fixation of displaced subcapital femoral neck fractures. Nyquist et al (1998) reviewed 512 consecutive male patients with intracapsular fractures, of whom 82 were registered as high alcohol consumers. No significant difference from other groups could be identified. Klenerman (1985) suggested that the complications of intracapsular fractures of the femoral neck in young patients were higher than in the elderly. Wu & Shih (1993) confirmed that this also held in a study of two groups of patients with intertrochanteric fractures treated with a dynamic hip screw. In the over 60s the incidence of complications was 0.67% (one deep infection), while in the under 60s the incidence of complications was 10% (two deep infections, three side plate breakages, one avascular necrosis of the femoral head, one non-union and one lag screw penetration).

The published results vary considerably, particularly in their assessment of the frequency of avascular necrosis and non-union. Protzman & Burkhalter (1976) reported a 59% incidence of non-union and an 86% incidence of avascular necrosis in 22 fractures in patients aged 22–40. Other reports, such as those of Kofoed (1982), Kulisch & Gustilo (1976), Askin & Bryan (1976) and Swiontkowski et al (1984), described a lower incidence of these complications than did Protzman & Burkhalter. All of these reports have adequate follow-up and criteria for avascular necrosis and non-union. The results are summarized in Table 11.21.

The Garden fracture classification is clearly outlined only in the work of Swiontkowski et al, Kofoed and Askin & Bryan. Protzman & Burkhalter (1976) commented that 'most were markedly displaced', but did not define the Garden stage for each patient. Analysis of the reports in which the Garden staging is clearly categorised has enabled the results in Table 11.22 to be produced.

These results merit emphasis of the following points:

■ They come from differing institutions with different approaches to documentation and treatment. The

Table 11.21 The incidence of avascular necrosis and non-union following intracapsular fractures of the neck of the femur in adults under the age of 50 (cases with associated medical problems and secondary osteoporosis excluded)

Reference	Number of cases	Avascular necrosis	Non-union
Protzman & Burkhalter (1976)	22	19	13
Kofoed (1982)	17	7	4
Kulisch & Gustilo (1976)	20	9	5
Swiontkowski et al (1984)	21	4	0
Askin & Bryan (1976)	16	3	3
Total	96	42 (44%)	25 (26%)

Table 11.22 The incidence of avascular necrosis and non-union according to Garden stage in patients under the age of 50

	Number	Avascular necrosis	Non-union
Garden stage I/II	14	2 (14%)	1 (7%)
Garden stage III/IV	40	12 (30%)	6 (15%)

poorest results (Protzman & Burkhalter 1976) were compiled from seven military hospitals and a wide variety of fixation devices were used. The best results (Swiontkowski et al 1984) emanate from a single centre with a specific interest in trauma, where the fractures were treated as emergencies (within 8 hours of injury) and were fixed with 6.5 mm cancellous screws after adequate reduction.

■ Although Protzman & Burkhalter (1976) comment that most of their fractures were markedly displaced, this does not help in the interpretation of their results according to Garden staging. This undoubtedly causes a bias in the results in Table 11.22, for if the Protzman & Burkhalter results could be included there would be a considerably higher incidence of avascular necrosis and non-union.

■ The question of the accuracy of reduction was addressed by Kofoed (1982). He found that when final reduction was good there was usually union without late segmental collapse (10 of 12 patients), whereas when there was malreduction (degree not specified), all five patients developed union with late segmental collapse.

Recent work by Chua et al (1998) states that the two most important predictors of fixation failure were varus reduction and perceived difficulty in achieving reduction. If the patient had a varus reduction or the surgeon had difficulty achieving a satisfactory reduction then fixation was 4.3 times more likely to fail. If the patient had a varus reduction and the reduction was difficult, fixation was 13.6 times more likely to fail. Under the latter scenario, 75% of fixations failed. They also found that women have a statistically higher rate of fixation failure (39.4% female v. 15.8% male).

An excellent follow-up study of intracapsular fractures in those aged under 50 was provided by Zetterberg et al (1982). Unfortunately, 38% of the 108 patients had concomitant disease leading to osteoporosis, and these patients are not identified in their results. The complication rate in this group has therefore not been reported here.

One interesting observation that the authors made concerned the working capacity of their patients. Of 48 patients who worked prior to their accident, only 27 (56%) were able to return to their former job; in other words, 44% had a reduced working capacity. In the military context, Protzman & Burkhalter (1976) found that only one of 21 patients with this injury was able to return to full duty.

Hulleberg & Finsen (1990) reported that many patients complain of pain after their hip fractures have healed. They report on 34 patients (27 intracapsular and seven extracapsular fractures) whose metal implants were removed. There was significant improvement in the pain in 64%, usually occurring within 3 months. Four out of nine patients with segmental collapse of the head of the femur improved.

Summary

■ In Garden stage I/II intracapsular fractures of the neck of the femur, union occurred in approximately 95% of patients at 12 months. Rates of early avascular necrosis are approximately 4%. Late segmental collapse occurred in 16–19.5% of cases at 3 years.

■ In Garden stage III/IV intracapsular fractures of the neck of the femur, union occurred in approximately 50% of patients at 12 months following reduction and internal fixation. By 24 months (with no further treatment) union occurred in 66–72% of patients.

■ In Garden stage III/IV intracapsular fractures of the neck of the femur, late segmental collapse occurred in 28% of women and 18% of men by 36 months, but not in the presence of non-union.

■ Although late segmental collapse occurred in 181 patients, it was disabling in only 53 (29%). In 32 of these (i.e. 18% of the total number with late segmental collapse) a salvage procedure was performed.

■ Hemiarthroplasty was associated with good results in 67%, fair results in 22% and poor results in 11% with follow-up of over 3 years in an elderly population.

■ Total hip replacement as a primary procedure for displaced fractures of the neck of the femur produces reliable relief of pain. Function is dependent on the pre-fracture status.

■ Primary hip replacement for fractured neck of the femur is associated with a high dislocation rate (9%), high infection rate (3%) and high incidence of early loosening (up to 54%).

■ The average failure rate of internal fixation is 24% and that of failed endoprosthesis 9%. The early clinical results of conversions to total hip replacements are similar to those for primary total hip replacements performed for osteoarthritis.

■ Failure due to sepsis (4.3%) is much higher in conversion operations than would be expected of a primary hip replacement for osteoarthritis (<1%).

■ Loosening of the prosthesis in conversion operations leading to re-operation (up to 15% at 5 years) is more common than that occurring following a routine hip replacement for osteoarthritis (less than 5% at 5 years). Prosthetic failure is more likely in the elderly and usually involves the femoral component.

- Stable intertrochanteric fractures of the femur united in 95–100% of patients irrespective of the type of implant used.
- Unstable intertrochanteric fractures were associated with a small incidence of non-union (0–2%, depending on the selection of implant). There was a higher risk of implant failure with unstable fractures. The lowest rate of implant failure (2.5–12.6%) was associated with the sliding screw-plate.
- In patients under the age of 50 with intracapsular fractures of the neck of the femur but with no associated osteoporosis, the overall incidence of avascular necrosis was 44% and of non-union 26%. There was evidence that this could be reduced by early emergency treatment, accurate reduction and rigid internal fixation.
- In patients under the age of 50 with intracapsular fractures of the neck of the femur, there was a 44% chance that their working capacity would be reduced as a result of the injury.

Fractures and dislocations about the hip in children

Fractures: proximal femoral

Fractures of the proximal femur are much less common in children than in adults. Lam (1971) reviewed the world literature on the subject and found 652 reported cases. Colonna (1929) described the most widely used classification of these fractures:

- type I—transphyseal
- type II—transcervical
- type III—basal cervical/cervicotrochanteric
- type IV—intertrochanteric

Some authors, such as Miller (1973) and Meyers (1985), have extended the classification to include subtrochanteric fractures, and these will be considered in Chapter 13. Most of the reports of these fractures give only a 5–6 year follow-up, although reports by Canale & Bourland (1977) and Leung & Lam (1986) gave a mean follow-up of 17–18 years, which is of great relevance when providing medicolegal reports. The classification of long-term results into good, fair and poor follows the criteria described by Ratliff (1962), as shown in Table 11.23.

Type I (transphyseal fractures)

As Meyers (1985), Miller (1973) and Ratliff (1962) stated, this diagnosis can be made only when there is a clear history of severe trauma; otherwise the diagnosis is of a slipped upper femoral epiphysis. There are insufficient numbers in the literature to allow comparison of different treatment methods. If there is severe displacement or associated hip joint dislocation the long-term results are poor. Canale & Bourland (1977) reported on five such patients, all of whom developed avascular necrosis; four also developed premature growth plate closure. The mean follow-up of those five patients was 30 years (range 18–43 years). Four had poor results, with severe arthritis or fibrous ankylosis, following avascular necrosis. Ng & Cole (1996) have recorded four cases of type I fractures and despite early reduction and fixation three developed avascular necrosis. Pforringer & Rosemeyer (1980) also had four documented cases. Two children had avascular necrosis with poor results and one had premature epiphyseal closure.

Miller (1973) reported on 11 patients, but the follow-up was much shorter (mean 3 years). In the three patients with severe displacement there were two poor results and one fair result. He described five patients with minimal displacement, their ages ranging from 7 weeks to

Table 11.23 Results of femoral neck fractures in children (after Ratliff 1962)			
	Good	**Fair**	**Poor**
Pain	None or patient ignores it	Occasional	Disabling
Movement	Full or only terminal restriction	Over 50%	Less than 50%
Activity	Normal or patient avoids games	Normal or patient avoids games	Restricted
X-ray	Normal or some deformity of femoral neck	Severe deformity of femoral neck and mild avascular necrosis	Severe avascular necrosis; arthritis; ankylosis

22 months; all subsequently had normal hips with no problems at follow-up (mean 18 months).

Type II (transcervical fractures)

Canale & Bourland (1977) provided the most comprehensive review of these fractures, reporting on 27 patients. There were 22 with displaced transcervical fractures with a mean follow-up of 19.5 years; their ages ranged from 2–16 years (mean 12.5). The majority (18) were treated by gentle closed reduction and fixation with Knowles pins. Fourteen (64%) developed avascular necrosis.

Ratliff (1962) described three distinct patterns of avascular necrosis and stated that it always appeared within 1 year of the injury. Four patients (18%) developed coxa vara (defined as a neck shaft angle of less than 135°). There were two cases of non-union (9%) and 16 patients (73%) suffered premature closure of the proximal femoral epiphysis; four (18%) required secondary operative procedures. At follow-up the result was good in eight patients (36%), fair in seven (32%) and poor in a further seven (32%).

In the five undisplaced transcervical fractures avascular necrosis, non-union and premature epiphyseal closure did not develop. There was one patient who developed coxa vara. At long-term follow-up the results were considered good in all five patients, and no secondary procedure had been performed.

The most important factor affecting the development of complications was the degree of displacement at the time of injury. Meyers (1985), Morrisey (1980) and Canale & Bourland (1977) observed that the incidence of avascular necrosis was related to displacement and the severity of the initial injury and was not influenced by the type of treatment. On the other hand, Canale & Bourland reported that closure of the growth plate was more common when threaded pins that penetrated the growth plate were used.

Type III (basal/cervicotrochanteric fractures)

Lam (1971) reported a follow-up of 18 patients and Canale & Bourland (1977) a follow-up of 22. Of these 40 fractures, 28 (70%) were displaced. In the undisplaced cases, conservative treatment yielded universally good results with neither avascular necrosis nor growth plate closure occurring. Considering the 28 cases with displacement, the complications were as listed in Table 11.24.

The data in Table 11.24 require further expansion. Most patients with displaced fractures in Canale & Bourland's 1977 series were treated by manipulation and fixation (14 of 17), whereas all the 11 patients with displaced fractures in Lam's 1971 series were treated conservatively, with manipulation and plaster hip spica. The complications related to the type of treatment are shown in Table 11.25.

From these results it appears that, as with transcervical fractures, the incidence of avascular necrosis is determined by the severity of the initial injury and is unaffected by the treatment. There was a higher incidence of premature growth plate closure in those cases undergoing internal fixation, which was recognised by Canale & Bourland

Table 11.24 Complications of displaced basal/cervicotrochanteric fractures in children (from Lam 1971 and Canale & Bourland 1977)

Complication	Number	%
Avascular necrosis	10/28	36
Coxa vara	15/28	54
Premature growth plate closure	15/28	54
Non-union	2/28	7

Table 11.25 Complications of basal (cervicotrochanteric) fractures in children related to the use of internal fixation (from Lam 1971 and Canale & Bourland 1977)

Complication	Treatment without internal fixation (n = 14)	Treatment with internal fixation (n = 14)
Avascular necrosis	5 (36%)	5 (36%)
Premature growth plate closure	6 (43%)	9 (64%)
Coxa vara	11 (79%)	2 (14%)
Non-union	2 (14%)	0

(1977) after penetration of the epiphysis with Knowles pins. There was a striking increase in the incidence of coxa vara in those cases treated without internal fixation. Lam (1971) recorded the degree of shortening in the four cases in which premature epiphyseal closure occurred. The ages of the children ranged from 7–15 years (mean 11 years) and the shortening ranged from 1.9–2.5 cm (mean 2.2 cm). Overall, Canale & Bourland (using Ratliff's 1962 grading) found that the long-term results of their displaced cervicotrochanteric fractures were 11 good (65%), three fair (17.5%) and three poor (17.5%). The follow-up in this group of children averaged 13.5 years.

Type IV (intertrochanteric fractures)

Meyers (1985) pointed out that fractures at the intertrochanteric level are the simplest and easiest of all children's hip fractures to treat. There is a low incidence of long-term problems and complications, and avascular necrosis is uncommon. Lam (1971) reported no avascular necrosis in his 13 intertrochanteric fractures, while Canale & Bourland (1977) had one case of an undisplaced intertrochanteric fracture (combined with premature epiphyseal fusion) treated with a hip spica. Jodoin et al (1980) reported no cases of avascular necrosis in 18 type IV fractures. Canale & Bourland (1977) described four displaced intertrochanteric fractures (two treated by abduction hip spica and two by operation); two of these developed coxa vara and one showed premature growth plate closure (following delayed Jewett nailing). The mean

follow-up in this group was 23.5 years (range 7–44 years). The long-term clinical results were good in three patients and fair in the other. There was no delayed union or non-union. Ovesen et al (1989) followed 17 fractures for an average of 18 years. Seven of these were type IV fractures. There were no cases of avascular necrosis and all results were classed as good. One patient had coxa vara.

In the undisplaced fractures the results appeared uniformly good, other than in the case reported by Canale & Bourland.

Significance of initial displacement

In all types of undisplaced fractures there is a high percentage of good results irrespective of the treatment. In displaced fractures the results are much more variable. Table 11.26 shows the final clinical result related to initial displacement from the series of Ratliff (1978), Lam (1971) and Canale & Bourland (1977), comprising 191 patients. Those patients in Lam's series who presented late are excluded, and his cases with minimal displacement are grouped with the undisplaced fractures. In the displaced fractures the fair and poor results are grouped together since in the large series of 170 fractures reported by Ratliff (1978) the fair and poor results were not separated.

Specific complications

Avascular necrosis

Canale & Bourland (1977) and Ratliff (1978) carried out a detailed analysis of those 98 cases in their series that were

Table 11.26 The relationship of initial displacement to the final clinical result (from the combined work of Ratliff 1978, Lam 1971 and Canale & Bourland 1977)

Displaced (n = 204)	
Good results	78 (38%)
Fair/poor results	126 (62%)
Undisplaced (or minimally displaced) (n=86)	
Good results	74 (86%)
Fair results	8 (9%)
Poor results	4 (5%)

Table 11.27 Long-term results of 98 patients with avascular necrosis (from Canale & Bourland 1977, Ratliff 1978)

Results	Number	%
Good	7	7
Fair	35	36
Poor	56	57

complicated by avascular necrosis. In all, 89 (91%) were displaced at the time of injury. Radiographic evidence of avascular necrosis was noted at an average of 9 months following injury by Canale & Bourland. The long-term results in these patients are shown in Table 11.27. The average follow-up was 17 years. The authors described seven patients within this group who showed radiological evidence of avascular necrosis with no evidence of remodelling. In five of these cases it was an average of 20 years before they complained of pain in the involved hip. The poor results in undisplaced fractures were all associated with severe avascular necrosis and, as Durbin (1959) pointed out, the prognosis must always be guarded, even in undisplaced fractures.

Ng & Cole (1996) studied the effect of early hip decompression on the rate of avascular necrosis, specifically in displaced type II and III fractures. Fractures in six of their patients who had no decompression were grouped with 48 similar cases of Canale & Bourland (1977). They combined 10 of their patients who had early decompression with 14 similar cases reported by Pforringer & Rosemeyer (1980) and six cases from Swiontkowski & Winquist (1986). Avascular necrosis was noted in 41% of hips that had not been decompressed and only 8% of those that had.

Pforringer & Rosemeyer (1980) retrospectively reviewed 52 fractures, separating children (aged 11 years and under) from adolescents (aged 12–18 years). Among children the overall rate of avascular necrosis was 19% (five of 27), for adolescents it was 30% (nine of 25). The authors consider children to have a better prognosis than adolescents with femoral neck fractures. The difference they demonstrate may be underestimated as the groups they observed had no type I fractures (conferring a poor prognosis) in the adolescent group (against four in the children's group) and only three (conferring a good prognosis) in the type IV group (against seven in the children's group).

Premature growth plate fusion
The relationship of premature growth plate closure to internal fixation has already been discussed. Canale & Bourland (1977) described 33 cases and attempted to correlate limb length discrepancy with premature closure of the subcapital femoral physis. Their results showed that there was a much higher incidence of significant shortening in patients with premature closure than those without. The 12 cases with shortening of more than 2 cm all had premature growth plate closure and avascular necrosis. Of 14 patients with less than 2 cm of shortening, only six had both avascular necrosis and premature closure, while eight had premature closure alone. Ratliff (1978) pointed out that premature closure may also occur in one of the growth plates of the knee on the side of the fracture. This compounds the shortening that may occur.

Coxa vara
A decrease in the neck shaft angle results in the hip operating at a mechanical disadvantage, because there is upward displacement of the greater trochanter and shortening of the leg, resulting in a Trendelenburg gait. Lam (1971) felt that this was the most common complication of hip fractures in children, but he believed that it was often compatible with a good clinical result. Ratliff (1978) reported an incidence of coxa vara of 15% (27 of 170), Canale & Bourland (1977) of 21% (13 of 61). The latter authors defined coxa vara as a neck shaft angle of less than 135°, Ratliff (1978) as of less than 120°. Of the 13 patients with coxa vara reported by Canale & Bourland, four (31%) had a good clinical result, six (46%) had a fair clinical result, and three (23%) a poor result.

Non-union
This complication occurred only in displaced fractures. In the series of Canale & Bourland (1977), Ratliff (1978) and Pforringer and Rosemeyer (1980) there were 226 displaced fractures and non-union developed in 25 (11%).

Fractures: acetabular
Acetabular fractures in children and adolescents are very rare. As Heeg et al (1989) pointed out, the child's pelvis differs markedly from the adult's in that:

- It is more malleable and the joints are more elastic, allowing a greater degree of displacement. As a result, single breaks in the pelvic ring can occur.
- The triradiate cartilage may be damaged in children, leading to growth disturbance in the acetabulum.

These authors reported a variety of fracture patterns in 23 patients below the age of 17. Mean follow-up was 8 years. They found that patients whose fractures were less than 2 mm displaced at the conclusion of treatment all had good or excellent functional and radiographic results. Eighteen patients were treated conservatively and five surgically.

Heeg et al had earlier (1988) reported on four patients with injuries to the triradiate cartilage. In three, premature fusion of the cartilage occurred, two developing acetabular deformity and subluxation of the hip. In all four patients with injuries of the triradiate cartilage the sacroiliac joint was injured; in two, the joint was completely disrupted, leading to fusion with growth disturbance of the ilium. The authors recommended that 'as injury of the triradiate cartilage is easily missed on the initial radiograph, it is advised that all patients with pelvic trauma should be followed clinically and radiographically for at least one year'.

Dislocations

The most comprehensive review of hip dislocations and their sequelae in both adults and children is Epstein's monograph (1980), with a mean follow-up of 6.5 years in 51 dislocations in children.

The main points of prognostic interest after these injuries are as follows:

- the risk of developing avascular necrosis of the femoral head
- the long-term clinical results

Anterior dislocations

Epstein (1980) reported on the follow-up of seven anterior dislocations; six had excellent clinical results, while one had a good result (Table 11.1). There were no fair or poor results. Barquet (1982) reported an incidence of 13% (two of 15) of avascular necrosis in anterior dislocations reduced within 24 hours of injury. If anterior dislocations were reduced more than 24 hours after the injury then the incidence of avascular necrosis increased to 86% (six of seven).

Posterior dislocations

In Epstein's 1980 series there were 38 simple posterior dislocations, with a mean follow-up of 6.5 years; 34 (89%) were associated with a good or excellent clinical result and four (11%) with a fair result. There are insufficient numbers of the other types of posterior dislocation to derive meaningful clinical results. The Pennsylvania Orthopedic Society (1968) reported on the status at skeletal maturity of 44 children who had sustained posterior dislocation of the hip. They found that 16 had an imperfect clinical result; of these 16 children, six had associated fractures about the hip joint, four had reduction delayed beyond 24 hours, and three had developed avascular necrosis. They felt that these three features carried a high risk of a poor clinical result in children.

Offierski (1981) followed 19 children with traumatic dislocations of the hip with an average follow-up of 10 years. Three patients (16%) had a poor result following avascular necrosis of the femoral head. Coxa magna was noted in 47% of patients, but this did not correlate to clinical outcome.

The incidence of avascular necrosis has been reported to be approximately 10% by the Pennsylvania Orthopedic Society (26 of 266 cases). Barquet (1982) has collected, both from his own practice and from the orthopaedic literature, 145 cases of avascular necrosis from a review of 1117 cases of traumatic hip dislocation in childhood. He felt that only in cases with a minimum of 2 years' clinical and radiological follow-up could avascular necrosis be confidently excluded. More recently avascular necrosis of the femoral head can be diagnosed much earlier with the use of isotope bone scans or magnetic resonance imaging. Using Barquet's strict criteria there were 145 cases of avascular necrosis in 412 cases with adequate follow-up (i.e. 35% incidence), whereas in the total group (145 from 1117) the incidence is approximately 13%. Barquet (personal communication) has recently claimed that he believes that the true incidence of avascular necrosis lies between 3% and 15% in dislocations that are reduced within 12 hours. He has looked carefully at factors that may influence the development of avascular necrosis and reached the following conclusions:

1. The incidence of avascular necrosis was much lower when the dislocation was reduced within the first 24 hours after the injury. Hougaard and Thomsen (1989) confirm this. They followed 13 cases with a mean follow-up of 14 years. There were 12 excellent results (all reduced within 6 hours) and one poor result with post-traumatic arthritis of the hip (reduced at 37 hours after dislocation).
2. The incidence of avascular necrosis was 11.5% in cases reduced within 24 hours. Barquet analysed the results within this period and found that the incidence in those cases reduced within 4 hours of injury was 6.25%; between 5 and 12 hours it was 12.8% and between 13 and 24 hours it was 13.5%.
3. There appears to be protection against avascular necrosis in children under the age of 6 years. Rieger and Penning et al (1991) would agree with this. They reported on three patients, all less than 6 years of age. None developed avascular necrosis despite one hip being reduced at 48 hours post injury.
4. The severity of the injury strongly influenced the result; in severe accidents the incidence of avascular necrosis was greater. The incidence was higher with an associated fracture.
5. Post-reduction immobilisation appeared not to influence the development of avascular necrosis in posterior dislocation without fracture.
6. The interval from dislocation to weight-bearing likewise appeared not to influence the development of avascular necrosis in posterior dislocation without fracture.

Pearson and Mann (1973) reported on 24 cases of traumatic hip dislocation in children. The most frequent complication they noted was a neurological injury (five of 24). There were four partial sciatic nerve injuries and one complete injury. Only one recovered fully.

Summary

- Transphyseal fractures of the hip are, in general, associated with a poor prognosis. Avascular necrosis is almost invariable if there is dislocation of the femoral head. Children under the age of 2 years with minimal displacement tend to suffer no long-term problems.

- Displaced transcervical fractures are associated with a poor prognosis, undisplaced transcervical fractures with a good prognosis (provided that they do not displace during treatment).

- Displaced cervicotrochanteric fractures are associated with good long-term clinical results in 65% of cases. The results vary according to the use of internal fixation; in particular, coxa vara is much more common in those treated without fixation. Premature growth plate closure is more common in those treated with internal fixation (Table 11.21). Undisplaced cervicotrochanteric fractures are associated with uniformly good results.

- Intertrochanteric fractures are generally associated with a good long-term result.

- A combination of avascular necrosis and premature growth plate closure carries a high risk of subsequent limb shortening.

- According to Ratliff (1978), avascular necrosis always occurs within 1 year of injury. Canale & Bourland (1977) found radiological evidence of avascular necrosis at an average of 9 months after injury.

- Avascular necrosis occurs in approximately 10% of posterior dislocations in children. The incidence may be as low as 6% if the dislocation is reduced within 4 hours of the injury.

References

Amstutz H C, Smith R K 1979 Total hip replacement following failed femoral hemiarthroplasty. Journal of Bone and Joint Surgery 61A: 1161–1166

Askin S R, Bryan R S 1976 Femoral neck fractures in young adults. Clinical Orthopaedics 114: 259–264

Asnis S E, Wanek-Sgaglione L 1994 Intracapsular fractures of the femoral neck. Journal of Bone and Joint Surgery 76A 12: 1793–1803

Austin R T 1971 Hip function after central fracture dislocation: a long term review. Injury 3: 114–120

Banks H H 1962 Factors influencing the results in fractures of the femoral neck. Journal of Bone and Joint Surgery 44A: 931–964

Barnes R, Brown J T, Garden R S, Nicoll E A 1976 Subcapital fractures of the femur: a prospective review. Journal of Bone and Joint Surgery 58B: 2–24

Barquet A 1982 Avascular necrosis following traumatic hip dislocation in childhood: factors of influence. Acta Orthopaedica Scandinavica 53: 809–813

Boardman K P, Charnley J 1978 Low friction arthroplasty after fracture-dislocations of the hip. Journal of Bone and Joint Surgery 60B: 495–497

Brav E A 1962 Traumatic dislocation of the hip; army experience over a 12 year period. Journal of Bone and Joint Surgery 44A: 1115–1134

Bray T J, Smith-Hoefer E 1988 The displaced femoral neck fracture. Clinical Orthopaedics 230: 127–140

Bridle S H, Patel A D, Bircher M, Calvert P T 1991 Fixation of intertrochanteric fractures of the femur. A randomised prospective comparison of the gamma nail and the dynamic hip screw. Journal of Bone and Joint Surgery 73B: 330–334

Canale S T, Bourland W L 1977 Fractures of the neck and intertrochanteric region of the femur in children. Journal of Bone and Joint Surgery 59A: 431–443

Chiu K Y, Pun W K, Luk K D K, Chow S P 1995 Primary total hip replacement for displaced subcapital femoral neck fracture. International Journal of Orthopaedic Trauma 5: 23–26

Christie J, Howie C, Armour P 1988 Fixation of displaced subcapital femoral fractures: compression screw fixation versus double divergent pins. Journal of Bone and Joint Surgery 70B: 199–201

Chua D, Jaglal B, Schatzker J 1998 Predictors of early failure of fixation in the treatment of displaced subcapital hip fractures. Journal of Orthopaedic Trauma 12, 4: 230–234

Coates R L, Armour P 1980 Treatment of subcapital femoral fractures by primary total hip replacement. Injury 11: 132–135

Colonna P C 1929 Delbet classification. In: Fractures of the neck of the femur in children. American Journal of Surgery 6: 795

Davis T R C, Sher J L, Horsman A, Simpson M, Porter B B, Checketts R G 1990 Intertrochanteric femoral fractures: Mechanical failure after internal fixation. Journal of Bone and Joint Surgery 72B: 26–31

Delamarter R, Moreland J 1987 Treatment of acute femoral neck fractures with total hip arthroplasty. Clinical Orthopaedics 218: 68–74

Dimon J H, Hughston J C 1967 Unstable trochanteric fractures of the hip. Journal of Bone and Joint Surgery 49A: 440

Dreinhofer K E, Schwarzkopf S R, Haas N P, Tscherne H 1994 Isolated traumatic dislocation of the hip: long term result in 50 patients. Journal of Bone and Joint Surgery 76B: 6–12

Dreinhofer K E, Schwarzkopf S R, Haas N P, Tscherne H 1996 Femoral head dislocation fractures. Long term outcome of conservative and surgical therapy. Unfallchirurg 99: 400–409

Drennan Lowell J 1980 Results and complications of femoral neck fractures. Clinical Orthopaedics 152: 162–172

Durbin F C 1959 Avascular necrosis complicating undisplaced fractures of the neck of the femur in children. Journal of Bone and Joint Surgery 41B: 758

Epstein H C 1980 Traumatic dislocation of the hip. Williams & Wilkins, Baltimore

Epstein H C, Wiss D A, Cozen L 1985 Posterior fracture dislocation of the hip with fractures of the femoral head. Clinical Orthopaedics 201: 9–17

Fassler P R, Swiontkowski M F, Kilroy A N, Routt M L 1993 Injury of the sciatic nerve associated with acetabular fracture. Journal of Bone and Joint Surgery 75A: 1157–1166

Franzen H, Nilsson L T, Stromqvist B, Johnsson R, Herrlin K 1990 Secondary total hip replacement after fractures of the femoral neck. Journal of Bone and Joint Surgery 72B: 784–787

Garden R S 1961 Low angle fixation in fractures of the femoral neck. Journal of Bone and Joint Surgery 43B: 647–663

Greenough C G, Jones J R 1988 Primary total hip replacement for displaced subcapital fracture of the femur. Journal of Bone and Joint Surgery 70B: 639–643

Harris W H 1969 Traumatic arthritis of the hip after dislocation and acetabular fractures: treatment by mould arthroplasty: an end result study using a new method of evaluation. Journal of Bone and Joint Surgery 51A: 737–755

Heeg M, Klasen H J, Visser J D 1989 Acetabular fractures in children and adolescents. Journal of Bone and Joint Surgery 71B: 418–421

Heeg M, Visser J D, Oostvogel H J M 1988 Injuries of the acetabular triradiate cartilage and sacroiliac joint. Journal of Bone and Joint Surgery 70B 1: 34–37

Heyse-Moore G H 1996 Fixation of intracapsular femoral neck fractures with a one-hole plate dynamic hip screw. Injury 27, 3: 181–183

Hinchey J J, Day P L 1964 Primary prosthetic replacement in fresh femoral neck fractures: a review of 294 consecutive cases. Journal of Bone and Joint Surgery 46A: 223–239

Holmberg S, Kalen R, Thorngren K G 1987 Treatment and outcome of femoral neck fractures. Clinical Orthopaedics 218: 42–52

Hougaard K, Thomsen P B 1987 Coxarthrosis following traumatic posterior dislocation of the hip. Journal of Bone and Joint Surgery 69A: 679–683

Hougaard K, Thomsen P B 1989 Traumatic hip dislocation in children: Follow up of 13 cases. Orthopaedics 12(3): 375–378

Hulleberg G, Finsen V 1990 Removal of osteosynthesis material from healed hip fractures: indications and prognosis. Annales Chirurgiae et Gynaecologiae 79: 161–164

Hunter G A 1969 Posterior dislocation and fracture dislocation of the hip: a review of 57 patients. Journal of Bone and Joint Surgery 51B: 38–44

Jodoin A, Duhaime M, Labelle P, Morton D 1980 Fractures of the hip in children. Journal of Bone and Joint Surgery 62B: 128

Johnson E E, Matta J M, Mast J W, Letourel E 1994 Delayed reconstruction of acetabular fractures. Clinical Orthopaedics 305: 20–30

Johnson J T H, Crothers O 1975 Nailing versus prosthesis for femoral neck fractures. Journal of Bone and Joint Surgery 57A: 686–692

Judet R, Judet J, Letournel E 1964 Fractures of the acetabulum: classification and surgical approaches for open reduction. Preliminary report. Journal of Bone and Joint Surgery 46A: 1615–1647

Klenerman L 1985 The young patient with a fractured neck of femur. British Medical Journal 290: 1928

Kofoed H 1982 Femoral neck fractures in young adults. Injury 14: 146–150

Kofoed H, Kofod J 1983 Moore prosthesis in the treatment of fresh femoral neck fractures: a critical review with special attention to secondary acetabular degeneration. Injury 14: 531–540

Koval K J, Friend K D, Aharonoff G B, Zuckerman J D 1996 Weight bearing after hip fracture: A prospective series of 596 geriatric hip fracture patients. Journal of Orthopaedic Trauma 10, 8: 526–530

Kulisch S D, Gustilo R B 1976 Fractures of the femoral neck in young adults. Journal of Bone and Joint Surgery 58A: 724

Lam S F 1971 Fractures of the neck of the femur in children. Journal of Bone and Joint Surgery 53A: 1165–1179

Letournel E 1980 Acetabular fractures: classification and management. Clinical Orthopaedics 151: 81–106

Letournel E, Judet R 1993 Fractures of the acetabulum. Translated and edited by R A Elson. Springer-Verlag, Berlin

Leung P C, Lam S F 1986 Long-term follow up of children with femoral neck fractures. Journal of Bone and Joint Surgery 68B: 537–540

Llinas A, Sarmiento A, Ebramzadeh, Gogoan W, McKellop H 1991 Total hip arthroplasty after failed hemiarthroplasty or mould arthroplasty. Journal of Bone and Joint Surgery 73B: 902–907

Lowell D 1979 External fixation: the current state of the art. Williams & Wilkins, Baltimore, p 119

Lu-Yao G, Keller R, Littenberg B, Wenberg J 1994 Outcomes after displaced fractures of the femoral neck: A meta-analysis of one hundred and six published reports. Journal of Bone and Joint Surgery 76A, 1: 15–25

Madsen J E, Naess L, Aune A K, Alho A, Ekeland A, Stromsoe K 1998 Dynamic hip screw with trochanteric stabilizing plate in the treatment of unstable proximal femoral fractures: a comparative study with the gamma nail and compression hip screw. Journal of Orthopaedic Trauma 12(4): 241–248

Marchetti M E, Steinberg G G, Coumas J M 1996 Intermediate term experience of Pipkin fracture dislocations of the hip. Journal of Orthopaedic Trauma 10 (7): 455–461

Matta J 1996 Fractures of the acetabulum: Accuracy of reduction and clinical result in patients managed operatively within three weeks after injury. Journal of Bone and Joint Surgery 78A: 1632–1645

Matta J M, Mehne D K, Roffi R 1985 Fractures of the acetabulum: early results of a prospective study. Clinical Orthopaedics 205: 241–250

McKee M D, Garay M E, Schemitsch E H, Kreder H J, Stephen D J 1998 Irreducible fracture dislocation of the hip: a severe injury with a poor prognosis. Journal of Orthopaedic Trauma 12 (4): 223–229

Meyers M H 1985 Fractures of the hip. Chicago Year Book, Chicago

Miller W E 1973 Fractures of the hip in children from birth to adolescence. Clinical Orthopaedics 92: 155–188

Morrisey R 1980 Hip fractures in children. Clinical Orthopaedics 152: 202–210

Ng G P K, Cole W G 1996 Effect of early hip decompression on the frequency of avascular necrosis in children with fractures of the neck of the femur. Injury 27(6): 419–421

Nilsson L T, Stromqvist B, Thorngren K G 1989 Secondary arthroplasty for femoral neck fracture complication. Journal of Bone and Joint Surgery 71B: 777–781

Nyquist F, Overgaard A, Duppe H, Obrant K 1998 Alcohol abuse and healing complications after cervical hip fractures. Alcohol and Alcoholism 33, 4: 373–380

Obrant K, Carlson A S 1987 Survival of hemiarthroplasties after cervical hip fractures. Orthopaedics 10: 1153–1156

O'Brien P J, Meek R N, Blachut P A, Broekhuyse H M, Sabharwal S 1995 Fixation of intertrochanteric hip fractures: gamma nail versus dynamic hip screw. A randomized, prospective study. Canadian Journal of Surgery 38(6): 516–520

Offierski O 1981 Traumatic dislocation of the hip in children. Journal of Bone and Joint Surgery 63B (2): 194–197

Ovesen O, Arreskov J, Bellstrom T 1989 Hip fractures in children: A long-term follow up of 17 cases. Orthopaedics 12(3): 361–367

Parker M J 1994 Parallel garden screws for intracapsular femoral fractures. Injury 25, 6: 383–385

Parker M J, Pryor G A 1993 Treatment of intracapsular fractures. In: Parker M J and Pryor G A Treatment of hip fractures. Blackwell, Oxford

Pearson D E, Mann R J 1973 Traumatic hip dislocation in children. Clinical Orthopaedics 92: 189–194

Pennal G F, Davidson J, Garside H, Plewes J 1980 Results of treatment of acetabular fractures. Clinical Orthopaedics 151: 115–123

Pennsylvania Orthopedic Society 1968 Final report of the scientific research committee on traumatic dislocation of the hip joint in children. Journal of Bone and Joint Surgery 590A: 79–88

Pforringer W, Rosemeyer B 1980 Fractures of the hip in children and adolescents. Acta Orthopaedica Scandanavica 51: 91–108

Pipkin G 1957 Treatment of grade IV fracture–dislocation of the hip. Journal of Bone and Joint Surgery 39A: 1027–1042

Protzman R R, Burkhalter M D 1976 Femoral neck fractures in young adults. Journal of Bone and Joint Surgery 58A: 686–694

Ratliff A H C 1962 Fractures of the neck of the femur in children. Journal of Bone and Joint Surgery 44B: 528–542

Ratliff A H C 1978 Fractures of the neck of the femur in children. In: Lloyd-Roberts G C, Ratliff A H C (eds) Hip disorders in children. Butterworths, London, pp 165–199

Regazzoni P, Reudi T H 1985 The dynamic hip screw implant system. Springer-Verlag, Berlin

Reusch P D, Holdener H, Ciaramitaro M, Mast J W 1994 A prospective study of surgically treated acetabular fractures. Clinical Orthopaedics 305: 38–46

Rieger H, Pennig D, Klein W, Grunert J 1991 Traumatic dislocation of the hip in young children. Archives of Orthopaedic and Trauma Surgery 110: 114–117

Rowe C R, Lowell D 1961 Prognosis of fractures of the acetabulum. Journal of Bone and Joint Surgery 43A: 30–59

Sarmiento A, Gerard F M 1978 Total hip arthroplasty for failed endoprostheses. Clinical Orthopaedics 137: 112–117

Sikorski J M, Barrington R 1981 Internal fixation versus hemiarthroplasty for the displaced subcapital fracture of the femur. Journal of Bone and Joint Surgery 63B, 3: 357–361

Sim F H Stauffer R N 1980 Management of hip fractures by total hip arthroplasty. Clinical Orthopaedics 152: 191–197

Skinner P, Riley D 1989 Displaced subcapital fractures of the femur: a prospective randomized comparison of internal fixation, hemiarthroplasty and total hip replacement. Injury 20: 291–293

Squires B, Bannister G 1999 Displaced intracapular neck of femur fractures in mobile independent patients: total hip replacement or hemiarthroplasty? Injury 30: 345–348

Stambough J L, Balderston R A, Booth R E, Rothman R H, Cohn J C 1986 Conversion to total hip replacement: a review of 140 hips with greater than 6 year follow-up study. Journal of Arthroplasty 1: 261–269

Steen Jensen J, Sonne-Holm S, Tondevold E 1980a Unstable trochanteric fractures: a comparative analysis of four methods of internal fixation. Acta Orthopaedica Scandinavica 51: 949–962

Steen Jensen J, Tondevold E, Sonne-Holm S 1980b Stable trochanteric fractures. A comparative analysis of four methods of internal fixation. Acta Orthopaedica Scandinavica 51: 811–815

Stromquist B 1983 Femoral head vitality after intracapsular hip fracture: 490 cases studied by intravital tetracycline labelling and tc-mdp radionuclide imaging. Acta Orthopaedica Scandinavica (suppl 200) 54: 5–71

Stromqvist B, Hansson L, Nilsson L, Thorngren K G 1984 Two year follow-up of femoral neck fractures: a comparison of osteosynthesis methods. Acta Orthopaedica Scandinavica 55: 521–525

Swiontkowski M 1994 Current concepts: Intracapsular fractures of the hip. Journal of Bone and Joint Surgery 76A 129–138

Swiontkowski M, Winquist R A 1986 Displaced hip fractures in children and adolescents. The Journal of Trauma 26(4): 384–388

Swiontkowski M, Winquist R A, Hansen S T 1984 Fractures of the femoral neck in patients between the age of 12 and 49 years. Journal of Bone and Joint Surgery 66A: 837–846

Taine W H, Armour P C 1985 Primary total hip replacement for displaced subcapital fractures of the femur. Journal of Bone and Joint Surgery 67B: 214–217

Thompson V P, Epstein H C 1951 Traumatic dislocation of the hip: a survey of 204 cases covering a period of 21 years. Journal of Bone and Joint Surgery 33A: 746–777

Tile M 1984 Fractures of the pelvis and acetabulum. Williams & Wilkins, Baltimore

Tile M, Kellam J F, Joyce M 1985 Fractures of the acetabulum: classification, management protocol and results of treatment. Journal of Bone and Joint Surgery 67B: 324–325

Turner A, Wroblewski B M 1984 Charnley low friction arthroplasty for the treatment of hips with late complications of femoral neck fractures. Clinical Orthopaedics 185: 126–130

Upadhyay S S, Moulton A 1981 The long term results of traumatic posterior dislocation of the hip. Journal of Bone and Joint Surgery 63B: 548–551

Weber M, Berry D J, Harmsden W S 1998 Total hip arthroplasty after operative treatment of an acetabular fracture. Journal of Bone and Joint Surgery 80A: 1295–1305

Wetherell R G, Hinves B L 1990 The Hastings bipolar hemiarthroplasty for subcapital fractures of the femoral neck. Journal of Bone and Joint Surgery 72B: 788–793

Whittaker R P, Abeshaus M M, Scholl H W, Chung S M K 1972 Fifteen years' experience with metallic endoprosthetic replacement of the femoral head for femoral neck fractures. Journal of Trauma 12: 799–806

Wilson J N 1982 Injuries of the hip. In: Watson Jones fractures and joint injuries. Churchill Livingstone, Edinburgh, p 931

Wu C C, Shih C H 1993 A comparison of intertrochanteric fractures in elderly and younger patients. Orthopaedics International Edition 1 (3): 216–220

Zetterberg G L, Irstam L, Anderson G B J 1982 Femoral neck fractures in young adults. Acta Orthopaedica Scandinavica 53: 427–435

The femur
Michael A. Foy

Introduction

There is some controversy concerning the merits of surgical and conservative treatment in all types of femoral fracture. Operative treatment of fractures is favoured where it is difficult to maintain reduction, e.g. displaced subtrochanteric fractures. However, the introduction of various types of locked nail over the last 20 years has considerably extended the place of surgery in the management of subtrochanteric and femoral shaft fractures. Non-operative treatment is preferred where good results can be expected without surgery, e.g. in children.

In the sections within this chapter, attempts will be made to consider the end-results in terms of both surgical and conservative treatment, where the appropriate information is available.

Subtrochanteric fractures

There is no classification of subtrochanteric fractures that correlates well with prognosis (Parker et al 1997). Boyd & Griffin (1949), Fielding et al (1974), Zickel (1976), Seinsheimer (1978) and Waddell (1979) have all suggested classifications. Velasco & Comfort (1978) and Delee (1984) rejected classification schemes for subtrochanteric fractures and recommended that each fracture should be assessed in terms of potential stability after internal fixation. As with fractures of the femoral neck, subtrochanteric fractures may be seen in two groups of patients—older patients suffering minor trauma to weakened bone and younger patients with normal bone who are subjected to high-velocity injury.

Delee (1984) pointed out that the two main problems arising from subtrochanteric fractures were malunion and delayed or non-union. The subtrochanteric area is composed mainly of cortical bone which may be comminuted in these fractures. The cortical bone vascularity and fracture surfaces are less than in the cancellous bone surfaces present in intertrochanteric fractures. There are also large biomechanical stresses in the subtrochanteric region, which may result in failure of internal fixation devices before bony union occurs.

Seinsheimer (1978) proposed a classification based on the number of major fragments and the location and shape of fracture lines. The classification is shown in Fig. 12.1. It identifies two types of fracture, which, in Seinsheimer's 1978 series, were associated with all the implant failures and non-unions. These were his type IIIA (a three-part spiral fracture in which the lesser trochanter is part of the third fragment) and the type IV (a comminuted fracture with four or more fragments).

When Velasco & Comfort (1978) analysed their unsatisfactory results they found that 19 out of 22 (86%) had a medial defect of more than 2 mm, while in those with satisfactory results only 15 of 50 (30%) had a medial defect greater than 2 mm. Velasco & Comfort defined a satisfactory result as follows:

- full pre-injury activity or job status, with slight or no pain
- hip flexion of over 90°, with less than 10° of rotational deformity
- no more than 10° varus
- less than 1.25 cm of shortening

The common feature throughout the various classifications is the importance of damage to the medial cortex of the femur and the less satisfactory results that occur if it is not reduced and stabilised to maintain a medial buttress.

Conservative treatment

The results of treatment in traction are fairly consistent in the literature, although the criteria for a satisfactory result vary slightly from series to series. These results are summarised in Table 12.1

The most common cause of an unsatisfactory result was a varus deformity in excess of 10° (13 out of 28 patients, i.e. 46%). Non-union or delayed union occurred in five out of 28 patients (18%), while shortening of more than 1.25 cm happened in four out of 28 patients (14%) and severe knee stiffness in three out of 28 patients (11%).

Delee et al (1981) described a treatment regime of preliminary traction followed by an ambulatory cast brace with a pelvic band for severely comminuted or open subtrochanteric fractures. In the 15 cases on which they reported they found no non-unions and 'no significant degree' of varus, rotation or shortening. They did stress that this treatment regime required exacting attention from the orthopaedic surgeon.

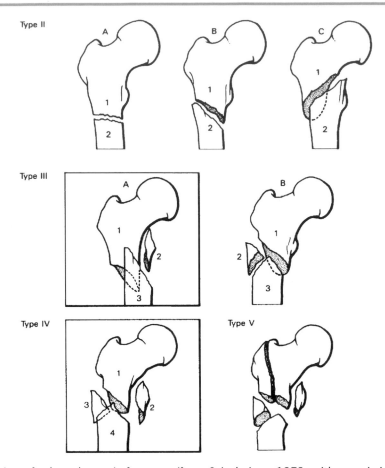

Fig. 12.1 Classification of subtrochanteric fractures (from Seinsheimer 1978, with permission).

Table 12.1 Results of subtrochanteric fractures treated by traction

	Number of cases	Satisfactory	Unsatisfactory
Waddell (1979)	18	10	8
Velasco & Comfort (1978)	22	11	11
Seinsheimer (1978)	8	3	5
Watson et al (1964)	8	4	4
Total	56	28	28

Therefore most orthopaedic/trauma surgeons would elect to operate on these difficult fractures unless there were some compelling reason for not doing so.

Surgical treatment

Most recent reviews of subtrochanteric fracture management advocate operative treatment. Trafton (1987) pointed out that there were significant complications after fixation with early hip implants such as the McLaughlin and Jewett devices. There are four major categories of operative treatment available:

1. Fixed angle nail and blade plates.
2. Sliding screws and plates, e.g. the DHS, DCS.
3. Rigid IM devices, e.g. gamma nail, GK, AO, Russell Taylor.
4. Flexible IM devices, e.g. Enders nails.

We will consider the results obtained following the use of devices commonly employed at the present time. There is some evidence from biomechanical studies (Curtis et al 1994) that intramedullary fixation is significantly stronger than that afforded by extramedullary devices.

Compression hip screws

The reported results are good, and this may reflect the familiarity of the implant to most orthopaedic surgeons. Waddell (1979) reported 24 cases with 21 satisfactory results, one implant failure and two non-unions. Wile et al (1983) reported 25 patients treated with a high-angle compression hip screw. There were no mechanical failures, delayed unions or non-unions. There were two instances of malunion in this series. Wile et al classified their fractures after Seinsheimer (1978) and found that the mean time to bony union was 3.6 months (range 1.3–6.9 months). In the series mentioned, the incidence of satisfactory results was 90% using the compression hip screw. Trafton (1987) reported that union without fixation failure was recorded in 95 to 100% of patients. Parker et al (1997) found an 8% implant failure rate with the sliding hip screw. However, they concluded that intramedullary nailing and sliding screw fixation were both equally effective.

AO condylar blade plate/Dynamic condylar screw

Trafton (1987) felt that the AO condylar blade plate was the only fixed-angle one-piece device that was still advocated for subtrochanteric fractures. Orthopaedic surgeons tend not to be as familiar with its use as they are with the compression hip screw. All authors emphasise the importance of reconstructing the medial cortical buttress when this device is used. More recently, the 95° DCS has been introduced by the AO group and its use has superceded that of the blade plate. In Waddell's 1979 series 40 patients were treated with the AO blade plate; 29 achieved a satisfactory result (72.5%). There were seven implant failures and four non-unions requiring further surgical treatment. Senter et al (1990) compared use of the angled blade plate and the DHS and found no difference in the result as long as the medial buttress was reconstituted.

Warwick et al (1995) reviewed 43 patients treated with the DCS. They concluded that the DCS can be used successfully in most subtrochanteric fractures although there was a considerable complication rate. They felt that this reflected the general condition of the patient and the biomechanics of the proximal femur.

Intramedullary devices

A variety of intramedullary devices have been used to fix subtrochanteric fractures internally. These include Enders nails, Zickel nail, Gamma nail and various types of second generation reconstruction nail. Both Edwards et al (2000) and van Doorn & Stapert (2000) found that the long Gamma nail gave a good functional result with acceptable complication rates. Condylocephalic (Enders) nails have been used, but complications—particularly early loss of fixation—are common (Trafton 1987).

Problems with predicting prognosis in subtrochanteric fractures

There is insufficient uniformity in classification (although Seinsheimer's is the most widely quoted) to enable results following application of the various fixation devices to be accurately correlated. The advent of the interlocking nail, reconstruction nail and the dynamic condylar screw may change the techniques of fixation of these fractures, and it may be a few more years before the situation is clear.

In Velasco & Comfort's 1978 series there were 50 fractures treated by operation, using the Jewett nail, the Massie nail, the AO blade plate and the Zickel nail. The results merit consideration as a general group as they were followed up using strict criteria for varus, shortening and rotational deformity. Of these, 39 patients (78%) achieved a good result while 11 (22%) achieved an unsatisfactory result. The reasons for the unsatisfactory results were varus deformity in two patients, shortening of more than 1.25 cm in three patients and non-union in one patient. Ten of the 11 failures (91%) occurred where there was a residual medial defect of more than 2 mm after fixation. However, Kinast et al (1989) point out that the medial reconstruction is desirable and advantageous only if it can be achieved without soft tissue stripping and devascularisation; under these circumstances they recommended indirect reduction and intraoperative pretensioning of the plate.

The subtrochanteric fracture appears *par excellence* to be a condition in which, if surgical treatment is contemplated, the prognosis is related to the familiarity of the surgeon with the implant to be used. The subtrochanteric fracture (particularly the Seinsheimer types IIIA and IV) is not a forgiving fracture. It is difficult, therefore, to formulate more than prognostic guidelines in this condition. Prospective trials, using accepted classifications, such as Seinsheimer's, or the newer AO are required to record accurate results and to clarify the prognosis. It should be recognised that each of the available implants may have advantages in certain types of subtrochanteric fracture, and implant selection should be made with reference to the fracture anatomy.

Summary

- There is no accepted classification of subtrochanteric fractures that correlates well with prognosis.
- The Seinsheimer type IIIA fracture (see Fig. 12.1) appears to be particularly associated with failure of internal fixation.

- Traction results in satisfactory results in 50% of cases. The cases selected for traction in the series studied tended to be undisplaced or comminuted, such that a stable internal fixation could not be contemplated.
- Operative treatment is favoured in the majority of cases but the choice of implant remains controversial. A high proportion of satisfactory results are reported with the compression hip screw (90–100%).

Femoral shaft fractures

The treatment of fractures of the femoral shaft may be operative or non-operative. Non-operative treatment is still the method favoured by some orthopaedic surgeons while, at the other extreme, most orthopaedic surgeons now feel that the advent of the interlocking and reconstruction nail has extended the indications for internal fixation.

Fractures of the femoral shaft reflect changes in lifestyle and developments in transport, with 85% resulting from motor vehicle accidents. The femur is the largest and strongest of the bones in the body and requires high energy force to break it. As a result of the high energy required, femoral fractures may be associated with other serious musculoskeletal or major organ injury. Costa et al (1988) found that 12% of their femoral fracture patients had associated vital organ injuries.

Mooney & Claudi (1984) suggested that femoral fractures should be classified as simple, butterfly fragment and comminuted/segmental. The butterfly fractures can be further subdivided into single butterfly fragments, two butterfly fragments and those with three or more intermediate fragments.

There is a large volume of literature on femoral shaft fractures. However, only a small number of reports carefully assess the functional, anatomical and social results in detail. The most comprehensive review is Kootstra's 1973 monograph.

Problems arise with analysis of the results because definition of the femoral shaft is either not specified or varies from series to series. Kootstra defined the shaft as extending from the lower edge of the lesser trochanter to a line which parallels the joint space of the knee at a distance equal to the width of the condyles. A small number of subtrochanteric fractures may fall within this definition, but the meticulous follow-up of Kootstra's work is so important that this small potential bias is accepted in this chapter.

Delayed union

Opinions differ over the definition of delayed union. Kootstra (1973) and Dencker (1965) identified it in 104 of 741 patients with femoral shaft fractures where union had not been achieved by 8 months. Dencker applied a second criterion; he wrote of delayed union if the attending surgeon had to perform an operation within 8 months to accelerate union.

Kootstra described 84% of 261 fractures healed by 6 months in patients treated by conservative and operative methods. Winquist et al (1984) reported that 87% of 442 femoral fractures treated by intramedullary nailing were united by 3 months. Winquist et al are experienced and skilled proponents of closed intramedullary fixation of femoral fractures. Cameron et al (1992) described a mean time to bony union of 20 weeks in a series of 84 patients with 88 acute traumatic femoral shaft fractures. Three patients had delayed or non-union (3.5%).

Kootstra (1973) identified delayed union in 16 of 261 patients and Dencker (1964) in 104 of 741 patients with femoral shaft fractures. Aggregation of these figures (i.e. 120 of 1002 fractures) suggests an incidence of 12% for delayed union of femoral shaft fractures following a variety of treatments—traction, intramedullary nailing, AO plating and cerclage wiring. Considering Dencker's second criterion for delayed union (see above) and its subjective nature, it may be that Kootstra's figure of 6% (16 of 261) is a clearer reflection of the incidence of delayed union in these fractures.

Kootstra used the radiological criteria of Charnley & Guindy (1961) to define osseous union: the presence of continuous bridging of bone at some part of the fracture, although not necessarily on all sides, combined with the absence of sclerosis. Fig. 12.2 is reproduced from his work and clearly shows the cumulative percentages of fracture unions per month using this definition. Kootstra attempted to define factors which influenced the rate of union. The duration of union following three different methods of treatment is summarised in Table 12.2.

Although the rate of union at 8 months is lower following AO plating, this is not statistically significant. Kootstra also found no significant difference in the duration of union in open and closed femoral fractures, but that it was significantly shorter in the 17–29 years age group when compared with those in the 30–70 years age group.

The criteria for osseous union outlined by Charnley & Guindy (1961) and used in Kootstra's work bear only limited relation to functional recovery. Rokkanen et al (1969) used functional results as the criteria for progress of fracture healing. In patients treated by operation they defined union according to the time elapsing between the accident and the time when the patient was able to walk without the aid of a stick, and subsequently to return to work. For

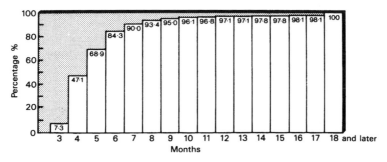

Fig. 12.2 Cumulative percentages of fracture unions per month (from Kootstra 1973, with permission).

Table 12.2 A comparison between three methods of treatment and their relation to delayed union (adapted from Kootstra 1973)

Month of union	Cumulative percentage united		
	Conservative	Intramedullary (K) nailing	AO plate
Third	13.4	4.2	5.4
Sixth	92.7	83.1	70.2
Eighth	95.1	94.4	86.5

patients treated conservatively, union was recorded as the time when immobilisation was discontinued. Using this criterion all fractures had healed within 12 months of the accident. The work of Rokkanen et al is discussed in more detail in the section on social and occupational factors.

Non-union

The incidence of non-union, compiled from several important reports, is summarised in Table 12.3.

Dencker's figures show a much higher incidence (3.7%) than other series. If these figures were excluded then the incidence of non-union would be 0.6% (8 of 1335). The incidence is probably around 1%, as described by Mooney & Claudi (1984).

Giannoudis et al (2000) looked in detail at the reasons for non-union in 32 patients with femoral shaft fracture non-unions. They compared these patients with 67 others (matched for age, sex, ISS and soft tissue injury) whose fractures had united. They found no relationship between the rate of union and the type of implant, mode of locking, reaming, distraction or smoking. They found fewer cases of non-union in comminuted fractures and in patients who were able to weight bear early. They found a marked association between non-union and the use of non steroidal anti-inflammatory drugs following the injury. Furlong et al (1999) reported a 96% union rate after

exchange nailing for aseptic non-union of femoral shaft fractures. Hak et al (2000) also advocated exchange nailing for non-union but found significantly worse results in smokers compared with non-smokers.

Refracture

The incidence of refracture in five large series is shown in Table 12.4. The overall incidence is 4.6%. In Dencker's series, 17 of the 20 refractures occurred within 1 year of the original injury. Breedeveld et al (1985) found that most of the refractures followed plate fixation.

In addition to refracture in the first year after injury, refracture after removal of rigid internal fixation devices is a problem because, under these circumstances, the bone has been protected from functional stresses.

Of the 15 refractures in Kootstra's series, nine occurred in 91 patients treated conservatively, three occurred in 43 patients treated by AO plating and three in 165 patients treated by intramedullary nailing. Hartmann & Brav (1954) and Seimon (1964) felt that approximately two-thirds of the refractures were avoidable. The avoidable cases occurred because of premature mobilisation, carelessness of the patient or early removal of implants.

Femoral shortening

Shortening following femoral shaft fractures may be due to overlapping of the fracture fragments or to angular

Table 12.3 The incidence of non-unions following femoral shaft fractures

Reference	Treatment	Non-unions
Dencker (1965)	Conservative/operative	31/837
Wickstrom et al (1968)	Intramedullary nailing	2/324
Rokkanen et al (1969)	Conservative/operative	0/154
Kootstra (1973)	Conservative/operative	1/261
Carr & Wingo (1973)	Conservative/operative	1/154
Winquist et al (1984)	Intramedullary nailing	4/442
Wolinsky et al (1999)	Intramedullary nailing	6/551
Total		45/2723 (1.65%)

Table 12.4 The incidence of refracture following femoral shaft fractures treated by conservative and operative methods

Reference	Treatment	Refracture rate
Hartmann & Brav (1954)	Conservative/operative	12/135
Dencker (1964)	Conservative/operative	20/837
Seimon (1964)	Conservative/operative	21/476
Kootstra (1973)	Conservative/operative	15/300
Breedeveld (1985)	Conservative/operative	19/148
Total		87/1896 (4.6%)

deformity. Assessment may be clinical or radiological. A myokinetic study by Morscher & Taillard (1965) showed that patients with 1 cm of shortening have a normal gait; likewise, many with 2 cm of shortening also have a normal gait and are free of symptoms. However, with shortening in excess of 2 cm, which can be detected clinically, the gait is almost always disturbed.

Shortening in the lower limb is an important consideration as far as insurance companies assessing compensation following trauma are concerned. Shortening of 2 cm or more was found in 37 of 323 (11.5%) patients reported by Rokkanen et al (1969) and Kootstra (1973). Treatment was by traction, intramedullary nailing (open and closed) and AO plating. The results from these two series are summarised according to method of treatment in Table 12.5.

Kootstra found that two of 53 (3.8%) patients treated conservatively developed shortening of 5 cm. Of the seven fractures in this series with shortening of 3 cm or more, six were comminuted and one was a spiral fracture with a butterfly fragment. Hardy et al (1979) reported a 31% incidence of shortening of more than 2 cm (i.e. similar to the conservative group shown in Table 12.5) in a series of 79 femoral shaft fractures treated by cast-bracing and early weight-bearing. Leg length in this series was assessed by scanogram, and the authors suggested that scanograms should be carried out routinely for medicolegal reasons. This is obviously a counsel of perfection and should not replace a full clinical assessment of the patient.

Clearly with the trend towards nailing of many femoral fractures, shortening only tends to be a significant problem in comminuted (multifragmentary) fractures where assessment of length peroperatively can be difficult. Braten et al (1995) reviewed 120 femoral fractures in 116 patients treated by intramedullary nailing and found shortening of 1 cm or more in 11 patients (9%). Only one patient had shortening of over 2 cm. Sojbjerg et al (1990) reviewed 40 comminuted/unstable femoral shaft fractures treated by locked intramedullary nailing and found that three (7.5%) had shortening of 1–2 cm and two (5%) had lengthening of 1 cm. Sharma et al (1993) found shortening of more than 1 cm in four of 81 patients with

Table 12.5 The incidence of shortening > 2 cm following femoral shaft fractures (from Rokkanen et al 1969, Kootstra 1973)

Method of treatment	Shortening >2 cm	
	Number	%
Conservative	23/81	28
Intramedullary nailing (open/closed)	13/209	6
AO plating	1/33	3.3
Overall	37/323	11.5

comminuted femoral shaft fractures treated by closed unlocked intramedullary nailing and functional cast bracing. Winquist & Hansen (1980) reviewed 245 comminuted femoral fractures (including segmental fractures) treated by intramedullary nailing and found shortening of more than 2 cm in seven cases (3%). Christovitsinos et al (1997) looked at the relatively newer technique of bridge plating of comminuted fractures and found shortening of 1–2 cm in four of 20 patients. However, this series included subtrochanteric fractures and three of the fractures were open.

It is not clear whether there is an increased incidence of osteoarthritis of the hip in association with femoral shortening. However, Hung et al (1996) studied the joint space prior to lengthening in 20 patients with a short femur due to a femoral fracture (15) or a distal femoral epiphyseal injury (five). The mean age at injury was 16 years (three to 27) and the mean shortening was 5.4 cm (1.1–14 cm). They found that the hip joint space of the shortened femur was significantly narrower than that on the normal side with a mean narrowing ratio of 15.5%. Interestingly, the narrowing ratio appeared to relate to the time spent non-weight bearing rather than the degree of shortening.

Angular deformities

Kootstra (1973) assessed varus, valgus and angular deformities in the sagittal plane in 232 patients with femoral shaft fractures. None of the patients with a varus deformity of less than 10° had symptoms referable to their deformity. Only two of nine patients with varus deformity in excess of 15° were symptomatic. Varus deformity of 10° or more occurred in 11 of 63 patients (17.5%) treated conservatively, six of 133 patients (4.5%) treated by intramedullary nailing and in none of 36 patients treated by AO plating. The long-term effect of varus deformity of the femur on the knee joint is unclear.

There were 30 patients with measurable valgus deformities in Kootstra's series, but none were symptomatic. The greatest degree of valgus was 15°. Valgus of 10° or

more was present in three of 63 patients (4.7%) treated conservatively, eight of 133 patients (6%) treated by intramedullary nailing and in none of 36 patients treated by AO plating.

Recurvation was present in 64 of 232 patients (27.5%), but none were symptomatic. Recurvation of 10° or more was present in six of 63 patients (9.5%) treated conservatively, five of 133 patients (3.7%) treated by intramedullary nailing and in none of 36 patients treated by AO plating. The opposite deformity of 'antecurvation' was less commonly found, but similarly gave no symptoms, even when it was 15° or more.

Rotational deformities

Nicod (1967) believed that significant clinical symptoms occurred with rotational deformities exceeding 20° and that external rotation deformities led to degenerative change in the lateral compartment of the knee joint, while internal rotation deformities led to degenerative changes in the medial compartment. Müller (1967) was of the opinion that rotational deformity in the femur could give rise to symptoms in the metatarsals and ankle joint. Kootstra (1973) assessed 206 of his patients for rotational deformities. The findings are summarised in Table 12.6.

Rokkanen et al (1969) reported a lower incidence of rotational deformity in their series; the deformity exceeded 10° in 10 to 11% of fractures treated by intramedullary nailing and in 4% of those treated conservatively. These authors do not give any information on subsequent progress of their patients.

Kootstra (1973) assessed 23 patients with external rotation deformity of 20° and found that eight (35%) were symptomatic, complaining of knee stiffness after walking, exertion fatigue in the leg and a tired feeling in the hip. There were assessments on 12 patients with external rotation deformity of 30° and six (50%) were symptomatic, complaining of fatiguability of the limb on exertion. Of two patients with an external rotation deformity of 40°, only one was symptomatic. In none of these patients (with a follow-up of from 2 to 11 years) was there radiological evidence of osteoarthritis of the knee or hip joint. One patient with a 50° external rotation deformity had unequivocal degenerative signs in the knee joint 8 years after the injury.

Of the five patients with internal rotation deformities of 20°, only one had symptoms of fatiguability of the leg; this patient had a coexistent valgus deformity. One patient with an internal rotation deformity of 30° suffered slight limitation of knee function, but was otherwise symptom-free. None of these patients had radiological evidence of osteoarthritis when assessed 2–11 years after injury.

A more recent review by Braten et al (1993) evaluated 110 patients who had been treated by intramedullary nailing. They found true torsional deformity (defined as an anteversion difference of 15° or more when compared to the normal side) in 21 patients (19%). However, only eight patients complained of symptoms. The authors felt that rotational deformities over 30° would cause serious complaint. They believed that most deformities were caused during surgery and rigorous attempts should be made to avoid this. They found an equal incidence of rotational deformities in locked and unlocked nails.

Knee function

Laubenthal et al (1972) suggested that the average knee motion required for sitting is 93°; for climbing stairs it is 100°; for tying shoelaces it is 106°; and for squatting to lift an object it is 117°. Laros & Spiegel (1979) concluded, on the basis of this work, that 125° or more of knee flexion will be required to enable normal function; 110–124° will permit shoelace tying in most cases; while 100–109° of flexion will generally allow patients to sit comfortably and to climb stairs. Laros & Spiegel believed that less than 100° of knee flexion resulted in difficulty with sitting and significant functional loss.

Laros & Spiegel (1979) summarised the results in terms of knee flexion in 1003 femoral shaft fractures from the literature. Their findings are shown in Table 12.7.

Other reports do not consider range of knee movements in these precise terms and cannot be directly compared. Nichols (1963) found that a range of knee flexion greater than 90° was obtained less frequently after comminuted fractures (58%) than after simple (78%) or compound (60%) fractures, irrespective of whether the treatment was by traction or intramedullary nailing.

Table 12.6 The frequency of rotational deformity exceeding 20° following femoral shaft fractures (adapted from Kootstra 1973)

Treatment	External rotation >20°	Internal rotation >20°
Conservative treatment	8/51 (15.7%)	2/51 (3.9%)
Intramedullary nailing	32/121 (26.4%)	4/121 (3.3%)
AO plating	1/34 (2.9%)	0/34

Table 12.7 The range of knee flexion following various methods of treatment for femoral shaft fractures (adapted from Laros & Spiegel 1979)

	Knee flexion (%)		
	0–90° Impaired function	91–120° Some impairment of function	>120° Normal function
Cast brace treatment	17	37	46
Traction	17	25	58
Open intramedullary nailing	5.5	94.5	
Closed intramedullary nailing	0	14	86
AO plating	0	6	94

McLaren et al (1990) reviewed data from 31 series that included 3243 femoral fractures treated by closed or open intramedullary nailing. They looked at the degree of flexion regained. Of patients who had closed nailing, 95% achieved over 90° of flexion compared with 89% of those who underwent open nailing.

Coexistent meniscal injuries

Vangness et al (1993) found a 27% incidence of meniscal tears in a series of 47 patients with closed, displaced, diaphyseal fractures of the femur. The tears were diagnosed by arthroscopy after femoral nailing. They emphasised that a high index of suspicion was necessary to identify the lesions.

Nerve injuries

The majority of nerve injuries are related to treatment. As intramedullary nailing is the commonest treatment for femoral fractures at the present time there has been increasing concern over traction injuries to the sciatic and pudendal nerves. Azer & Rankin (1994) describe a 1 to 2% incidence of sciatic nerve injury due to excessive intraoperative traction during reduction. Brumbach et al (1992) prospectively assessed 106 patients who underwent static interlocking nailing. They found that 10 patients (9.5%—six men and four women) had a pudendal nerve palsy. Nine had sensory changes only and one had erectile dysfunction. The symptoms had resolved at the 3 month follow-up in all patients except for one man who complained of dysaesthesia 6 months postoperatively.

Social and occupational factors

In this section we will consider two factors—duration of unfitness to work and change of occupation. These factors are influenced not just by the type of fracture and its treatment but also by the nature of the patient's employment, the patient's age, associated injuries, the patient's personality and the labour market in general.

Duration of unfitness to work

As might be expected, hospitalisation is less in those cases treated operatively compared to those treated non-operatively. Reviewing the work of Nichols (1963), Rokkanen et al (1969), Bilcher Taft & Hammer (1970) and Kootstra (1973), the mean duration of unfitness to work was approximately 9 months (with a range from 2–24 months) after femoral shaft fractures. Nichols (1963) and Kootstra (1973), found that patients were able to return to work approximately 2 months earlier (i.e. after 7 months) following intramedullary nailing. Cameron et al (1992) reported a mean time to return to work of 31 weeks following intramedullary nailing of femoral shaft fractures; however, three-quarters of their patients were able to return earlier than this.

Carr & Wingo (1973) analysed the duration of unfitness to work according to fracture type. In simple, transverse or oblique fractures (72 patients treated by open (42) and closed (30) methods) the mean time for return was 9.5 months. In fractures with a butterfly fragment (33 patients treated by open (15) and closed (18) methods) the mean time was 10.5 months. In segmental or severely comminuted fractures (11 cases treated by open (5) and closed (6) methods) the mean time for return to work was 13.5 months.

Change of occupation

There is little information in the literature on the effect of a femoral shaft fracture on subsequent employability. Numerous factors affect occupation after femoral shaft fracture; the most important are the nature of the patient's job and the development of complications of the fracture or complications of its treatment. In a series of military personnel, Nichols (1963) reported that 28% of patients with femoral shaft fractures were subsequently invalided out of the service. Of this group 50% had fractures of the patella or tibia in the same limb.

Kootstra (1973) found that only two of 200 patients were unable to work after a femoral fracture solely because of the femoral fracture, while 12 of 202 patients (6%) were unable to work because of associated injuries. He was able to identify only five out of 202 patients (2.5%) who had to change their occupation as a result of their femoral fracture. Moulton et al (1984) considered the influence of associated injuries in two matched series of femoral shaft fractures; they concluded that the presence of an associated injury increased the chance of permanent disability, as measured in terms of knee flexion less than 90°, shortening of more than 2.5 cm and angulation of more than 15°.

Implant failure

When any metal implant is inserted to facilitate fracture healing, it is a 'race' between the bone healing and the implant failing. The loads taken through a major bone like the femur are immense and if the fracture fails to heal the load through the bone will cause the implant to break. Webb et al (1986) reported 15 broken or bent nails in 105 delayed unions and non-unions. Wolinsky et al (1999) had breakage of one nail and 13 locking bolts in 551 fractures in 515 patients treated by locked intramedullary nailing. Ruedi & Luscher (1979) analysed 126 comminuted femoral shaft fractures treated by plating and found a 9% incidence of implant failure.

Removal of implants

Removal of implants following fracture healing is essentially a quality of life issue. It is generally accepted that if all implants were removed after their insertion, orthopaedic and trauma surgeons would have little time to do anything else. The work load involved was discussed in detail by Bostman and Pihlajamaki (1996) in a review of the impact on a large university orthopaedic and trauma unit. Brown et al (1993) reviewed 297 operations where internal fixation for fractures or joint injuries had occurred. Implant removal was undertaken in 42% of these cases and complications occurred in 19%. Patients need to be warned of the risks of refracture, infection and nerve injury.

Ryf et al (2000) point out that implants are usually left in place for 1–2 years before removal is considered. They state that if implants are removed contact sports and heavy work should be deferred for two to four months.

Summary

- Delayed union, as defined by failure of full union to occur by 8 months, occurs in 6–12% of patients.
- Non-union occurs in approximately 1% of femoral shaft fractures.
- Refracture occurs in approximately 4% of femoral shaft fractures. The literature suggests that two-thirds of these are avoidable.
- Shortening of 2 cm or more occurs in approximately 11% of patients with femoral shaft fractures. It is more common after conservative treatment (28%) than after intramedullary nailing (6%). Shortening in excess of 2 cm is usually associated with gait impairment.
- Angular deformities, except where associated with shortening of more than 2 cm, were not usually symptomatic.
- In Kootstra's 1973 series 40% of patients with external rotation deformities of 20° or more were symptomatic, while only one of the five patients with internal rotation deformities of 20° or more was symptomatic. In none of the patients with rotational deformities was there evidence of osteoarthritis of the knee joint (follow-up 2–11 years).
- The incidence of impaired knee function (flexion less than 90°) is higher after conservative treatment (17%) than after operative treatment (0–5%).
- The average time lost from work following a femoral fracture was 9 months. It was slightly less (7 months) in those patients who underwent operative treatment.
- Following severely comminuted or segmental femoral fractures the mean time lost from work was 13.5 months.
- Only 1% of patients were unable to return to work, while 2.5% were forced to change their job as a result of their femoral fracture.

Supracondylar/intercondylar fractures

Hohl (1986) pointed out that fractures of the supracondylar and intercondylar regions of the femur inevitably lead to some functional sequelae ranging from loss of knee movement to instability, pain, weakness and traumatic arthritis. The AO classification (Müller et al 1990) is most commonly used to categorise these fractures.

Laros (1979) reviewed the literature up to that time on the clinical results following supracondylar fractures of the femur. He carefully analysed the available reports to enable comparison of results to be made from series to series. Results were graded as acceptable if they fell within the excellent—good—fair rating of Schatzker et al (1974), as follows:

- excellent:
  - full extension
  - flexion loss less than 10°
  - no varus, valgus or rotational deformity
  - no pain
  - perfect joint congruity
- good–not more than *one* of the following:
  - loss of length not more than 1.2 cm
  - less than 10° varus or valgus
  - flexion loss not more than 20°
  - minimal pain
- fair–any *two* criteria from the good category

Failures (i.e. unacceptable results) were those with 90° or less flexion, varus or valgus deformity greater than 15°, joint incongruity and disabling pain, no matter how perfect the X-ray.

These figures give an indication of the *overall* incidence of acceptable results, but there are significant variations from series to series. The results of AO internal fixation are significantly better in experienced centres where the AO principles are rigidly adhered to, as pointed out by Schatzker & Lambert (1979). These authors also point out that, even in centres of excellence, if the AO principles are not rigidly adhered to the results are much less satisfactory. Some of the less satisfactory results of operative treatment analysed by Laros (1979) covered the period 1940–1960, when attitudes to open reduction and available implants were less sophisticated than those currently in use.

The overall incidence of acceptable results in 535 cases reviewed by Laros (1979) was 62%. The best results (100% acceptable) were reported by Schatzker & Lambert (1979) following operative fixation with rigid adherence to AO principles. The worst results (31% acceptable) were reported by Neer et al (1967) following internal fixation using blade plates, Rush nails, plates and bolts and various combinations of wire, bolts and screws. The overall incidence of acceptable results was 64% of 254 patients treated operatively and 60% of 281 patients treated conservatively in this review. The overall incidence of non-union in this group of patients was 6%, with no significant difference between operative and non-operative treatment.

Egund & Kolmert (1982) carried out a detailed analysis of the late results in 62 patients with distal femoral fractures. Their paper is worth referring to in an attempt to predict the future outlook for individual patients. Their conclusions were as follows:

- The most significant predictor of osteoarthritis was a step in the articular surface exceeding 3 mm. The relationship of angular deformity to osteoarthritis was not clear.
- Osteoarthritis most commonly affected the patellofemoral joint (14 of 62 cases, 22%) rather than the tibiofemoral joint (3 of 62 cases, 5%).

The patellofemoral joint requires careful assessment at follow-up and in medicolegal reports.

Behrens et al (1986) emphasised the importance of reconstructing the articular surface, and found a much lower incidence of osteoarthritis in articular fractures where there had been surgical reconstruction of the joint surface, compared to those treated non-operatively. However, their criteria for the diagnosis of osteoarthritis and degree of articular incongruity in the non-operatively treated cases are not reported. A more recent article (Leung et al 1991) described closed intramedullary nailing and, where appropriate, percutaneous lag screws in the treatment of supracondylar and intercondylar fractures of the distal femur in 35 patients. They assessed functional results with the modified knee rating system of the Hospital for Special Surgery and found that 94% of their patients had a good or excellent result at an average follow-up of 20 months.

An overview of the situation (with the exception of Leung et al's paper) suggests that two-thirds of the patients have acceptable results (as defined by Laros) following supracondylar fractures of the femur. However, in favourable circumstances, particularly with articular (intercondylar) fractures, strict application of AO principles can lead to a higher proportion of acceptable results. The literature suggests that patients with comminuted fractures do less well and that older patients with osteoporotic bone have less satisfactory long-term results. Seinsheimer (1980) found that patients aged 60 or over, regardless of fracture type or treatment, consistently achieved less knee flexion than those under 60.

Summary

- The overall incidence of acceptable results (see text) following supracondylar or intercondylar fractures of the femur treated by a variety of methods is approximately 60%.
- The most significant predictor of osteoarthritis is the congruity of the articular surface. Incongruity of more than 3 mm is associated with a significantly increased risk of osteoarthritis.
- The patellofemoral joint requires careful assessment following supracondylar or intercondylar fractures of the femur, as osteoarthritis may occur there in up to 20% of cases.

Femoral Fractures in children
Subtrochanteric fractures

Velasco & Comfort (1978) reported on 10 subtrochanteric fractures in children. They were all treated conservatively and eight out of 10 had good results. The two unsatisfactory results were due to a fixed rotational deformity in one child and shortening of 2.5 cm in another. The authors classed a good result as follows:

- full pre-injury activity achieved
- minimal or no pain
- hip flexion of 90° or more
- rotational deformity of 10° or less
- shortening of 1.25 cm or less

Ireland & Fisher (1975) described 20 subtrochanteric fractures in children; 19 were treated non-operatively. They found that angular or rotational deformity occurred but caused no functional problem. Three children (15%) had shortening in excess of 1.25 cm and this was felt to be a particular problem in older children. A 13-year-old female with 5 cm of shortening required a contralateral femoral shortening procedure.

Femoral shaft fractures

Staheli (1984) pointed out that length malunion was th most common problem in the management of femoral shaft fractures in children. The rate of overgrowth is related to the patient's age when the femoral fracture occurs. Growth stimulation is less predictable in infancy and most active between the ages of 2 and 10 (Ogden 1987). Staheli (1984) pointed out that shortening was more common in children over the age of 10. The rate of growth following a femoral fracture is illustrated in Fig. 12.3: growth stimulation is most active in the first 6 months after injury but may persist for 2 years or more.

Shapiro (1981) found a mean femoral overgrowth of 0.92 cm in 74 patients with femoral shaft fractures, while Clement & Colton (1986) reported an average overgrowth of 0.81 cm in 44 femoral shaft fractures. The latter authors found that overgrowth was more common in boys than girls. However, Staheli (1984) believed that as long as the leg lengths were within 1 cm of each other there would be no noticeable difference, while if there was a disparity of 1–2 cm it may be noticeable to the family but not the child. It is only if the leg length inequality exceeds 2 cm that both parents and child are aware of it.

There is no study encompassing all the interacting factors following the childhood femoral shaft fracture and relating these to leg lengths at skeletal maturity. Final leg length is a function of the age of the child, the type of fracture and particularly the degree of overlap accepted on traction during treatment of the fracture. The long-term effects of minor degrees of limb length inequality are not clear, but, as pointed out by Staheli (1984), it seldom produces structural scoliosis but may produce a slight asymmetry of gait and aggravate the common back pain problem of adult life. Malkawi et al (1986) reported an incidence of 2% (3 of 141) leg length inequality of over 1 cm in a group of patients followed up for 2–10 years after treatment on skin traction.

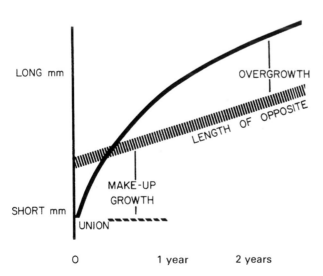

Fig. 12.3 The rate of growth following femoral shaft fracture in children. The fractured femur is initially short from overriding at union. Growth acceleration results in 'make-up' growth and in some cases overgrowth occurs (from Staheli 1984, with permission).

Acceptable amounts of angular malunion in children's femoral fractures are controversial. Malkawi et al (1986) accepted 20° of initial angulation in the frontal (coronal) plane and 30° of initial angulation in the lateral (sagittal) plane in the expectation that remodelling would occur. Using the classification of Anderson (1967) that 0–5° of final angulation is excellent alignment, 5–10° of final angulation is satisfactory alignment and over 10° is unsatisfactory alignment, they found that 74% of their 141 cases had excellent alignment, 18% had satisfactory alignment and 8% had unsatisfactory alignment at final assessment 2–10 years after injury. Wallace & Hoffman (1992) reviewed 28 children with unilateral middle third fractures of the femoral shaft who had an angular deformity, after union, of 10–26°. They concluded that in children under the age of 13, malunion of as much as 25° in any plane will remodel enough to gain normal alignment of the joint surfaces.

Brouwer et al (1981) considered the long-term incidence of rotational deformities following femoral shaft fractures in childhood, with a 27–32 year follow-up. They studied 50 cases and found a persistent rotational difference of more than 10° between the normal and the affected side in six cases, and in these cases it was asymptomatic. Davids (1994) followed up a series of seven children who had rotational deformity of over 10° with serial CT scans and found little potential for the deformity to correct. Moreover, in the long-term follow-up there was no evidence that persistent rotational deformity led to premature osteoarthritis.

Non-union or delayed union is very uncommon in childhood femoral fractures and, as Blount (1955) pointed out, when they occur they are usually seen in patients who have had open procedures complicated by infection.

Epiphyseal damage can result from treatment. Anterior proximal tibial growth arrest with secondary recurvatum deformity has been reported following tibial skeletal traction (Van Meter & Branick 1980). Coxa valga can occur if intramedullary nailing is carried out in the child with an open greater trochanteric epiphysis (Staheli 1984).

Fractures involving the distal physis

Riseborough et al (1983) recognised that fracture separation of the distal femoral physis could lead to lower limb length discrepancy, angular deformity and reduced knee movement. It may also result in acute vascular or neurological injury. Ogden (1987) and Czitrom et al (1981) reported that growth at this physis contributes 40% to overall leg length.

Roberts (1984) believed that the prognosis for separation of the distal femoral physis was usually excellent. Czitrom et al (1981) reviewed 41 cases and found that results were good or excellent in 28 (68%). Good or excellent results implied minimal or no symptoms, minimal loss of motion, no ligamentous laxity, angular deformity of less than 5° and shortening of less than 1.5 cm.

Riseborough et al (1983) studied 66 children, but did not feel that their incidence of complications was a true reflection because many were referred secondarily with growth problems. The authors reported that growth problems correlated well with the severity of the trauma, and they were seen in each of the Salter–Harris groups (Salter & Harris 1963). They found that fractures in the age group 2–11 years were associated with the most severe trauma and the poorest prognosis. Injuries in patients over the age of 11 were usually caused by less extensive trauma—often sports injuries—and were associated with a lesser incidence of growth disturbance. Children under the age of 2 years did not develop severe growth problems in this series.

Roberts (1984) reviewed the recent literature on this injury and found a 19% incidence of angular deformity greater than 5°, a 24% incidence of leg length discrepancy greater than 2 cm and a 16% incidence of knee stiffness (although the precise criteria for knee stiffness were not defined).

Controversy exists over the predictive value of the Salter–Harris classification. Czitrom et al (1981) found it useful, while Lombardo & Harvey (1977) felt that it was not valuable.

The final prognosis in these injuries is influenced by the mechanism and severity of injury, the amount of initial displacement, the adequacy of reduction, the classification of the injury and the time remaining to physeal closure.

Summary

- Subtrochanteric fractures in children are usually managed conservatively and good results occur in over 80% of cases. The incidence of shortening in excess of 1.25 cm is approximately 13%.
- Long-term results of femoral shaft fractures in children are usually good, with a 2% incidence of leg length inequality greater than 1 cm and an 8% incidence of angular deformity in excess of 10°. Rotational deformities in excess of 10° occurred in 12% of patients, but were not symptomatic and did not appear to predispose the hip or knee joint to premature degenerative change when followed up for 27–32 years.
- Approximately two-thirds of patients with injuries involving the distal femoral physis achieve good or excellent results (see text). Long-term results tend to be poorer in children aged between 2 and 11 years who sustain severe trauma.

Special groups
Femoral shaft fracture with ipsilateral hip injury
Kootstra (1973) suggested that injury to the ipsilateral hip occurred in approximately 5% of femoral shaft fractures and stressed the importance of obtaining pelvic X-rays routinely in all cases of femoral shaft fractures.

Associated hip injuries may be of three types: proximal femoral fracture, acetabular fracture or hip dislocation. In Kootstra's series proximal femoral fracture occurred in 11 of 329 patients (3.4%), while acetabular fracture occurred in five of 329 patients (1.5%) and hip dislocation occurred in one of 329 (0.3%).

The additional variable of further injury with added treatment options and the small numbers of cases reported in the literature make it difficult to give clear prognostic guidelines. There is no doubt that the single most important factor is early recognition of the hip injury. Swiontkowski et al (1984) found that one-third of associated femoral neck fractures were missed at initial assessment. Dehne & Immermann (1951) found that nine of 16 (56%) hip dislocations were missed at initial assessment when associated with a femoral shaft fracture. This correlates with Lyddon & Hartmann's 1971 observation that 50 to 54% of dislocations were initially unrecognised.

In these combined injuries, prognosis has to be given on the basis of the individual injuries, with due consideration made for the increased incidence of complications which may occur following late recognition of a hip dislocation or subcapital fracture (see Chapter 11).

Swiontkowski (1987) reviewed the orthopaedic literature and found 176 cases with proximal femoral fractures in association with femoral shaft fractures. He found an incidence of only 5% of avascular necrosis of the femoral head, and suggested that this relatively low percentage was because the majority of energy causing the fracture was dissipated at midshaft level. This incidence may be falsely low, as the follow-up in some series was only 1 year and Swiontkowski suggested that the true incidence is probably 10 to 15%.

Femoral shaft fracture with fracture of the ipsilateral patella
Ipsilateral patellar fracture was found in 1.7% of Dencker's 1963 large series and 5.8% of Kootstra's 1973 series. Treatment methods are diverse (i.e. fixation versus patellectomy) and there are insufficient numbers to draw firm conclusions on the prognosis. The conclusion from Kootstra's work is that the results are less satisfactory

when femoral shaft and patellar fracture are combined than when either occurs in isolation.

Femoral shaft fracture with fracture of the ipsilateral tibia (floating knee)

Again it is possible only to generalise on prognosis following combined tibial and femoral injuries because of the large number of variables involved and the small number of reports on the subject. Karlstrom & Olerud (1977) and Fraser et al (1978) reported follow-up on 87 patients using the same criteria for assessment of end-results, as shown in Table 12.8.

Both groups found that the worst results occurred in patients who had conservative treatment of both fractures, agreeing with the earlier work of Ratliff (1968). The 87 patients were divided into three groups according to their treatment:

- group I—both fractures rigidly internally fixed
- group II—one fracture rigidly fixed and the other treated, conservatively
- group III—both fractures treated conservatively

The mean follow-up of Karlstrom & Olerud (1977) was 2 years 9 months, while Fraser et al (1978) reported a mean follow-up of 5 years. Patients in group I were reported to be back at work in a mean time of 6 months by Karlstrom & Olerud and in 11 months by Fraser et al. Patients in group III returned to work in 15 and 21 months respectively in the two reports. The end-results in these patients are summarised in Table 12.9.

The overall incidence of good or excellent results is 40%, with 62% good or excellent in group I and 28 to 33% good or excellent in groups II and III. Fraser et al (1978) pointed out that there was a higher incidence of chronic

Table 12.8 Criteria for the assessment of end-results in ipsilateral femoral and tibial fractures (after Karlstrom & Olerud 1977, with permission)

Criterion	Excellent	Good	Acceptable	Poor
Subjective symptoms from thigh or leg	Nil	Intermittent slight symptoms function	More severe symptoms impairing	Considerable impairment at rest
Subjective symptoms from knee or ankle joint	Nil	Same as above	More severe symptoms impairing function	Considerable impairment at rest
Walking ability	Unimpaired	Same as above	Walking distance restricted	Cane, crutches or other support
Work and sports	Same as before accident	Given up some sport; work as before accident	Change to less strenuous work	Permanent disability
Angulation, rotational deformity, or both	0	<10°	10–20°	>20°
Shortening	0	<1 cm	1–3 cm	>3 cm
Restricted joint	0	<10° at ankle;	10–20° at ankle;	>20° at ankle;
mobility (hip, knee or ankle)	<20° at hip, knee or both	20–40° at hip, knee or both	>40° at hip, knee or both	

Table 12.9 End-results after ipsilateral femoral and tibial fractures in 87 patients reported by Karlstrom & Olerud (1977) and Fraser et al (1978): results according to the criteria of Karlstrom & Olerud (see Table 12.8)

	Excellent	Good	Acceptable	Poor
Group I (24)	7	8	8	1
Group II (31)	3	7	16	5
Group III (30)	0	9	13	8
Total (85)	10 (12%)	24 (28%)	37 (43%)	14 (16%)

osteomyelitis in patients who had both fractures internally fixed.

Bohn & Durbin (1991) reviewed a group of children and adolescents with ipsilateral fractures of the femur and tibia. They were able to follow up 19 patients by personal examination and X-ray. Only seven of these had normal function without major problems. The remainder had a compromised result due to limb length discrepancy, angular deformity or knee ligament instability.

Yokoyama et al (2000) published an extensive review of 65 patients with 66 floating knee injuries. Of the 66 femoral fractures, 29% (19) were open and 43 of the tibial fractures were open. Ninety-five percent of the patients were treated operatively (interlocked nails, plates, Enders nails, external fixation). The major determinant of outcome appeared to be the severity of the damage to the knee joint and compounding of the femoral fracture. However, follow-up in this series was only 16.6 months (range 12–50).

Summary

- Early recognition of ipsilateral hip injury requires a high level of clinical suspicion. The incidence of avascular necrosis of the femoral head following associated femoral neck fracture is probably 5–15%.

- In ipsilateral femoral and tibial fractures the overall incidence of good/excellent results is 40% (see Table 12.9). Better results (62% good/excellent) were seen in patients who had internal fixation of both fractures.

References

Anderson R L 1967 Conservative treatment of fractures of the femur. Journal of Bone and Joint Surgery 49A: 1371–1375

Azer S N, Rankin E A 1994 Complications of treatment of femoral shaft fractures In: Epps C H (ed) Complications in orthopaedic surgery, 3rd edn. J B Lippincott, Philadelphia, pp 487–524

Behrens F, Ditmanson P, Hartleben P, Comfort T H, Gaither D W, Denis F 1986 Long term results of distal femoral fractures. Journal of Bone and Joint Surgery 68B: 848

Bilcher Taft M, Hammer A 1970 Treatment of fractures of the femoral shaft. Acta Orthopaedica Scandinavica 41: 341

Blount W 1955 Fractures in children. Williams & Wilkins, Baltimore

Bohn W W, Durbin R A 1991 Ipsilateral fractures of the femur and tibia in children and adolescents. Journal of Bone and Joint Surgery 73A: 429–439

Bostman O, Pihlajamaki H 1996 Routine implant removal after fracture surgery: a potentially reducible consumer of hospital resources in trauma units. Journal of Trauma 41(5): 846–849

Boyd H, Griffin L 1949 Classification and treatment of trochanteric fractures. Archives of Surgery 58: 853–866

Braten M, Terjesen T, Rossvoli I 1993 Torsional deformity after intramedullary nailing of femoral shaft fracture: measurement of anteversion angles in 110 patients. Journal of Bone and Joint Surgery 75B: 799–803

Braten M, Terejesen T, Rossvoli I 1995 Femoral fractures treated by intramedullary nailing. A follow up study focusing on problems relating to the method. Injury 26(6): 379–383

Breedeveld R S, Patka P, Von Mourik J C 1985 Refractures of the femoral shaft. Netherlands Journal of Surgery 37(4): 114–116

Brouwer K J, Molenaar J C, Van Linge 1981 Rotational deformities after femoral shaft fractures in childhood: a retrospective study 27–32 years after the accident. Acta Orthopaedica Scandinavica 52: 81–89

Brumbach R J, Scott Ellison T, Molligan H, Molligan D J, Mahaffey S, Schmidhauser C 1992 Pudendal nerve palsy complicating intramedullary nailing of the femur. Journal of Bone and Joint Surgery 74A: 1450–1455

Cameron C D, Meek R N, Blachut P A, O'Brien P J, Pate G C 1992 Intramedullary nailing of the femoral shaft: a prospective, randomised study. Journal of Orthopaedic Trauma 6: 448–451

Carr C W, Wingo C H 1973 Fractures of the femoral diaphysis: a retrospective study of the results and costs of treatment by intramedullary nailing and by traction and spica cast. Journal of Bone and Joint Surgery 55A: 690–700

Charnley J, Guindy A 1961 Delayed operation in the open reduction of fractures of long bones. Journal of Bone and Joint Surgery 43B: 664

Christovitsinos J P, Xenakis T, Paoajiaruswa K G, Skaltsoyannis N, Grestas A, Soucacos P N 1997 Bridge plating osteosynthesis of 20 comminuted fractures of the femur. Acta Orthopaedica Scandinavica (Supp 1) 275: 72–76

Clement D A, Colton C L 1986 Overgrowth of the femur after fracture in childhood: an increased effect in boys. Journal of Bone and Joint Surgery 68B: 534–536

Costa P, Carretti P, Giancecchi F K, Rostini R, Tartaglia I 1988 The locked Grosse Kempf in the treatment of diaphyseal and metaphyseal fractures of the femur and tibia. Italian Journal of Orthopaedics 14: 475

Curtis M J, Jinna R H, Wilson V, Cunningham B W 1994 Proximal femoral fractures: A biomechanical study to compare intra- and extramedullary fixation. Injury 25(2): 99–104

Czitrom A A, Salter R B, Willis R B 1981 Fractures involving the distal epiphyseal plate of the femur. International Orthopedics 4: 269–277

Davids J R 1994 Potential deformity and remodeling after fracture of the femur in children. Clinical Orthopaedics 302: 27–35

Dehne E, Immermann E W 1951 Dislocation of the hip combined with fracture of the shaft of the femur on the same side. Journal of Bone and Joint Surgery 33A: 731–745

Delee J C, Clanton T O, Rockwood C A Jr 1981 Closed treatment of subtrochanteric fractures of the femur in a modified cast brace. Journal of Bone and Joint Surgery 63A: 773–779

Delee J C 1984 Fractures and dislocations of the hip. In: Rockwood C A Jr, Green D P (eds) Fractures in adults, 2nd edn, vol 2, J B Lippincott, Philadelphia

Dencker H M 1963 Fractures of the shaft of the femur. Orstadius Boktryckeri, Gothenborg

Dencker H M 1964 Refracture of the shaft of the femur. Acta Orthopaedica Scandinavica 35:158

Dencker H M 1965 Shaft fractures of the femur: a comparative study of the results of various methods of treatment in 1003 cases. Acta Chirurgica Scandinavica 130: 173–184

Edwards S A, Pandit H G, Clarke H J 2000 The long gamma nail: A DGM experience. Injury 31(9): 701–709

Egund N, Kolmert L 1982 Deformities, gonoarthrosis and function after distal femoral fractures. Acta Orthopaedica Scandinavica 53: 963

Fielding J W, Cochran G, Van B, Zickel R E 1974 Biomechanical characteristics and surgical management of subtrochanteric fractures. Orthopedic Clinics of North America 5: 629–649

Fraser R D, Hunter G A, Waddell J P 1978 Ipsilateral fracture of the femur and tibia. Journal of Bone and Joint Surgery 60B: 510–515

Furlong A J, Giannoudis P V, De Boer P, Mathers S J, MacDonald D A, Smith R M 1999 Exchange nailing for femoral shaft aseptic non union. Injury 30 (4): 245

Giannoudis P V, MacDonald D A, Matthews S J, Smith R M, Furlong A J, De Boer P 2000 Non union of the femoral diaphysis. The influence of reaming and non-steroidal anti-inflammatory drugs. Journal of Bone and Joint Surgery 82(5): 655–658

Hak D J, Lee S S, Goulet J A 2000 Success of exchange reamed intramedullary nailing for femoral shaft non union or delayed union. Journal of Orthopaedic Trauma 14(3): 178–182

Hardy A E, White P, Williams J 1979 The treatment of femoral fractures by cast brace and early walking: a review of 79 patients. Journal of Bone and Joint Surgery 61B: 151–154

Hartmann E R, Brav E A 1954 The problem of refracture in fractures of the femoral shaft. Journal of Bone and Joint Surgery 36A: 1071–1079

Hohl M 1986 Complications of treatment of fractures and dislocations of the knee. Ch 19, Section 1: Complications of fractures. In: Epps C H Jr (ed) Complications in orthopaedic surgery, 2nd edn, vol 1. J B Lippincott, Philadelphia, pp 537–556

Hung S C, Kurokawa T, Nakamura K, Matsushita T, Shiro R 1996 Narrowing of the joint space of the hip after traumatic shortening of the femur. Journal of Bone and Joint Surgery 78(5): 718–721

Ireland D C R, Fisher R L 1975 Subtrochanteric fractures of the femur in children. Clinical Orthopaedics 110: 157–166

Karlstrom G, Olerud S 1977 Ipsilateral fracture of the femur and tibia. Journal of Bone and Joint Surgery 59A: 240–243

Kinast C, Bolhofner B R, Mast J W, Ganz R 1989 Subtrochanteric fractures of the femur. Results of treatment with the 95° condylar blade plate. Clinical Orthopaedics 238: 122–130

Kootstra G 1973 Femoral shaft fractures in adults: a study of 329 consecutive cases with statistical analysis of different methods of treatment. Van Gorcum, Assen, The Netherlands

Laros G S 1979 Supracondylar fractures of the femur: editorial comments and comparative results. Clinical Orthopaedics 138: 9–12

Laros G S, Spiegel P G 1979 Femoral shaft fractures: editorial comment and comparative results. Clinical Orthopaedics 138: 5–9

Laubenthal R N, Smidt G L, Kettelkamp D B 1972 A quantitative analysis of knee motion during daily living. Physical Therapy 52: 32

Leung K S, Shen W Y, So W S, Mui L T, Grosse A 1991 Interlocking intramedullary nailing for supracondylar and intercondylar fractures of the distal part of the femur. Journal of Bone and Joint Surgery 73A: 332–346

Lombardo S J, Harvey J P 1977 Fractures of the distal femoral epiphysis: factors influencing prognosis, a review of 34 cases. Journal of Bone and Joint Surgery 59A: 742–751

Lyddon D W Jr, Hartmann J T 1971 Traumatic dislocation of the hip with ipsilateral femoral fracture. Journal of Bone and Joint Surgery 53A: 1012–1016

Malkawi H, Shennak A, Hadidi S 1986 Remodelling after femoral shaft fractures in children treated by the modified Blount method. Journal of Paediatric Orthopaedics 6: 421–429

McLaren A C, Roth J N, Wright C 1990 Intramedullary rod fixation of femoral shaft fractures: Comparison of open and closed in section techniques. Canadian Journal of Surgery 33: 286

Mooney V, Claudi B F 1984 Fractures of the shaft of the femur. In: Rockwood C A Jnr, Green D P (eds) Fractures in adults, vol 2. J B Lippincott, Philadelphia

Morscher E, Taillard W 1965 Beinlangenunterschiede. Karger, Basel

Moulton A, Upadhyay S S, Fletcher M, Bancroft G 1984 Does an associated injury affect the outcome of a fracture of the femoral shaft? A statistical analysis. Journal of Bone and Joint Surgery 66B: 285

Müller M E 1967 Vorwortin Posttraumatische Aschenfehistellungen an den unteren Extremitaten. Hans Huber Verlag, Bern, pp 7–8

Müller M E, Nazarian S, Koch P, Schatzker J 1990 The AO classification of fractures. Springer Verlag, Berlin, Heidelberg, New York

Neer C S, Grantham S A, Shelton M L 1967 Supracondylar fractures of the adult femur: a study of 110 cases. Journal of Bone and Joint Surgery 49A: 591–613

Nichols P R 1963 Rehabilitation after fractures of the shaft of the femur. Journal of Bone and Joint Surgery 45B: 96–102

Nicod L 1967 Effects cliniques et pronostics des defauts d'axe du membre inferieur chez l'adulte, a la suite dune consolidation vicieuse dune fracture du membre inferieur. Posttraumatische Ashenfehlstellungen an den unteren Extremitaten. Hans Huber Verlag, Bern, pp 57–78

Ogden J A 1987 Pocket guide to pediatric fractures. Williams & Wilkins, Baltimore

Parker M J, Dutta B K, Sivaji C, Pryor G A 1997 Subtrochanteric fractures of the femur. Injury 28920: 91–95

Ratliff A H C 1968 Fractures of the shaft of the femur and tibia in the same limb. Proceedings of the Royal Society of Medicine 61: 906–908

Riseborough E J, Barrett I R, Shapiro F 1983 Growth disturbance following distal femoral epiphyseal fracture separations. Journal of Bone and Joint Surgery 65A: 885–893

Roberts J M 1984 Fractures and dislocations of the knee. In: Rockwood C A Jr, Wilkins K E, King R E (eds) Fractures in children, vol 3. J B Lippincott, Philadelphia

Rokkanen P, Slatis P, Vankka E 1969 Closed or open intramedullary nailing of femoral shaft fractures? A comparison with conservatively treated cases. Journal of Bone and Joint Surgery 51B: 313–323

Ruedi T P, Luscher J N 1979 Results after internal fixation of comminuted fractures of the femoral shaft with DC plates. Clinical Orthopaedics 138: 74

Ryf C, Weymann A, Matter P 2000 Post operative management: general consideration in AO principles of fracture management. Eds Colton, Fernandez, Dell'Oca, Holz, Kellam, Ochsner. Thieme, Stuttgart, New York, pp 719–727

Salter R B, Harris W R 1963 Injuries involving the epiphyseal plate. Journal of Bone and Joint Surgery 45A: 587–622

Schatzker J, Horne G, Waddell J 1974 The Toronto experience with the supracondylar fracture of the femur 1966–1972. Injury 6: 113

Schatzker J, Lambert D C 1979 Supracondylar fractures of the femur. Clinical Orthopaedics 138: 77–83

Seimon L P 1964 Refracture of the shaft of the femur. Journal of Bone and Joint Surgery 46B: 32–39

Seinsheimer F 1978 Subtrochanteric fractures of the femur. Journal of Bone and Joint Surgery 60A: 300–306

Seinsheimer F 1980 Fractures of the distal femur. Clinical Orthopaedics 153: 169–179

Senter B, Kendig R, Savoie F H 1990 Operative stabilisation of subtrochanteric fracture of the femur. Journal of Orthopaedic Trauma 4(4) 399–405

Shapiro F 1981 Fractures of the femoral shaft in children: the overgrowth phenomenon. Acta Orthopaedica Scandinavica 52: 649–655

Sharma J C, Gupta S P, Mathur N G, Kalla R, Aseri M K, Biyani A, Arora A 1993 Comminuted femoral shaft fractures treated by closed intramedullary nailing and functional cast bracing. Journal of Trauma 34(6): 786–791

Sojbjerg J O, Eiskjaer S, Moller-Larsen F 1990 Locked nailing of comminuted and unstable fractures of the femur. Journal of Bone and Joint Surgery 72(1): 23–25

Staheli L T 1984 Fractures of the shaft of the femur. In: Rockwood C A Jr, Wilkins K E, King R E (eds) Fractures in children, vol 3. J B Lippincott, Philadelphia

Swiontkowski M F 1987 Ipsilateral femoral shaft and hip fracture. Orthopedic Clinics of North America 18: 73–84

Swiontkowski M F, Hansen S T, Kellam J 1984 Ipsilateral fractures of the femoral neck and shaft: a treatment protocol. Journal of Bone and Joint Surgery 66A: 260–268

Trafton P G 1987 Subtrochanteric-intertrochanteric femoral fractures. Orthopedic Clinics of North America 18: 59–71

van Doorn R, Stapert J W 2000 The long gamma nail in the treatment of 329 subtrochanteric fractures with major extension into the femoral shaft. European Journal of Surgery 166(3): 240–246

Van Meter J, Branick R 1980 Bilateral genu recurvatum after skeletal traction. Journal of Bone and Joint Surgery 62A: 837–839

Vangness T C, De Campos J, Merritt P O, Wiss D A 1993 Meniscal injury associated with femoral shaft fracture. An arthroscopic evaluation of incidence. Journal of Bone and Joint Surgery 75B: 207–209

Velasco R U, Comfort T H 1978 Analysis of treatment problems in subtrochanteric fractures of the femur. Journal of Trauma 18: 513–523

Waddell J P 1979 Subtrochanteric fractures of the femur: a review of 130 patients. Journal of Trauma 19: 582–592

Wallace M E, Hoffman E B 1992 Remodelling of angular deformity after femoral shaft fractures in children. Journal of Bone and Joint Surgery 74B: 765–769

Warwick D J, Crichlow T P, Langmaker V G, Jackson M 1995 The dynamic condylar screw in the management of subtrochanteric fractures of the femur. Injury 26(4): 241–244

Watson H K, Campbell R D, Wade P A 1964 Classification and complications of adult subtrochanteric fractures. Journal of Trauma 4: 457–480

Webb L X, Winquist R A, Hansen S T 1986 Intramedullary nailing and reaming for delayed union or non union of the femoral shaft: a report of 105 consecutive cases. Clinical Orthopaedics 212: 133

Wickstrom J, Corban M S, Vise G T 1968 Complications following intramedullary nailing of 324 fractured femurs. Clinical Orthopaedics 60: 103–113

Wile P B, Paniabi M M, Southwick W O 1983 Treatment of subtrochanteric fractures with a high angle compression hip screw. Clinical Orthopaedics 175: 72–78

Winquist R A, Hansen S T 1980 Comminuted fractures of the femoral shaft treated by intramedullary nailing. Orthopedic Clinics of North America 11(3): 633–648

Winquist R A, Hansen S T Jr, Clawson D K 1984 Closed intramedullary nailing of femoral fractures: report of 520 fractures. Journal of Bone and Joint Surgery 66A: 529–539

Wolinsky P R, McCarty E, Shyr Y, Johnman K 1999 Reamed intramedullary nailing of the femur: 551 cases. Journal of Trauma 46(3): 392–399

Yokoyama K, Nakamura T, Shindo M, Tsukamoto T, Saita Y, Aoki S, Homan N 2000 Contributing factors influencing the functional outcome of floating knee injuries. American Journal of Orthopaedics 29(9): 721–729

Chapter 13

The knee

Philip Wilde

Introduction

The knee is one of the most complex joints in the body. Function relies on a balance between flexibility and stability which is provided by a combination of bony anatomy, powerful muscles, strong ligaments and meniscal cartilages. All of these can be injured either separately or in combination.

Knee injuries are common and can be caused either by direct force being applied to the knee or indirectly from forcible contraction of the strong quadriceps and hamstring muscles. One of the commonest causes of a knee injury is a twisting or angular deforming force sustained while playing sport. This has led to what some people describe as a modern epidemic of ligament injuries.

However, the knee is also somewhat vulnerable in the seated position and is therefore often damaged in road traffic accidents. Direct force to the anterior aspect to the knee can damage the patello-femoral joint as well as causing major fractures or ligamentous injuries. The knee is thus vulnerable to injury from a wide variety of sources.

The pattern of injury also changes with age. Fractures are more common in the extremes of life and soft tissue injuries more prevalent in the middle years. Isolated ligament injuries in those over 60 years of age are rare as the bones are relatively weaker and, therefore, fracture is more likely in this age group.

There is also a difference in incidence of injury between the sexes. With the increasing number of women enjoying high level sporting participation, studies have shown that the incidence of anterior cruciate ligament and meniscal injury in women undertaking sport is significantly greater than in men undertaking similar activities (Arenadt & Dick 1995).

The complexity of the knee makes long-term prediction of outcome difficult but important. Long-term symptoms can be quite disabling and certain injuries predispose to osteoarthritic change in later life.

Before proceeding to review the outcome from individual injuries, it is helpful to consider some general aspects of knee function and, in particular, identify the common symptoms attributable to knee injuries.

General considerations

The outcome of a knee injury depends upon the restoration of normal function. The knee is essentially a complex hinge joint which allows motion in one plane. Some rotation occurs at the knee, however, to allow changes of direction and twisting movements.

The function of the knee depends, to a large extent, on the strength of the muscles around it. In particular, adequate strength of the quadriceps muscles is essential for restoration of knee function. It is also recognised that the hamstring muscles are important in controlling stability of the knee. Strength in these muscles is thus important in compensating for certain ligament injuries, in particular injuries to the anterior cruciate ligament.

The ligaments of the knee are primarily responsible for controlling motion and limiting instability. There is a significant normal variation within the population with some people having so-called 'physiological laxity' related to hypermobile joints. Examination of the knee, therefore, must always be compared with the contralateral, 'normal' side before ligament laxity can be quantified.

When discussing symptoms of ligamentous injuries, it is also vitally important to differentiate between ligament laxity, which is a clinical sign detected on examination, and knee instability, which is a symptom complained of by the patient. Instability can be due to factors other than laxity and the presence of ligamentous laxity does not necessarily mean that the patient will have symptoms of instability.

Symptoms of knee injury
Pain

Pain is a common complaint following knee injuries and in most cases is activity related and eased by rest. Anterior knee pain, however, can be severe even at rest, particularly if the knee is held bent for any period of time.

In general, ligament injuries do not, themselves, cause symptoms of pain except following acute episodes of instability. They may, however, be associated with other lesions which are responsible for the continuing discomfort.

One of the commonest sources of pain in the knee is the patello-femoral joint. Severe wasting of the quadriceps muscles, for whatever reason, frequently gives rise to patello-femoral discomfort, which is made worse by physical activity. Discomfort on weight bearing with the knee flexed, as commonly experienced on climbing stairs, should immediately raise suspicion of patello-femoral involvement.

Pain on twisting movements of the knee is more likely to be emanating from the tibio-femoral joint and is most commonly caused by meniscal injuries. This type of pain also occurs once degenerative changes have become established.

Restricted movement

The knee has a normal range of movement from 0° (full extension) to approximately 140° of flexion. There is a certain physiological variance, however, with some patients having between 5° and 10° of hyperextension at the knee. Flexion is also often limited in the obese patient.

Loss of range of movement can be somewhat disabling. Injuries which disrupt the tibio-femoral joint may lead to loss of full extension. Although not, in itself, functionally disabling, this has far-reaching consequences. It is quite possible to walk with the knee slightly flexed and mobility can be maintained with some fixed flexion. This action, however, causes relative overloading of the patello-femoral joint as the quadriceps muscles cannot relax in full extension. This leads to altered mechanics of the patello-femoral joint and is a potent source of pain. In addition it is difficult to maintain adequate quadriceps strength when the knee will not fully extend and there is rapid wasting of the quadriceps muscles in this situation. Loss of full extension, therefore, commonly leads to patello-femoral pain, which can be severe and disabling.

Loss of flexion can also be disabling. Full flexion of the knee is required in order to kneel on the floor and, therefore, loss of flexion can prevent this activity. Although a number of patients tolerate this restriction well, in patients where kneeling is required for either social or religious reasons, it can be a significant impediment. Knee flexion of at least 110° is required to rise from the seated position. As long as one knee bends to greater than 110° then it is usually possible to compensate for stiffness in the other. If both knees have restricted flexion, however, then rising from the seated position is impossible without help.

Instability

Patients often complain that their knee gives way. This can have a number of causes, the most common being laxity of the ligaments, weakness of the quadriceps muscles, meniscal tears and patello-femoral pain.

Any ligament injury can give rise to symptoms of instability in the knee. Different ligament injuries give rise to different patterns of instability. An anterior cruciate ligament tear generally gives rise to symptoms only during changes of direction or if landing on a slightly flexed knee. It is, therefore, more common to get instability during sport with this type of injury. Other types of ligament injury, particularly more severe combined injuries, can give rise to symptoms of instability during normal walking.

Instability from ligamentous laxity is usually sudden and unexpected and often causes the patient to fall. There is rarely sufficient warning of the knee collapsing for the patient to save himself. This condition should be differentiated from patello-femoral giving-way, where the initial feeling is frequently of discomfort and reflex muscle inhibition, causing the knee to collapse. In these circumstances, the patient often has sufficient warning to prevent himself from falling.

Locking

Patients often complain of locking, although this symptom covers a wide variety of conditions. True locking in a medical sense relates to an inability to extend the knee fully, when compared to the contralateral side. This can have a number of causes which can be either pain related or mechanical. Locking is commonly seen with meniscal injuries and anterior cruciate ligament tears.

Patients' descriptions of locking may relate to 'jamming up' of the knee in certain positions. This in turn can be related to meniscal lesions but is more commonly seen with patello-femoral pain. This so-called 'pseudo-locking' occurs during straightening of the knee, often after the leg has been relaxed. The patient experiences acute pain in the knee and has an inability to move the leg. This is generally relieved by rubbing the front of the knee and gently allowing it to straighten, after which time the knee returns to normal. This is to be differentiated from true mechanical locking which is usually more prolonged and often does not resolve spontaneously.

Summary

- Knee function requires a combination of flexibility and stability.
- Adequate muscular strength, particularly of the quadriceps muscles, is essential for normal knee function.
- When considering outcome, it is important to differentiate between knee instability (a symptom) and ligament laxity (a clinical sign).
- Loss of extension produces overloading of the patello-femoral joint and is a potent source of knee pain.

■ The symptoms following knee injury usually fall into one of four categories, namely pain, reduced movement, instability or locking.

Injuries to the meniscus

Injuries to the meniscus are common and often occur from a twisting injury to a flexed knee. The tear in the meniscus can have variable morphology but, in general, tears can be divided into the bucket handle tears with displacement and various split tears. These splits can be either radial, horizontal or a combination of the two. This latter group are often referred to as degenerate type tears.

Most studies of the late results following meniscal surgery have looked at all meniscal tears together. Some studies have tried to differentiate between the outcome from a buckle handle tear and a split tear, although most studies do not have sufficient numbers to allow this differentiation. The long-term data, therefore, relate to all types of meniscal tears.

In general, most studies of meniscal injuries relate to the late results of meniscectomy (meniscal removal). This is principally because the meniscus was thought to be expendable and techniques of repair of a torn meniscus have only recently been popularised.

Evolution of treatment

Fifty years ago the standard form of treatment for meniscal problems was total open meniscectomy. This involved removal of the entire meniscus via an open approach. Once it was realised that this may be harmful, some surgeons practised partial meniscectomy whereby only the torn part of the meniscus was removed. This, again, was performed by an open approach.

In the early 1960s the arthroscope was introduced to clinical practice. The technique of arthroscopy of the knee has developed rapidly over the last 30 years and is now a standard form of treatment for meniscal injuries. Today total open meniscectomy is rarely performed and most meniscal lesions are treated by arthroscopic partial meniscectomy, with a significantly faster recovery time.

More recently, with the advent of magnetic resonance imaging (MRI), pre-operative diagnosis has become much easier. This has dramatically reduced the number of diagnostic arthroscopies required in centres that have access to this form of imaging.

Timing of surgery

Very little hard data exist regarding the role of an untreated torn meniscus and the development of secondary damage to the knee. Tapper & Hoover (1969) suggested that the timing of surgery for a meniscal tear did not affect the

ultimate outcome. This finding was somewhat contradicted by Johnson et al (1974) when he suggested that the duration of symptoms and the frequency of re-injury prior to surgery affected the long-term result. Both of these series included patients with ligamentous laxity and cannot, therefore, be reliably used to predict outcome from isolated meniscal tears.

Fahmy et al (1983) examined 150 knees at autopsy and showed that meniscal tears could be present without osteoarthritis having been induced in the knee and that also osteoarthritis could be present without significant meniscal pathology. Their conclusion was that there was little evidence that degenerate meniscal tears caused osteoarthritis.

It would, therefore, seem sensible that treatment for meniscal injuries should be based upon symptoms rather than concerns regarding the long-term outcome. Meniscal tears giving severe pain or repeated giving-way should be treated, whereas those that are found incidentally and are not associated with symptoms can be left without harm.

Osteoarthritis following meniscectomy

The earliest report of radiological changes occurring following meniscectomy was by Fairbank in 1948. His paper was a pure radiological study with a variable length of follow-up. The importance of his paper lies in his identification of three radiological changes commonly found following meniscectomy and which have continued to be used in most recent publications. He described the following three radiological abnormalities:

■ Formation of an anterior/posterior ridge on the margin of the femoral condyle (this represents peri-articular osteophyte formation).
■ Narrowing of the joint space of the affected tibio-femoral compartment.
■ Flattening of the relevant femoral condyle.

These abnormalities have commonly been referred to in subsequent publications, although Fairbank (1948) does not suggest that they occur in any sequential order. His report suggested that radiological signs of osteoarthritis occurred in up to 67% of patients undergoing medial meniscectomy. He did not, however, relate this to clinical outcome.

Tapper & Hoover (1969) reviewed 255 patients at least 10 years following total, open meniscectomy. They showed that 85% of patients had radiological osteoarthritis at between 10 and 30 years following meniscectomy and 55% had some symptoms from the operated knee. Despite being one of the largest studies available, these results are of limited value, however, as it is a highly selective retrospective study and patients with ligamentous instability were not excluded.

Johnson et al (1974) reviewed 99 patients at an average of 17.5 years post menisectomy. Again this series was selective and did not exclude patients with ligamentous laxity. Johnson found that 74% of patients had radiological signs of osteoarthritis, which were severe in 40% of cases. He makes the point that ligamentous laxity is associated with a poor outcome, although does not analyse the data of the isolated meniscal injuries.

These early studies, then, form the basis of our knowledge of the incidence of late osteoarthritis following total open menisectomy.

More recently, some prospective work has been undertaken. Hede et al (1992) followed up 200 patients who were randomised to receive partial or total menisectomy as an open procedure. Patients were reviewed at 1 year and an average of 8 years following surgery. Their compliance rate is excellent, with 95% of patients being available for the late review and 90% of patients agreeing to undergo radiological analysis. The authors found that, at 1 year following surgery, 90% of patients after partial menisectomy and 80% after total menisectomy were symptom free. At 8 years these figures had dropped to 62% and 52% respectively. Patients with partial menisectomy also had a higher functional score.

Hede et al (1992) found no significant difference in the incidence of osteoarthritis when partial menisectomy was compared to total menisectomy. The overall incidence of radiological osteoarthritis was 46% at 8 years; 13% of patients had significant complaints relating to their knee and 5% had either stopped work or changed employment as a result of their menisectomy. This study is important, as it is well constructed and patients with symptomatic chondromalacia patella, osteochondritis or ligamentous laxity were excluded from the investigation.

The above study, although useful, was however, undertaken on patients undergoing open menisectomy. Similar studies have been performed following arthroscopic menisectomy. Fauno & Nielsen in 1992 reviewed 136 patients following isolated arthroscopic menisectomy. Length of follow-up was on average 8.5 years and other diagnoses had been excluded. The study was undertaken prospectively and 87% of patients attended for follow-up. The authors found that, on average, patients had some symptoms following surgery for up to 14 weeks but the average period of absence from work was only 4 weeks.

With regard to the incidence of osteoarthritis, overall Fauno & Nielsen found that 55% of their patients had radiological osteoarthritis at second review, between 7 and 11 years post surgery. There was no significant difference

between bucket handle tears and split tears. They also looked at the relationship of postoperative osteoarthritis to physiological alignment of the knee, and found a significantly greater incidence of osteoarthritis in both the operated and the non-operated knee in patients with a varus alignment, particularly if they had undergone medial menisectomy. The combination of a medial menisectomy in a varus knee produced an osteoarthritis rate of 76% at 8 years.

Medial versus lateral menisectomy

Debate continues regarding the difference between medial and lateral menisectomy in the aetiology of outcome and, in particular, osteoarthritis. A number of authors have addressed this difference and Johnson et al (1974) suggested that the outcome in lateral menisectomy was significantly worse than that following medial menisectomy. Heda (1992), in his excellent prospective study, has suggested that total lateral menisectomy was associated with a worse outcome, but that partial lateral menisectomy was no more severe than partial medial menisectomy. Fauno & Nielsen (1992), in their study of arthroscopic menisectomy, confirmed these findings, with no greater incidence of late problems following partial lateral menisectomy when compared with partial medial menisectomy. They did make the point, however, that in a valgus knee, partial lateral menisectomy can give rise to an increased incidence in degenerative change similar to that found following medial menisectomy in a varus knee. It would therefore seem that modern techniques with preservation of the meniscal rim have removed any difference between medial and lateral menisectomy with regard to the incidence of late degenerative change.

Summary

- Menisectomy is associated with radiological post-traumatic osteoarthritis. The incidence with modern techniques is approximately 55% at 8 years.
- The functional outcome following partial menisectomy is better than total menisectomy, although the incidence of radiological osteoarthritis is no different.
- Following arthroscopic menisectomy, the average period of absence from work is 4 weeks. However, some symptoms commonly continue for up to 3 months

Patello-femoral injuries
Patello-femoral dislocations

Dislocation of the patello-femoral joint can occur at any age but is much commoner in children than adults. The patella usually dislocates laterally, although medial dislocations can occur.

Treatment is generally non-operative, with splintage of the leg for 6 weeks followed by physiotherapy to regain strength and movement in the knee. Some authors recommend early operative treatment (Vainionpaa et al 1990), although most restrict surgical management to those dislocations causing osteochondral injuries.

There is a relative lack of good quality long-term data on the results from patello-femoral dislocations, although some medium-term data are available.

Re-dislocation rate

A number of authors have looked at the re-dislocation rate following acute dislocation of the patella. Maenpaa & Lehto (1997) followed 100 patients treated non-operatively for an average of 13 years, 44% having had at least one re-dislocation. When he looked at the re-dislocation group he found that their average age at initial dislocation was 17.5 years compared with a mean age of 23 years in the overall group, and he suggested that age was an important factor in re-dislocation rate. This was supported by Larsen & Lauridsen (1982), who found a 15-fold increased in re-dislocation in patients under 20 years of age, when compared with older patients.

Cash & Hughston (1988) studied 100 patients for an average of 18 years and found that no one who was 28 years of age or older, at the time of their initial dislocation, suffered a recurrence. They further divided the patients into those who had what they described as congenital risk factors, and those that did not. The risk factors thought important were found by examining the uninjured knee. They felt that hypermobility, weakness of the vastus medialis, a high or laterally riding patella and a history of dislocation in the unaffected knee were important. If these factors were considered, the overall re-dislocation rate was 36% in the group showing these findings in the uninjured knee, compared with only 15% of those where the uninjured knee was deemed normal.

Functional result

Function following acute dislocation of the patella has been assessed by a small number of studies. Potential symptoms following this injury are persistent patello-femoral pain and/or a reduced range of movement. Most authors report that approximately 80% of patients obtain a satisfactory outcome.

Patello-femoral pain

The rate of persistent patello-femoral pain does not appear to be dependent on treatment. In the published series, there appears to be a relatively consistent incidence of long-term patello-femoral discomfort following dislocation of between 15 and 25%. In Cash & Hughston's

1988 study, they found that, in patients with predisposing factors in the contralateral knee, the incidence of patello-femoral discomfort rose to 52%.

Loss of movement

Most patients regain adequate mobility following patellar dislocation when treated by plaster immobilisation or operation. Maenpaa & Lehto (1997) showed that 27% of patients had lost at least 5° of flexion, although this did not appear to be a major functional impediment. He found that the restriction of flexion was slightly less in patients treated without significant immobilisation, although this was at the expense of an increased re-dislocation rate.

Osteochondral fractures

Osteochondral fractures of the patella and distal femur are known to occur following acute patello-femoral dislocation. The standard textbooks suggest that their overall incidence is in the region of 5%. However, it appears that this may be an underestimate as more recent studies, especially those involving operative exploration of acute patello-femoral dislocations, have suggested that the figure can be as high as 50% (Cash & Hughston 1988, Vainionpaa et al 1990). Most authors agree that if a significant osteochondral fracture is identified then it should be removed. This usually requires either arthroscopic or open exploration. When surgical exploration is undertaken, then the long-term results are similar to those following acute patello-femoral dislocations without osteochondral fracture.

In Cash & Hughston's 1988 series of 100 patients, an osteochondral fracture was identified radiologically in the case of nine patients at the initial presentation but was treated non-operatively. Five of these nine ultimately had a poor result. In the patients in the series treated by early operative removal, 80% had a good or excellent result, which was identical to those without an osteochondral fracture.

In a study of 55 patients treated by open exploration and repair of an acute patellar dislocation, Vanionpaa et al (1990) found a 50% incidence of osteochondral fractures. There were three patients with large (15 mm × 15 mm) fragments which were repaired and all the others were removed. The author found no difference in outcome at 2 years between the group sustaining an osteochondral fracture and those without.

Late osteoarthritis

There is no good quality long-term data to quantify the incidence of late osteoarthritis following an acute patellar dislocation. Larsen & Lauridsen in 1982 performed a clinical and radiological examination of 78 patients at a mean of 6 years post injury. They did not report significant radiological osteoarthritis. Maenpaa & Lehto (1997), in a clinical review at 13 years, found a 61% incidence of patello-femoral crepitus after an acute dislocation, although they did not comment on it the incidence in the uninjured knee. They related this to degradation of the articular cartilage, although it did not relate to symptoms. It is, therefore, not possible accurately to quantify the incidence of patello-femoral osteoarthritis after a single acute patellar dislocation.

There is also controversy regarding the incidence of osteoarthritis following recurrent patellar dislocation. McNabb (1964) suggested that severe osteoarthritis could develop following recurrent dislocation of the patella whereas Crosby & Insall (1978) suggested that this was rarely seen. Clearly, long-term prospective studies are required but, to date, are not available.

Summary

- Up to 44% of patients will suffer at least one recurrent dislocation of the patella following an initial injury.
- Age is the most important factor in determining recurrence, with younger patients having a significantly increased risk.
- Anatomical abnormalities in the uninjured knee significantly increase the incidence of re-dislocation.
- Persistent patello-femoral pain occurs in approximately 20% of patients following an acute patello-femoral dislocation.
- Approximately one-quarter of patients will have some permanent loss of flexion of the affected knee, although this rarely produces functional problems.
- Osteochondral fractures may occur in up to 50% of acute patellar dislocations.
- Surgical removal of radiologically visible osteochondral fragments is advisable and does not prejudice the long-term result.
- Of patients with radiologically identifiable osteochondral fractures treated non-operatively, half will have a poor result.
- The true incidence of late osteoarthritis following acute dislocation of the patella is unknown.

Extensor mechanism injuries

Rupture of the extensor mechanism can occur with separation of the soft tissue of the quadriceps or the patellar tendons. In either case, operative repair is required, followed by protection of the repair to allow healing. Siwek & Rao (1981) looked at the demographics of the injury and found that there was a 6:1 male to female ratio in ruptures of the extensor mechanism. They also found that ruptures of the patellar tendon occurred almost exclusively in the

under 40 age group and three-quarters of the quadriceps ruptures were in patients over the age of 40. They concluded that early surgical repair of both injuries produced excellent results.

Patellar tendon rupture

Because of the anatomy it is usually possible to protect the repaired tendon with a wire loop, thereby allowing early movement. It is very easy to shorten the patellar tendon but it is essential that normal length is maintained, for shortening gives rise to patella bahja (low riding patella) and significantly compromises the result. If the tendon is repaired early and correct orientation obtained, then the results are uniformly excellent (Siwek & Rao 1981). If the diagnosis is delayed then results are less predictable, with only one-third of patients obtaining an excellent result.

Quadriceps tendon rupture

Rupture of the quadriceps tendon requires surgical repair followed by splintage of the leg in full extension for 6 weeks. Siwek & Rao in 1981 studied 34 patients with quadriceps tendon rupture, in two of whom it occurred bilaterally. They found that in all patients undergoing early repair, the ultimate result was good or excellent. They commented that it was usually at least 6 months before the patient made a satisfactory recovery, however, and loss of the last 10–15° of knee flexion was common. In the delayed treatment group, where the diagnosis had been missed initially, the result was significantly less good with an average knee flexion of only 90°.

In a separate study of quadriceps tendon rupture, Vainionpaa et al (1985) reviewed 12 patients at an average of 5 years post injury. All had been treated by early repair followed by splintage. One patient suffered a re-rupture at 8 weeks post injury with a poor result. However, the remainder of the patients went on to achieve good results, although three had some minor activity-related symptoms and loss of flexion. Once again, the author concluded that early surgical repair produced a uniformly excellent result in this injury.

Summary

- Patellar tendon ruptures occur at a younger age than those with quadriceps tendon ruptures.
- Early surgical repair gives uniformly good results.
- Full recovery often takes up to 6 months.
- Slight loss of flexion is often seen, particularly following a quadriceps tendon rupture.

Patellar fractures

Patellar fractures usually occur following a direct blow to the front of the knee. Occasionally, an insufficiency type fracture can occur in the older patient. Many classification systems have evolved, although none reliably predicts outcome. Nummi (1971) reviewed one of the largest series of patellar fractures with late review and suggested that only two factors were important in identifying long-term prognosis. These were fragmentation of the articular surface and disruption of the quadriceps mechanism. Both of these gave a worse prognosis.

General considerations

Patellar fractures have been treated by a number of methods over the years. Undisplaced fractures are generally treated by splintage followed by physiotherapy. It is universally agreed that significant displacement of the fracture fragments, particularly if the quadriceps mechanism is disrupted, necessitates surgical intervention. There are basically three surgical options, namely internal fixation of the patellar fragment, partial excision of the patella followed by repair of the ligamentous structures or total excision of the patella (patellectomy). Series have been published with all methods of treatment, although true comparative studies are rare.

To obtain an overall view on the incidence of long-term symptoms following patellar fractures, Nummi's 1971 study of 707 patients provides the most useful data, 391 of his patients being reviewed at between 4 and 8 years following injury. He found that disability continued for a significant period following patellar fracture, only 78% in his series returning to work within 4 months of injury. He divided his group into undisplaced and displaced fractures and found that 94% of patients treated for an undisplaced fracture were back at work within 4 months whereas this figure dropped to 45% for displaced injuries. At 6 months post fracture, 93% of all patients had returned to some form of employment.

In his late review at between four and eight years, Nummi found that 87% of all patients had regained their pre-injury occupation without significant problems. The subjective assessment at this stage showed that 34% of these had no complaints, 38% had some persistent aching on physical activity and 37% had a feeling of weakness in the leg when loaded. Nummi's objective assessment of the same patients showed that 26% could be classified as excellent, 34% good, 32% satisfactory and 8% poor. He also mentioned that improvement in objective assessment continued for between 3 and 4 years following injury. He therefore recommended that final assessment be delayed until this point to assess long-term outcome.

Nummi also looked at the fracture pattern and found that this did affect outcome. In transverse fractures 62% were good or excellent at 4–8 years, whereas in fragment-

ed fractures this dropped to only 50%. This large series allows general quantification of outcome following a patellar fracture. Nummi's conclusion, however, was that significant fragmentation of the articular surface produced a worse result, as did disruption of the quadriceps mechanism. He attributed this, in part, to the necessity for surgical reconstruction and also to the potential damage to the blood supply of the patella caused by tearing of the patellar retinaculae.

The above data give us general information regarding outcome from patella fractures. There is also some data available on specific treatment methods although some studies are quite small.

Undisplaced fractures

Almost all authors define an undisplaced fracture as one with less than 1–2 mm of displacement of the articular surface. These are almost always treated by non-operative means with splintage of the knee, followed by physiotherapy. The results are uniformly good. Sorenson (1984) found that 70% of patients were symptom free at 20 years following an undisplaced fracture. These results were confirmed by Bostrom (1972) and Edwards et al (1989).

Displaced fractures
Internal fixation

In general, the results of internal fixation relate to the quality of the reduction and fixation. Marya et al (1987) looked at the results of internal fixation for two- and three-part fractures of the patella. The author found that 93% of patients were graded good or excellent, of which 80% were symptom free. The follow-up was between 2 and 5 years. Bostman et al (1981) looked at fragmented fractures of the patella with displacement. Where the patella could be adequately reconstructed and stabilised, he found that 43% could be considered excellent, 43% good and only 14% poor when reviewed 2 years after injury.

Levack et al (1985) also reviewed the results of internal fixation and found that broadly one-third were good, one-third fair and one-third poor. He commented, however, that the majority of fixation methods used were circumferential wires rather than anterior tension band wires, and suggested that with the latter better results could be obtained. This hypothesis was supported by Marya (1987), who had 93% good or excellent results at between 2 and 5 years using this technique.

Partial patellectomy

Removal of part of the patella has been suggested for the treatment of fragmented patellar fractures. Most authors agreed with Duthie & Hutchinson (1958) that at least 60% of the patella must be maintained in order to preserve function. If this can be achieved then the results are better than for total patellectomy but inferior to those for successful internal fixation. Bostman et al (1981) reported that at 2 years only 21% had excellent results after partial excision, although a further 60% were classified as good with only minimal symptoms.

All authors support the hypothesis of Duthie & Hutchinson (1958) that technical aspects of partial patellectomy are important. If, on postoperative radiographs, the patella is seen to be tilting towards the articular surface of the femur, then this will predispose to a poor result. It is important, therefore, to investigate knees radiologically following partial patellectomy to look for abnormal alignment. This also has a significant effect on post-traumatic osteoarthritis, as discussed below.

Total patellectomy

Historically, total patellectomy has been recommended for fractures of the patella. Most recent authors still recommend it for fractures in which adequate reconstruction is not possible, although there is abundant evidence that the result from patellectomy is not as good as that following successful internal fixation.

Numerous studies have looked at the long-term effects of patellectomy. Einola et al (1976) considered 38 patients at an average of 7.4 years. He found that they had been off work for between 1 and 6 months following their patellectomy and all patients had measurable quadriceps atrophy. When assessed biomechanically at least three-quarters of them had lost 25% or more of their quadriceps power. Sutton et al (1976) specifically looked at the effect of patellectomy on function. They found, on average, patients had 2.2 cm of quadriceps atrophy and had lost 50% of their quadriceps strength. Most had also lost at least 20° of knee flexion as a result of their patellectomy. The authors also noted that complete patellectomy caused an abnormal walking pattern and function was particularly reduced when going up and down stairs.

Jakobsen et al (1985) looked at the 20 year follow-up of patients undergoing patellectomy. Two-thirds of these patients had significant quadriceps weakness with the average wasting being approximately 2 cm of circumference. They also commented that the average quadriceps power was only 50% of the contralateral limb.

There is, therefore, no doubt from the literature that patellectomy does produce a permanent reduction in knee function when assessed objectively. A few studies have also looked at the overall function following patellectomy for fracture. Marya et al (1987) found that only 50% of patients following patellectomy could be classified as having an excellent result, with 27% being good and 21% fair.

The predominant complaints were of aching and stiffness, loss of flexion and reduced quadriceps power. Jakobsen et al (1985), in his 20 year follow-up of patients, found that 12 were excellent, 10 were good and six were fair. Three out of 28 patients had changed their occupation as a result of their patellectomy but only one patient had deteriorated significantly over the 20 years of the study.

The incidence of osteoarthritis following patellar fracture

The development of late osteoarthritis following patellar fracture has been covered extensively in the literature. The results, however, can seem somewhat contradictory.

Nummi (1971) conducted the largest study with 391 patients being followed up for 8 years. He reported that 56% of these patients had radiological osteoarthritis at late review, although this rose to 76% in those with more severe injuries treated by operative means. He did not, however, compare this to the uninjured knee. This group of patients encompassed all methods of treatment.

Sorensen (1984) reported on a 20 year follow-up of patients with patellar fractures. He noted a 70% incidence of radiological patello-femoral osteoarthritis in the injured knee, compared with only 31% on the uninjured side. He also looked at osteoarthritis in the tibio-femoral joint and showed no statistical difference between the injured and the uninjured knee. He therefore concluded that there was a definite increase in the chances of developing patello-femoral osteoarthritis following patellar fracture. Interestingly, of the 70% of patients with radiological osteoarthritis, only half had significant symptoms, and no patient had symptoms sufficient to require further surgical treatment. However, he did report that 12% of patients had had to change their occupation as a result of worsening symptoms.

Significant debate continues as to the role of patellectomy in producing osteoarthritis. Animal studies suggested that patellectomy could produce tibio-femoral osteoarthritis, although this had never been substantiated in humans. Jakobsen et al (1985) found an incidence of tibio-femoral osteoarthritis of 14% at 20 years. Eionola (1976) found that the incidence was 22% at 7 years, although his results were compromised by inadequate initial data in the majority of his patients. None of these studies compares the incidence of osteoarthritis with the contralateral leg.

There is thus no convincing evidence that total patellectomy leads to tibio-femoral osteoarthritis and the long-term results would suggest that the situation does not change significantly from that found at 1–2 years.

The same is not true, however, of partial patellectomy. Considerable debate exists in the literature as to the exact technique of partial patellectomy, but agreement is uniform that at least three-fifths of the patella needs to be retained. It is also of vital importance to assess the alignment of the retained fragment. Duthie & Hutchinson (1958) suggested that after partial patellectomy, the incidence of post-traumatic osteoarthritis was as high as 72%. They related this to angulation of the patellar fragment. This is reinforced by all authors when discussing this technique. Hung (1989) looked at patients following partial patellectomy for fracture and found that 70% had radiological signs of osteoarthritis at 2 years post injury. The longitudinal studies however, do not suggest that function is dramatically reduced as long as patellar alignment is satisfactory. Partial patellectomy, therefore, gives an improved result when compared with total patellectomy if normal alignment can be maintained.

Summary

- The two most important factors in predicting outcome from patellar fractures are fragmentation of the articular surface and disruption of the extensor mechanism.
- Undisplaced fractures when treated non-operatively give uniformly good results with few late complications.
- The best results from patellar fracture are obtained by reconstruction of the articular surface with up to 93% good or excellent results reported in simple fracture patterns.
- Some long-term symptoms are common, although severe functional impairment is rare.
- There is a definite increased incidence of patellofemoral osteoarthritis following patellar fractures, although this is not seen following patellectomy.
- The functional outcome following preservation of the patella is better than following patellectomy, even in the presence of radiological osteoarthritis.
- Partial patellectomy is technique dependent and can give rise to an increased incidence of osteoarthritis.

Tibial plateau fractures
Introduction

Intra-articular fractures of the proximal tibia can be caused by a wide variety of injuries. In the older patient they can be associated with minimal violence, whereas in younger patients high energy injuries are more common. A number of classification systems have been suggested, of which Schatzker's (1979) has become the most commonly used. He describes six types of fracture depending on the amount of joint depression and the anatomical site of the main fracture lines.

The treatment of these injuries remains controversial although there is a modern trend towards operative intervention. It is by no means clear, though, that this definitely gives improved results. Schatzker, himself a proponent of operative intervention, was keen to point out that the results of failed surgical reconstruction are worse than those of failed non-operative management. The essential element, therefore, is to avoid complications in whatever type of treatment is suggested.

The overriding principle of treatment, then, is to preserve normal alignment of the knee, as this is critical to the end result. Joint depression, per se, if it is not associated with malalignment, does not necessarily cause poor results.

Associated injuries

Fractures of the tibia can be associated with injuries to both the menisci and the collateral ligaments. Recent advances in MRI scanning have identified that injuries to both these structures are more common than has previously been appreciated. Most authors agree that ligament injuries occurring with tibial plateau fractures rarely need repair unless associated with major instability. In general, restoration of bony architecture is the most important factor in restoring knee stability.

Late results following tibial plateau fracture
Clinical results

Apley (1956) published a review of 60 cases treated by traction and early mobilisation. This paper is often quoted and records a good or excellent result in 78% of cases. Critical analysis of the paper, however, shows that there was only a 45% follow-up rate in his study and the fracture pattern was extremely varied. Both these factors significantly undermine the review's validity.

More recent studies have been better controlled and are much more powerful. DeCosta et al (1987) published a ten year follow-up of 30 patients treated by cast brace and early mobilisation for tibial plateau fractures. All of the patients who were alive at the time of the late review (90% of the original sample) were examined. He recorded that 61% had what was classed as a good or excellent result using the Iowa Knee Score. The average range of movement was 117° in the affected knee compared with 135° on the contralateral side, and 67% of patients recorded no pain or mild activity related aching whereas 33% had significant and disabling pain on occasion.

Jensen et al (1990) reviewed 109 patients at an average of 6 years post injury. Treatment was either by internal fixation or traction and early movement. He reported a 65% good or excellent rate, although noted that five of the original 109 patients had required either knee arthroplasty or arthrodesis. He looked at factors which might determine the overall outcome and noted that in the split fracture group without joint depression, 74% had a good or excellent result. In fractures where the joint surface was depressed, if this was less than 4 mm then 70% had a good or excellent result. Depression of the joint surface by more than 4 mm, however, reduced the proportion with a good or excellent result to 56%. Jensen commented that instability in the knee was associated with a poor clinical result.

Rasmussen & Sorensen (1973) published a study of 260 patients with tibial plateau fractures treated by operative or non-operative means. His study had an average follow-up of 7.3 years and he noted that 60% of patients had what could be considered to be an acceptable result and 40% had significant long-term symptoms. The same group of patients were reviewed at 20 years by Lansinger et al (1986), but unfortunately only 50% of the original group were available for follow-up. It is difficult to draw accurate conclusions from this paper, although it would appear that patients with persistent joint instability and significant central joint depression had a worse outcome. It is not possible accurately to quantify this any further, however.

Radiological result

The incidence of radiological osteoarthritis following tibial plateau fractures remains somewhat controversial. Apley (1956) stated that in these fractures 'radiographic appearances do not, however, correspond in any way with loss of function or with pain'. As only 45% of his patients were available for follow-up this may be a questionable conclusion. Certainly, more recent studies would tend to contradict his statement.

DeCosta et al (1987) showed that radiological osteoarthritis correlated well with the clinical result. He found radiological changes in 32% of patients at an average of 10 years and 33% of his group had significant or disabling pain. He felt that the degree of displacement of fracture pattern had a significant effect upon the incidence of late osteoarthritis. In undisplaced fractures, he found that the incidence was negligible whereas in bi-condylar fractures 72% of patients had significant radiological osteoarthritis and symptoms. No patient in his study had required further surgery at review 10–13 years from fracture, however.

Jensen et al (1990) looked at 106 patients at an average of 6 years. Five of his patients had required salvage surgery. He found that 43% had no radiological evidence of osteoarthritis; 37% had what he describes as minimal changes and 20% had moderate to severe radiological

signs. Twenty percent of this severe group had undergone salvage surgery. He also felt that there was a close correlation between radiological osteoarthritis and the clinical result.

Rasmussen & Sorensen (1973) also looked at radiological osteoarthritis at an average of 7.3 years. He reported the overall incidence as being 17% in his group of 260 fractures, although in bi-condylar injuries it was 42%. The size of his study allowed him to assess risk factors further in developing osteoarthritis. The most potent risk factor he found was alignment of the knee. In patients with normal alignment, the incidence of radiological osteoarthritis was 13%. With valgus deformity it rose to 31% but with a varus deformity of the knee the incidence was 79%. He also commented that the radiological findings had a close association with the clinical outcome. Unfortunately, when the same group of patients were reviewed at 20 years no radiological study was undertaken and no comment was made regarding radiological osteoarthritis.

Summary

- The treatment of tibial plateau fractures can be either operative or non-operative with relatively uniform results.
- In all fractures, 60–65% of patients will achieve a good or excellent result clinically.
- Undisplaced fractures without joint depression give a uniformly good result with minimal incidence of late osteoarthritis.
- Joint alignment and instability is the most important factor in deciding long-term outcome.
- Joint depression in a stable knee is not necessarily associated with a poor result, although depression of more than 4 mm does have an effect on outcome.
- There is a close correlation between the clinical result and radiological signs of osteoarthritis.
- The rates of osteoarthritis vary according to the fracture pattern and the alignment of the knee.
- A satisfactory clinical outcome at 2 years in a stable knee is unlikely to show significant late deterioration.

Ligamentous injuries of the knee
Introduction

The development of arthroscopic surgery over the last 35 years and, more recently, the advent of accurate MR imaging of the knee, has led to an improvement in the diagnosis of ligamentous injuries. The incidence of anterior cruciate ligament rupture is estimated at 0.3 per thousand patient years in the modern population. There is also evidence that injury rates are increasing at a greater rate in women than in men (Arendt & Dick 1995).

Although tears of the anterior cruciate ligament appear to be the commonest injury they are often combined with other ligament damage, Daniel et al (1994) showing that up to 49% of anterior cruciate ligament injuries have an associated meniscal tear.

Historically, injury patterns were described upon clinical grounds and divided into a number of rotatory or straight instabilities. More recently, accurate diagnosis has meant that emphasis has changed towards instability created by rupture of specific ligaments, although the overall clinical picture, particularly in combined injuries, remains important.

In general, the prognosis in these injuries is related to the degree of clinical instability, although joint laxity may also be important. As a general rule, late deterioration following ligamentous injuries is related to the onset of degenerative osteoarthritis and the clinical result is usually reflected in the radiological appearance.

Collateral ligament injuries

In assessing the long-term outcome from a collateral ligament injury, it is essential to assess the integrity of the cruciate ligaments as prognosis is markedly different when they are involved. Medial collateral ligament injury is often associated with an anterior cruciate ligament tear and lateral collateral ligament injury with an injury to the posterior cruciate ligament.

Isolated lateral collateral ligament injuries

The lateral collateral ligament is an extremely strong structure and represents one of the primary supporting structures resisting varus displacement of the knee. True isolated injury to the lateral collateral ligament is extremely rare (Insall 1984). This is probably because significant violence is required to rupture it and secondary damage to the cruciate ligament usually follows.

As lateral collateral ligament injury is most commonly associated with damage to the cruciate ligaments it is most important to assess these ligaments when offering a prognosis in this type of injury. If the cruciate ligaments are definitely intact then good recovery is to be expected. Persistent varus deformity of the knee, however, is known as a potent cause of medial compartment osteoarthritis and the overall alignment of the knee should thus be taken into consideration.

Most studies of collateral ligament injuries do not exclude combined cruciate injuries. There are, therefore, no long-term studies of true isolated lateral collateral ligament injuries to provide accurate data on long-term outcome.

Isolated medial collateral ligament injuries

Injury to the medial collateral ligament is more common than to the lateral. True isolated injury of this structure can occur but damage to the anterior cruciate ligament must always be suspected. Isolated injuries are commonly treated non-operatively by bracing and early movement although some surgeons still advocate surgical repair.

Lundberg & Messner (1996) published a 10 year clinical and radiological evaluation of isolated medial collateral ligament ruptures. They found that patients were able to return to a normal level of sport and/or work and had no clinical instability. However, on clinical examination, slight laxity was detectable on the side of the injury. On radiological follow-up there was no significant difference in the incidence of osteoarthritis between the injured and the uninjured knee. In addition, they found that over the 10 year period of the study there was a similar incidence of further ligament or meniscal injury in the injured and contralateral knee suggesting that there was no greater potential for injury following isolated medial collateral rupture.

This would suggest that true isolated medial collateral injury can lead to slight laxity on clinical examination but does not give rise to significant symptoms, functional impairment or radiological osteoarthritis at 10 years.

Anterior cruciate ligament (ACL) rupture

The rupture of the anterior cruciate ligament (ACL) of the knee has a significant and long-term effect upon future knee function. Accurate diagnosis is, therefore, important when offering a prognosis following knee ligament injuries. Careful clinical examination will usually detect some laxity in the anterior/posterior direction and MRI scanning is becoming increasingly sensitive at detecting abnormalities in the ligament. Arthroscopy depends on the skill of the surgeon and an inexperienced arthroscopist can easily pass a torn ligament as normal.

The long-term outcome following ACL rupture has attracted considerable attention. The situation is complicated by the need for an accurate diagnosis and the fact that meniscal tears commonly co-exist with these injuries. It is well known that isolated injury to the meniscus requiring meniscectomy increases the incidence of osteoarthritis in the knee and this must be borne in mind when interpreting studies of these ruptures.

Incidence of further injury

Most authors agree that in a patient with an ACL injury who continues to undertake normal activity including sport, there is an increased risk of subsequent meniscal injury. The incidence reported in the literature is between

10 and 24% at 5 years (Hawkins et al 1986, Andersson et al 1991, Daniel et al 1994). Sommerlath et al (1991) found an incidence of 16% at an average of 12 years post injury. Patients in these studies had been treated by a variety of techniques including early surgical repair, although primary ligament reconstruction had not been undertaken.

More recently, prospective studies of patients undergoing ligament reconstruction using modern arthroscopic techniques have suggested that the incidence of meniscal tear can be significantly reduced by this procedure. Webb et al (1998) studied 82 patients with intact menisci following ACL reconstruction for an average of 2 years and no subsequent meniscal injuries were identified.

Long-term outcome following ACL injury

Considerable data have been published on the outcome following ACL injury both with and without reconstruction. Treatment has changed significantly over the last 30 years, particularly with the advent of arthroscopic techniques and therefore any true long-term studies, may not be relevant to patients treated by modern methods. They do, however, provide useful data on the outcome following this injury.

Daniel et al (1994) followed almost 300 patients over a 5 year period post injury. Patients were treated based upon their symptoms with those with significant instability or high demands undergoing reconstruction. The author found that in all patients, regardless of treatment, the level and time spent in sporting participation decreased although no patient changed occupation because of the knee injury. Symptoms were significantly less in the patients who had undergone reconstruction.

The incidence of osteoarthritis following ACL injury

Gillchrist and Mesner (1999) produced an excellent review dealing with the incidence of long-term osteoarthritis following ACL injury. They concluded that the incidence of post-traumatic osteoarthritis was multi-factorial but there was a definite increase in incidence following ACL rupture. Their results are summarised in Table 13.1. They furthermore suggested that patients at between 10 and 20 years following ACL injury may not have major symptoms, often being able to continue their pre-injury occupation although sporting participation was affected. The authors also suggested that the progression of arthritis was somewhat more rapid in patients who sustained injury when over 30 years of age.

The role of ACL reconstruction in limiting osteoarthritis remains controversial. Despite studies suggesting that it can reduce subsequent meniscal injury (Webb et al 1998) no long-term data are available to confirm the effects of modern reconstruction techniques on the late development of osteoarthritis. However, Daniel, in his 1994 study, specifically looked at the incidence of radiological osteoarthritis in patients with intact menisci undergoing early reconstruction for ACL tear. Somewhat alarmingly, he found that the incidence of radiological osteoarthritis was higher in patients undergoing reconstruction than in similar patients treated non-operatively.

Most authors, therefore, agree that there is no hard evidence to suggest that ACL reconstruction alters the long-term incidence of osteoarthritis, although there are data to suggest that it reduces the incidence of meniscal injury.

The exact reason for the incidence of osteoarthritis despite reconstruction is not clearly understood. It is postulated that the severity of the initial injury may be responsible for damage to the articular surface of the knee. Fowler (1994) reviewed the incidence of so-called occult bone lesions in ACL injury as diagnosed by MRI scanning. He found that over 80% of ACL tears had what he described as occult micro-fracturing of the lateral tibial plateau, which is not visible on plain radiographs.

It has been suggested that this may be sufficient damage to initiate post-traumatic osteoarthritis, although 80% of the occult fractures occur in the lateral compartment and osteoarthritis following ACL injury is equal in both medial and lateral compartments. The link between the two, therefore, is far from clear.

To summarise the situation, it appears that the initial injury, for whatever reason, is a major determinant of the late incidence of osteoarthritis. It is thus not possible to avoid late sequelae completely no matter what treatment is undertaken.

Table 13.1 Incidence of radiological osteoarthritis at 10–20 years post injury (Gillquist & Messner 1999)

General population	1–2%
Isolated ACL injury	15–20%
ACL injury and meniscectomy	50–70%

Posterior cruciate ligament (PCL) injury

Injury to the posterior cruciate ligament (PCL) can be either isolated or combined with other ligamentous damage. It is most commonly combined with lateral collateral ligament injuries or damage to the postero-lateral corner. Despite considerable violence being required to rupture the PCL, it is often undiagnosed, Fanelli et al (1994) suggesting that up to one-third of multiply injured patients with a knee injury had a late diagnosed rupture.

The late results of PCL injuries have been studied in some detail. As surgical treatment is a relatively recent trend, a considerable amount of data on the untreated posterior cruciate deficient knee are available. Boynton & Tietjens (1996) studied 38 patients for an average of 13.5 years. They found that the isolated PCL deficient knee had a relatively good outcome. Twenty-six percent of patients were symptom free at follow-up and 37% were playing sport, albeit at a reduced capacity to their pre-injury status. Fifteen per cent, however, had moderate pain on walking and 50% of the study group had patello-femoral type pain on climbing stairs.

Torg et al in 1989 also recorded a high incidence of patello-femoral pain in patients with a PCL rupture and they suggested that this was one of the indicators of a poorer result following this injury. This was also concluded by Cross & Powell (1984) in their longitudinal study.

The incidence of osteoarthritis following PCL injury

The incidence of late osteoarthritis has also been studied. Torg et al (1989) suggested a close link between the symptomatic outcome and radiological signs of osteoarthritis. In patients with few symptoms it was rare to find radiological degenerative change.

Boynton & Tietjens (1996) specifically looked at the incidence of osteoarthritis. They found that at a mean of 13.5 years, 65% of patients had radiological signs of osteoarthritis. In patients with a Grade III posterior draw, however, this rose to 80% and in patients who had undergone meniscal surgery at the time of their initial injury the incidence was 88%. The distribution of the osteoarthritis was predominantly in the medial compartment. Fifty-three percent of patients had medial osteoarthritis, 20% lateral compartment osteoarthritis and 13% patello-femoral osteoarthritis. The authors also noted that the development of osteoarthritis was time related. All patients who were more than 20 years from injury had some radiological signs of osteoarthritis.

The effect of PCL reconstruction on the late results is, as yet, unproved. No true comparative studies are available and, as with the ACL, there is no evidence yet that reconstruction alters the development of post-traumatic osteoarthritis.

Severe combined injuries

Severe combined injuries or dislocation of the knee is fortunately rare. It is a severe injury, however. Neurovascular complications are common with up to 10% of patients having an associated popliteal artery injury and 40% damage to the common peroneal nerve (Sisto & Warren 1985). Treatment can be either non-operative or surgical, although the current trend is towards operative repair of the ligaments followed by early mobilisation. Postoperative stiffness is a significant and somewhat disabling sequelae.

Accurate data on the long-term results are difficult to find although some studies are available. Taylor et al (1972) suggested that approximately half of the patients would obtain at least 90° of knee flexion and little in the way of pain. The remainder, however, would have less than 90° of flexion and some continuing instability in the knee.

Sisto & Warren (1985), in a study of operative treatment, reported somewhat better results. In their series, however, there was a high incidence of bony avulsion of the cruciate ligaments which allowed accurate reconstruction by bony reattachment. Despite this, pain and limitation of movement were frequent sequelae. Pain was a significant complaint in 46% of patients and the average range of knee flexion was only 110°. The authors concluded that knee dislocation was a serious injury with significant long-term sequelae.

The incidence of late osteoarthritis following knee dislocation has not been studied in isolation. However, one can infer the incidence from the studies of ACL and PCL ruptures, as most dislocations have ruptures of both cruciate ligaments. As with other ligamentous injuries, there are no data as yet to suggest that early surgery or reconstruction alters the incidence of long-term osteoarthritis.

Summary

- Isolated injury to the collateral ligaments is a benign injury with uniformly good results at 10 years.
- ACL injury has a significant and permanent impact upon knee function. The late incidence of osteoarthritis in isolated ACL injury is 15–20%, rising to 50–70% where meniscal damage has occurred.
- There is no evidence that ligament reconstruction alters the long-term incidence of osteoarthritis.
- Untreated isolated PCL injury of the knee can be associated with good functional outcome.
- Knee dislocation is a severe injury which is likely to give rise to permanent limitation of function.

References

Andersson C, Odensten M, Gillquist J 1991 Knee function after surgical or nonsurgical treatment of acute rupture of the anterior cruciate ligament: A randomized study with a long-term follow-up period. Clin Orthop 264: 255–263

Apley A G 1956 Fractures of the lateral tibial condyle treated by skeletal traction and early mobilisation. Journal of Bone and Joint Surgery 38B: 699–707

Arendt E, Dick R 1995 Knee injury patterns among men and women in collegiate basketball and soccer. NCAA data and review of literature. American Journal of Sports Medicine 23(6): 694–701

Böstman O, Kiviluto O, Nirhamo J 1981 Comminuted displaced fractures of the patella. Injury 13: 196–202

Bostrom A 1972 Fracture of the patellar: a study of 422 patellar fractures. Acta Orthopaedica Scandinavica (Suppl) 143

Boynton M D, Tietjens B R 1996 Long-term followup of the untreated isolated posterior cruciate ligament-deficient knee. American Journal of Sports Medicine 24(3): 306–310

Cash J D, Hughston J C 1988 Treatment of acute patellar dislocation. American Journal of Sports Medicine 16(3): 244–249

Crosby E B, Insall J 1978 Recurrent dislocation of the patella. Journal of Bone and Joint Surgery 58A: 9

Cross M J, Powell J F 1984 Long term follow-up of posterior cruciate ligament rupture: A study of 116 patients. American Journal of Sports Medicine 12: 292

Daniel D M, Stone M L, Dobson B E, Fithian D C, Rossman D J, Kaufman K R 1994 Fate of the ACL-injured patient. A prospective outcome study. American Journal of Sports Medicine 22(5): 632–644

DeCosta T A, Nepola J V, El-Khoury G Y 1987 Cast brace treatment of proximal tibial fractures. Clinical Orthopaedics 231: 196–204

Duthie H L, Hutchinson J R 1958 The results of partial and total excision of the patella. Journal of Bone and Joint Surgery 40B: 75–81

Edwards B, Johnell O, Redlund-Johnell I 1989 Patellar fractures: a 30-year follow up. Acta Orthopaedica Scandinavica 60: 712–714

Einola S, Aho A J, Kallio P 1976 Patellectomy after fracture. Acta Orthopaedica Scandinavica 47: 441–447

Fahmy N R M, Williams E L, Noble J 1983 Meniscal pathology and osteoarthritis of the knee. Journal of Bone and Joint Surgery 65B: 24

Fairbank T J 1948 Knee joint changes after meniscectomy. Journal of Bone and Joint Surgery 30B: 664–670

Fanelli G C, Giannotti B F, Edson C J 1994 Current concepts review. The posterior cruciate ligament arthroscopic evaluation and treatment. Arthroscopy 10(6): 673–688

Fauno P, Nielsen A B 1992 Arthroscopic partial meniscectomy. A long-term follow-up. Arthroscopy 8(3): 345–349

Fowler P J 1994 Current concepts. Bone injuries associated with anterior cruciate ligament disruption. Arthroscopy 10(4): 453–460

Gillquist J, Messner K 1999 Anterior cruciate ligament reconstruction and the long term incidence of gonarthrosis. Sports Medicine 27: 143–156

Hawkins R J, Misamore G W, Merritt T R 1986 Follow-up of the acute non-operated isolated anterior cruciate ligament tear. American Journal of Sports Medicine 14: 205–210

Hede A, Larsen E, Sandberg H 1992 Partial versus total menisectomy. A prospective, randomised study with long term follow-up. Journal of Bone and Joint Surgery 74B: 118–121

Hung L K 1989 Partial patellectomy. Thesis M Ch (Orth) University of Liverpool

Insall J N (ed.) 1984 Surgery of the knee. Churchill Livingstone, pp 286–290

Jakobsen J, Christensen K S, Rasmussen O 1985 Patellectomy—A 20 year follow-up. Acta Othopaedica Scandinavica 56: 430–432

Jensen D B, Rude C, Duus B, Bjerg-Nielson A 1990 Tibial plateau fractures: a comparison of conservative and surgical treatment. Journal of Bone and Joint Surgery 72B: 49–52

Johnson R J, Kettelkamp D B, Clark W, Leaverton P 1974 Factors affecting late results after meniscectomy. Journal of Bone and Joint Surgery 56A: 719–729

Lansinger O, Bergman B, Korner L, Anderrson G B J 1986 Tibial condyle fractures. A twenty year follow-up. Journal of Bone and Joint Surgery 68A: 13–19

Larsen E, Lauridsen F 1982 Conservative treatment of patella dislocations. Influence of evident factors on the tendency to redislocate and the therapeutic result. Clinical Orthopaedics and Related Research 171: 131–136

Levack B, Flannagan J P, Hobbs S 1985 Results of surgical treatment of fractures of the patella. Journal of Bone and Joint Surgery 67B: 416–419

Lundberg M, Messner K 1996 Long term prognosis of isolated partial medial collateral ligament ruptures. American Journal of Sports Medicine 24: 160–163

Maenpaa H, Lehto M U K 1997 Patellar dislocation. The long-term results of nonoperative management in 100 patients. American Journal of Sports Medicine 25(2): 213–217

Marya S K, Bhan S, Dave P K 1987 Comparative study of knee function after patellectomy and osteosynthesis with a tension band wire following patellar fractures. International Surgery 72: 211–213

McNabb I 1964 Recurrent dislocation of the patella. Journal of Bone and Joint Surgery 46B: 498

Nummi J 1971 Fractures of the patella. A clinical study of 707 fractures. Ann Chir Gynaecol Fenn 60 (suppl 179): 5–85

Rasmussen P S, Sorensen S E 1973 Tibial condylar fractures. Injury 4: 265

Schatzker J, McBroom R, Bruce D 1979 The tibial plateau fracture. Clinical Orthopaedics 138: 94–104

Sisto D J, Warren R F 1985 Complete knee dislocation. Clinical Orthopaedics 198: 94–101

Siwek C W, Rao J P 1981 Ruptures of the extensor mechanism of the knee joint. Journal of Bone and Joint Surgery 63A: 932–937

Sommerlath K, Lysholm J, Gillquist J 1991 The long-term course after treatment of acute anterior cruciate ligament ruptures. A 9 to 16 year followup. American Journal of Sports Medicine 19(2): 156–162

Sorenson K H 1984 The late prognosis after fracture of the patella. Acta Orthopaedica Scandinavica 34: 198–212

Sutton F S, Thompson C U, Lipke J, Kettelkamp D B 1976 Effect of patellectomy on knee function. Journal of Bone and Joint Surgery 58A: 537–540

Tapper E M, Hoover N W 1969 Late results after meniscectomy. Journal of Bone and Joint Surgery 51A: 517–526

Taylor A R, Arden G P, Rainey H A 1972 Traumatic dislocation of the knee. Journal of Bone and Joint Surgery 54B: 96–102

Torg J S, Barton T M, Pavlov H, Stine R 1989 Natural history of the posterior cruciate ligament deficient knee. Clinical Orthopaedics 246: 208–216

Vainionpaa S, Bostman O, Patiala H, Rokkanen P 1985 Ruptue of the quadriceps tendon. Acta Orthopaedica Scandinavica 56: 433–435

Vainionpaa S, Laasonen E, Silvennionen T, Vasenius J, Rokkanen P 1990 Acute dislocation of the patella. A prospective review of operative treatment. Journal of Bone and Joint Surgery 72B: 366–369

Webb J M, Corry I S, Clingeleffer A J, Pinczewski L A 1998 Endoscopic reconstruction for isolated anterior cruciate ligament rupture. Journal of Bone and Joint Surgery 80B: 288–294

The tibia and fibula

Andy Cole

Introduction

Fractures of the tibial shaft are the most common of the long bone fractures (Russell 1996). Treatment remains controversial and proponents can be found for treatment with casts, functional braces, external fixation, plates and intramedullary nailing (locked or unlocked/reamed or unreamed).

A recurrent problem in the orthopaedic literature is the lack of standardisation for reporting results and complications. In an attempt to aid treatment decisions and prognosis of tibial fractures a number of classification systems have been devised. A major difficulty is that outcome has often been evaluated in terms of physical measurements such as average time to union, risk of delayed union, infection and deformity. Even with regard to these variables there are marked differences in their interpretation since the definitions of delayed union, non-union and malunion are arbitrary (Goulet & Templeman 1997). Although these are relatively objective criteria that can be measured by the surgeon, often little regard is paid to functional criteria and patient satisfaction.

This problem of analysis of the literature is highlighted in a recent meta-analysis of the treatment of closed tibial shaft fractures (Littenberg et al 1998) in which 2372 reports of comparative trials and uncontrolled studies were evaluated. Even with this wealth of data, due to the inconsistencies within these studies, there was insufficient data to evaluate any aspect of functional status, level of pain, or other patient-related outcomes.

It is difficult to compare older series of tibial and fibular fractures to current reviews because of the mixture of open and closed fractures and the lack of uniformity in classification and outcome; however, they do give insight into the natural history and outcome of these injuries.

Prognostic factors

Nicoll (1964) was the first orthopaedic surgeon to describe the 'personality of the fracture'. He identified inherent factors that would affect the prognosis regardless of the method of treatment. Analysing the results of over 700 tibial fractures he identified four prognostic indicators:

- The amount of initial displacement.
- The degree of comminution (fragmentation).
- The degree of soft tissue damage.
- The presence of infection.

Ellis (1958a) was one of the first investigators to appreciate that the severity of the initial injury affected the speed of healing and outcome in tibial fractures. He looked at three variables: namely, fracture displacement, extent of the open wound and the severity of fragmentation. Ellis classified the fractures into three degrees of severity:

- *Minor*—undisplaced or angulated fragments (may be minor fragmentation or minor open wound).
- *Moderate*—completely displaced fragments (may be minor fragmentation or minor open wound).
- *Major/severe*—displaced fractures complicated by major fragmentation or a major open wound.

Reviewing 343 fractures in adults largely treated non-operatively (98%), Ellis found that the *severity* of the injury as judged by complete displacement, severe soft tissue injury and severe *fragmentation* significantly and adversely affected the times to union (Table 14.1).

Table 14.1 Relating severity of fracture and outcome (modified from Ellis 1958)

Severity of fracture	No. patients	Time to union Weeks	Delayed union >20 weeks
Minor	98	10	2 (2%)
Moderate	200	15	22 (11%)
Severe	45	23	27 (60%)
Total	343		

Ellis (1958a,b) further related his classification to functional outcome. Eighty-six percent had an excellent clinical and anatomical result. Almost 6% had shortening of 1–2 cm, 6% overall had limitation of foot and ankle movements with this occurring in 1% of minor injuries, 5% of moderate injuries and 22% of major severity fractures. This was invariably a source of disability. The follow-up study ranged from 1–6 years and drew important conclusions on functional end-results of non-operative cast management. Since then other authors have confirmed that the severity of the injury has an effect on outcome (Nicoll 1964, Johner & Wruhs 1983, Waddell & Reardon 1983) and others have looked more specifically at the effects of displacement, fragmentation, fibular fractures and soft tissue injury.

Displacement

The prognostic significance of initial displacement is not clear. Russell (1996) states that it may be underestimated and may give a useful insight into the amount of soft tissue disruption and thus the prognosis for healing. Johner & Wruhs (1983), however, developed a classification based on fracture morphology and felt that the displacement detected on the radiographs was unreliable because reduction may occur prior to the investigation.

In a review of 780 tibial shaft fractures treated with a functional brace (Sarmiento et al 1989), displacement of more than one-third was associated with prolonged healing times except when associated with gun shot injuries. Non-displaced and minimally displaced fractures demonstrated no difference in healing times, while fractures with a moderate displacement (34–67%) and severe displacement (68–100%) took the same time to unite.

Similar conclusions were reached by Digby et al (1983), who found that in a series of 100 tibial shaft fractures treated non-operatively the healing time was directly related to the degree of displacement (Table 14.2).

Nicoll (1964) found that delayed union was three times more common in displaced fractures and Weissman (1966) demonstrated that displacement of less than a fifth resulted in healing at 3 months compared with 6 months in completely displaced fractures.

It would therefore appear that displacement is one of the indicators of the severity of the injury. It is directly related to fracture union but there is little evidence that displacement per se affects the long-term clinical outcome.

Fragmentation

Fragmentation is another feature of high velocity injury and is likely to be associated with a more significant soft tissue injury or open fracture. In reviewing the healing parameters of 780 tibial fractures, Sarmiento (1989) found that fragmentation was associated with an increased incidence of delayed union for all fracture groups except closed fractures with an intact fibula. One-third of fragmented closed and grade I/II open fractures resulted in a delayed union. Johner & Wruhs (1983) noted that the degree of fragmentation greatly influenced the rate of local complications, healing time and final result based on their evaluation criteria (Tables 14.3 and 14.4).

Nicoll (1964) distinguished four types of fragmentation and compared fractures with no or slight fragmentation with moderate and severe fragmentation. He found that the risk of delayed and non-union was almost double in the latter group, with an incidence of 30% compared with 18%. Other authors have found similar correlations of healing times and outcomes with increasing fragmentation. It is likely that fragmentation, as with displacement, is associated with injuries of greater energy and hence a less satisfactory outcome.

Many of the studies relating displacement and fragmentation to outcome are based on closed methods of treatment. Recently, Gaston et al (2000) reviewed a num-

Table 14.2 Relationship between displacement and time to union (from Digby et al 1983)

Displacement	Number	Healing time Weeks
Nil	21	15.3
1/4 shaft diameter	26	16.9
1/4–1/2 diameter	19	18.4
1/2 diameter	8	18.3
Severe comminution	8	22.6

Table 14.3 Complication rates related to fracture type (modified from Johner & Wruhs 1983)

	A Simple	B Butterfly fragments	C Comminuted
Local complications	9.5%	18.1%	48.3%
WB at 11 weeks	46%	28%	9%
Hospitalisation	14d	17d	42d
Inability to work	109d	168d	185d
Malalignment	7%	10%	42%
Excellent/good	89%	88%	69%
Fair	8%	9%	14%
Poor	3%	3%	17%

Table 14.4 Criteria for evaluation of final results after tibial shaft fractures (modified from Johner & Wruhs 1983)

	Excellent (left = right)	Good	Fair	Poor
Non-union, osteitis, amputation	None	None	None	Yes
Neurovascular disturbances	None	Minimal	Moderate	Severe
Varus/valgus	None	2–5°	6 10°	>10°
Anteversion/recurvation	0–5°	6–10°	11–20°	>20°
Rotation	0 5°	6–10°	11–20°	>20°
Shortening	0 5 mm	6–10 mm	11–20 mm	>20 mm
Mobility				
Knee	Normal	>80%	>75%	<75%
Ankle	Normal	>75%	50%	<50%
Subtalar joint	>75%	>50%	<50%	
Pain	None	Occasional	Moderate	Severe
Gait	Normal	Normal	Insignificant limp	Significant limp
Strenuous activities	Possible	Limited	Severely limited	Impossible

ber of factors, including AO fracture classification, Winquist–Hansen grade, open and closed injuries, displacement (AP and lateral), Tscherne Score, location and associated fibular fracture in an attempt to predict outcome in fractures treated with an intramedullary nail. They did not find a significant correlation between displacement/fragmentation and outcome. Although these factors are important predictors of final outcome in closed treatment, Gaston et al (2000) felt that if modern treatment methods are used, fragmentation and initial displacement of fragments are unreliable indicators of outcome when these fractures are treated with intramedullary nails.

Soft tissue injury

Ellis (1958a,b) recognised the importance of the degree of soft tissue injury and the natural history of these fractures. In his review of the disabilities after tibial shaft fractures he found that increasing soft tissue injury resulted in an increase in ankle and foot stiffness.

Closed fractures

Tscherne & Gotzen (1984) have classified the soft tissue injury associated with closed fractures:

C0 Simple fracture configuration with little or no soft tissue injury.

C1 Superficial abrasion, mild to moderate soft tissue damage or severe fracture configuration.

C2 Deep contaminated abrasion with local damage to skin or muscle. Moderate to severe fracture configuration.

C3 Extensive contusion or crushing of skin or destruction of muscle. Severe fracture configuration.

Court-Brown et al (1990), in a review of 132 tibial fractures of which 124 were closed, and all of which were treated by intramedullary nailing, found a correlation between healing times and the Tscherne & Gotzen classification with a mean time to union of 12.5 weeks in C0 and 23.7 weeks in C3 injuries. In their prospective review of the predictors of outcome in intramedullary nailing of the tibia (Gaston et al 2000) found that the Tscherne classification of closed fractures was the best for predicting outcome (compared with displacement, AO fracture classification, Winquist–Hansen grade, location and associated fibular fracture) and correlated with time to walking, running, jumping, climbing ladders and return to sporting activities.

Open fractures

In 1976 Gustilo & Anderson reported on a prognostic classification scheme for open fractures based on wound size, and then in 1984 further subclassified the type III fractures based on prognosis (Gustilo et al 1984). Sarmiento (1989) noted a difference in average healing times comparing closed fractures (18.7 weeks) and open fractures (21.7 weeks). They found that grades II and III required substantially longer periods to heal.

Caudle & Stern (1987), in a review of 62 Gustilo type III injuries (11 IIIa, 42 IIIb and nine IIIc), demonstrated the significant prognostic value of this classification. Type IIIa fractures had a non-union rate of 27% with no deep infection or subsequent amputations. Type IIIb fractures had much worse results with a 43% non-union rate, 29% deep infection and 17% secondary amputation rate. Type IIIc fractures had the worst prognosis with all patients having major complications (100% non-union rate, 57% infection rate and 78% secondary amputation rate). However, this was a heterogeneous group of patients and included all types of primary bone stabilisation.

Overall, there are a number of studies showing increasing times to union and increasing requirement for secondary surgery using the Gustilo Grading (Court Brown et al 1990, 1991).

More recent studies looking at one form of skeletal stabilisation only have also confirmed the trend of worsening outcome with increasing severity of Gustilo grading (Bonatus et al 1997, Keating et al 1997). The incidence of ankle and subtalar joint stiffness was related to the severity of the original injury and was significantly higher in grade IIIb injuries (Table 14.5).

Fibular fractures

The evidence that associated fibular fractures affect the outcome is conflicting. It has been suggested that an intact fibula holds the tibial surfaces apart, contributing towards complications—particularly non-union and varus malunion. This was supported by Tietz et al (1980), who found that in patients older than 21, where there was no associated fibular fracture, there was a 26% incidence of delayed or non-union and a 26% varus malunion rate. Sarmiento (1989) states that fractures with an intact fibula require close observation, as they are prone to drift into varus.

There is also evidence to the contrary. Nicoll (1964), Weissman et al (1966) and Hoaglund & States (1967) all found that the absence of a fibular fracture was associated with a better prognosis because the injury was associated with less severe trauma. Further evidence supporting this

Table 14.5 Relationship of grade of open injury and functional results (from Keating et al 1997)

Grade fracture	Time to union	Non-union	Deep infection	Ankle stiffness	Subtalar stiffness
I (31)	29	1 (3%)	0	4%	4%
II (38)	32	2 (5%)	4 (10%)	17%	14%
IIIa (23)	34	3 (13%)	—	7%	7%
IIIb (20)	39	3 (17%)	2 (11%)	32%	26%

comes from other large studies such as Digby et al (1983) and Oni et al (1988), who reported more rapid healing and lower rates on delayed union in those without fibular fractures. In a prospective review looking at basic descriptive criteria and functional outcome after tibial nailing, Gaston et al (2000) found that the incidence of fibular fracture does not predict outcome other than an earlier return to sporting activities.

Age

There is little evidence that age effects the prognosis of tibial fractures occurring over the age of 16 years. Nichol (1964) suggested that adults over the age of 60 might show prolonged times to healing, although there were relatively few elderly patients in his series. Sarmiento (1989) failed to demonstrate any correlation between age and fracture union in either closed or open fractures. However, Gaston et al (2000) found that age did seem to influence both time to union and full weight bearing with increased times to union with age. The authors felt that this was the first report of such a correlation and therefore it warrants further investigation.

Location of fracture

Allum & Mowbray (1980) have suggested that location of the fracture plays a significant role in the rate of healing. Nicoll (1964) took into account fracture morphology and location and found a slightly higher risk of delayed union in middle third fractures compared with those in the lower third. Gaston et al found that the location of the fracture within the diaphysis of the tibia correlated well with the time to weight bearing but not fracture union, malunion or non-union. However, the number of proximal third fractures was very small in this study. Sarmiento (1989) also confirmed that anatomical location did not significantly affect union, although segmental fractures take an average 1 month longer to unite.

There is some evidence that the anatomical position of the fracture has an influence over malunion rate following nailing. In a series of fractures stabilised with an unreamed nail, Singer et al (1995) found significantly more malunions in those fractures around the junction of the proximal and middle thirds.

Summary

- The severity of the injury and 'personality' of the fracture are very important prognostic indicators.
- The patient's age, presence of fibular fracture and anatomical position of the fracture have little effect on the prognosis.

Non-operative treatment

Plaster immobilisation

The clinical results of Ellis (1958a,b) have been described above. They show that 86% of 343 fractures treated by plaster immobilisation achieved excellent functional and anatomical results. There was increasing evidence of ankle and foot stiffness with increasing severity of injury.

Nicoll (1964) reported a 26% incidence of significant joint stiffness in tibial fractures treated by immobilisation in plaster. Significant stiffness was defined as follows:

- Knee—any loss of extension; loss of more than 10° of flexion.
- Ankle—loss of more than 25% of flexion or extension.
- Subtalar joint—loss of more than 25% of inversion or eversion.

Within this group of patients Nicoll found that one-third (9%) had severe, disabling stiffness. This was defined as follows:

- Knee—loss of 15° or more of extension; loss of more than 30° of flexion.
- Ankle—loss of more than 50% of flexion or extension.
- Subtalar joint—loss of more than 50% of inversion or eversion.

The frequency of significant joint stiffness can be related to fracture personality.

Nicoll (1964) also assessed the residual deformity in 671 of the patients and found that 8.6% had a significant deformity as defined by angulation of more than 10° in any plane or shortening of 2 cm or more.

Weismann et al (1966), in their review of 200 consecutive tibial fractures, found that 90% had a perfect clinical recovery, although 12% developed delayed union; 23.5% had a step-off deformity but they claimed that this had no bearing on the functional result.

In many of these earlier reports a full length plaster cast was applied with the knee in 20–45° of flexion to help control rotation; however, this precluded early weight bearing.

Functional bracing

The importance of early weight bearing was not emphasised in the work of Ellis (1958a,b) or Nicoll (1964), but it was reported in 1961 by Dehne et al. Later, Sarmiento (1967), Brown (1974) and Sarmiento & Latta (1981) all confirmed the benefit of functional bracing with early weight bearing. Sarmiento et al (1989) produced a detailed anatomical analysis of the results in 780 tibial fractures.

However, they did not give a breakdown of the functional results in these patients.

In fact, many of the studies regarding functional bracing have failed to provide details of functional results and they have often combined open and closed fractures, making comparison difficult (Table 14.6).

Operative treatment
Plating/Nailing

Enthusiastic supporters of rigid internal fixation have reported very good results after operative treatment of the tibial shaft (Ruedi et al 1976, Allgower & Perren 1980). However, most authors now list tibial shaft fractures associated with displaced intra-articular fractures and metaphyseal fractures as the prime indications for open reduction and internal fixation.

Ruedi et al (1976) reported on the outcome of 418 fractures of the tibial shaft treated with dynamic compression plating. Of the 323 closed fractures, 93% achieved excellent or good results (full anatomical/functional restoration or minimal symptoms) and 2% had moderate results, 6% had complications, 3% delayed union, 1% non-union and there was infection in 1%.

Bilat et al (1994) reported their early and late complications in 245 tibial fractures. Of the 185 closed fractures there were 94% excellent or good results. There was a 7% delayed union rate and a 1.7% infection rate. Of the open fractures 93% were good or excellent, 10% developed a delayed union and there was a 6.8% infection rate.

Johner & Wruhs (1983) produced a thorough appraisal of the results of internal fixation, producing a set of criteria for evaluation and a morphological classification of the fracture type (table 14.3 and 14.4). They reported a significant increase in complications as progressively higher energy fractures were treated by open reduction and internal fixation. They reported 291 fractures, 97% of which were followed for up to 8 years. In this group 67% were treated by plating, 30% by intramedullary nailing and 3% with external fixation. Complication rates increased from 9.5% for group A, 18% group B and 48% in group C fractures. The infection rate rose from 2% in group A to 10% in group C. The number of excellent and good results decreased from 89% in group A to 69% in group C. Twice as many non-unions and five times as many cases of infection were seen in open compared with closed fractures. Karlstrom & Olerud (1974) recorded even higher complication rates of internal fixation (19%).

Intramedullary nailing has gained popularity. Court Brown et al (1990) described closed intramedullary nailing of 125 patients with displaced closed and grade I compound tibial fractures. The average time to bony union was 16.7 weeks. The average time for return to work in those patients without multiple injuries was 84 days. Court Brown et al (1991) have also recommended the use of locked nails for grade II and III open fractures. They found that the rate of union and infection was similar to previous series describing treatment with external fixation, but that the incidence of malunion was less and fewer patients required bone grafting.

Table 14.6

Author	Mix	Number	Healing time	Shortening mm None	1–5,	6–10	11–15	>15	Malunion varus/ valgus	Ant/ Post	Non-union	Delayed union
Sarmiento 1967	O and C	780	17.4/ 21.7	40%		27.9%	21.9%	6.3%	3.3%	25%		2.5%	
Pun et al 1991	O and C	98	17.4 +/−5.4	76.8%	7.4%	11.6%	4.2%		23.7%	20.6%	—	7.2%
Oni et al 1988	Closed	100	81% at 20 weeks				5.3%		21%	13%		19%
Sarmiento 1967	Closed	960	18.1						1.4%	10.8%	5%	6%

Results of cast bracing.
O—open fractures.
C—closed fractures.

Complications

Non-union and malunion

The definitions of non-union and malunion are arbitrary and therefore careful attention by the reviewer is needed in the interpretation of series comparing these outcomes. Non-union has been defined as a condition in which, in the opinion of the operating surgeon, further non-surgical management will fail to unite the fragments (Nicoll 1964).

Delayed union is defined as the state in which the expected progression to union has not been observed at a specific time. Failure to see evidence of union on radiographs at various times ranging from 20–26 weeks has been the criterion used by several authors (Nicoll 1964, Jones 1965, Rosenthal et al 1977, Skelley 1981).

Many factors have been associated with delayed union and non-union. The incidence increases with the severity of open fractures. The presenting factors contributing to non-union or delayed union include fracture displacement, bone loss, associated fibular fractures, fragmentation and infection (Nicoll 1964, Ellis 1958, Urist 1954, Watson Jones 1943).

A direct correlation exists between the energy absorbed by the bone and soft tissues and the complications of wound healing, including delayed union, non-union and skin problems (Hoaglund & States 1967, Cierney et al 1983).

Destruction of the endosteal blood supply is most extensive when the fracture occurs in the middle third but Nicoll (1964) has shown that the distribution of non-unions among proximal, middle and distal segments appears equal. However, periosteal stripping contributes significantly to delayed and non-unions of the tibial shaft (Goulet et al 1997).

Nicoll (1964) found that 78% of 674 fractured tibias had united by 20 weeks. These fractures were treated in long leg plasters and no emphasis was placed on early weight bearing. The author showed quite clearly that the incidence of delayed union (and non-union) increased with moderate to severe displacement (36%) and moderate to severe fragmentation (30%). If Nicoll's results are analysed according to fracture personality, it is clear that a higher frequency of delayed union and non-union occurs in the poor personality fractures.

Ellis (1958a) made similar observations in a series of 343 tibial fractures, 85% of which had united by 20 weeks. The incidence of delayed union was 2% in the minor severity injuries, 11% in the moderate severity injuries and 60% in the major severity injuries (see Prognostic factors, earlier in this chapter, for the definition of the injury severity groups). The treatment of patients in this group was similar to that in Nicoll's 1964 series.

Ruedi et al (1976) reported a 3% incidence of delayed union in closed fractures, and a 7% incidence in open fractures. All fractures were treated by AO dynamic compression plating. In the same series, the incidence of non-union was 1% in closed fractures and 5% in open fractures.

Johner & Wruhs (1983) described 283 tibial shaft fractures (both open and closed) and reported a 1% incidence of non-union. All fractures in this group were treated operatively by dynamic compression plating, intramedullary nailing or, rarely, external fixation.

Sarmiento et al (1989) reported a 2.5% non-union rate in a large series of 780 open and closed tibial shaft fractures treated by early weight-bearing and functional bracing. Court Brown et al (1990) described delayed union in two of 125 patients (1.6%) treated by IM nailing. The two patients were treated by exchange nailing and went on to unite.

Open fractures may be expected to have higher complication rates. Table 14.7 shows the non-union, delayed union, malunion and infection rates for open fractures stabilised with intramedullary nails.

A recent meta-analysis of closed fractures of the tibial shaft (Litterman et al 1999), reviewing 2372 comparative trials (only 19 reports met inclusion criteria), found that the median time to union for intramedullary nailing was 20 weeks, cast immobilisation 15 weeks and 13 weeks for open reduction and internal fixation. There was no difference in the numbers reaching union in 20 weeks or the rates of non-union. However, the authors urge caution in interpreting these data, as the methods for determining or reporting rates of union were not uniform.

Malunion

Malunion of tibial shaft fractures can result in:

- Angular deformity.
- Rotational deformity.
- Shortening.

The criteria for determining malunion of the tibial shaft that requires operative intervention are not clearly defined (Russell 1996).

Angular malunion

The importance of residual angular deformity after tibial fractures is still uncertain. It has been suggested that angular deformity of more than 5° in any direction could lead to late degenerative changes in the adjacent joints (Sarmiento & Latta 1981). Russell (1996) suggested that malalignment of more than 15–20° may require corrective osteotomy.

Table 14.7

Author	Number	I	II	Infection rates IIIa	IIIb	IIIc	Malunion	Delayed union	Non-union
Sanders et al 1994	64	0/10	0/16	1/17	5/21	0/0	0	26%	1.5%
Stegemann et al 1995	41	0/15	1/12	1/14	0/0	0/0	NR	5%	0
Whittle et al 1992	50	0/3	0/13	1/22	3/12	0/0	0	50%	4%
Keating et al 1997[†]	112	1/31	4/38	0/23	2/20	—	6%	—	8%
Bonatus et al 1997	72	0/27	1/22	1/11	1/12	—	3%	15%	17%
Court-Brown et al 1991[†]	41	0/0	1/14	0/14	3/13		7%	31% required exchange nailing	
Singer & Kellam 1993	43	1/6	1/11	1/16	2/9	0/1	49%	NR	2.5%

Outcome of intramedullary nailing of open fractures.

NR—not recorded.

[†] Reamed nailing.

Kristensen et al (1989) re-examined patients after low energy trauma at a minimum of 20 years following the fracture. Of 92 patients identified, 17 had angular deformity of more than 10°. Only seven of these had symptoms of ankle discomfort and none showed any radiographic changes of arthritis. The authors concluded that there was no evidence that an angular deformity of less than 15° will lead to arthrosis of the ankle.

Merchant & Dietz (1996) retrospectively evaluated 37 patients, 29 years after sustaining a closed or open grade I tibial injury. They were unable to find any correlation between the degree of malunion and the clinical outcome or incidence of osteoarthritis.

Van der Schoot (1996) holds the opposite opinion. From the author's study of 88 patients followed up clinically and radiologically 15 years after injury, it was concluded that the incidence of arthritic change was higher in the knee and ankle in those patients with an angular deformity and that a relationship existed between tibial malalignment and degenerative change.

Puno et al (1991) studied the long-term effects of tibial angular malunion on the knee and ankle joints in 27 patients with 28 fractures at an average of 8.2 years from injury. They demonstrated that increasing malalignment at the ankle joint level correlated significantly with symptoms and the functional outcome. Poorer scores were associated with radiographic changes of degenerative arthritis. However, they were unable to demonstrate a critical angle of malalignment resulting in a poor result. They also failed to show any correlation between the knee scores and knee malalignment. The authors concluded that a relationship between malalignment and functional result did exist, although they could not provide a critical limit of malalignment of the ankle above which degenerative arthrosis was a certainty. It was clear that there was a higher probability of having good/excellent results with lesser degrees of malalignment.

Rotational deformity

Most reports fail to consider this problem. Russell (1996) believed that external rotation was better tolerated than internal rotation and that internal rotation of more than 10° may cause gait disturbance

Nicoll (1964) found only two patients with a rotational abnormality of over 10° (0.3%) in 671 conservatively treated patients. Gamble et al (1972) described a 3% incidence of rotational deformity in a series of tibial fractures treated by plaster fixation and early weight bearing.

Shortening

Nicoll (1964) reported a 2.5% incidence of shortening of over 2 cm in 671 tibial shaft fractures treated by plaster immobilisation. Ellis (1958a) found a 5.5% incidence of shortening of between 13 and 19 mm in a group of 343 patients treated by similar methods. Weissman et al (1966) reported a 3% incidence of shortening of over 1 cm in 140 patients treated in plaster.

Supporters of early weight bearing (Dehne et al 1961, Sarmiento 1967) believed that physiological shortening allowed impaction and that this favoured early union. Sarmiento reported an average shortening of 6.4 mm, with a maximum of 2 cm, in his patients treated by functional bracing with early weight bearing.

Johner & Wruhs (1983) described a 1.4% incidence of shortening of 5 mm in 283 patients treated almost exclusively by rigid internal fixation.

Compartment syndrome

Compartment syndrome is a well-recognised complication of fractures of the tibial shaft. If left untreated it can result in nerve and muscle dysfunction, infection, myoglobinuria, renal failure and even amputation. Despite the development of various techniques for measurement of intracompartmental pressure it is not appropriate to rely solely on this. There is no reliable objective method to determine when a fasciotomy is required and the fundamental problem is the inability to identify the pressure at which nerve and muscle become ischaemic (Tornetta & Templeman 1997).

Tile (1987) outlined the value of early diagnosis and recognition of compartment syndromes, stressing the importance of prompt treatment in the prevention of ischaemic muscle damage.

Nicoll (1964) found only five patients with ischaemic contractures in 671 tibial shaft fractures (0.75%), and Ellis (1958b) found an incidence of 4% in 225 fractures. More recently Court-Brown et al (1990) quoted a 1.6% incidence in 125 grade I and closed fractures undergoing intramedullary nailing. In a study of 622 diaphyseal fractures, McQueen et al (1996) noted an overall incidence of 4% with a 1.2% incidence in open fractures. Rorabeck & Macnab (1975) suggested that open fractures will allow decompression of muscle compartments; however, McQueen et al found no difference in the pressures generated in open and closed fractures. They also found a significant strong correlation between the intracompartmental pressures generated and the severity of the soft tissue injury grade measured by the Oestern & Tscherne grading.

DeLee & Stiehl (1981) reported an incidence of 6% in 104 open fractures and others have quoted an incidence as high as 9% (Blick et al 1986). However, these series may quote incidences that are falsely high in terms of prognosis as they used routine pressure monitoring. The true incidence probably lies between this range of figures and is likely to be closer to Ellis' figure of 4% as he was specifically looking for the sequelae of ischaemia in his patients.

Joint stiffness

Opinion is divided as to the cause of joint stiffness with some believing that it results from prolonged immobilisation and others to the soft tissue injury initially sustained. Joint stiffness may be a cause of significant morbidity. Nicoll (1964) reported that 9% of his patients had disabling joint stiffness. He defined this as loss of more than 50% of movement compared to the normal side. This mainly affected the ankle and subtalar joints, although three cases of disabling knee stiffness were recorded. Stiffness is related to the personality of the fracture.

Ellis (1958b) found a 2.5% incidence of reduced knee flexion and a 6% incidence of reduced ankle flexion after tibial shaft fractures. In the group with ankle stiffness, 11 had heavy jobs and only two were able to return to work as a consequence of their stiff ankles. The incidence of significant stiffness was greater as the severity of the fracture increased.

Ruedi et al (1976) described six cases with reduced movement of 20–30° in 323 patients with closed tibial fractures treated by AO plating (2%). The incidence of reduced movement rose to 8% in open fractures in this group of patients. Assessment in this series took into account total reduced movement in knee, ankle and subtalar joints.

Many of the current operative treatment methods encourage early motion of the joints and state this as an advantage. Lucas & Todd (1973), however, found that although patients treated with compression plating had better function at 8 months after injury, by 12 months their functional status was not significantly different from those who had been treated with cast immobilisation.

Pun et al (1991) specifically assessed joint stiffness at an average of 1.86 years after treatment with functional bracing of diaphyseal tibial fractures. The majority of patients did not have a full range of movement of the ankle and subtalar joints when the brace was removed. The stiffness decreased with time, but at 1.86 years 68.4% had normal ankle motion and 60% had normal subtalar motion. This increased to 75.5% and 71.1% respectively at 2 years or more. Merchant & Dietz (1989), using regression analysis, were unable to demonstrate any correlation between the duration of immobilisation and the final range of movement of the knee and ankle.

Re-fracture

The incidence of re-fracture has been reported as 3% in tibial fractures treated in plaster (Chrisman & Snook 1968). Ruedi et al (1976) reported a 0.5% incidence of refracture after AO plating in a series of 388 patients. However, higher refracture rates have been reported after AO plating, ranging from 1.9–6% (Solheim 1960, Karlstrom & Olerud 1974).

Post-phlebitic syndrome

Recent reports have highlighted the importance of the post-phlebitic syndrome after fractures of the tibia (Aitken et al 1987, Wolfe 1987). Wolfe found that post-phlebitic symptoms occurred more commonly after tibial fractures than after femoral fractures. He also found that this syndrome was less common in patients under the age of 25.

Aitken et al (1987) emphasised the medico-legal importance of this condition. They particularly stressed that it may take 5–10 years before significant clinical features of chronic venous insufficiency develop. They described other reports which revealed an increasing incidence of post-phlebitic limbs with the passage of time—13%, 35% and 39% at 3, 9 and 14 years respectively, following tibial shaft fractures. The authors advise patients and their legal representatives to be cautious in settlement of Personal Injury claims following tibial shaft fractures, for it may be that an early 'full and final settlement' will leave the patients with no redress if a post-phlebitic limb should develop later.

In the series of Aitken et al (1987), 11 of 60 limbs with femoral and/or tibial fractures (18%) had clinically disabling post-phlebitic symptoms, including venous ulceration.

Reflex sympathetic dystrophy

Sarangi et al (1993) carried out a prospective study of the incidence and natural history of reflex sympathetic dystrophy and associated changes in bone mineral density in the ankles and feet of 60 consecutive patients who had suffered unilateral fractures of the tibial shaft. At the time of bone union, 18 (30%) showed signs of reflex sympathetic dystrophy. Its development was independent on the type of fracture management and of the severity of the injury. In most cases the symptoms resolved within 6 months of fracture union, but in four patients they were still present at 1 year, and two of these had still not returned to work.

Complications related to internal fixation

Plate fixation

Complications include implant failure, irritation from the implant and deep infection. Ruedi et al (1976) comprehensively reviewed the results of 418 diaphyseal fractures of which 323 were closed and 95 open. In the closed group 6% had a significant complication including fracture of the plate, infection, non-union and delayed union. In the open fracture group this rose to 31.5%.

Intramedullary nailing

In a review of the complications of nailing in 102 closed tibial fractures, Williams et al (1995) found that 37% exhibited one or more components of malunion; 18% required further operative procedures to achieve union or correct malalignment, and 19% developed new peroneal nerve lesions of which 4% were permanent; 7% developed an acute compartment syndrome.

Koval et al (1991), in a retrospective analysis of acute fractures treated with reamed nailing, found a 10% incidence of intra-operative complications including propagation of the fracture and poor hold of the locking bolts. A haematoma developed in 6.7%, 13% developed a malunion and 30% developed neurological deficits, although 89% settled spontaneously. Up to 22% developed tenderness around the insertion site, and overall 58% developed some complication related to the procedure. However, most were minor and did not affect the long-term clinical outcome.

Summary

- Delayed union occurs in 15–22% of tibial shaft fractures treated by plaster immobilisation without weight bearing.
- 2–5% non-union rate with cast bracing.
- Delayed union occurs in 3–7% of tibial fractures treated by plating.
- Non-union occurs in 1–10% of tibial fractures treated by plating.
- 1–9% will develop an acute compartment syndrome and 1–4% develop an ischaemic contracture.
- 2–9% develop significant stiffness of the knee or ankle.
- The post-phlebitic syndrome may be a clinically significant factor after tibial shaft fracture. It may take 5–10 years for symptoms to develop fully.

Tibial fractures in children

Tibial and fibular fractures are the third most common paediatric long bone injury (15%) after femoral and forearm fractures. Fifteen percent occur in the distal third and

39% in the middle third; 35% are oblique, 32% comminuted, 20% transverse and 13% spiral. Approximately 9% of paediatric tibial fractures are open (Heinrich 1996).

Proximal tibial physis

Ogden (1987) pointed out that this fracture was uncommon because of the local anatomy, particularly the anterior overhang of the tibial tuberosity. Neer & Horwitz (1965) described an incidence of 0.8% in 2500 consecutive physeal fractures.

The two largest series reporting injuries to the proximal tibial physis were from Shelton & Canale (1979) and Burkhart & Peterson (1979). Shelton & Canale described follow-up to skeletal maturity in 28 physeal injuries in 27 patients. Burkhart & Peterson reported 26 injuries; five of these were compound lawnmower injuries and all five had a uniformly poor prognosis.

Shelton & Canale (1979) classified their results as satisfactory or unsatisfactory. A result was considered unsatisfactory if any of the following was present:

- Leg length discrepancy of 2.5 cm or more.
- Angular deformity of more than 7°.
- Incongruity of the joint with secondary traumatic arthritis or pain.
- Neurovascular compromise with resultant loss of function in the limb.

Treatment of patients in these two groups consisted of cast immobilisation in the Salter–Harris types I and II injuries and open reduction and internal fixation for displaced Salter–Harris types III and IV injuries (Salter & Harris 1963). Average follow-up was 7 years in the patients reported by Shelton & Canale (1979) and 2.5 years in Burkhart & Peterson's 1979 series. Nine of the 49 patients in these series had unsatisfactory results according to Shelton & Canale's criteria, an incidence of 18%.

The lawnmower injuries reported by Burkhart & Peterson (five cases) had a very poor prognosis. Four of the patients developed significant angulation (12–30°) and two developed leg length discrepancy of over 3.5 cm. One patient developed osteomyelitis after open reduction and internal fixation and one a severed peroneal nerve. All results were unsatisfactory.

In these two series the Salter–Harris classification was not a reliable predictor of growth disturbance. Indeed, in Shelton & Canale's series all of the seven patients exhibiting growth abnormalities were Salter–Harris type I or II injuries. Roberts (1984) believed that this was due to longitudinal compression causing damage to the deeper proliferative zone of the growth plate in these patients.

Poulsen et al (1989) reviewed 15 patients with proximal tibial epiphyseal fractures. They found that type III Salter–Harris lesions were often accompanied by ligamentous injuries (eight of 15 patients), a frequency similar to that of Bertin & Goble (1983). They also found that Salter–Harris IV and V injuries correlated with symptoms at follow-up and the development of degenerative changes was confined to those patients with these injuries. They concluded that close attention should be paid to these ligamentous injuries and that they should be repaired if possible.

Fractures of the proximal metaphysis

These injuries usually occur in children aged 3–6 years and most commonly from a force applied to the lateral aspect of the extended knee causing the medial cortex to fail in tension. They occur with an incidence of approximately six tibial metaphyseal fractures per 100 000 children per year (Skak et al 1987).

The most common sequelae of these injuries is a valgus deformity and this is most commonly associated with greenstick and complete fractures (Robert et al 1987, Skak et al 1987). As a result, these fractures need to be carefully monitored (Heinrich 1996). The incidence of this complication is unclear. Salter & Best (1973) reported an incidence of 62% with angulation of between 11 and 22° in 21 patients on removal of the cast. On follow-up this increased to 18–25°. Roberts et al (1987) studied 25 children, 48% of whom developed valgus deformity, and Skak et al (1987) reported an incidence of 10%. A number of theories have been put forward as possible aetiologies including asymmetric medial physeal activity, the tethering effect of the fibula, inadequate reduction, soft tissue interposition and early weight bearing.

It would seem from the evidence of Ogden et al (1995) that the valgus deformity that develops is usually not a complication of the initial reduction but is more likely secondary to differential growth between the medial and lateral aspects of the proximal tibial epiphysis.

It is now accepted that the valgus deformity will stabilise and then improve with growth and development. The deformity usually occurs within 5 months of injury, reaching a maximum within 18–24 months, stabilises and then improves. Unfortunately, there are no data indicating how much improvement can be expected. (Thompson & Behrens 1998).

Tibial tuberosity fractures/avulsions

Ogden et al (1980) reported 15 fractures of the tibial tuberosity in 14 adolescents. Hand et al (1971) reported seven avulsion fractures in adolescents.

Ogden et al concluded that complications were rare after this injury, and that the theoretical possibility of the subsequent development of genu recurvatum appeared unlikely, since most of these injuries occurred when the physis of the tuberosity was undergoing normal closure.

Both of these reports stressed the importance of accurate reduction if the tibial tuberosity was displaced.

Tibial shaft fractures

Blount (1955) believed that the treatment of fractures of the tibia in children was gratifying because the fractures had a short healing time, a low complication rate and there were no cases of non-union or delayed union, if surgery was omitted. The major problems with fracture of the tibial shaft are shortening, angulation, malrotation and valgus deformities. Allum & Mowbray (1980) confirmed the rapid healing of tibial fractures in children. Weissman et al (1966) reported normal function and absence of subjective complaints in 60 children under the age of 16 following tibial shaft fractures.

Hansen et al (1976) described the subjective and objective findings in 85 children under 15 years of age at 2 years from their tibial shaft fracture. Six patients (7%) experienced pain after major exertion. The authors did not find any gait abnormalities and observed symmetrical hip, knee and ankle movements in all patients. They found restriction of subtalar movements in two patients (2%).

Thompson & Behrens (1998) have suggested that in general, non-operative management of uncomplicated closed tibial and fibular shaft fractures results in uniformly satisfactory results. The fractures heal rapidly, depending on age, and minor discrepancies in length and angulation may correct spontaneously. Union can be expected in 2–18 weeks (Hansen et al 1976) with a mean of approximately 37 days (Shannak et al 1988).

Angular deformity

Greater angular remodelling can be expected:

- In the younger child.
- With increasing proximity to the physis.
- With smaller degrees of angulation.
- With angulation in the plane of the joint.

Swaan & Oppers (1971) believed that the capacity for children to correct angular deformity diminished with increasing age. However, even in the youngest age groups angular correction did not exceed 5°. Hansen et al (1976) estimated that the overall spontaneous correction of angular deformity in tibial fractures in children was 13.5%. They found only 14% correction of angular deformity. It ceased after 18 months from injury and was independent of age. They concluded that more than 10%

correction should not be expected after the conclusion of treatment.

Dias (1984) summarised the literature on the potential for the tibia to correct angular malalignment in children. He concluded that the maximum angulation that should be accepted during treatment was 10° of recurvatum and 5° of varus or valgus. Shannak (1988), in a review of 117 children with tibial shaft fractures treated in above knee casts, reported that 41% had residual varus or valgus angulation. In 25 it was 1–10°, in 18 it was more than 10° but less than 22°. At follow-up of almost 4 years, 91 had no angulation, 20 had angulation of 1–10° and six had angulation of more than 10°, i.e. a third of these fractures with greater than 10° of angulation had a persistent deformity. Deformities in two planes did not remodel as completely as those in one plane. The least correction occurred in posteriorly angulated fractures followed by fractures with valgus malalignment.

There is general agreement that rotational deformity in the tibia will not correct spontaneously. The incidence of rotational malunion is low, ranging from 3–6% (Hansen et al 1976, Shannak et al 1988).

Leg length discrepancy

Approximately 25% of children with tibial and fibular shaft fractures will have minor tibial length inequalities. The amount of growth acceleration after tibial fractures is less than after femoral fractures in children of comparable age (Heinrich 1996). Shannak et al (1988) have shown that the average growth acceleration of a child's tibia after fracture is approximately 4 mm. Swann & Oppers reported that younger children have a greater chance for overgrowth than older children. Hansen et al (1976) suggested that accelerated growth after tibial fractures occurs in children younger in age than 10 and that older children may have growth inhibition. Comminuted fractures with ipsilateral femoral shaft fractures have the greatest risk of accelerated growth and overgrowth.

Open fractures

Open fractures are invariably the result of high velocity trauma, they are serious injuries and they have high complication rates. Incidence varies between 2–14% of all tibial fractures, that of associated injuries between 15–74% (Thompson & Behrens 1988).

In 1990 Buckley et al reviewed 42 open fractures followed until healing; 42% of them had associated injuries. They reported that children with open fractures have an incidence of vascular injury, compartment syndrome, infection and delayed union similar to that in adults. Tibial overgrowth, however, was associated with severe open fractures.

Thompson & Behrens summarised the recent available literature on 323 open fractures in children. Type II fractures were the most common, at 42%, type I accounted for 30% and 28% were type III; 50% were associated with other injuries. There was a 3% incidence of amputation and of compartment syndrome. Infection occurred in 13%, delayed union in 14% and non-union in 5%; 6% develop a malunion and 2% a leg length discrepancy.

Levy et al studied 40 open fractures in children with an average age of 10 years and at an average follow-up of 26 months (18–84 months). They found that the children surveyed missed an average of 4.1 months of school and 33% had to repeat the year, 25% complained of nightmares and, despite solid union, 30% complained of chronic pain.

Summary

- Over 80% of children with injuries to the proximal tibial epiphysis achieve a satisfactory result.
- Complications are rare after injuries to the tibial tuberosity in adolescents.
- Most children with tibial shaft fractures achieve a normal clinical result. Even in young children, the evidence suggests that angular correction of more than 5–10° does not occur.
- In open fractures, despite solid union, 30% continue to experience pain.

References

Aitken R J, Mills C, Immelman E J 1987 The post-phlebitic syndrome following shaft fractures of the leg: a significant late complication. Journal of Bone and Joint Surgery 69B: 775–778

Allgower M, Perren S M 1980 Operating on tibial shaft fractures. Unfallheilk/Traumatology 83: 214–218

Allum R L, Mowbray M A S 1980 A retrospective review of the healing of fractures of the shaft of the tibia with special reference to the mechanism of injury. Injury 11: 304–308

Bertin K C, Goble E M 1983 Ligament injuries associated with physeal fractures about the knee. Clinical Orthopaedics 177: 188–195

Bilat C, Leutenegger A, Ruedi T 1994 Osteosynthesis of 245 tibial shaft fractures: early and late complications. Injury Aug 25(6): 349–358

Blick S S, Brumback R J, Poka A, Burgess A R, Ebraheim N A 1986 Compartment syndrome in open tibial fractures. Journal of Bone and Joint Surgery 68A: 1348–1353

Bonatus T, Olson S A, Lee S, Chapman M W 1997 Nonreamed locking intramedullary nailing for open fractures of the tibia. Clinical Orthopaedics Jun (339): 58–64

Brown P W 1974 Early weight bearing treatment of tibial shaft fractures. Clinical Orthopaedics 105: 165–178

Buckley S L, Smith G, Sponseller P D et al 1990 Open fractures of the tibia in children. Journal of Bone and Joint Surgery 72A: 1462–1469

Burkhart S S, Peterson H A 1979 Fractures of the proximal tibial epiphysis. Journal of Bone and Joint Surgery 61A: 996–1002

Caudle R J, Stern P J 1987 Severe open fractures of the tibia. Journal of Bone and Joint Surgery 69A: 801–807

Chrisman O D, Snook G A 1968 The problem of refracture of the tibia. Clinical Orthopaedics 60: 217–219

Cierny G 3d, Byrd H S, Jones R E 1983 Primary versus delayed soft tissue coverage for severe open tibial fractures. A comparison of results. Clinical Orthopaedics Sept (178): 54–63

Court-Brown C M, Christie J, McQueen M M 1990 Closed intramedullary tibial nailing: its use in closed and type I open fractures. Journal of Bone and Joint Surgery 72B: 605–611

Court-Brown C M, McQueen M M, Quater A A, Christie J 1991 Locked I M nailing of open tibial fractures. Journal of Bone and Joint Surgery 73B: 959–964

Dehne E, Metz C W, Deffer P, Hall R 1961 Non-operative treatment of the fractured tibia by immediate weight bearing. Journal of Trauma 1: 514–535

DeLee J C U, Stiehl J B 1981 Open tibia fracture with compartment syndrome. Clinical Orthopaedics Oct (160): 175–184

Dias L S 1984 Fractures of the tibia and fibula. In: Rockwood C A Jr, Wilkins K E, King R E (eds) Fractures in children, vol 3. J B Lippincott, Philadelphia

Digby J M, Holloway G M, Webb J K 1983 A study of function after tibial cast bracing. Injury Mar 14(5): 432–439

Ellis H 1958a The speed of healing after fracture of the tibial shaft. Journal of Bone and Joint Surgery 40B: 42–46

Ellis H 1958b Disabilities after tibial shaft fractures. Journal of Bone and Joint Surgery 40B: 190–197

Gamble W E, Clayton M L, Leidholt J D, Cletsher J O 1972 Complications following treatment of tibial fractures with weight bearing. Journal of Bone and Joint Surgery 54A: 1343

Gaston P, Will E, McQueen M M, Elton R A, Court-Brown C M 2000 Analysis of muscle function in the lower limb after fracture of the diaphysis of the tibia in adults. Journal of Bone and Joint Surgery 82B: 326–331

Goulet J A, Templeman D 1997 Delayed union and non union of tibial shaft fractures. AAOS Instructional Course Lectures Vol 46 28: 281–291

Gustilo R B, Anderson J T 1976 Prevention of infection in the treatment of one thousand and twenty-five open fractures of long bones: retrospective and prospective analyses. Journal of Bone and Joint Surgery 58A: 453–458

Gustilo R B, Mendoza R M, Williams D N 1984 Problems in the management of type III (severe) open fractures: a new classification of type III open fractures. Journal of Trauma 24(8): 742–746

Hand W L, Hand C R, Dunn A W 1971 Avulsion fractures of the tibial tubercle. Journal of Bone and Joint Surgery 53A: 1579–1583

Hansen B A, Greiff J, Bergmann F 1976 Fractures of the tibia in children. Acta Orthopaedica Scandinavica 47: 448–453

Heinrich S D 1996 Fractures of the shaft of the tibia and fibula. In: Rockwood C A, Wilkins K E, Beaty J H (eds) Fractures in children. Lippincott-Raven, Philadelphia

Hoaglund F T, States J D 1967 Factors influencing the rate of healing in tibial shaft fractures. Surgery, Gynecology and Obstetrics 124: 71–76

Johner R, Wruhs O 1983 Classification of tibial shaft fractures and correlation with results after rigid internal fixation. Clinical Orthopaedics 178: 7–25

Jones K G 1965 Treatment of infected nonunion of the tibia through the posterolateral approach. Clinical Orthopaedics 43: 103–109

Karlstrom G, Olerud S 1974 Fractures of the tibial shaft: a critical evaluation of treatment alternatives. Clinical Orthopaedics 105: 82–115

Keating J F, O'Brien P I, Blachut P A, Meek R N, Broekhuyse H M 1997 Reamed interlocking intramedullary nailing of open fractures of the tibia. Clinical Orthopaedics May (338): 182–391

Koval K J, Clapper M F, Brumback R J, Ellison P S Jr, Poka A, Bathon G H, Burgess A R 1991 Complications of reamed intramedullary nailing of the tibia. Journal of Orthopaedic Trauma 5(2): 184–189

Kristensen K D, Kiaer T, Blicher J 1989 No arthrosis of the ankle 20 years after malaligned tibial-shaft fracture. Acta Orthopaedica Scandinavica Apr 60(2): 208–209

Leach R E 1984 Fractures of the tibia and fibula. In: Rockwood C A, Green D P (eds) Fractures in adults, vol 2. J B Lippincott, Philadelphia

Levy A S Wetzler M, Lewars M, Bromberg J, Spoo J, Whitelaw G P 1997 The orthopaedic and social outcome of open tibial fractures in children. Orthopaedics 20 (7): 593–598

Littenberg B, Weinstein L P, McCarren M, Mead T, Swiontkowski M F, Rudicel S A, Heck 1998 Closed fractures of the tibial shaft. A meta-analysis of three methods of treatment. Journal of Bone and Joint Surgery 80A: 174–183

Lucas K, Todd C 1973 Closed adult tibial shaft fractures. Journal of Bone and Joint Surgery 55B: 878

McQueen M M, Court-Brown C M 1996 Compartment monitoring in tibial fractures. The pressure threshold for decompression. Journal of Bone and Joint Surgery 78B: 99–104

McQueen M M, Christie J, Court-Brown C M 1996 Acute compartment syndrome in tibial diaphyseal fractures. Journal of Bone and Joint Surgery 78B: 95–98

Merchant T C, Dietz F R 1989 Long-term follow-up after fractures of the tibial and fibular shafts. Journal of Bone and Joint Surgery America 71A: 599–606

Neer C S, Horwitz B S 1965 Fractures of the proximal humeral epiphyseal plate. Clinical Orthopaedics 41: 24–31

Nicoll E A 1964 Fractures of the tibial shaft: a survey of 705 cases. Journal of Bone and Joint Surgery 46B: 373–387

Ogden J A 1987 Pocket guide to paediatric fractures. Williams & Wilkins, Baltimore

Ogden J A, Ogden D A, Pugh L et al 1995 Tibia valga after proximal metaphyseal fractures in childhood. A normal biologic process. Journal of Pediatric Orthopaedics 15: 489–494

Ogden J A, Tross R B, Murphy M J 1980 Fractures of the tibial tuberosity in adolescents. Journal of Bone and Joint Surgery 62A: 205–214

Oni O O, Hui A, Gregg P J 1988 The healing of closed tibial shaft fractures. The natural history of union with closed treatment. Journal of Bone and Joint Surgery 70B: 787–790

Poulsen T D, Skak S V, Jensen T T 1989 Epiphyseal fractures of the proximal tibia. Injury Mar 20 (2): 111–113

Pun W K, Chow S P, Fang D, Ip F K, Leong J C, Ng C 1991 A study of function and residual joint stiffness after functional bracing of tibial shaft fractures. Clinical Orthopaedics Jun (267): 157–163

Puno R M, Vaughan J J, Stetten M L, Johnson J R 1991 Long-term effects of tibial angular malunion on the knee and ankle joints. Journal of Orthopaedic Trauma 5(3): 247–254

Rang M 1974 Children's fractures. J B Lippincott, Philadelphia

Robert M, Khouri N, Carlioz H, Alain J L 1987 Fractures of the proximal tibial metaphysis in children: Review of a series of 25 cases. Journal of Pediatric Orthopaedics 7: 444–449

Rorabeck C H, Macnab I 1975 The pathophysiology of the anterior tibial compartment syndrome. Clinical Orthopaedics (113): 52–57

Rosenthal R E, MacPhail J A, Oritz J E 1977 Non-union in open tibial fractures. Journal of Bone and Joint Surgery 59A: 244–248

Ruedi T, Webb J K, Allgower M 1976 Experience with the dynamic compression plate (DCP) in 418 recent fractures of the tibial shaft. Injury 7: 252–265

Russel T A 1996 Fractures of the tibia and fibula. In: Rockwood C A, Green D P, Bucholz R W, Heckman D (eds) Fractures in adults, 4th ed. Lippincott-Raven, Philadelphia

Salter R B, Best T 1973 The pathogenesis and prevention of valgus deformity following fractures of the proximal metaphyseal region of the tibia in children. Bone Joint Surgery 55A: 1324

Salter R B, Harris W R 1963 Injuries involving the epiphyseal plate. Journal of Bone and Joint Surgery 45A: 587–622

Sanders R, Jersinovich I, Anglen J et al 1994 The treatment of open tibial shaft fractures using an interlocked intramedullary nail without reaming. Journal of Orthopaedic Trauma 8: 504–510

Sarangi P P, Ward A J, Smith E J, Staddon G E, Atkins R M 1993 Algodystrophy and osteoporosis after tibial fractures. Journal of Bone and Joint Surgery 75B: 450–452

Sarmiento A 1967 A functional below-the-knee cast for tibial fractures. Journal of Bone and Joint Surgery 49A: 855–875

Sarmiento A, Gersten L M, Sobol P A, Shankwiler J A, Vangsness C T 1989 Tibial shaft fractures treated with functional braces. Journal of Bone and Joint Surgery 71B: 602–609

Sarmiento A, Latta L L 1981 Closed functional treatment of fractures. Springer-Verlag, Berlin

Shannak A O 1988 Tibial fractures in children: Follow up study. Journal of Pediatric Orthopaedics 8(3): 306–310

Shelton W R, Canale S T 1979 Fractures of the tibia through the proximal tibial epiphyseal cartilage. Journal of Bone and Joint Surgery 61A: 167–173

Singer R W, Kellam Jr 1993 Open tibial diaphyseal fractures. Results of unreamed locked intramedullary nailing. Clinical Orthopaedics 315: 114–118

Skak S V, Toftgard T, Torben D P 1987 Fractures of the proximal metaphysis of the tibia in children. Injury 18: 149–156

Skelley J W, Hardy A E 1981 Results of bone grafts in the treatment of tibial fractures. Clinical Orthopaedics Jul–Aug (158): 108–110

Solheim K 1960 Disabilities after shaft fractures of the bones of the leg: a clinical and radiographic follow-up study of 131 patients after approximately 15 years. Acta Chirurgica Scandinavica 119: 280

Stegemann P, Lomo M, Soriano R et al 1995 Management protocol for unreamed interlocking tibial nails for open tibial fractures. Journal of Orthopaedic Trauma 9: 117–120

Swaan J W, Oppers V M 1971 Crural fractures in children. Archivum Chirurgicum Neerlandicum 23: 259–272

Teitz C C, Carter D R, Frankel V H 1980 Problems associated with tibial fractures associated with intact fibulae. Journal of Bone and Joint Surgery 62A: 770–776

Thompson G H, Behrens F 1998 Fractures of the tibia and fibula. In: Neil E. Green and Marc F Swiantkowski (eds) Skeletal trauma in children. Philadelphia, WB Saunders

Tile M 1987 Fractures of the tibia. In: Schatzker J, Tile M (eds) The rationale of operative fracture care. Springer-Verlag, Berlin

Tornetta P 3rd, Templeman D 1997 Compartment syndrome associated with tibial fracture. Instructional Course Lecture 46: 303–308 (review)

Van der Schoot D K, Den Outer A J, Bode P J, Obermann W R, van Vugt A B 1996 Degenerative changes at the knee and ankle related to malunion of tibial fractures. 15-year follow-up of 88 patients. Journal of Bone and Joint Surgery Sept 78(5): 722–725

Waddell J P, Reardon G P 1983 Complications of tibial shaft fractures. Clinical Orthopaedics 178: 173–178

Weissman S L, Herold H Z, Engelberg M 1966 Fractures of the middle two-thirds of the tibial shaft. Journal of Bone and Joint Surgery 48A: 257–266

Whittle A P, Russel T A, Taylor J C et al 1992 Treatment of open fractures of the tibial shaft with the use of interlocking nailing without reaming. Journal of Bone and Joint Surgery 74A: 1162–1171

Williams J, Gibbons M, Trundle H, Murray D, Worlock P 1995 Complications of nailing in closed tibial fractures. Journal of Orthopaedic Trauma 9(6): 476–481

Wolfe J H N 1987 Post-phlebitic syndrome after fractures of the leg. British Medical Journal 295: 1364–1365

Chapter 15

The ankle

Michael A. Foy

▉ Introduction

Buhr & Cooke (1959) found that ankle fractures accounted for 11% of all fractures. Willenegger (1961) and Phillips et al (1985) reported that the ankle was the most commonly injured weight bearing joint. Ankle fractures may follow falls, sporting injuries or road traffic accidents. They may be the subject of personal injury litigation. Management may be conservative or operative. There is controversy regarding the tolerance of the ankle joint to minor degrees of incongruity.

Ligament injuries

Injuries to the lateral ligament complex of the ankle joint are diverse. There is no reliable information on the incidence of instability, or on the potential for the ankle to develop osteoarthritis.

Current treatment policy of lateral ligament injuries has been outlined by Lightowler (1984). Recurrent instability of the ankle joint may follow lateral ligament rupture. It has not been possible to identify the incidence of recurrent instability following these injuries. The incidence is related to the severity of the initial injury, and also to the method and duration of treatment. A meta-analysis by Pijnenburg et al (2000) looked at time lost from work, residual pain and giving way. They observed operative repair, functional treatment and cast immobilisation. They found that the risk of giving way was reduced after operative treatment and felt that a 'no treatment' strategy led to more residual symptoms.

Coltart (1951), Harrington (1979), Glasgow et al (1981) and Bauer (personal communication) suggested that long-term chronic lateral instability of the ankle joint may lead to osteoarthritis. This was said to be due to unbalanced loading of the medial joint space. Harrington (1979) reported on 36 patients with lateral ligament instability which had been present for at least 10 years. X-ray examination and arthroscopy revealed arthritic changes in all cases.

No statistics can be given for the risk of developing osteoarthritis from the present published reports. However, the available evidence suggests that there may be a tendency for osteoarthritis to develop in chronic lateral ligament instability.

Isolated injury to the medial ligament is much less common than isolated lateral ligament injury. Chronic medial ligament instability is rare. Medial ligament injuries tend to occur as part of more complex ankle fracture patterns, particularly abduction injuries.

Summary

- Injuries to the lateral ligament are common and may lead to ankle instability. There is evidence to suggest that chronic instability may predispose the ankle joint to develop osteoarthritis.
- Isolated injuries to the medial (deltoid) ligament are uncommon and rarely lead to long-term problems.

Ankle fractures
Classification

The most comprehensive and widely used classification of ankle fractures is the genetic system described by Lauge-Hansen (1948). He assigned double names to each fracture type. The first part defined the position of the foot, and the second defined the direction of the injuring force. There have been criticisms of this classification, but it is the most useful one in terms of prognosis. Four major groups were defined:

1. Supination–adduction fractures.
2. Supination–eversion (external rotation) fractures.
3. Pronation–abduction fractures.
4. Pronation–eversion (external rotation) fractures.

Details of this classification are given in Figs 15.1–15.4. The injuries occur in stages, as shown, and these stages reflect the progressive severity of the injury.

Danis (1949) described a classification which was later used by Weber (1972). In this classification, fractures were divided into three groups, A, B and C, according to the level of the fibular fracture and its relationship to the tibiofibular syndesmosis. This classification was adopted by the AO group and is widely recognised. More recently the AO group have introduced a very comprehensive numerical

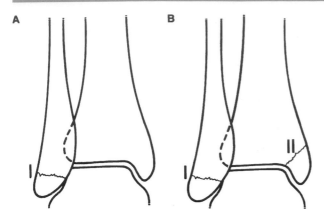

Fig. 15.1 (A)   Stage I supination–adduction injury with a lateral malleolar fracture below the ankle joint (or a lateral ligament injury). **(B)** Stage II supination–adduction injury with a vertical or oblique fracture through the medial malleolus.

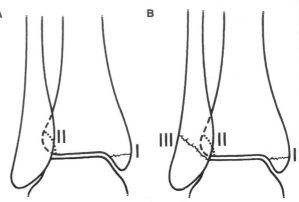

Fig. 15.3 (A)   Stage I and II pronation–abduction injuries. Stage I is an avulsion fracture of the medial malleolus. Stage II is an injury to the anterior tibiofibular ligament. **(B)** Stage III pronation–abduction injury superimposed on Fig. 15.3 (A). This is a short oblique fracture of the fibula just above the level of the ankle joint.

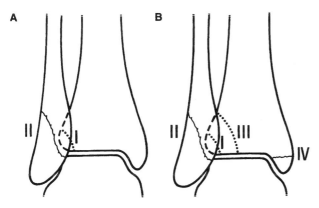

Fig. 15.2 (A)   Stage I and II supination–eversion injuries. Stage I is an injury to the anterior tibiofibular ligament with either a bony avulsion or insubstance rupture. Stage II is an oblique fracture of the fibula at the level of the joint. **(B)** Stage III and IV supination–eversion injuries superimposed on Fig. 15.2 (A). Stage III is a fracture of the posterior tibial malleolus. Stage IV is a 'pull-off' fracture through the medial mallelous or a deltoid ligament rupture.

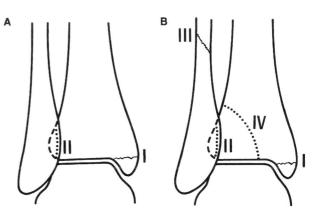

Fig. 15.4 (A)   Stage I and II pronation–eversion injuries. Stage I is an avulsion fracture of the medial malleolus. Stage II is an injury to the anterior tibiofibular ligament. **(B)** Stage III and IV pronation–eversion injury superimposed on Fig 15.4 (A). Stage III is a torsional fracture of the fibular shaft, well above the level of the ankle joint. Stage IV is a fracture of the posterior tibial malleolus.

classification, that if widely used in research may replace the Lauge–Hansen classification as a predictor of outcome.

The Danis–Weber classification is not detailed enough to make it valuable in the prediction of prognosis. This view is supported by the work of Neithard & Plaüe (1977), Zenker & Nerlich (1982) and Bauer (1985). Cedell (1967), for example, described the frequency of post-traumatic arthritis in stage II supination–eversion fractures as 2.6%, compared to an incidence of 23.5% for stage IV supination–eversion fractures. This difference in the severity of the injuries would not have been recognised from the Danis–Weber classification.

Assessment of the end-results of ankle fractures may be difficult. Phillips & Spiegel (1979) reported that the correlation between X-ray appearances and clinical symptoms was often poor. Difficulties arose in comparing results following open reduction and closed manipulation because the adequacy of reduction was not defined. Phillips & Spiegel (1979) summarised the problem well: 'The degree of tolerance permissible between an *exact* anatomic reduction and an *acceptable or adequate* reduction remains undefined'.

Incidence of osteoarthritis

According to Phillips & Spiegel (1979), although the ankle is the most frequently injured weight bearing joint, it has the lowest incidence of degenerative joint disease. In medico-legal reporting the risk of the patient developing post-traumatic osteoarthritis is of importance in the assessment of damages.

It is difficult accurately to predict the risk of a patient developing osteoarthritis after an ankle fracture. Wilson (1984) reported that it occurred in 20 to 40% of ankle fractures 'regardless of the method of treatment', but this is still a controversial issue. There is agreement between orthopaedic surgeons that an anatomical reduction should be the aim of treatment. The controversy surrounds the influence of open reduction and internal fixation, compared to successful closed manipulation, on the incidence of osteoarthritis.

The only prospective randomised trial which attempted to answer this question was reported by Phillips et al (1985). They studied grade IV supination–eversion and pronation–eversion fractures and used a complex scoring system to assess their results. Their criteria for a satisfactory closed reduction are shown in Table 15.1. The only significant difference between open reduction with internal fixation and closed manipulation was seen in the adequacy of reduction, based on radiographic measurements. When reduction was satisfactory, there was no significant difference in the clinical results or in the incidence of osteoarthritis.

Bauer (1985) reviewed 27 reports in the orthopaedic literature, and found that the frequency of post-traumatic arthritis ranged from 18 to 86% in patients treated conservatively, and from 7 to 70% in patients treated by internal fixation. Colton (personal communication) pointed out that this may reflect unfairly on the operatively treated patients, because the methods of internal fixation in some of the quoted series would be unacceptable when judged by current standards.

Minor degrees of osteoarthritis may cause no symptoms. There is more agreement regarding the occurrence of subjective symptoms following ankle fractures. Bauer (1985) reported that after 7 years approximately one-third of patients with supination–eversion fractures (Danis–Weber B) complained of residual discomfort. Magnusson (1944), Klossner (1962) and Cedell (1967) described similar results, with no difference between operative and conservatively treated patients.

There are many variables influencing the development of osteoarthritis following ankle fractures. The conclusions from the orthopaedic literature are unclear and frequently contradictory. The report from Phillips et al (1985) attempted to clarify the situation. Unfortunately, only 51% of their patients returned for follow-up. The authors were unable to prove that open reduction and internal fixation were superior to adequate manipulative treatment, as defined in Table 15.1, in terms of clinical results and development of osteoarthritis.

It is possible only to emphasise those factors that make the development of osteoarthritis more likely. In current orthopaedic practice, Wilson's 1984 assessment of a 20 to 40% incidence, irrespective of treatment, is reasonable.

Table 15.1 Criteria for a satisfactory closed reduction of an ankle fracture (from Phillips et al 1985, with permission)

1. Medial clear space not more than 2 mm wider than the space between the tibial plafond and the dome of the talus

2. Less than 2 mm of displacement of the medial malleolus in any direction

3. Less than 2 mm of lateral displacement of the distal end of the fibula at the fracture

4. Less than 5 mm of posterior displacement of the distal end of the fibula

5. Less than 25% of the anteroposterior length of the tibial articular surface, as seen on the lateral radiograph, included in the posterior fracture fragment, or less than 2 mm of displacement of a posterior fragment that includes more than 25% of the anterior–posterior length of the articular surface

Factors influencing the development of osteoarthritis

Severity of initial injury

In the studies of Cedell (1967), Neithard & Plaüe (1977) and Zenker & Nerlich (1982) good correlation was found between the development of osteoarthritis and the number of single lesions, as reflected in the Lauge-Hansen stages (1948).

The presence of a posterior tibial fragment indicates a more severe injury. Olerud (1981) pointed out that a posterior tibial fragment, even if radiographically well reduced, 'implies a substantially increased risk of arthritis, and thus a poorer prognosis'. Bauer (1985) described 12 other scientific reports supporting this view. In the Lauge-Hansen (1948) classification the presence of a posterior tibial fragment reflects a later stage in the injury sequence, usually III or IV. Neithard & Plaue (1977) found that even the smallest flake fragment posteriorly doubled the rate of post-traumatic arthritis.

Lindsjø (1981) considered the clinical and radiological result in 174 patients with posterior tibial fragments. The clinical results were poorer when there was a large articular fragment. Arthritis occurred in 34% of patients with a posterior articular fragment, but in only 17% of patients with a posterior non-articular fragment. If the articular fragment was not anatomically reduced, then the incidence of arthritis was 44%. All the patients in this study were surgically treated using AO principles. The criteria for a diagnosis of arthritis were based on reduction of the joint space as described by Magnusson (1944) and, later, Cedell (1967).

A posterior tibial fragment indicates a more severe injury and a greater risk of developing osteoarthritis.

The posterior tibial fragment occurring in these stage III and IV injuries should not be confused with the much less common isolated fracture of the posterior tibial margin which follows hyperplantarflexion injuries. According to Bauer (personal communication) these isolated injuries have a good prognosis.

Macko et at (1991) carried out a cadaveric study under simulated clinical conditions to determine the effect of increasing the size of the posterior malleolar fragment on the contact area of the ankle joint and on the distribution of joint pressure. They concluded that any inaccuracy in the reduction or fixation of the posterior fragment in a non-anatomical position will increase the risk of post-traumatic arthritis.

Adequacy of the reduction

Lindsjø (1981) reported on a series of over 300 ankle fractures treated by open reduction and internal fixation. On the postoperative X-rays residual displacement was assessed. Lindsjø paid particular attention to the presence of small displaced fragments, incongruity between the articular surfaces, irregularity of the articular surface and articular defects. He found that there was a significant difference in the clinical results between accurately and inadequately reduced fractures. This is illustrated in Table 15.2.

Lindsjø (1981) defined osteoarthritis in terms of reduction of the joint space of the ankle. He found a statistically significant relationship between the degree of arthritis and the clinical result: this is shown in Table 15.3.

Table 15.2 The adequacy of reduction related to the treatment result (from Lindsjø 1981, with permission)

	Excellent–good results (%)
Accurately reduced fractures (*n* = 217)	86.6
Inadequately reduced fractures (*n* = 89)	68.5

Table 15.3 The relationship of osteoarthritis of the ankle joint to the clinical result (from Lindsjø 1981, with permission)

	Frequency of excellent–good clinical results (%)
No arthritis	82
Slight joint space narrowing	76
Joint space reduced to at least half	42
Joint space virtually eliminated	0

Bauer (1985) supported the view that accurate reduction led to a better clinical result. He found that this opinion was supported in 23 other publications dealing with the results of ankle fractures.

There is strong evidence and opinion to support the accurate reduction of ankle fractures. This improves the long-term results. When considering long-term clinical results, and the development of osteoarthritis, there is no conclusive evidence that satisfactory open reduction and internal fixation are better than satisfactory closed manipulation.

Age and sex of patient

Lindsjø (1981) found that the worst overall results—in both clinical and radiographic terms—occurred in females aged from 45–64 years. Beauchamp et al (1983) reported that patients over the age of 50 had less satisfactory results after displaced ankle fractures.

Radiographic indicators

Residual displacement on X-ray, and its implications for prognosis, have already been discussed.

Phillips et al (1985) considered several radiographic measurements in an attempt to find a reliable predictor of satisfactory and unsatisfactory results. The only reliable indicator proved to be the talocrural angle, as described by Sarkisian & Cody (1976). This is shown in Fig. 15.5. Two lines are drawn, one between the tips of the malleoli and one parallel to the tibial plafond, on an anteroposterior

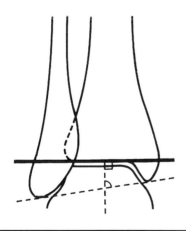

Fig. 15.5 The talocrural angle, as described by Sarkisian & Cody (1976). One line is drawn parallel to the tibial plafond and a second between the tips of the malleoli on a true anteroposterior (mortise) X-ray. The talocrural angle is the superomedial angle subtended when a perpendicular is dropped from the line parallel to the plafond (see text for further details).

X-ray in internal rotation (the mortise view). A perpendicular is taken from the line of the tibial plafond. The talocrural angle is the superomedial angle, where the perpendicular intersects the line joining the tips of the malleoli.

The normal range of the talocrural angle in adults is $83 \pm 4°$. The difference in the angle between two ankles in a normal individual is less than 2°. Phillips et al (1985) classified a difference of over 5° as abnormal, because this was the smallest angle that they could reliably measure. They found significantly better overall results when the talocrural angles were within 5° of each other. Sarkisian & Cody (1976) proposed that fibular rotation led to shortening and this altered the talocrural angle.

Other radiographic measurements have been studied, but have not proved to be reliable predictors of prognosis.

Time taken for arthritis to develop

This is an important consideration when deciding on the timing of medico-legal reports. Willenegger (1961) and Lindsjø (1981) found that the majority of arthritic change occurred in the first 12–18 months from injury. Lindsjø (1981) examined his patients at mean periods of 18 months and 4 years from their injury. There was no significant difference in the incidence of osteoarthritis at these times. Between these two follow-up appointments, both subjective and objective results tended to improve rather than deteriorate.

It is wise to delay a final medical report until 18 months after the ankle fracture. If osteoarthritis is going to develop, radiographic evidence should be apparent at this stage.

Social/occupational factors

Lindsjø (1981) considered the functional results in 305 patients treated surgically according to AO principles. In all, 90% were able to continue in the same occupation; 82% were able to continue sports and other physical activities at the same level. There was no significant difference in working, sports and walking capacity between male and female patients.

Lindsjø (1981) found that sick leave following operative treatment of ankle fractures ranged from 13–18 weeks. He also assessed further sick leave, usually associated with implant removal. The combined duration of primary and secondary sick leave in this series averaged 22.5 weeks. Solonen & Lauttamus (1968) reported slightly shorter sick leave periods for conservatively treated patients (4.3 months) than for surgically treated patients (4.5 months). Cedell (1967) reported sick leave periods for 355 supination–eversion fractures. For fractures with a higher grade in the Lauge-Hansen classification, the sick leave periods were longer. The average for a supination–eversion type II fracture was 14 weeks, while that for a type IV fracture was 20 weeks. These patients were treated surgically, but not using AO techniques.

Sick leave periods should be interpreted with great caution. Social conditions, occupation, patient motivation and health insurance are probably more relevant than methods of treatment in the timing of return to work. These figures represent a very general guide.

Non-union

Bauer (1985) reported that the incidence of non-union of the medial malleolus was from 5 to 20% in conservatively treated patients. Wilson (1984) gave the incidence of medial malleolar non-union as 10 to 15% in conservatively treated patients. Lindsjø (1981) reported only one non-union of the medial malleolus in 314 fractures treated operatively by AO techniques (0.3% incidence). Opinions vary regarding the significance of a medial malleolar non-union. Mendelsohn (1965) and Sneppen (1971) suggested that non-union did not influence the long-term prognosis, Cox & Laxson (1952) that non-union predisposed to the development of osteoarthritis.

Non-union of the lateral malleolus is rare, Bauer (1985) reporting the incidence to be around 0.1%. He found no lateral malleolar non-unions in 51 patients treated surgically and 200 patients treated conservatively. Lindsjø (1981) noted one lateral malleolar non-union in 314 fractures treated operatively.

Summary

- The incidence of osteoarthritis after ankle fractures is probably 20–40%.
- When there is anatomical reduction of the ankle fracture, and this is maintained until healing, internal fixation and closed treatment show similar clinical results and similar risks of developing osteoarthritis.
- Approximately one-third of patients experience discomfort in their ankle when followed up for 5 years or more. This occurs equally in both operatively and non-operatively treated patients.
- The presence of a posterior tibial fragment represents a more severe injury, in terms of the Lauge-Hansen classification. It is associated with an increased risk of developing arthritis.
- The talocrural angle (Fig. 15.5) is the only reliable radiographic indicator of prognosis.
- Final medical reports should be delayed until 18 months after ankle fractures. If osteoarthritis is going to develop, radiographic evidence should be apparent at that time.

Tibial plafond/pilon fractures

Pilon fractures have usually been classified according to Ruedi & Allgower (1969). They recognised three fracture types, as shown in Fig. 15.6. However, in the new AO classification they are listed as code 43 injuries.

Bone (1987) reported that in experienced hands, open reduction and internal stabilisation with plate fixation gave the best results for this difficult fracture. Dillin & Slabaugh (1986) offered a cautionary warning on the hazards of inexperienced surgeons operating on these fractures.

Ruedi (1973) reported good and excellent functional results in 74% of patients treated operatively, according to the principles of the AO group (Müller et al 1979).

Ruedi & Allgower (1979) assessed a group of 75 patients in a city hospital to see whether these results were reproducible. These patients were treated according to AO principles. At an average of 6 years postoperatively, 80% of the patients were able to use the injured limb normally. Only 15% complained of disability or discomfort. Some 5% underwent arthrodesis for severe osteoarthritis. Over half (54%) of the patients went back to playing sport, and 63 patients (84%) had returned to the same job. Twelve patients (16%) had to find a new job as a result of their injury, some with lower income. Objective assessment revealed normal movement or restriction of movement of less than 10° in 69% of patients.

Ovadia & Beals (1986) reviewed 145 fractures of the tibial plafond. The mean follow-up was 57 months, with a minimum of 24 months. These authors extended the classification into five groups. Their types I and II are equivalent to Ruedi & Allgower's type I; their type III is equivalent to Ruedi & Allgower's type II, and their types IV and V correspond to Ruedi & Allgower's type III, as shown in Fig. 15.6.

The results of rigid internal fixation (80 cases) were compared to the results of other treatment (65 cases). The final clinical results of treatment by open reduction and rigid internal fixation were better than the results for those treated by other methods. Some 35 (54%) of the 65 fractures treated by other methods had good or excellent final clinical results; 59 (74%) of the 80 fractures treated by rigid internal fixation achieved a good or excellent final clinical result. This difference is statistically significant. Ovadia & Beals (1986) also found that 55 (69%) of patients treated by rigid internal fixation returned to their pre-injury employment, compared with 28 (43%) of the patients who were treated by other methods. This difference is also statistically significant.

An excellent clinical result was defined by Ovadia & Beals (1986) as follows: absence of pain; the patient having

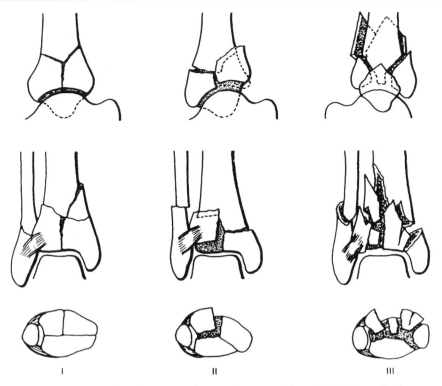

Fig. 15.6 The AO classification of pilon fracture. I, fissure fracture without significant displacement. II, fissure fracture with significant articular incongruity; III, compression fracture with displacement of the weight-bearing cancellous segments of the metaphysis (from Müller et al 1979, with permission).

returned to the same job; and the patient being able to carry out normal recreational activities and having no limp. A good result indicated that the patient had mild pain following strenuous exercise, had returned to the same job, had undertaken mild moderation of recreational activities and had no limp.

Ovadia & Beals (1986) considered the variables affecting the clinical results. They found that there were four main prognostic indicators:

- fracture type
- quality of reduction
- treatment method
- associated medical problems

Ovadia & Beals showed that prognosis correlates well with fracture type. This point is illustrated in Fig. 15.7.

The quality of reduction is closely related to the fracture type and the method of treatment. Better reduction was obtained in types I and II (Ruedi & Allgower's type I) fractures and in those fractures treated by rigid internal fixation. The quality of the reduction correlated well with

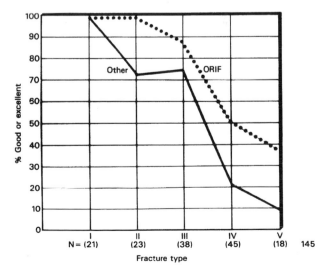

Fig. 15.7 Correlation of the pilon fracture type with the prognosis (from Ovadia & Beals 1986, with permission). ORIF, open reduction internal fixation.

the clinical result. Of the patients whose reduction was rated as good using Ovadia & Beals' criteria (shown in Table 15.4), 89% had an excellent or good final clinical result. All of the 18 patients who had a poor reduction also had a poor final clinical result. Another variable related to fracture reduction was the presence of a gap in the articular surface. One or more gaps in the articular surface, measuring 1–4 mm on the post-reduction X-ray, were identified in 35 of 83 patients who were otherwise judged to have a good reduction. In this subgroup of 83 patients with a good reduction, the clinical results were good or excellent in 98%, where there was no articular defect. In the group with a good reduction, but one or more persisting articular defects, the incidence of good or excellent clinical results was 80%. This difference was statistically significant and emphasises the importance of closing articular defects.

The only concomitant medical problem that appeared adversely to affect the clinical results was alcoholism. Alcoholics appeared to show significantly worse clinical results.

Summary

- The quality of the clinical result is related to the quality of reduction of the articular surface.
- Good or excellent clinical results may be achieved in 75% of patients treated by rigid internal fixation in experienced hands.
- Good or excellent clinical results were found in 50–55% of patients treated by a variety of methods, other than rigid internal fixation.

Ankle fractures in children

Spiegel et al (1978) analysed 184 patients with epiphyseal fractures of the distal end of the tibia and fibula. They reported significant skeletal complications in 14% of patients. The majority of the complications (23 of 26) involved the tibial growth plate. The authors identified three risk groups according to the likelihood of developing shortening, angular deformity or joint incongruity. The risk groups are defined in Table 15.5. The fracture types refer to the classification of Salter & Harris (1963).

There are four types of complication which may follow ankle fractures in children—angular deformity, rotational deformity, leg length discrepancy and joint surface incongruity.

Angular deformity

This may result from asymmetrical growth plate closure or malunion.

Dias (1984) considered that varus deformity was the most common angular deformity associated with asymmetric closure of the tibial growth plate. He reviewed 101 Salter–Harris type III and IV fractures from the literature and found that varus deformity occurred in 14%. He stated that varus deformity was rarely associated with a Salter–Harris type II fracture.

Spiegel et al (1978) identified five cases in their series, with over 5° of varus angulation due to asymmetric growth plate closure. Two of these were Salter–Harris type III fractures, but the others were Salter–Harris type II.

Table 15.4 A classification of reduction of tibial plafond fractures (from Ovadia & Beals 1986, with permission)

	Good	Fair	Poor
Malleolus Lateral Anatomical or	<1 mm displacement	2–5 mm displacement	>5 mm displacement
Medial	<2 mm displacement	2–5 mm displacement	>5 mm displacement
Posterior	Proximal displacement	Proximal displacement	Proximal displacement
Mortise widening	<0.5 mm	0.5–2.0 mm	>2 mm
Talus Tilt	<0.5 mm	0.5–1.0 mm	>1 mm
Displacement	<0.5 mm	0.5–2.0 mm	>2 mm

The authors found that only one patient, with varus angulation of 15°, required additional surgical treatment.

Dias (1984) reported that valgus deformity was uncommon following asymmetric growth plate closure. Spiegel et al (1978) found only one case with significant valgus deformity (15°). This occurred in a Salter–Harris type II fracture which was inadequately reduced and subsequently developed asymmetric growth plate closure. Dias (1984) pointed out that complete arrest of the distal fibular growth plate could lead to fibular shortening and valgus deformity. Spiegel et al (1978) described 21 cases of Salter–Harris type I and II fractures of the fibula. Three type I fractures developed premature closure of the fibular growth plate, two with shortening. However, none had angular deformities.

Rotational deformity

Rotational deformity is uncommon following ankle fractures in children. Cooperman et al (1978) reported follow-up on 12 children with triplane fractures. Three of these patients had external rotation deformity of 5–10°. Spiegel et al (1978) did not describe rotational deformity in their follow-up series.

Leg length discrepancy

Dias (1984) reported that leg length discrepancy occurred in 10 to 30% of patients with injuries to the distal tibial growth plate. Chadwick & Bentley (1987) described growth retardation in eight out of 28 (29%) children with distal tibial growth plate injuries, and Spiegel et al (1978) 17 patients (9%) with growth retardation of 0.4–1.3 cm in their series of 184 children.

The incidence of leg length discrepancy is related to the Salter–Harris fracture type, as shown in Table 15.6. In the majority of these cases the shortening was less than 2 cm and required no treatment.

Table 15.5 The risk of development of skeletal complications following distal epiphyseal injuries of the tibia and fibula (from Spiegel et al 1978)

Risk	Type of fracture
Low risk (6.7% incidence of complications)	Type I and II fibular fractures Type I tibial fractures Type III and IV tibial fractures with less than 2 mm displacement Epiphyseal avulsions
High risk (32% incidence of complications)	Type III and IV tibial fractures with more than 2 mm displacement Juvenile Tillaux fractures Triplane fractures Comminuted epiphyseal fractures
Unpredictable risk (16.7% incidence of complications)	Type II tibial fractures

Table 15.6 Leg length discrepancy following injuries of the distal tibial epiphysis: its relationship to the Salter–Harris classification (from Spiegel et al 1978 and Chadwick & Bentley 1987)

	Cases with shortening	Number of cases	%
Salter–Harris type			
I	1	28	3.5
II	11	78	14
III	3	45	6.5
IV	6	11	54
V	1	2	50
Triplane fractures	3	20	15
Overall	25	184	13.5

Joint surface incongruity

Joint surface incongruity is determined partly by the nature of the injury and partly by the approach to treatment. There is evidence from Lindsjø's 1981 work that articular incongruity predisposes to osteoarthritis in adults. Spiegel et al (1978) demonstrated that there was a higher incidence of skeletal complications when articular steps of 2 mm or more were present. However, Landin et al (1986) found no cases of arthrosis in 59 physeal fractures examined at a mean of 9 years from the injury.

Summary

- Significant skeletal complications occur in approximately 15% of children with epiphyseal fractures of the distal end of the tibia and fibula. Risk groups related to fracture type have been identified by Spiegel et al (1978) (see Table 15.5).
- Growth arrest may be delayed following epiphyseal injury. Follow-up should continue for at least 1 year before a final prognosis is given.
- Varus deformity occurs more commonly than valgus deformity as a complication of ankle fractures in children.
- Leg length discrepancy occurs in 10–30% of children with injuries to the distal tibial growth plate. It appears to be more common after Salter–Harris type IV injuries. In the majority of cases, it is less than 2 cm and requires no treatment.

References

Bauer M 1985 Ankle fractures: with special reference to post-traumatic arthrosis. MD Thesis, Lund University, Malmo

Beauchamp C G, Clay N R, Thexton P W 1983 Displaced ankle fractures in patients over 50 years of age. Journal of Bone and Joint Surgery 65B: 329–332

Bone L B 1987 Fractures of the tibial plafond. Orthopedic Clinics of North America 18: 95–104

Buhr A J, Cooke A M 1959 Fracture patterns. Lancet, vol 1, 14 March: 531–536

Cedell C 1967 Supination—outward rotation injuries of the ankle. Acta Orthopaedica Scandinavica (suppl) 110

Chadwick C J, Bentley G 1987 The classification and prognosis of epiphyseal injuries. Injury 18: 157–168

Coltart W D 1951 Sprained ankle. British Medical Journal ii: 957–961

Cooperman D R, Spiegel P G, Laros G S 1978 Tibial fractures involving the ankle in children: the so-called triplane epiphyseal fracture. Journal of Bone and Joint Surgery 60A: 1040–1046

Cox F J, Laxson W W 1952 Fractures about the ankle joint. American Journal of Surgery May: 674–679

Danis R 1949 Théorie et pratique de l'osteosynthése. Desouer et Masson, Liège

Dias L S 1984 Fractures of the tibia and fibula. In: Rockwood C A Jr, Wilkins K E, King R E (eds) Fractures in children, vol 3. J B Lippincott, Philadelphia

Dillin L, Slabaugh P 1986 Delayed wound healing, infection and non union following open reduction and internal fixation of tibial plafond fractures. Journal of Trauma 26: 1116–1119

Glasgow M, Jackson A, Jamieson A M 1981 Instability of the ankle after injury to the lateral ligament. Journal of Bone and Joint Surgery 62B: 196–200

Harrington K D 1979 Degenerative arthritis of the ankle secondary to long standing lateral ligament instability. Journal of Bone and Joint Surgery 61A: 354–361

Klossner O 1962 Late results of operative and non operative treatment of ankle fractures. Acta Chirurgica Scandinavica (suppl) 293

Landin L A, Danielsson L G, Jonsson K, Pettersson H 1986 Late results in 65 physeal ankle fractures. Acute Orthop Scand 57(6): 530–534

Lauge-Hansen N 1948 Fractures of the ankle. Analytic-historic survey as the basis of a new experiment, roentgenologic and clinical investigations. Archives of Surgery 56: 259–317

Lightowler C D R 1984 Injuries to the lateral ligament of the ankle. British Medical Journal 289: 1274

Lindsjø J 1981 Operative treatment of ankle fractures. Acta Orthopaedica Scandinavica 52 (suppl) 189

Macko V W, Matthews L S, Zwirkoski P, Goldstein S A 1991 The joint contact area of the ankle: the contribution of the posterior malleolus. Journal of Bone and Joint Surgery 73A: 347–351

Magnusson R 1944 On the late results in non-operated cases of malleolar fractures: a clinical, roentgenological, statistical study. I. Fractures by external rotation. Acta Chirurgica Scandinavica (suppl) 84

Mendelsohn H A 1965 Non-union of malleolar fractures of the ankle. Clinical Orthopaedics 42: 103–118

Müller M E, Allgower M, Schneider R, Willenegger H 1979 Manual of internal fixation. Springer-Verlag, Berlin

Neithard F V, Plaüe R 1977 Das linters tibiakantenfragment als prognostisches kriterium. Archiv für Orthopaedische und Unfailchirurgie 87: 213–221

Olerud S 1981 Foreword to operative treatment of ankle fractures. Acta Orthopaedica Scandinavica 52 (suppl) 189

Ovadia D N, Beals R K 1986 Fractures of the tibial plafond. Journal of Bone and Joint Surgery 68A: 543–551

Phillips W A, Schwartz H S, Keller C S et al 1985 A prospective randomised study of the management of severe ankle fractures. Journal of Bone and Joint Surgery 67A: 67–78

Phillips W A, Spiegel P G 1979 Evaluation of ankle fractures: non-operative v operative. Clinical Orthopaedics 138: 17–20

Pijneburg A C, Van Dijk C N, Bossuyt P M, Marti R K 2000 Treatment of ruptures of the lateral ankle ligament: a meta-analysis. Journal of Bone and Joint Surgery 83A: 761–773

Ruedi T 1973 Fractures of the lower end of the tibia into the ankle joint: results 9 years after open reduction and internal fixation. Injury 5: 130–134

Ruedi T, Allgower M 1969 Fractures of the lower end of the tibia into the ankle joint. Injury 1: 92–99

Ruedi T, Allgower M 1979 The operative treatment of intra-articular fractures of the lower end of the tibia. Clinical Orthopaedics 138: 105–110

Salter R B, Harris W 1963 Injuries involving the epiphyseal plate. Journal of Bone and Joint Surgery 45A: 587–622

Sarkisian J S, Cody S W 1976 Closed treatment of ankle fractures: a new criterion for evaluation—a review of 250 cases. Journal of Trauma 16: 323–326

Sneppen O 1971 Treatment of pseudarthrosis involving the malleolus: a post-operative follow up of 34 cases. Acta Orthopaedica Scandinavica 42: 201–216

Solonen K A, Lauttamus L 1968 Operative treatment of ankle fractures. Acta Orthopaedica Scandinavica 39: 223–237

Spiegel P G, Cooperman D R, Laros G S 1978 Epiphyseal fractures of the distal end of the tibia and fibula. Journal of Bone and Joint Surgery 60A: 1046–1050

Weber B G 1972 Die verletzunger des oberen sprugglenkes. Aktuelle probleme in der chirurgie. Band 3. Verlag Hans Huber, Bern

Willenegger H 1961 Die behandlung der luxationsfrakturen des oberen sprunggelenkes nach biomechanischen gesichtspunkten. Helvetica Chirurgica Acta 28: 225–239

Wilson F C 1984 Fractures and dislocations of the ankle. In: Rockwood C A Jr, Green D P (eds) Fractures in adults, vol 11. J B Lippincott, Philadelphia

Zenker H, Nerlich M 1982 Prognostic aspects in operated ankle fractures. Archives of Orthopaedics and Traumatic Surgery 100: 237–241

Chapter 16

The foot
Roger M. Atkins

◾ Introduction

In the USA, for every 300 men working in heavy industry, 15 working days are lost per month as a result of foot problems. Of these, 65% result from trauma (Hillegass 1976). The National Safety Council (1972) estimated that over US$500 million were paid in compensation in 1971 in the USA as a result of work-related leg and foot injuries.

Fractures and ligamentous injuries involving the foot are common and it is increasingly recognised that they cause significant long-term morbidity, which may be out of proportion to severity of the injury.

General assessment of disability

Disability due to foot injury should be assessed both functionally and clinically.

Functional assessment of disability
Pain

The presence and severity of pain at rest, during activity and at night must be assessed. The nature, site and quality of the pain combined with other clinical information will indicate its origin. This will allow an assessment of prognosis. For example, generalised burning pain may indicate reflex sympathetic dystrophy or complex regional pain syndrome.

Walking

Limitations in the patient's ability to walk, run, climb and descend stairs and use ladders compared to the situation prior to the injury must be documented. This would include any specific limitation in traversing rough ground and problems with ascending or descending hills. Certain functional limitations are strongly associated with the specific injuries, for example difficulty in crossing rough ground is often associated with the dysfunction of the subtalar joint.

Shoeware

Limitations in shoeware are common and often permanent. Female patients may complain of an inability to wear high heels, which is particularly irksome for shorter individuals. Persistent swelling or deformity may necessitate a larger shoe size or lace-up shoes. Rigidity of the foot and toe deformity may limit the patient to flat unfashionable shoes with a wide toe box. In an extreme case, difficulties with shoeware by themselves may prevent patients from returning to their pre-accident occupation. For example, inability to wear shoeware with protective toecaps may disbar a worker from an industrial site.

The majority of patients who have suffered significant foot injury and who remain symptomatic should have orthotics, which may need to be custom-made. The cost of shoeware modification and orthotics, which may be required for the remainder of the patient's life, should not be underestimated.

Work

Foot injuries can cause a functional disability that is apparently out of proportion to the severity. For example, an athlete may be unable to function properly after a fracture of the fifth metatarsal bone. Furthermore, injuries to the foot frequently occur at work to people who rely on excellent foot function for their employment. Thus a roofer may fall at work and suffer a calcaneus fracture that prevents him returning to this occupation, although for everyday activities his foot is satisfactory. Where return to work is possible, there may be limitation in particular tasks and pain by the end of the day. These minor limitations may in time lead to early retirement.

Driving

Many injuries, particularly when the left foot is involved, limit the ability to drive a motor vehicle with a heavy clutch. This may necessitate the provision of an automatic car, and in the case of a heavy goods vehicle driver, for example, continued employment may be severely curtailed or impossible.

Hobbies

Active individuals may often find that their leisure activities are significantly curtailed following an injury to the foot. Characteristically, activities that entail walking on rough ground or climbing ladders are limited and this may affect DIY or gardening. Where a patient has in the past enjoyed an athletic pursuit he may find that he is no longer able to perform to the level to which he could aspire prior to the accident and therefore his pleasure in the sport is diminished and he may abandon it.

The inability to undertake a hobby may lead to financial loss as for example if a decorator or gardener has to be employed.

Timing of disability assessment

Minor injuries to the foot, for example a sprain, will settle completely over 3–6 months. More serious injuries, such as a fracture of the calcaneus, will take 18 months to 2 years to reach a stable state. Injuries that produce biomechanical abnormalities of the foot, such as a displaced calcaneus fracture treated nonoperatively, or that lead to marked joint instability, for example a midfoot subluxation, may cause symptoms which plateau after a year or so only to worsen inexorably due to secondary changes.

Functional improvement and reconstruction

Disability following foot injury may be substantially improved by the provision of appropriate orthotics or by reconstructive operations. Although the necessary surgery may be complex, as for example a bone block distraction arthrodesis for a calcaneal mal-union, this is not necessarily the case, and for instance a marked functional improvement may result from a simple correction of hammer toes that are the result of a compartment syndrome.

Specific injuries

Specific, severe foot injuries are often rare, the exception being the calcaneus fracture. Therefore in order to give guidelines concerning the outcome of this fracture, the results of several series will be combined throughout this discussion.

Fractures and dislocations about the talus
Fractures of the neck of the talus

Fractures of the talus are relatively rare injuries and the most common is the neck fracture. Hawkins' classification (1970) is widely employed and is useful prognostically. Fractures are divided into three types:

- type I—undisplaced fracture
- type II—displaced fracture with subtalar joint subluxation
- type III—displaced fracture with dislocation of the body of the talus from both the subtalar and ankle joints

Canale & Kelly (1978) described a case in which the talonavicular joint was also dislocated, and which has been termed a type IV fracture.

The main fracture complications are delayed union, mal-union, avascular necrosis of the body of the talus and osteoarthritis of the subtalar and ankle joints. The frequency and severity of complications are directly proportional to the degree of displacement of the fracture and prompt, exact anatomic reduction with rigid internal fixation is associated with optimal long-term results (Comfort et al 1985; Szyskowitz et al 1985; Heckman 1996).

Delayed union/non-union

Peterson et al (1977) defined delayed union as occurring when there was no evidence of healing at 6 months. Since talar neck fractures occur through cancellous bone, non-union is almost unknown. The incidence of delayed union increases with initial displacement. The combined series of Hawkins (1970), Peterson et al (1977) and Lorentzen et al (1977) provides 216 cases with 14 delayed or non-union (6%; for further analysis see Table 16.1).

Mal-union

A complex bony and ligamentous ring is formed by the talus, the talo-navicular joint, the midfoot, the calcaneo-cuboid joint, the body of the calcaneus and the posterior facet of the subtalar joint. The hindfoot is analogous to the forearm in this respect. Just as in the forearm an isolated, displaced fracture of one bone is associated with a dislocation, causing a Monteggia or Galleazi fracture, so too in the hind foot the ring cannot be broken in one place only. The weakest link in the ring is the posterior facet of the subtalar joint. Therefore any displacement of a talar

Table 16.1 The incidence of delayed union or non-union in talar neck fractures (from Hawkins 1970, Lorentzen et al 1977 and Peterson et al 1977)

Hawkins type	Delayed or non-union	Number of fractures	%
I	1	68	1.5
II	7	96	7
III	6	52	11.5
Overall	14	216	6

neck fracture, however slight, is associated with a subluxation of the posterior facet of the subtalar joint which leads to secondary degenerative arthritis. In this respect types I and II fractures form a continuum, while type III and IV fractures are a different entity. Tile (1987) believed that mal-union was of greater clinical significance than avascular necrosis because of subsequent hind foot arthritis and alteration in hind foot biomechanics.

Mal-union occurred in 18 of the 123 patients described by Lorentzen et al (1977). Fifteen of these cases occurred in the 53 type II fractures (28%). Canale & Kelly (1978) found 18 mal-unions in 71 talar neck fractures, the majority in type II fractures. Some caution is necessary in interpreting these figures. By definition a type I fracture is not associated with displacement and cannot lead to a mal-union. Plain radiographs are, however, insensitive and subtle degrees of displacement will pass unnoticed unless CT scanning is undertaken.

Avascular necrosis

The blood supply to the talus is profuse. However, owing to the fact that the talus is totally covered with cartilage, it is very vulnerable to damage due to displacement of fracture fragments and subluxation of joints. Avascular necrosis is therefore a common complication of talar neck fractures and its incidence increases with fracture displacement and number of joints subluxed from 3% in type I fractures to 77% in type III (Table 16.2). A combination of three series (Table 16.3) shows that 28% of cases with avascular necrosis achieved a good or excellent final clinical result. This is due either to the necrosis being partial or to its recovery without collapse. Whether or not long-term avoidance of weight bearing contributes to a good result in a case with avascular necrosis is controversial (Canale & Kelly 1978; Norgrove, Penny & Davis 1980).

The finding of subchondral osteoporosis on an antero-posterior ankle radiograph 6–8 weeks after

Table 16.2 The incidence of avascular necrosis following talar neck fractures (Hawkins' 1970 classification)

Reference	Number of cases (avascular necrosis in brackets)			Follow-up (years)
	Type I	Type II	Type III	
Peterson et al (1977)	8 (0)	19 (3)	9 (3)	6
Lorentzen et al (1977)	54 (2)	53 (13)	16 (11)	2
Hawkins (1970)	6 (0)	24 (10)	27 (20)	Not known
Norgrove Penny & Davis (1980)	5 (0)	11 (2)	11 (11)	6
Canale & Kelly (1978)	15 (2)	30 (15)	23 (19)	13
Coltart (1952)	37 (0)	38 (12)	15 (14)	Not known
Total	125 (4)	175 (55)	101 (78)	
Rate of AVN	3%	31%	77%	

Table 16.3 Results in patients with avascular necrosis after talar neck fractures (Hawkins' 1970 criteria)

Reference	Number of cases with a vascular necrosis	Excellent	Good	Fair	Poor
Hawkins (1970)	24	1	2	12	9
Norgrove Penny & Davis (1980)	13	0	2	3	8
Canale & Kelly (1978)	23	4	8	5	6
Total	60	5	12	20	23
			28%		72%

fracture may exclude significant avascular necrosis (Hawkins 1970; Heckman 1984). Canale & Kelly (1978) reviewed 49 cases. In 23 patients with subchondral osteoporosis, one (4%) developed avascular necrosis. In contrast, in 26 patients without this sign, 20 (77%) developed avascular necrosis.

Osteoarthritis

This may affect primarily the ankle joint, the subtalar joint or both. Other midfoot joints may have secondary involvement. It may be due to avascular necrosis with articular collapse, mal-position leading to mal-union, joint subluxation or the severity of the initial trauma. The incidence increases with fracture displacement and joint subluxation and a quarter of the patients will develop arthritis involving both joints (Lorentzen et al 1977; Table 16.4).

Clinical results

Most series employ the classification of Hawkins (1970; see Table 16.5), which is heavily weighted for pain. An excellent result can be achieved only when pain is absent. The presence of avascular necrosis is associated with a worse outcome, as is an increasing Hawkins grade—a type I fracture showed a 72% good or excellent result, whereas a type III fracture was associated with a 76% fair or poor outcome (Table 16.6).

Syzszkowitz et al (1985) and Grob et al (1985) described operative treatment of displaced talar fractures. Fracture classification and assessment of the results differed from the series already described in which conservative treatment predominated. There are insufficient numbers to allow comparison of differing methods of operative treatment or the influence of rigid fixation and early mobilisation on the long-term outcome. Accurate anatomic reduction and rigid internal fixation should obviate mal-union and its sequelae. However, when the neck of the talus fractures there is usually some comminution, and, owing to the superior curve of the bone, it may be extremely difficult to match the two sides of the fracture accurately even when the region is displayed surgically.

Fractures of the body of the talus

These are rare fractures with many similarities to those of the talar neck. Sneppen et al (1977) described 31 cases. Shearing fractures (17 of 31) may involve subluxation of the subtalar joint, while in compression fractures (10 of 31) only the superior articular surface of the talus is involved. In a crush fracture (four of 31), the body of the talus is severely comminuted. The fracture is usually displaced with concurrent subluxation or incongruity of the ankle and subtalar joints. Assessment of joint involvement may require CT scanning.

The outcome of these fractures is often poor with a high incidence of avascular necrosis, mal-union and arthritis. In Sneppen's series, the patients were assessed by the Directorate of Employment Accident Insurance in Copenhagen and all had disability. In 17 (55%) it was greater than 12%. Nineteen (61%) developed osteoarthritis of the ankle joint, subtalar joint or both. Only 11 patients (35%) were able to return to their previous job; 12 (39%) were forced to obtain lighter work and eight (25%) were unable to continue working due to their persisting disability. Eight patients (26%, three of the four crush fractures) developed avascular necrosis. This is less likely to occur if there is an associated ankle fracture which protects the soft tissue attachments of the talus. Other series also report avascular necrosis. Coltart (1952) found one in 22 cases and Kenwright & Taylor (1970) described two cases of avascular necrosis among six patients with talar body fractures in a series of 58 patients with major talar injuries.

Manipulation and long-term plaster immobilisation were the most common method of treatment in this group and although the final results were not closely correlated to the degree of residual displacement, it is suggested (Szyszkowitz et al 1985) that exact open reduction and internal fixation will improve the outcome.

Head of the talus

This is a rare fracture. Coltart (1952) found only six cases in 228 injuries of the talus, and Kenwright & Taylor

Table 16.4 The incidence of osteoarthritis following fractures of the talar neck (from Lorentzen et al 1977)

Hawkins type	Number of patients	Ankle joint arthritis	Subtalar joint arthritis
I	54	8 (15%)	13 (24%)
II	53	19 (36%)	35 (66%)
III	16	11 (69%)	10 (63%)
Total	123	38 (31%)	58 (47%)

Table 16.5 Evaluation of results using Hawkins' 1970 criteria

	Points
Pain	
None	6
After activity	3
Continuous	0
Limp	
Absent	3
Present	0
Ankle range of motion	
Full	3
Limited	2
Fused	1
Fixed deformity	0
Subtalar range of motion	
Full	3
Limited	2
Fused	1
Fixed deformity	0
Excellent result	13–15
Good result	10 12
Fair result	7–9
Poor result	6 or less

Table 16.6 Clinical results in 108 talar neck fractures (from Hawkins 1970, Peterson et al 1977 and Norgrove Penny & Davis 1980)

Hawkins type	Number of patients	Excellent	Good	Fair	Poor
I	18	7	6	4	1
		72%		28%	
II	48	7	11	12	18
		37.5%		62.5%	
III	42	2	8	16	16
		24%		76%	

(1970) just two cases in 58 talar injuries, indicating an incidence of approximately 3% of all talar injuries. No particular long-term difficulties are reported with this fracture. When undisplaced it unites satisfactorily and displaced fractures are best treated by open reduction and internal fixation. Comminuted fractures may require removal of smaller fragments. Increasing displacement and fracture comminution are associated with greater long-term symptoms and talo-navicular osteoarthritis (Heckman 1996).

Fractures of the talar processes

The lateral and posterior processes of the talus may fracture in isolation or as part of another injury. Isolated fractures are reported rarely and the long-term outcome is poorly described.

Lateral process of the talus

The fracture usually occurs in a dorsiflexion and inversion injury (Hawkins 1965; Mukherjee et al 1974) and has been reported increasingly in snowboarding accidents (Nicholas et al 1994). Occasionally the fragment may involve up to a third of the articular surface of the posterior facet of the subtalar joint. Stress fractures may occur in athletes (Motto 1993; Black & Ehlert 1994). The best results occur in small, undisplaced fractures, which unite following non-operative treatment, isolated larger fragments treated by internal fixation and comminuted fractures treated by primary excision. Long-term symptoms are common, due to the intimate relationship between the fracture fragment and the subtalar joint. Approximately 25% of patients are symptom free and a further 50% have minor symptoms that require no treatment. The remaining 25% of patients have persisting pain in the subtalar joint, which may require late subtalar arthrodesis.

Posterior process of the talus

The most posterior part of the talus is termed the posterior process and it arises from a single secondary centre of ossification that usually fuses to the rest of the talar body at about 12 years. It consists of a larger, more frequently fractured lateral tubercle separated from the medial tubercle, situated medially and inferiorly by a groove for the flexor hallucis longus tendon. This lies immediately posterior to a similar feature on the sustentaculum tali. The os trigonum is a relatively common (64 of 1000 feet; Grogan et al 1990) accessory bone situated behind the lateral tubercle. An elongated lateral tubercle may be described as a 'fused os trigonum'. The lateral process is usually fractured by a forced equinus injury to the ankle and an acute lateral tubercle fracture can be distinguished from the os trigonum radiographically by its irregular outline (Wilson 1982) but it may be difficult to differentiate an old fracture. Radiography of the opposite ankle may help since the os trigonum is bilateral in 60% of cases (Heckman 1996). Trauma can, however, render a previously asymptomatic os trigonum painful and a symptomatic lateral tubercle non-union or a painful os trigonum usually responds to excision.

Fractures of the medial tubercle of the posterior process are rare and usually arise by forced pronation of the foot avulsing the tubercle with part of the deltoid ligament (Cedell 1974). Symptomatic non-union may be treated satisfactorily by excision.

Osteochondral fractures of the dome of the talus

These injuries may occur on the medial or lateral side of the talar dome. A lateral lesion is usually associated with a history of inversion trauma, with or without a fibular fracture. The medial osteochondral lesion less commonly has a defi-

nite history of injury but is thought to arise from impaction of the medial side of the talus against the ankle mortise. The lesion is often invisible on the initial X-rays and a high index of suspicion is necessary for diagnosis. MRI scanning is the investigation of choice. It will visualise the bone fragment, surrounding bone bruising, healing fibrocartilage and the extent of articular cartilage damage. Classification is as follows (Berndt & Harty 1959):

- type I—subchondral bone compression without occult acute fracture
- type II—incomplete fracture
- type III—complete fracture without displacement
- type IV—complete fracture with displacement

The literature is confused concerning the outcome of these injuries. There is widespread agreement that the radiographic stage of the lesion is the major determinant of outcome with type 1 and 2 lesions having a greater number of good and excellent results than type 3 and 4. Bony healing is poorly correlated with clinical outcome and a stable fibrous non-union is consistent with a good long-term result. With surgical treatment, type 3 and 4 lesions may yield good results in up to 88% of cases (Canale & Belding 1980; Pritsch et al 1986; Pettine & Morrey 1987; Van Buecken et al 1987). However, fragment excision must be performed early to minimise the risk of post-traumatic arthritis (Davidson et al 1967; Newberg 1979; O'Farrell & Costello 1982; Pettine & Morrey 1987).

Pettine & Morrey (1987; see Table 16.7) reported on 71 osteochondral fractures in 68 patients after an average of 7.5 years. Most type III and IV lesions were treated by excision and in only five cases was the fragment re-attached. Overall, 75% of patients continued to experience some pain and 22% had constant pain. The results in type III and IV lesions were worse. The majority of patients stabilised approximately 1 year after definitive treatment.

Late osteoarthritis may occur and is seen most frequently in types III and IV injuries. The rate and severity of deterioration reflect the lesion size and its position as well as the patient's weight and activities. Furthermore, results may deteriorate with time (Canale & Belding 1980; Pettine & Morrey 1987). Angermann & Jensen (1989) reported 85% satisfactory short-term results; however, after 9 years, 60% of patients had pain on activity, 33% noted stiffness, 40% complained of swelling and 90% showed mild radiographic arthritis of the ankle.

Dislocation about the talus

In the majority of cases, dislocation or subluxation of the joints around the talus occurs as part of a fracture.

Table 16.7 Results of treatment in osteochondral fractures of the talus (adapted from Pettine & Morrey 1987)

Type of fracture (Berndt & Harty 1959)	Number of patients	Results					
		With operation			Without operation		
		Good	Fair	Poor	Good	Fair	Poor
I	5	0	0	0	3	1	1
II	16	2	0	1	11	2	0
III	27	6	4	4	3	5	5
IV	17	2	2	7	0	0	6

Occasionally, however, associated fractures are minimal or nonexistent in which case one of two broad categories of dislocation will occur.

Subtalar dislocation (peritalar dislocation)

Subtalar dislocation (also more appropriately called peritalar dislocation) implies the simultaneous dislocation of the subtalar and talo-navicular joints. The ankle joint is not affected. The dislocation may occur in any direction but is most commonly medial. Prompt, anatomic reduction is essential for a satisfactory outcome and open reduction may be necessary.

In the case of a simple, uncomplicated subtalar dislocation treated by prompt anatomic reduction either closed or open, the outcome is usually good with minimal long-term functional impairment. Limitation of subtalar joint movement is common and this may be associated with difficulty in walking on rough ground (Smith 1937; Larson 1957; Grantham 1964; Buckingham 1973). Review of the results in 62 patients reported by Dunn (1974), Christensen et al (1977), Monson & Ryan (1981) and Delee & Curtis (1982) shows that the outcome is not always satisfactory (Table 16.8). A poorer outcome is seen in patients with significant associated soft tissue injuries or fractures, lateral dislocations and injuries associated with higher violence (Delee & Curtis 1982; Lancaster et al 1985). Avascular necrosis occurred in only 5% of cases, presumably because the intact ankle mortise maintains an adequate blood supply to the talus (Dunn 1974; Christensen et al 1977; Heppenstall et al 1980), but radiographic osteoarthritis of the ankle or subtalar joint occurred in over half of the patients. (Table 16.9)

Total dislocation of the talus

Total dislocation of the talus implies a peritalar dislocation with a super-added dislocation of the ankle joint. It is very rare and usually results from a continuation of a peritalar dislocation. It is a devastating injury with very high rates of infection, avascular necrosis, talar collapse, osteoarthritis of the hind foot and consequent disability (Coltart 1952; Dettenbeck & Kelly 1969; Heckman 1996). Treatment will often include long periods without weight bearing, talectomy and tibio-calcaneal fusion. However, results are poor.

Fractures of the calcaneus
Introduction

The calcaneus is the most commonly fractured bone in the foot, accounting for 2% of all fractures. The incidence has probably not changed with the advent of the mechanical age (Cave 1963). The calcaneus is a very complex bone with many functions. For example, it provides the insertion point for the tendo Achilles, which is the major plantarflexor of the foot. It includes the heel strike point of the hind foot and takes part in the articulation of the subtalar joint, which is one of the major weight-bearing joints of the body. It is therefore not surprising that significant fractures of the calcaneus are often associated with long-term morbidity. 'Ordinarily speaking, the man who breaks his heel burden is "done" so far as his industrial future is concerned' (Cotton & Wilson 1908).

There remains considerable controversy regarding the classification, management and prognosis of calcaneal fractures (Kenwright 1993); however, the use of CT scanning has allowed an improved understanding of the nature of the different fracture types. This has facilitated the development of rational treatment methods, with the majority of displaced fractures now being treated safely by open reduction and anatomic internal fixation. Scientific evidence is accumulating that this gives better results than conservative treatment.

Classification

There exist a number of different types or families of calcaneus fractures with differing management and prognosis.

Table 16.8 Subjective results after subtalar dislocation. The criteria are based upon the level of pain, as follows:

- good—no pain
- fair—mild pain, or pain only when walking on uneven ground
- poor—severe pain

Reference	Number of patients	Good	Fair	Poor	Follow-up
Dunn (1974)	7	4	2	1	15 months
Christensen et al (1977)	30	9	16	5	23 months
Monson & Ryan (1981)	8	3	4	1	28 months
Delee & Curtis (1982)	17	8	6	3	35 months
Overall	62	24	28	10	26 months
		(39%)	(45%)	(16%)	

Table 16.9 The incidence of avascular necrosis and osteoarthritis after subtalar dislocations

Reference	Number of patients	Medial	Lateral	Avascular necrosis	Osteoarthritis
Dunn (1974)	7*	5	1	1	N/A
Christensen et al (1977)	30	26	4	2	19
Monson & Ryan (1981)	8	7	1	0	5
Delee & Curtis (1982)	17*	12	4	0	7
Total	62	50	10	3 (5%)	31/55 (56%)

* One anterior and one posterior dislocation included.

The usual initial classification is into extra-articular and intra-articular fractures (Heckman 1996). In adults, the ratio of intra-articular and extra-articular fractures is about 3:1 (Wilson 1982).

Extra-articular fractures

Five types are recognised (Heckman 1996): anterior process, tuberosity, medial process, sustentaculum tali and body.

Anterior process fracture

Two distinct isolated fractures of the anterior process occur. The more common, which may account for up to 15% of all calcaneal fractures (Carey 1965), is the avulsion fracture, which usually occurs in women. A small anterolateral part of the calcaneus occasionally including a small part of the calcaneo-cuboid joint is avulsed by the bifurcate ligament or extensor digitorum brevis in a low energy injury. This fracture is typically treated non-operatively by immobilisation. The acute symptoms may take up to 9 months to settle but long-term disability is rare.

In contrast, the rare compression fracture is a high energy abduction injury, typically seen in a motor-cycle accident (Hunt 1970). The displaced fragment is large and involves a substantial part of the calcaneo-cuboid joint. This fracture requires open reduction and internal fixation to restore the congruency of the joint. Treated non-operatively, the displaced fragment may block subtalar motion and require late excision. Despite operative treatment long-term symptoms are common.

Tuberosity fractures

The extra-articular tuberosity fracture represents an avulsion of the tendo Achilles insertion and occurs principally in elderly or unfit patients. In this patient group, the fracture usually follows a trip. If displaced it requires internal fixation. Provided that a satisfactory reduction is obtained with sound bone union, normal function is usually restored. Residual displacement causes a heel boss, which can lead to difficulty with shoeware. In addition, weakness of plantarflexion may cause problems with walking. Rowe et al (1963) reported this injury in six (4%) of 146 patients. All had good or excellent results following closed or open reduction.

Fractures of the medial calcaneal process

This rare injury may represent an avulsion of the plantar fascia (Bohler 1931) or a vertical shear injury. Treated non-operatively it rarely gives rise to symptoms; however, a symptomatic mal-union has been reported (Rowe et al 1963; Heckman 1996). It is important not to confuse either an extra-articular tuberosity fracture or a medial process fracture with the more serious intra-articular tuberosity fracture.

Fractures of the sustentaculum tali

This represents an intra-articular fracture of the calcaneal bone in which the primary fracture line is placed so far medial that it misses the posterior facet of the subtalar joint. Provided it is undisplaced, this fracture produces few long-term symptoms (Carey et al 1965), but occasional symptomatic non-union may necessitate excision of the sustentacular fragment or late internal fixation. If displaced, the fracture requires reduction and internal fixation to restore hindfoot biomechanics. Under these circumstances the outcome is usually good.

Fractures of the body (tuberosity) not involving the subtalar joint

Older series report a high preponderance of this fracture (for example, Rowe et al 1963 found 19.5%). More modern reports suggest that this is a less frequent injury, which probably reflects increasing accuracy of diagnosis using CT scanning. Generally speaking, these fractures give rise to few long-term symptoms unless they are severely displaced. However, weather aching may persist for up to 2 years following injury (Heckman 1996).

Intra-articular fractures

Intra-articular fractures of the calcaneus comprise 60% of all tarsal injuries and 75% of all calcaneal fractures (Cave 1963). The fracture usually results from a fall of between 10 and 20 ft and the great majority follow a single basic fracture pattern with wide variations; however, approximately 5% of cases are totally different. Very high violence, usually the result of a road traffic accident or a fall from a cliff, may result in fractures which are severely comminuted and difficult to classify. These fractures fare particularly badly if treated non-operatively.

A brief description of the usual fracture patterns provides a background to the bewildering area of fracture classification and serves as a useful introduction to a discussion of disability.

In an injury that causes a calcaneal fracture, the point of impact is the inferior surface of the body of the calcaneus. The first fracture line to develop (*the primary fracture line*; Essex-Lopresti 1952; Eastwood & Atkins 1993a) splits the posterior facet of the subtalar joint longitudinally and divides the bone in a roughly sagittal plane (although the line is rather more medial posteriorly and inferiorly), creating a two-part fracture. Sanders' 1993 classification is based on the number and position of primary fracture lines as they cross the subtalar joint. He demonstrated that operative fixation is more difficult and the outcome less favourable with increasing comminution of the subtalar joint (Sanders type 4 fracture). The two-part fracture exists, although it is rare. When undisplaced the outcome is good following non-operative treatment. Usually, however, in a two-part fracture the lateral fragment dislocates lateral to the talus and impinging upon the lateral malleolus, fractures it and rebounds, subluxing the ankle joint (Eastwood & Atkins 1993c). Treated by operative reduction and fixation, the outcome of this fracture is good with very few long-term limitations. Unfortunately, the fracture occurs following a minor trauma (usually in a middle-aged woman) and the signs on plain X-ray are subtle. The fracture is therefore not infrequently missed and the opportunity for primary fixation is lost. If a two-part fracture dislocation is treated non-operatively, initial recovery is slow. The patient gradually regains the ability to walk; but after a year or so the severe biomechanical derangement of the hind foot leads to a progressive deterioration in symptoms with progressive midfoot arthritis and eventually a midfoot break.

In the majority of cases (Essex-Lopresti 1952), two further fracture lines occur together. The coronal secondary fracture line splits the calcaneus along the sinus tarsi, while the longitudinal secondary fracture line arises on the lateral wall at the level of the peroneal tubercle and passes posteriorly and upwards to rejoin the primary fracture behind the subtalar joint. The calcaneus has now been split into five fragments. The body fragment, containing the heel strike point and the insertion of the tendo Achillis, lies lateral and inferior to the primary fracture line and behind the secondary fracture lines. The lateral joint fragment, containing the lateral part of the subtalar joint, is between the primary fracture line and the longitudinal secondary fracture line. The sustentacular fragment, containing the medial part of the subtalar joint, is medial to the primary fracture line and behind the coronal fracture line. The antero-lateral fragment, which lies in front of the coronal secondary fracture line and lateral to the primary fracture line, contains the lateral part of the calcaneo-cuboid joint. The anteromedial fragment line is medial to the primary fracture line and anterior to the coronal secondary fracture line. It contains the medial part of the calcaneo-cuboid joint.

Two significant variations occur in the secondary fracture lines. The longitudinal secondary fracture line make it either skirt the subtalar joint creating a central joint compression lateral joint fragment or pass round the back of the calcaneus forming a larger tongue type fragment (Essex–Lopresti 1952). In approximately 25% of cases the coronal fracture line stops medially at the primary fracture line and the anteromedial fragment is not separate from the sustentacular fragment. This creates a four-part rather than a five-part fracture (for this classification, see Zwipp et al 1993).

Usually the body fragment is wedge shaped and pushes upwards between the sustentacular fragment and the lateral joint fragment, rotating them outwards, creating an angular displacement of the subtalar joint. Occasionally, in osteoporotic or high energy fractures, the lateral joint fragment impacts into the body fragment and is depressed away from the subtalar joint, creating a Malgaine or Atkins type 3 fracture (Eastwood & Atkins 1993a). This is an important variant because treated non-operatively this fracture type leads to greater disability than the more common wedge type of fracture.

Approximately 5% of intra-articular fractures have a primary fracture line in the coronal plane. Treated non-operatively, recovery is slow with marked bossing of the heel, difficulty with shoeware and weakened plantar-flexion (the intra-articular tuberosity fracture; Squires & Atkins 2000).

Outcome of intra-articular fractures

This discussion will concentrate on the usual pattern of intra-articular fracture. Undisplaced fractures have a good prognosis. Thoren (1964) reviewed 13 cases; all achieved excellent or good results. Essex-Lopresti (1952) found excellent or good results in 84% of 32 patients.

Results following conservative and non-operative treatment

The results following conservative treatment of displaced intra-articular fractures can be classified into three groups (Lindsay & Dewar 1958; Lance et al 1963; Rowe et al 1963; Thoren 1964; Pozo et al 1984):

- Excellent/good: the patient felt that the foot was entirely normal or experienced only minor symptoms.
- Fair: the patient could resume previous or similar work but had to limit recreational activities. There was moderate pain and swelling.
- Poor: the patient continued to suffer moderate to severe pain and had limited employability. Patients requiring major secondary surgery are included in this group.

If those patients treated by primary subtalar arthrodesis and internal fixation are excluded, then 210 of 338 patients (62%) achieved an excellent or good result. Lindsay & Dewar (1958) and Pozo et al (1984) did not distinguish clearly between the fair and the poor results. The other authors made this distinction, and 47 of 234 patients (20%) had a fair result and 57 of 234 (24%) a poor result. These figures are unbalanced because the two studies which did not categorise fair and poor results showed the highest incidence of good and excellent results (Table 16.10).

Table 16.10 Results after non-operative treatment of displaced intra-articular fractures of the calcaneus

Reference	Number of cases	Excellent/ good	Fair	Poor
Pozo et al (1984)	21	17		4
Lindsay & Dewar (1958)	83	63		20
Thoren (1964)	75	43	18	14
Rowe et al (1963)	62	32	15	15
Lance et al (1963)	97	55	14	28
Total	338	210/338 (62%)	47/234 (20%)	57/234 (24%)

These reports may be criticised because their outcome scoring systems are less rigorous than those employed in more modern studies. Thus Paley & Hall (1993) found that, using the criteria of Rowe and of Lindsay & Dewar, their patients had 65 to 75% of good/excellent/satisfactory results, while using their own (more rigid) criteria the figure was only 60%. This problem was more fully investigated by Kerr et al (1996), who devised a simple rational scoring system.

A further criticism is that the precise nature of the fractures being reported in the early studies is not clear owing to the lack of CT scans. Crosby & Fitzgibbon (1990) reported a series of 30 fractures with 14 good or excellent results using a modern rigorous outcome scoring system. When analysed using CT scanning, 12 of 13 undisplaced fractures had a good or excellent result. In contrast, the results in 80% of cases showing subtalar joint displacement of 2 mm or more and all cases with subtalar comminution were unacceptable.

Overall, the literature supports the view that if a calcaneal fracture is treated non-operatively, increasing deformity and displacement are associated with increasing long-term symptoms. Janzen et al (1992) investigated the influence of plain X-ray and CT findings on the outcome of displaced fractures treated non-operatively. They found that the best determinant of outcome was Bohler's angle followed by loss of congruity of the subtalar joint.

Results following open reduction and internal fixation

Modern techniques for calcaneal fracture fixation are safe and the results are better than the reported results of non-operative treatment (Stephenson 1987, 1993; Benirschke & Sangeorzan 1993; Bezes 1993; Letournel 1993; Sanders et al 1993; Zwipp et al 1993; Freeman 1996; Melcher 1995). Overall, these studies showed good or excellent results in the majority of cases. The surgery is difficult and surgeon experience and anatomic reduction are important for optimal outcome (Buckley & Meek 1992; Janzen et al 1992; Sanders et al 1993). Stephenson (1987, 1993) recorded good results in 75%. Melcher et al (1995) reported on 16 cases followed up after 10 years and found excellent or good results in the majority despite radiographic evidence of post-traumatic arthritis of the subtalar joint. Thordarson & Krieger (1996) reviewed a study of 30 displaced cases randomised prospectively into ORIF or non-operative treatment. They found a large and significant improvement in the group treated operatively (average outcome score 86.7 in the ORIF group compared to 55.0 in the non-operated group, p<0.01).

Sources of residual disability and timing of reports

In general, it takes 18–36 months for symptoms to reach a plateau following intra-articular fractures of the calcaneus (Essex-Lopresti 1952; Lindsay & Dewar 1958; Nade & Monahan 1973), but Kenwright (1993) reported that improvement had been noted in some patients up to 6 years after the injury. Following open reduction and internal fixation the plateau is reached by approximately 1 year to 18 months. After the initial plateau has been reached, symptoms may worsen in cases where an anatomic or near anatomic reduction has been achieved because of the development of osteoarthritis of the subtalar joint, due to the severity of the initial fracture damage. This process is normally established by 18 months following fracture.

Stabilisation of symptoms takes longer in cases of severe residual displacement and a gradual deterioration in function is not infrequently seen after the initial plateau has been reached due to the onset of hind foot and midfoot arthritis secondary to joint mal-alignment and alteration in biomechanics. In view of the time taken for symptoms to reach a plateau, final medico-legal reports should not be given until at least 2 years after the injury and then the prognosis must take careful account of the nature of the fracture and residual deformity.

The use of orthotics and specialist shoeware may minimise symptoms and reconstructive surgery may be possible. Myerson & Quill (1993) retrospectively reviewed the results of 43 patients with calcaneal fractures who had required surgical reconstruction an average of 26 months after their fracture because of a poor clinical result. Pain was partially relieved in 90%, function was improved in 83% and 76% returned either to work or to their pre-injury level of activity.

Disability after fracture
Introduction

Owing to the pivotal role of the calcaneus in foot function, the complexity of the bone and the frequency of the fracture, disability following calcaneus fracture is an important and complex subject. Disability is due to a combination of pain, deformity, stiffness and swelling (McLaughlin 1963) which will limit walking ability and derange lifestyle. The assessment and treatment of disability are made difficult by the multiple possible sources of symptoms, which cause overlapping syndromes. For example, causes of pain include subtalar osteoarthritis, peroneal tendonitis, calcaneofibular abutment due to lateral wall bulging, plantar fascitis, a bony spur and nerve entrapment. A careful, detailed clinical assessment backed by extensive radiological investigation will usually reveal one or more of the following problems.

Subtalar joint derangement
Angular mal-alignment
Angular mal-alignment of the posterior facet of the subtalar joint is an inevitable consequence of displacement of the fragments of a calcaneal fracture (Eastwood, Gregg & Atkins 1993). In the early time course following a fracture, mal-alignment produces few if any symptoms, in contrast to subtalar joint depression, which is invariably severely symptomatic. The more severe the mal-alignment and the greater the comminution of the subtalar joint, the more likely it is that the patient will develop degeneration of the joint at a later stage. This causes a characteristic syndrome of pain on walking, which is particularly intrusive when negotiating uneven ground. As the condition progresses, rest pain becomes a significant feature. In the presence of normal hindfoot biomechanics, subtalar joint symptoms are not usually a significant problem unless the patient has a job which entails regular rough walking such as in the building trade. In this case a simple subtalar joint fusion will alleviate the problem. Where subtalar joint arthritis is associated with abnormal hindfoot biomechanics, in situ subtalar fusion may worsen the situation by removing the compensatory mechanism of subtalar movement and reconstructive arthrodesis may be required.

Subtalar joint depression
True lateral joint fragment depression as described by Malgaine (Essex-Lopresti 1952) is rare (Eastwood, Gregg & Atkins 1993), tending to occur in more severely displaced or atypical fractures which follow high energy impacts or in older, osteoporotic patients. The patients are invariably seriously disabled and although this may relate to the general disorganisation of the hindfoot, a characteristic syndrome is seen.

The patient complains of a sense of insecurity and giving way within the foot when trying to take a step, as if walking on water. Weight bearing is associated with severe pain deep within the foot and laterally. With time night pain becomes increasingly intrusive. In addition to the usual features of a severely displaced calcaneal fracture, examination, particularly in the latter stages, will reveal tenderness laterally and a valgus hindfoot. On walking, the heel may collapse visibly into valgus because the sustentaculum tali remains in place with a small medial part of the subtalar joint, while the lateral part of the joint is deficient.

Alterations of hindfoot biomechanics
In the large majority of symptomatic calcaneal fractures, abnormalities of hindfoot biomechanics are a significant underlying factor. They are mainly due to movement of the body fragment, which contains the bulk of the bone, the insertion of the tendo Achilles and the heelstrike point of the foot. During fracture, the body fragment moves in relation to the talus upward, forwards and laterally while it rotates into varus and internal rotation. Three types of abnormality are commonly seen.

Heelstrike medial
Where the movement of the body fragment has carried the heelstrike point medial to the axis of the hindfoot, the unloaded hindfoot will lie in varus and this is accentuated when the foot is weight bearing. There is a secondary cavus midfoot and in a severe case the patient will be unable to put weight on the medial ray of the forefoot. At toe off, when the plantarflexors of the foot contract, the varus will be further accentuated because of the medial mal-alignment of the insertion of the tendo Achilles. This combination of abnormalities is often sufficiently severe to cause the foot to give way into supination and in some cases the patient will actually walk on the outer border of the foot. In addition, because of the close association of the tendon of flexor hallucis longus to the primary fracture line, function of this muscle is frequently impaired, further deranging the gait pattern.

These patients complain of severe difficulty in walking or standing for any length of time. The foot tends to collapse into supination, which the patient interprets as giving way, and this is both frightening and painful. In an attempt to avoid this, they try to pronate the foot as far as possible and this pushes the damaged subtalar joint into maximal and painful eversion. In order to produce eversion, patients contract the peroneal muscles, which are themselves at a disadvantage because of involvement of the course of the tendons in the fracture and damage of the insertion of peroneus brevis. Excessive activity of the peroneal muscles produces calf pain.

Clinical examination shows a varus and internally rotated heel but there is usually a lateral boss, which all but obliterates the normal outline of the lateral malleolus. The heel is broadened because of movement of the body fragment and splaying of the lateral wall, which combine to narrow the gap between the lateral wall of the calcaneum and the fibula, producing 'fibular impingement' and a prominent lateral calcaneal wall.

Initially the patients experience pain only on weight bearing, located deep within the foot and laterally; however, in these severely deranged feet, secondary degenerative changes in the joints of the ankle and mid-foot occur relatively rapidly, and with time rest pain occurs. In addition, the regular collapse strains the lateral ligaments, causing hindfoot instability.

Conservative treatment of these feet is of little use. An outer iron may help to prevent the giving way but the author has yet to find a patient who regarded this as sufficient. The only satisfactory solution is surgical reconstruction of the heel and this is made particularly difficult by the varus position of the hindfoot.

Heelstrike lateral

This is more benign than heelstrike medial but it is unfortunately less common. The position of the body fragment produces a heelstrike lateral to the axis of the foot, causing a valgus heel and a secondary planus midfoot. When the foot is load bearing the situation is accentuated, and because the damaged subtalar joint is being forced into eversion it becomes painful. The patient will often contract the invertors of the hindfoot excessively in order to limit the heel valgus, causing calf pain. The valgus movement of the heel during walking is effectively limited by the lateral malleolus, so that 'fibular impingement' is a feature. However, resection of the lateral bony boss may make matters worse by allowing the heel to collapse further into valgus. Likewise, in situ fusion of the subtalar joint will destroy the compensatory effect of subtalar inversion and may make matters worse.

Treatment by a medial shoe-raise and supporting insole is often extremely effective in these cases. Operative treatment to reconstruct the hindfoot biomechanics and fuse the subtalar joint is easier than in the case of heelstrike medial.

Short heel

Following a displaced calcaneal fracture, the heel is always shortened and broadened in relation to the extent of the displacement. However, when the heelstrike is displaced medially or laterally, the symptoms from this shortening are usually masked by those more intrusive problems.

The short broad heel causes problems with shoeware and sometimes the broadening is sufficient to cause lateral pain beneath the fibula. The major problem, however, is weakness of plantarflexion due to reduction of the moment arm of the gastrocnemius–soleus complex. In order to compensate for the short heel the ankle is held in dorsiflexion, and if the problem is severe there may be an overall apparent equinus deformity of the foot. The abnormal posture of the ankle may lead to secondary arthritis with typically an anterior impingement lesion. The

patient characteristically complains of weakness of the foot and limping, while in a severe case the equinus may lead to catching the foot. Later ankle arthritic pain becomes a feature.

Treatment is by provision of a heel raise to restore the ankle to neutral and protect it. However, the patient often finds that this makes matters symptomatically worse by exaggerating the weakness of the plantarflexors. Operative treatment is by hindfoot reconstruction. If treatment is delayed until ankle arthritis supervenes, the situation is difficult to recover.

Anterior calcaneal syndromes

Owing to its attachment to the bifurcate ligament, the anterior part of the anteromedial fragment is rarely displaced following a fracture. The posterior part is attached to the talus and may ride upwards compared to the posterior facet of the subtalar joint. Although the displacement is seldom great, even this small mal-alignment may contribute to blocking subtalar joint movement. In contrast, the anterolateral fragment will often tip upwards because of its attachment to the inferior peroneal retinaculum. As it does so its postero-superior border fills in the crucial angle of Gissane, preventing eversion and in severe cases causing a fixed inversion deformity (Langdon, Langkamer & Atkins 1993). When this is combined with a medial translation of the heel due to body fragment movement, the resulting disability is severe.

The anterolateral fragment syndrome is seen in untreated isolated compression fractures or in inadequately treated fractures where the crucial angle of Gissane has not been correctly addressed. The patient complains of pain, initially only on attempted eversion. Gradually the pain becomes more intrusive, occurring first on walking on rough ground, then on any walking, on standing and finally, as arthritic changes occur, at rest. Rarely a late spontaneous fusion will occur. Before degenerative changes occur, excision of the displaced bone may produce a satisfactory result. At a late stage fusion combined with reconstruction of the hindfoot is necessary.

Heelpad syndrome

The specialised weight-bearing tissues of the heelpad are undoubtedly damaged acutely in a calcaneal fracture. With satisfactory fracture healing, these changes disappear within a year (Kuhns 1949) and the heelpad is usually asymptomatic. Heelpad pain does however occur when a piece of bone is left protruding into the plantar fascia, almost exclusively where non-operative treatment has been used. These patients are always severely disabled clinically. They walk with a severe limp and great pain, although rest pain is rare. Treatment is very difficult.

Thick bespoke insoles which relieve the load on the tissues under pressure are of some help but reconstructive surgery is usually required. Resection of the bony spur is surprisingly difficult and symptoms may be improved but are rarely abolished.

Fibular impingement *(peroneal tendon impingement)*

The anatomic relationship between the lateral wall of the calcaneus, the peroneal tendons and the distal fibula is inevitably disturbed in a displaced calcaneal fracture. The normal situation will be restored by anatomic internal fixation. In a mildly displaced calcaneus fracture, the lateral wall bulges outward, narrowing the gap between it and the lateral malleolus and compressing the peroneal tendons which are constrained by their retinacular attachment to the fibula. In more severe cases the entire distal fibula may be surrounded by displaced bone from the calcaneus and the peroneal tendons may be dislocated anteriorly. Thoren (1964) found that broadening of more than 1 cm occurred in approximately 50% of intra-articular fractures and was correlated with the functional result. If broadening of the heel compared to the other side was less than 1 cm, 84% of patients (37 of 44) achieved a good or excellent result. If there was broadening of 1 cm or more, only 46% of patients (21 of 46) achieved a good or excellent result.

It is important to differentiate static fibular impingement described above from dynamic impingement where a valgus hind foot mal-alignment causes the calcaneus to twist laterally on load bearing. Static fibular impingement may be due to bursting of the lateral wall, in which case it is readily treated by lateral wall resection. Alternatively, it may be due to lateral migration of the body fragment, which will require hind foot reconstruction for correction. Dislocated peroneal tendons may be reduced and stabilised in situ at the time of reconstruction.

Mid-tarsal fracture–dislocations

Main & Jowett (1975) reviewed a large series of midfoot injuries and described the treatment and results in 73 patients. In 30 (41%) the diagnosis was delayed. That delay in diagnosis continues to be a feature of this injury is due to its relative rarity compared to simple ankle sprain, the subtlety of radiographic features in less displaced cases and the bewildering number of varieties of injury. The authors classified the injuries into five types, medial, longitudinal, lateral, plantar and crush, based on the direction of the presumed causative violence. Each type of injury was then further divided according to its extent, based on whether it was a sprain, characterised

by flake fractures of the dorsal margins of the talus or navicular and of the calcaneus and cuboid, an isolated dislocation or subluxation, a fracture dislocation or a crushing injury. Not surprisingly the extent of the injury is more closely correlated with the prognosis than is the direction of the causative force. They reported 90% good or excellent results from midfoot sprains with or without associated flake fractures. Isolated dislocations yielded acceptable outcomes in 60% of cases. In contrast only 20% of fracture dislocations achieved good or excellent results (Table 16.11). Main & Jowett noted a high incidence of poor results where a closed reduction failed to improve the position and better results were associated with accurate reduction being maintained until healing occurred.

The modern view concerning these injuries is that anatomic reduction must be obtained by closed or if necessary open means and then maintained until bone and ligamentous healing has occurred by the use of screws or wires, which are then removed. With this treatment the degree of residual disability will depend on the extent of the initial disruption of the foot. Sprains and isolated dislocations will give good results although occasional recurrent subluxation will be seen. Fracture dislocations will also give good results provided that bone union is obtained rapidly in an anatomic position. Stiffness of the midfoot is common following injury, particularly where open reduction and internal fixation are required. Mild degrees of stiffness usually cause no symptoms but severe stiffness may mean difficulty in walking, particularly over rough ground. Radiographic features of osteoarthritis may occur in disrupted joints, but apart from stiffness it does not normally cause significant disability. Occasionally, progressive symptomatic osteoarthritis occurs. This will usually be established by 18 months after injury and local fusion may be required.

This optimal form of management may not be possible if the injury is missed initially or it is not possible to obtain an anatomic reduction due to crushing of bone. In these cases residual mal-alignment and instability may cause significant symptoms with progressive midfoot arthritis. Fusion may be required.

Fractures of the navicular bone
Avulsion fractures

Forced plantarflexion and eversion injuries may cause an avulsion fracture of the dorsal aspect of the navicular bone. The piece of bone is usually small and contains little articular surface, in which case the injury is normally of no long-term significance. Occasionally, a prominent

Table 16.11   Results after injury to the mid-tarsal joint (adapted from Main & Jowett 1975)

- excellent—no symptoms or signs
- good—trivial symptoms and signs, insufficient to impair function
- fair—residual symptoms and signs, with some disability
- poor—marked symptoms and limitation of function, with subsequent arthrodesis or a request for further treatment from the patient

Injury	Number	Excellent	Good	Fair	Poor
Fracture sprains	20	13 (65%)	5 (25%)	2 (10%)	0
Fracture–dislocation	32	1 (3%)	6 (19%)	13 (41%)	12 (37%)*
Dislocations (including swivel dislocations)	10	1 (10%)	5 (50%)	1 (10%)	3 (30%)*
Crush fractures	4	0	1 (25%)	3 (75%)	0
Isolated navicular fractures	5	4 (80%)	1 (20%)	0	0

* Of the patients with poor results, 11 underwent mid-tarsal or triple arthrodesis.

fragment causes irritation on shoeware and may require excision. Very rarely, the avulsed fragment contains a significant amount of the articular surface of the talo-navicular joint. If an anatomic position has been obtained the long-term prognosis is good but in the presence of significant joint mal-alignment, local osteoarthritis may supervene. If this produces significant long-term symptoms fusion may be necessary.

Tuberosity fracture

An acute eversion injury of the foot may cause an avulsion of the medial navicular tuberosity with its attached insertion of tibialis posterior. Displacement is normally minimal. This injury must be differentiated from an accessory navicular bone. The latter is usually bilateral and has a smooth well-corticated outline. Occasionally, an accessory navicular bone may fracture. These injuries rarely cause long-term symptoms apart from some local prominence of the bone. Occasionally, a symptomatic non-union requires excision.

Stress fractures
Fracture of the body of the navicular bone

Fractures of the navicular bone usually occur with other midfoot injuries. In these cases the prognosis is that of the overall injury. Occasionally, an isolated, displaced fracture occurs and these have been classified by Sangeorzan et al (1989), based on a series of 21 cases:

- type I: fracture is in the coronal plane with no angulation of the forefoot

- type II: the major fracture line is dorsolateral to plantar medial and the forefoot is displaced medially
- type III: the fracture is comminuted and the forefoot is displaced laterally

Undisplaced fractures of all types treated non-operatively give good long-term results. In contrast, closed reduction of displaced fractures of whatever type does not lead to a stable, satisfactory reduction and the outcome is poor with persistent forefoot mal-alignment and disability (Eichenholtz & Levine 1964; Greenberg & Sheehan 1980).

Displaced type I fractures are readily treated by open reduction and screw fixation. Sangeorzan obtained good results in all four patients.

It is more difficult to maintain an adequate reduction in a type II fracture. Where anatomic reduction is maintained, which may necessitate the use of the medially placed external fixator, the outcome was good. Continued fracture displacement was associated with midfoot deformity, arthritis and continuing disability.

Despite aggressive surgical treatment, only one of Sangeorzan's type III fractures obtained a good result.

Fracture of the cuboid bone

Lateral subluxation of the midtarsal joint can lead to a compression fracture of the cuboid bone. When displacement is minimal conservative treatment generally leads to a good outcome. Where there has been considerable crushing of the bone with loss of length of the lateral column, a distraction arthrodesis of the calcaneocuboid joint may be necessary to restore foot function.

Tarsometatarsal fracture–dislocations

The incidence of injury of the tarsometatarsal joints (Lisfranc's injury) is controversial. Aitken & Poulson (1963) found only 16 cases in a review of some 80 000 fractures over a 15 year period. In contrast, more modern works suggest a higher incidence either due to an increasing prevalence of the injury with mechanisation or because a significant number of less displaced injuries were overlooked in the earlier, retrospective series (Heckman 1996). The complexity of the tarsometatarsal articulation leads to a wide variety of injury types. The fundamental anatomic features that determine the manner of injury to this region are the recession of the second metatarsal base between the medial and lateral cuneiform bones, the deficiency of the plantar metatarsal ligament between the first and second metatarsal heads, the presence of Lisfranc's ligament and the relative weakness of the dorsal metatarsal ligament. The trapezoidal shape of the bases of the medial three metatarsal bones also helps to prevent plantar dislocation. Thus when this joint complex is disrupted the metatarsal heads tend to migrate dorsally and the first ray may separate from the others. The usual classification is that of Quenu & Kuss (1909), who described three basic types:

■ Isolated (partial incongruity injury): in which the first ray alone dislocates
■ Homolateral (total incongruity injury): in which all five metatarsals deviate laterally

■ Divergent (total incongruity injury): in which the first ray dislocates medially and the lesser four rays dislocate laterally

The isolated first ray injury was the most common in all series.

There is controversy regarding the importance of accurate reduction of these injuries. Aitken & Poulson (1963), for example, reported good results even in cases where a persistent dislocation caused obvious long-term deformity. This finding must raise concern about the sensitivity of the method of assessment of disability. The majority of series support the view that anatomic reduction combined with the stabilisation of the reduced joint complex until sound bony and ligamentous healing have occurred gives the best results. Poor reduction is, however, consistent with a satisfactory outcome (Key & Conwell 1956; Wilson 1972; Wilpulla 1973; Hardcastle et al 1982; Myerson et al 1986; Arntz & Hansen 1987; Brunet & Wiley 1987). The combined results of these series, comprising 132 cases, showed that 55% of patients achieved a good result (Table 16.12). The outcome was worse in those patients in whom the diagnosis was missed (Myerson et al 1986). Not surprisingly, there was a tendency for an isolated first ray injury to give better results than the more severe homolateral and divergent injuries. Thus Brunet & Wiley (1987) found that half of the group with total incongruity had functionally unsatisfactory results, compared with only one unsatisfactory result in 23 patients with partial incongruity. Overall, however, persisting displacement was more important for long-term outcome than the type of dislocation. Brunet & Wiley (1987) suggested that a persistent gap between the first and second metatarsal heads had little bearing on the final result as far as pain and function were concerned. In contrast, Myerson et al (1986) suggested that a

Table 16.12 Clinical results after tarsometatarsal fracture–dislocations. Criteria are:

■ good—no pain (or trivial pain), could stand on tiptoe, normal gait and no deformity
■ fair—moderate pain on activity, difficulty standing on tiptoe and a limp
■ poor—marked continuous pain, inability to stand on tiptoe, limp and deformity

Reference	Number of patients	Good	Fair	Poor	Mean follow-up
Wilpulla (1973)	26	9	9	8	5 years
Hardcastle et al (1982)	68	46	16	6	18 months to 12 years
Myerson et al (1986)	55	27	13	15	4.2 years
Total	149	82 (55%)	38 (25%)	29 (20%)	

persistent gap of more than 5 mm between the base of the first and second metatarsals was associated with a less satisfactory clinical result.

Myerson et al (1986) compared simple immobilisation in plaster after reduction with fixation by percutaneous pinning or screws and found a better clinical result in those treated by pin or screw fixation.

Symptoms reach a stable level after an average of 1.3 years although improvement can continue for as long as 5 years (Brunet & Wiley 1987). This is an important consideration for the timing of medicolegal reports.

Osteoarthritis is relatively common after these injuries but it may be asymptomatic. Brunet & Wiley (1987) observed arthritis in 25 of 32 patients (78%). This was mild in all cases. Only 20 to 25% of patients with osteoarthritis had symptoms that affected their work or social activities. In view of the length of follow-up in this series, these figures are of considerable value in predicting the prognosis, and also in assessing the effect of osteoarthritis after these injuries.

In Brunet & Wiley's 1987 series, 76% of patients were able to return to their original job (10 had been labourers and 16 were involved in office or clerical work). The other patients were forced to seek lighter work due to persistent foot discomfort.

Fractures of the metatarsals

The metatarsal bones are usually injured as a result of direct trauma, as for example when a heavy weight drops on the foot. Indirect injuries may cause spiral fractures of the central metatarsals and the base of the fifth metatarsal bone is normally fractured as part of an inversion injury. Occasionally, fractures of several metatarsals are part of a midfoot injury.

Metatarsal shaft fractures

Undisplaced and minimally displaced metatarsal shaft and neck fractures produce little or no long-term disability (Johnson 1976) unless they are immobilised in plaster for an excessive period, which may lead to permanent stiffness.

Owing to the first metatarsal's major role in load bearing, residual displacement in fractures is poorly tolerated. Similar considerations apply with somewhat less force to fractures of the fifth metatarsal shaft. In contrast, displacement of fractures of the second, third or fourth metatarsals in the coronal plane produces little or no disability (Heckman 1996). However, displacement of these bones in a sagittal plane is more serious. It produces a

dorsal boss, which mal-interfere with shoeware and the plantarflexed metatarsal head can cause painful metatarsalgia. Even with anatomical reduction and early mobilisation, there may be some residual symptoms that are not severely intrusive (Joplin 1958; Spector et al 1984).

Fractures of the base of the fifth metatarsal

For a common fracture, the literature on this injury is remarkably confusing. At least two and possibly three separate fracture patterns occur at this site. Three separate fracture zones have been described (Dameron 1975; Lawrence & Botte 1993).

Zone 1 is the common avulsion fracture caused by sudden inversion of the foot. It is due to avulsion of the lateral cord of the plantar aponeurosis (Richli & Rosenthal 1984). The fracture is almost always extra articular but occasionally the articulation with the cuboid is involved. Treatment is invariably symptomatic and long-term disability is very rare, the acute symptoms usually settling within a month to 6 weeks. Non-union may occur but is usually asymptomatic. Persistent symptomatic non-union is best treated by excision of the fragment. Entrapment of a branch of the sural nerve with local irritation and dysaesthesia has been reported (Gould & Trevino 1981). The rare displaced intra-articular fracture requires open reduction and internal fixation to avoid local arthritic symptoms.

Zone 2 is an acute fracture at the junction of the metaphysis and diaphysis, similar to the original Jones (1902) fracture. This is a more troublesome injury than that in Zone 1. Dameron (1975) reported 20 cases and found that 12 (60%) united in 2–12 months and three within 21 months with conservative treatment. Five (25%) required a surgical procedure to achieve union. Not all non-unions of this fracture were asymptomatic.

Zone 3 is a stress fracture of the proximal 1.5 cm of the metatarsal shaft. This is not an acute injury and the patients, who are often young, fit and athletic, have prodromal symptoms. Radiographic signs of repetitive stress injury are present.

Torg et al (1984) preferred to consider all transverse fractures of the proximal metatarsal (that is, zone 2 and zone 3 injuries, including the Jones fracture) as one fracture type. They subdivided this injury into:

- Acute fracture: a definite acute history of injury and no radiographic or clinical evidence of stress lesion.
- Delayed union: a history of previous injury or fracture with some evidence of medullary sclerosis and cortical resorption.

- Non-union: a history of recurrent symptoms with radiographic sclerosis and obliteration of the medullary canal.

Torg et al (1984) reported 43 patients with such transverse fractures with an average follow-up of 40 months. Twenty-five were acute injuries, 10 of which were treated with immobilisation and early weight bearing. Only four (40%) of these went on to uneventful union, the remainder requiring surgery for symptomatic delayed or non-union. The other 15 patients were treated by plaster immobilisation and non-weight bearing; 14 (43%) healed uneventfully and the other patient required surgical treatment for a symptomatic non-union. The authors recommended that acute transverse fractures should be treated in a below-knee, non-weight-bearing plaster for 6 weeks.

Kavanaugh et al (1978) described 23 patients with Jones fractures. Follow-up in these patients averaged 3.5 years. Forty percent had a delayed or non-union and approximately half of these fractures had not united 6 months after injury.

In summary, fractures of the base of the fifth metatarsal bone represent a spectrum, with the fractures becoming increasingly difficult to treat as the fracture line passes distally from the simple minor avulsion fracture through to the stress lesion of the proximal diaphysis. The minor avulsion fracture (zone 1) resolves with symptomatic treatment and the acute Jones fracture (zone 2) will usually unite following a period of non-weight-bearing immobilisation. In contrast, the chronic lesion (zone 3) requires surgical fixation with compression to achieve union (Delee et al 1983; Lawrence & Botte 1993). Internal fixation usually leads to prompt union of the fracture, although bone grafting may be required and the metal work may irritate and require removal. Once union has been achieved, disability is usually slight or absent.

From a medicolegal viewpoint it is clearly essential to establish whether the patient is suffering from an acute fracture attributable to an individual episode of trauma or a delayed or non-union which may be the result of repetitive minor injuries.

Fractures and dislocations of the metatarsophalangeal joints and phalanges
Metatarsophalangeal dislocations
Traumatic dislocations of these joints are much less common than those occurring as a manifestation of degenerative disease. The majority heal well, causing little long-term disability (Heckman 1996).

Interphalangeal dislocations
These injuries are more frequent than metatarsophalangeal dislocation. Reduction is usually easy. In fracture dislocations exact reduction may be unnecessary in the lesser toes but desirable in the hallux (Wilson 1982). There are no long-term results reported in the literature but the overall outcome appears to be good.

Phalangeal fractures
Intra-articular fractures in the hallux should be reduced in order to avoid painful non-union which is an uncommon complication (Heckman 1996). There is no mention in the literature of any significant long-term complications after lesser phalangeal fractures.

Sesamoid fractures
Fracture of the sesamoid is an uncommon injury, which may result from direct trauma, avulsion or repetitive stress. The medial sesamoid is more frequently involved than the lateral and acute fracture must be differentiated from a bipartate bone. The latter is bilateral in 85% and has smooth sclerotic edges. Persistent discomfort may result from this injury and require surgical excision, which is usually curative (Elleby & Marcinko 1985; Heckman 1996).

Traumatic partial amputations of the foot
Millstein et al (1988) reviewed 169 partial amputations of the foot following trauma. Follow-up ranged from 1 to 68 years, with a mean of 16 years (Table 16.13). A total of 118 initial amputations in 113 patients had been retained and the remaining 49 partial amputations were later revised to a Symes or below-knee amputation because the patient was unable to tolerate the partial foot amputation. Revisions were rated good in 43%, fair in 38% and poor in 19%.

The primary amputations were classified as digital, transverse or longitudinal. Transverse amputations were further classified as metatarsophalangeal if all toes were removed, transmetatarsal, Lisfranc or Chopart. Longitudinal amputations were in the sagittal plane and involved resection of either the medial or the lateral side of the foot.

Preservation of length in the foot was unimportant for functional outcome compared with the provision of stable, durable, sensate skin cover preferably from the plantar surface. A fracture proximal to the amputation was associated with a poor result but when internal fixation was employed, the effect was less marked. Patients without skin grafts showed better results and plantar and

Table 16.13 The outcome of 167 partial traumatic amputations of the foot (adapted from Millstein et al 1988). Method of assessment:

- good—same (or similar) employment as before accident; no restriction of function or gait; no ulceration or pain
- fair—change of occupation required; moderate pain; recurrent callosities and shoe modifications; restriction of function
- poor—persistent pain; severe limitation of function and gait; recurrent ulceration; unable to work or had retired prematurely

Initial level of amputation	Number	Revised	Good	Fair	Poor
Digital					
Transverse	34	5 (15%)	14 (41%)	7 (21%)	8 (23%)
Metatarsophalangeal	13	4 (31%)	4 (31%)	5 (38%)	0
Transmetatarsal	54	15 (28%)	11 (20%)	17 (32%)	11 (20%)
Lisfranc	20	5 (25%)	7 (35%)	7 (35%)	1 (5%)
Chopart	23	14 (61%)	6 (26%)	3 (13%)	0
Longitudinal					
Medial	12	6 (50%)	4 (33%)	2 (17%)	0
Lateral	11	0	5 (45%)	4 (36%)	2 (19%)
Total	167	49 (29%)	51 (30%)	45 (27%)	22 (13%)

terminal grafts had significantly fewer good results than dorsal grafts. The use of flap cover was disappointing. Of 10 cases, only two were rated good. Overall, good results were associated with fewer operations; amputation performed sooner after injury (average 2 months vs. 8 months for poor results); and if revision was required to a more proximal level in the foot, this was performed earlier (average 2.5 months vs. 4.4 years).

Failure and re-amputation were associated with a more severe or crushing injury, poor quality of the final soft tissue cover, especially with regard to plantar or terminal skin grafts, infection, late deformity due to non-union or malunion of fractures and incongruity and arthritis of joints. Other factors leading to a poor result included persistent pain in the stump, skin problems such as callosities and ulceration, and unsuitable footwear and orthotic devices.

Patients with a good result returned to work within 9 months of injury. Those with poor results who were able to return to work took 17 months.

Compartment syndrome of the foot

The compartments of the foot are an area of controversy and rapidly expanding knowledge. It was originally believed that the muscles of the foot lay in four separate compartments, medial, lateral, central and interosseous. More recently, studies by Manoli (1990) and Manoli & Weber (1990) have increased the number to nine and this is becoming widely accepted.

The compartments and their contents are:

- Medial containing abductor hallucis and flexor hallucis brevis
- Superficial central containing the lumbrical muscles and flexor digitorum brevis
- Lateral containing flexor digiti minimi brevis and abductor digit minimi
- Abductor containing abductor hallucis
- Four separate compartments containing the interosseous muscles
- Deep central (or calcaneal) containing the quadratus plantae muscle

From a functional viewpoint, the four separate interosseous compartments are sometimes considered as one.

Although the deep posterior compartment is small and contains only one muscle, its importance is that it communicates directly with the deep posterior compartment of the leg so that it may be secondarily involved. Furthermore, it contains the posterior tibial neurovascular bundle.

Compartment syndromes are usually caused by crushing injury, where the prevalence has been reported as being as high as 27% (Myerson et al 1994). In these cases there is frequently massive swelling and the diagnosis is obvious provided that the surgeon is aware of the possibility of compartment syndrome. In other cases, however, the diagnosis may be considerably more subtle and indeed only one compartment may be involved (Myerson & Berger 1995). The incidence following calcaneal fracture has been reported as 7% and in these cases the deep posterior compartment is mainly affected. Silas et al (1995) have reported compartment syndrome of the foot in children following crushing injuries. In the younger children there were no bone injuries. Early fasciotomy was undertaken and closure without skin grafting was possible at 5 days. Good or excellent results were achieved in all cases.

In adult patients, the outcome of a compartment syndrome when decompressed acutely is probably not as favourable as in a child. When, as is frequently the case, there is some delay in diagnosis, some muscle damage with consequent fibrosis is usual. Continuing disability will occur due to clawing of the toes and contracture and, where skin grafting has been required, the poor quality of the soft tissues. These problems may cause significant functional limitation.

Crushing injury of the foot

This devastating injury occurs commonly, especially in blue collar workers. In assessing the injury and its outcome, the foot must be viewed as a whole and the individual fractures may not be particularly important. The long-term outcome will depend on the extent of the initial injury, the adequacy of initial treatment and the extent to which it has been possible to restore anatomic alignment to the foot (Heckman 1996). The foot will probably be permanently substandard and this may have significant implications for working ability.

Injuries of the foot in children
Introduction

There are a number of differences between fractures of the foot in children and in adults. These include the possibility of growth plate damage giving rise to progressive late deformity and difference in fracture types, due presumably to a combination of the difference in bone strength

between adults and children and differences in the trauma experienced. Furthermore, children seem to have a remarkable ability to recover from an injury which in an adult might cause serious long-term disability, possibly due in part to bony growth and remodelling. Significant fractures of the foot probably occur less frequently in children than in adults and the long-term outcome is not always well described. Where the literature is sufficiently comprehensive to give a separate account of a childhood fracture it is included here. For those fractures which are not covered separately, the long-term prognosis is likely to be similar to that for the fracture in an adult, with the provisos given above.

Fractures of the calcaneus

In contrast to the adult situation, extra-articular fractures of the calcaneus are more common than intra-articular fractures in children (Schmidt & Weiner 1982; Schanz & Rasmussen 1987). Of a total of 133 cases, 63% were extra-articular and 37% intra-articular.

Extra-articular fractures seem to do well regardless of treatment, with the possible exception of fractures of the anterior process. The anterior process appears radiographically at about 10 years and is usually injured by plantarflexion and inversion, being avulsed by the bifurcate ligament. The distal part of the fracture fragment involves the calcaneo-cuboid joint. Degan et al (1982) reported 25 patients with fractures of the anterior process of the calcaneus. Eighteen healed with non-operative management and became asymptomatic, while seven patients underwent excision of the fracture fragment for treatment of non-union and pain. The injury was often missed initially and was associated with a prolonged period of disability (Backman & Johnson 1953) if the fragment was large, when open reduction and internal fixation might be required.

Schanz & Rasmussen (1986) examined the prognosis of displaced intra-articular fractures in children. They reported on 15 cases treated conservatively initially with no attempt to improve the position of the fracture at an average of 12 years after injury. No patient had any functional limitation. Nine had slight inconvenience and deformity as a result of their injury. All had heel broadening and reduction of Bohler's angle on X-ray. The authors concluded that the prognosis in children was better than in adults. Wiley & Profitt (1984) reviewed 34 calcaneal fractures treated conservatively in 32 children after an average follow-up of 33 months and found a favourable outcome, although three of 20 cases did report mild symptoms. Schmidt & Weiner (1982) concluded that calcaneal fractures treated conservatively had a benign prognosis in children. Thomas

(1969) reported on five children with calcaneal fractures, all of whom had a satisfactory clinical result. In four cases, there was some loss of Bohler's angle, indicating displacement and 'depression' of the particular surface of the posterior facet of the subtalar joint. However, the inferior articular facet of the talus appeared to remodel the subtalar joint in order to restore its exact congruity, so producing an excellent result despite some initial residual subtalar joint mal-alignment. The extent of this remodelling will clearly depend on the patient's age. Marti (1980) suggested that displaced intra-articular fractures of the calcaneus should be reduced and internally fixed. The three patients described by him were 12–15 years of age and it seems likely that a greater degree of displacement may be tolerated in a younger child.

Ogden (1987) mentioned the possibility of growth arrest and subtalar arthritis as potential complications of calcaneal fractures in children. There is no evidence in the orthopaedic literature to suggest that these complications occur commonly, however.

Matteri & Frymoyer (1973) reported on three infants aged 16–30 months and found minimal disability in comparison to the adult situation; however, their follow-up was relatively short.

Fractures of the talus

Gross (1984) described avascular necrosis as the most significant complication of a fracture of the talus in a child and prognosis probably depends on the location of the fracture line and the degree of displacement (Marti 1980), with undisplaced fractures having a better prognosis. However, Letts & Gibeault (1980) reported three cases of avascular necrosis in 12 children with undisplaced fractures of the talar neck and Canale & Kelly (1978) described two similar cases in a group of five children. These figures suggest a 28% incidence of avascular necrosis in Hawkins type I fractures of the neck of the talus in children, which is similar to that quoted by Linhart & Höllwarth (1985). This is higher than the incidence in similar fractures in adults (see Table 16.2). In contrast, none of 11 patients with undisplaced talar neck fractures reported by Jensen et al (1994) developed avascular necrosis. Of the three children reported by Letts & Gibeault (1980) who developed avascular necrosis, two were under 2 years of age. Both of these children developed flattening of the talus with marked ankle stiffness. Overall, some degree of remodelling appears to be possible, particularly in younger patients who may achieve an acceptable long-term result despite initial residual displacement (Gross 1984).

Mid-tarsal injuries

Gross (1984) pointed out that isolated fractures of the mid-foot were extremely uncommon in children, and that when they occurred were usually uncomplicated. Richards et al (1984) described fracture of a calcaneo-navicular bar in a tarsal coalition; Ogden (1987) cited recurrent pain as a possible complication of this rare injury.

Tarsometatarsal joint injuries

Wiley (1981) described 18 children under 16 years of age who had sufferred tarsometatarsal joint injuries. Seven required manipulation. Complications were relatively uncommon. After a relatively short follow-up of 8–12 months four had minor residual symptoms

Metatarsal fractures

Fractures of the metatarsal shaft and neck are common in children (Gross 1984) and generally heal well with no long-term sequelae. When metatarsal fractures occur as a result of crushing injuries, complications are more likely to arise from the soft tissue and vascular injury rather than the bony injury.

Avulsion fractures of the base of the fifth metatarsal are relatively common in children, but they should be differentiated from the Jones fracture. Ogden (1987) described non-union as a possible complication of these injuries. No figures are available on the incidence of this potential complication in children.

Crush injury of the foot

A crushed or mangled foot is a common injury in a child and is often caused by a lawnmower. These injuries, as in adults, often result in long-term symptoms, and premature physeal closure, particularly of the first metatarsal, may occur (Gross 1984; Ogden 1987).

■ References

Aitken A P, Poulson D 1963 Dislocations of the tarsometatarsal joint. Journal of Bone and Joint Surgery 45A: 246–260

Angermann P, Jensen P 1989 Osteochondritis dissecans of the talus: long-term results of surgical treatment. Foot and ankle 10: 161–163

Arntz C T, Hansen S T 1987 Dislocations and fracture–dislocations of the tarsometatarsal joints. Orthopedic Clinics of North America 18: 105 114

Backman S, Johnson S R 1953 Torsion of the foot causing fracture of the anterior calcaneal process. Acta Scandinavica Chirurgica 105: 460–466

Benirschke S K, Sangeorzan B J 1993 Extensive intra-articular fractures of the foot. Surgical management of calcaneal fractures. Clinical Orthopaedic Rel Res 292: 128–134

Berndt A L, Harty M 1959 Transchondral fractures of the talus. Journal of Bone and Joint Surgery 41A: 988–1020

Bezes H, Massart P, Delvaux D, Fourquet J P, Tazi F 1993 The operative treatment of intra-articular calcaneal fractures. Clinical Orthopaedic Rel Res 290: 55–59

Bohler L 1931 Diagnosis, pathology, and treatment of fractures of the os calcis. Journal of Bone and Joint Surgery 13: 75–89

Black K P, Ehlert K J 1994 A stress fracture of the lateral process of the talus in a runner. A case report. Journal of Bone and Joint Surgery 60A: 441–443

Brunet I A, Wiley J J 1987 The late results of tarsometatarsal joint injuries. Journal of Bone and Joint Surgery 69B: 437–440

Buckingham W W 1973 Sub-talar dislocation of the foot. Journal of Trauma 64A: 753–756

Buckley R E, Meek R N 1992 Comparison of open versus closed reduction of intraarticular calcaneal fractures. A matched cohort study in workmen. Journal of Orthopaedic Trauma 6: 216–222

Canale S T, Belding R H 1980 Osteochondral lesions of the talus. Journal of Bone and Joint Surgery (Am) 62A: 97–102

Canale S T, Kelly F B 1978 Fractures of the neck of the talus: long term evaluation of 71 cases. Journal of Bone and Joint Surgery (Am) 60A: 143–156

Carey E J, Lance E M, Wade P A 1965 Extra articular fractures of the os calcis. Journal of Trauma 5: 362–372

Cave E F 1963 Fractures of the os calcis. The problem in general. Clinical Orthopaedic Rel Res 30: 64–66

Cedell C A 1974 Rupture of the posterior talar tibiali ligament with the avulsion of a bone fragment from the talus. Acta Orthopaedica Scandinavica 45: 454–461

Christensen S B, Lorentzen J E, Krogsoe O, Sneppen O 1977 Subtalar dislocation. Acta Orthopaedica Scandinavica 48: 707–711

Coltart W D 1952 Aviator's astragalus. Journal of Bone and Joint Surgery 34B: 545–567

Comfort T H, Behrens F, Gaither D W, Denis F, Sigmond M 1985 Long term results of talar neck fractures. Clinical Orthopaedic Rel Res 199: 81–87

Cotton F J, Wilson L T 1908 Fractures of the os calcis. Boston Medical and Surgical Journal 159: 559–565

Crosby L A, Fitzgibbon T 1990 Computerised tomography scanning of acute intra-articular fractures of the calcaneus: a new classification system. Journal of Bone and Joint Surgery (Am) 72A: 852–859

Dameron T B 1975 Fractures and anatomical variations of the proximal portion of the fifth metatarsal. Journal of Bone and Joint Surgery (Am) 57A: 788–792

Davidson A M, Steele H D, MacKenzie D A 1967 A review of twenty-one cases of transchondral fracture of the talus. Journal of Trauma 7: 378–413

Degan T J, Morrey B F, Braun D P 1982 Surgical excision for anterior process fractures of the calcaneus. Journal of Bone and Joint Surgery (Am) 64A: 519–524

Delee J C, Curtis R 1982 Subtalar dislocation of the foot. Journal of Bone and Joint Surgery (Am) 64A: 433–437

Delee J C, Evans J P, Julian J 1983 Stress fracture of the fifth metatarsal. American Journal of Medicine Sports 11: 349–353

Dettenbeck L C, Kelly P J 1969 Total dislocation of the talus. Journal of Bone and Joint Surgery (Am) 51A: 283–288

Dunn W A 1974 Peritalar dislocation. Orthopedic Clinics of North America 5: 7–17

Eastwood D M, Gregg P J, Atkins R M 1993 Intra-articular fractures of the calcaneum: Part I. Pathological anatomy and classification. Journal of Bone and Joint Surgery 75B: 183–188

Eastwood D M, Langmaher V G, Atkins R M 1993 Intra-articular fractures of the calcaneum: Part II. Open reduction and internal fixation by the extended lateral transcalcaneal approach. Journal of Bone and Joint Surgery 75B: 189–195

Eastwood D M, Maxwell-Armstrong C A, Atkins R M 1993 Fracture of the lateral malleolus with talar tilt. Primarily a calcaneal fracture *not* an ankle injury. Injury 24: 109–112

Eichenholtz S N, Levine D B 1964 Fractures of the tarsal navicular bone. Clinical Orthopaedic Rel Res 4: 142–157

Elleby D H, Marcinko D E 1985 Digital fractures and dislocations. Clinics in Podiatry 2: 233–245

Essex-Lopresti P 1952 The mechanism, reduction technique and results in fractures of the os calcis. British Journal of Surgery 39: 395–419

Freeman B J, Duff S, Atkins R M 1998 The extended lateral approach to the hindfoot. Anatomical basis and surgical implications. Journal of Bone and Joint Surgery 80: 139–142

Gould N, Trevino S 1981 Sural nerve entrapment by avulsion fracture of the base of the fifth metatarsal bone. Foot and Ankle 2: 153–155

Grantham S A 1964 Medial sub-talar dislocation. Five cases with a common aetiology. Journal of Trauma 2: 845–849

Greenberg M J, Sheehan J J 1980 Vertical fracture dislocation of the tarsal navicular. Orthopaedics 3: 254–255

Grob D, Simpson L A, Weber B G, Bray T 1985 Operative treatment of displaced talus fractures. Clinical Orthopaedics 199: 88–96

Grogan D P, Walling A K, Ogden J A 1990 Anatomy of the os trigonum. Journal of Paediatric Orthopaedics 10: 618–622

Gross R H 1984 Fractures and dislocations of the foot. In: Rockwood C A, Wilkins W E, King R E (eds) Fractures in children, vol 3. J B Lippincott, Philadelphia

Hardcastle P H, Reschauer R, Kutscha-Lissberg E, Schoffman W 1982 Injuries to the tarsometatarsal joint. Journal of Bone and Joint Surgery 64B: 349–356

Hawkins L G 1965 Fracture of the lateral process of the talus: a review of 13 cases. Journal of Bone and Joint Surgery 47A: 1170–1175

Hawkins L G 1970 Fractures of the neck of the talus. Journal of Bone and Joint Surgery 52A: 991–1002

Heckman J D 1996 Fractures and dislocations of the foot. In: Rockwood C A, Green D P (eds) Fractures in adults, vol 11. J B Lippincott, Philadelphia. 4th ed.

Heppenstall R B, Farahvar H, Balderston R, Lotke P 1980 Evaluation and management of sub-talar dislocations. Journal of Trauma 20: 494–497

Hillegass R C 1976 Injuries to the mid foot. In: Bateman J E (ed.) Foot science. W B Saunders, Philadelphia

Hunt D D 1970 Compression fracture of the anterior articular surface of the calcaneus. Journal of Bone and Joint Surgery (Am) 52A: 1637–1642

Janzen D L, Connell D G, Munk P L, Buckley R E, Meek R N, Schechter M T 1992 Intra-articular fractures of the calcaneus: value of CT findings in determining prognosis. American Journal of Roentgenology 158: 1271–1274

Jensen I, Wester J U, Rasmussen F, Lindquist S, Schantz K 1994 Prognosis of fracture of the talus in children. Acta Orthopaedica Scandinavica 65: 398–400

Johnson V S 1976 Treatment of fractures of the forefoot in industry. In: Bateman J E (ed.) Foot science. W B Saunders, Philadelphia, pp 257–265

Jones R 1902 Fracture of the base of the fifth metatarsal bone by indirect violence. Annals of Surgery 35: 697–700

Joplin R J 1958 Injuries of the foot. In: Cave C F (ed.) Fractures and other injuries. Year Book Publishers, Chicago

Kavanaugh J H, Brower T D, Mann R V 1978 The Jones fracture revisited. Journal of Bone and Joint Surgery 60A: 776–782

Kenwright J 1993 Fractures of the calcaneum. Journal of Bone and Joint Surgery 75B: 176–177

Kenwright J, Taylor R G 1970 Major injuries of the talus. Journal of Bone and Joint Surgery 52B: 36–48

Kerr P S, Prothero D, Atkins R M 1996 Assessing outcome after calcaneal fracture: a rational scoring system. Injury: 27: 35–39

Key J A, Conwell H E 1956 The management of fractures, dislocations and sprains, 6th ed. C V Mosby, St Louis

Khuns J G 1948 Changes in elastic adipose tissue. Journal of Bone and Joint Surgery 31A: 541–547

Korn R 1942 Der bruch durch das lintere obere drittel des fersenbeines. Achiv far Orthopädische und Unfall-Chirurgie 41: 789

Lancaster S, Horowitz M, Alonso J 1985 Sub-talar dislocation. A prognosticating classification. Orthopaedics 8: 1234–1240

La Tourette G, Perry J, Patzakis M J 1980 Fractures and dislocations of the tarso-metatarsal joint. In: Bateman J E, Trott A W (eds) The foot and ankle. Brian C Decker, New York

Lance E M, Carey K J Jr, Wade P A 1963 Fractures of the os calcis: treatment by early mobilisation. Clinical Orthopaedics 30: 76–90

Larson H W 1957 Sutastragalar dislocation. A follow-up report of eight cases. Acta Chirurgica Scandinavica 113: 380–392

Lawrence S J, Botte M J 1993 Jones' fractures and related fractures of the proximal fifth metatarsal. Foot and Ankle 14: 358–365

Letournel E 1993 Open treatment of calcaneal fractures. Clinical Orthopaedics 290: 60–67

Letts R M, Gibeault D 1980 Fractured talus in children. Foot and Ankle 1: 74–77

Leung K S, Yuen K M, Chen W S 1993 Operative treatment of displaced intra-articular fractures of the calcaneum: medium term results. Journal of Bone and Joint Surgery 75B: 196–201

Lindsay W R N, Dewar F P 1958 Fractures of the os calcis. American Journal of Surgery 95: 555–575

Linhart W E, Höllwarth O N 1985 Talusfrakturen beei Kindern. Unfallchirurg 88: 168–174

Lorentzen J E, Bach Christensen S, Krogsoe O, Sneppen O 1977 Fractures of the neck of the talus. Acta Orthopaedica Scandinavica 48: 115–120

Lowy M 1969 Avulsion fractures of the calcaneus. Journal of Bone and Joint Surgery 51B: 494–497

Main B J, Jowett R L 1975 Injuries of the mid-tarsal joint. Journal of Bone and Joint Surgery 57B: 89–97

Manoli A 1990 Compartment syndromes of the foot: current concepts. Foot and Ankle 10: 340–344

Manoli A, Weber T G 1990 Fasciotomy of the foot: an anatomical study with special reference to release of the calcaneal compartment. Foot and Ankle 10: 267–268

Marti R 1980 Fractures of the talus and calcaneus. In: Weber B G, Brunner C, Freuler F (eds) Treatment of fractures in children and adolescents. Springer-Verlag, New York

Matteri R E, Frymoyer J W 1973 Fracture of the calcaneus in young children. Journal of Bone and Joint Surgery 55A: 1091–1094

McLaughlin H L 1963 Treatment of late complications after os calcis fractures. Clinical Orthopaedics 30: 111–115

Melcher G, Degonda F, Leutenegger A, Ruedi T 1995 Ten-year follow-up after operative treatment for intra-articular fractures of the calcaneus. Journal of Trauma 38: 713–716

Millstein S G, McCowan S A, Hunter G A 1988 Traumatic partial foot amputation in adults: a long term review. Journal of Bone and Joint Surgery 70B: 251–254

Monsey R D, Levine B P, Trevino S G, Kristiansen T K 1995 Operative treatment of acute displaced intra-articular calcaneus fractures. Foot and Ankle International 16: 57–63

Monson S T, Ryan J R 1981 Subtalar dislocation. Journal of Bone and Joint Surgery 63A: 1156–1158

Motto S G 1993 Stress fracture of the lateral process of the talus. A case report. British Journal of Sports Medicine 27: 275–276

Mukherjee S K, Pringle P M, Baxter A D 1974 Fracture of the lateral process of the talus: a report of 13 cases. Journal of Bone and Joint Surgery 56B: 263–273

Mutschler W, Mittlemeier T, Bauer G 1993 Operative treatment of intra-articular fractures of the calcaneus. Orthopaedics International 1(4): 297–305

Myerson M, Quill G E 1993 Late complications of fractures of the calcaneus. Journal of Bone and Joint Surgery 75A: 331–341

Myerson M S, Berger B 1995 Isolated medial compartment syndrome of the foot. Foot and Ankle International 17: 183–185

Myerson M S, Fisher R T, Burgess A R, Kenzora J E 1986 Fracture dislocation of the tarsometatarsal joints: end results correlated with pathology and treatment. Foot and Ankle 6: 225–242

Myerson M S, McGarvey W C, Henderson M R, Hakim J 1994 Morbidity after crush injuries to the foot. Journal of Orthopaedic Trauma 8: 343–349

Nade S, Monahan P R W 1973 Fractures of the calcaneum. A study of the long term prognosis. Injury 14: 200–207

National Safety Council 1972 Accident facts, cited in: Kleiger B, Work-related injury of the foot and ankle. In: J E Bateman (ed.) Foot Science. W B Saunders, Philadelphia, pp 254–256

Newberg A H 1979 Osteochondral fractures of the dome of the talus. British Journal of Radiology 52: 105–109

Nicholas R, Hadley J, Paul C, James P 1994 Snowboarders fracture: fracture of the lateral process of the talus. Journal of American Board of Family Practitioners 7: 130–133

Norgrove Penny J, Davis L A 1980 Fractures and dislocations of the neck of the talus. Journal of Trauma 20: 1029–1037

O'Farrell D A, O'Byrhe J M, McCabe J P, Stephens M M 1993 Fracture of the os calcis: improved results with internal fixation. Injury 24: 263–265

O'Farrell T A, Costello B G 1982 Osteochondritis dissecans of the talus: late results of surgical treatment. Journal of Bone and Joint Surgery 64B: 494–497

Ogden J A 1987 Pocket guide to paediatric fractures. Williams & Wilkins, Baltimore

Paley D, Hall H 1993 Intra-articular fractures of the calcaneus: a critical analysis of results and prognostic factors. Journal of Bone and Joint Surgery 75A: 342–354

Peterson L, Goldie I F, Irstam L 1977 Fractures of the neck of the talus: a clinical study. Acta Orthopaedica Scandinavica 48: 696–706

Pettine K A, Morrey B F 1987 Osteochondral fractures of the talus: a long term follow up. Journal of Bone and Joint Surgery 69B: 89–92

Pozo I L, Kirwan E O'G, Jackson A M 1984 The long term results of conservative management of severely displaced fractures of the calcaneus. Journal of Bone and Joint Surgery 66B: 386–390

Pritsch M, Horoshouski H, Farine I 1986 Arthroscopic treatment of osteochondral lesions of the talus. Journal of Bone and Joint Surgery 68A: 862–865

Quenu E, Kuss G 1909 Etude sur les luxations du metatarse. Revue Chirurgicale 39: 231–336, 720–791, 1093–1134

Richards R R, Evans J G, McGoey P F 1984 Fracture of a calcaneo-navicular bar: a complication of tarsal coalition. Clinical Orthopaedics 185: 220–221

Richli W R, Rosenthal D J 1984 Avulsion fracture of the fifth metatarsal: experimental study of pathomechanics. AJR 143: 889–891

Rowe C R, Sakellarides H T, Fasman P A, Sorbie C 1963 Fractures of the os calcis: a long term follow up study of 146 patients. Journal of the American Medical Association 184: 920–923

Sanders R P, Fortin 1993 'Operative treatment in 120 displaced intraarticular calcaneal fractures. Results using a prognostic computed tomography scan classification.' Clinical Orthopaedics 290: 87–95

Sangeorzan B J, Benirschke S K, Mosca V V, Mayo K A, Hansen S T 1989 Displaced intra-articular fractures of the tarsal navicular. Journal of Bone and Joint Surgery 71A: 1504–1510

Schanz K, Rasmussen F 1986 The prognosis of displaced intra-articular fractures of the calcaneus in children. Acta Orthopaedica Scandinavica 57: 471

Schanz K, Rasmussen F 1987 Calcaneal fractures in the child. Acta Orthopaedica Scandinavica 58: 504–506

Schmidt T L, Weiner D S 1982 Calcaneal fractures in children: an evaluation of the nature of the injury in 56 children. Clinical Orthopaedics 171: 150–155

Silas S I, Herzenberg J, Myerson M S, Sponsellor P 1995 Compartment syndrome of the foot in children. Journal of Bone and Joint Surgery 77A: 356–371

Smith H 1937 Subastragalar dislocation. A report of seven cases. Journal of Bone and Joint Surgery 10: 373–380

Sneppen O, Bach Christensen S, Krogsoe O, Lorentzen J 1977 Fractures of the body of the talus. Acta Orthopaedica Scandinavica 48: 317–324

Spector F C, Karlin J M, Scurran B L, Silvani S L 1984 Lesser metatarsal fractures: incidence, management and review. Journal of the American Podiatry Association 74: 259–264

Squires B, Atkins R M 2000 Tuberosity fractures of the calcaneum. Journal of Bone and Joint Surgery (in press)

Stephenson J R 1993 Surgical treatment of displaced intra-articular fractures of the calcaneus. A combined lateral and medial approach. Clinical Orthopaedic Rel Res 290: 68–75

Stephenson J R 1987 Treatment of displaced intra-articular fractures of the calcaneum using medial and lateral approaches, internal fixation and early motion. Journal of Bone and Joint Surgery 69A: 115–130

Szyszkowitz R, Reschauer R, Seggi W 1985 Eighty-five talus fractures treated by ORIF with 5 to 8 years of follow up: study of 69 patients. Clinical Orthopaedics 199: 97–107

Thomas H M 1969 Calcaneal fracture in childhood. British Journal of Surgery 56: 664–666

Thordarson D B, Krieger L E 1996 Operative vs. nonoperative treatment of intra-articular fractures of the calcaneus: a prospective randomized trial. Foot and Ankle International 17: 2–9

Thoren O 1964 Os calcis fractures. Acta Orthopaedica Scandinavica (suppl) 70: 1–116

Tile M 1987 Fractures of the talus. In: Schatzker J, Tile M (eds) The rationale of operative fracture care. Springer-Verlag, Berlin

Torg J S, Baldvinis F C, Zelko R R, Pavlov H, Pet T C, Das M 1984 Fractures of the base of the fifth metatarsal distal to the tuberosity. Journal of Bone and Joint Surgery 66A: 209–214

Van Buecken K, Barrack R L, Alexander A H et al 1989 Arthroscopic treatment of transchondral talar dome fractures. American Journal of Sports Medicine 17: 350–356

Vestad E 1968 Fractures of the calcaneum: open reduction and bone grafting. Acta Chirurgica Scandinavica 134: 617–625

Weber B G, Bruner C, Freuler F 1980 Treatment of fractures in children and adolescents. Springer-Verlag, New York, p 375

Wiley J J 1981 Tarso-metatarsal joint injuries in children. Journal of Pediatric Orthopedics 1: 255–260

Wiley J J, Profitt A 1984 Fractures of the os calcis in children. Clinical Orthopaedics 188: 131–138

Wilpulla E 1973 Tarso-metatarsal fracture-dislocation. Acta Orthopaedica Scandinavica 44: 335–345

Wilson D W 1972 Injuries of the tarsometatarsal joints. Journal of Bone and Joint Surgery 54B: 677–686

Wilson D W 1982 Fractures of the foot. In: Klenerman L (ed.) The foot and its disorders. Blackwell, Oxford

Zwipp H, Tscherne H, Thermann H, Weber T 1993 Osteosynthesis of displaced intraarticular fractures of the calcaneus. Clinical Orthopaedics 290: 76–86

Section 4

Results following fractures of the axial skeleton

Chapter 17

The pelvis
Michael A. Foy

Introduction

A satisfactory classification of pelvic fracture patterns is fundamental to any attempt to interpret complications and long-term results. Generally, pelvic fractures may be classified into stable and unstable types. The Pennal classification (Pennal & Sutherland 1961, Pennal et al 1980) was an important contribution to a logical understanding of pelvic fractures. It utilised easily reproducible X-ray views (such as a standard anteroposterior view of the pelvis, a pelvic inlet view and a pelvic outlet view at 90° to the inlet view).

This classification has been modified by Tile (1984, 1988) as shown in Table 17.1. Tile made the point that there was a spectrum of stability, and if the anteroposterior or lateral compression force was of sufficient severity, then the posterior sacroiliac ligamentous complex may be disrupted, resulting in an unstable situation. Macdonald (1980) pointed out that pelvic ring distortion at the time of impact may be gross, but some pelvic injuries (particularly symphysis pubis and sacroiliac injuries) may spontaneously reduce during transfer of the patient to hospital, and the severity of the original injury may not be appreciated on X-ray assessment. These factors cause difficulties in assessing the severity of pelvic injuries and hence predicting prognosis.

Tile's modification of the Pennal classification combines two interrelated factors; namely, stability and direction of the injuring forces. A brief look at the fracture patterns which follow these injury mechanisms may help in relating them to prognosis. For a detailed interpretation of fracture patterns the reader is referred to Tile (1984).

Anteroposterior compression

There are two typical injuries which follow anteroposterior compression:

- the open-book disruption (Fig. 17.1)
- the isolated four-rami (straddle or butterfly) fracture (Fig. 17.2)

The degree of symphyseal separation in open-book disruptions may be divided into those with less than 2.5 cm (Tile's stage I) and those with more than 2.5 cm (Tile's stage II). If the anteroposterior compression force contains

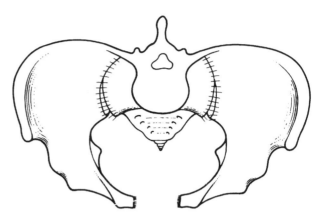

Fig. 17.1 The open-book disruption.

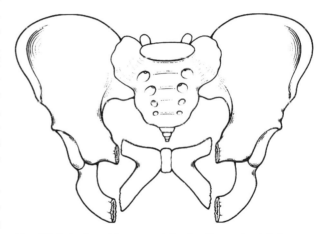

Fig. 17.2 Isolated four-rami (butterfly or straddle) fracture.

a shearing element then the posterior ligaments may be disrupted, resulting in a vertically unstable fracture.

Four-rami fractures may also result from a lateral compression or vertical shearing force; Tile believed that this was a more common cause.

Lateral compression

A lateral compression force may cause several types of injury. Most will be stable, because the lateral compression force causes impaction of the posterior pelvic complex, leaving the posterior ligaments intact. The common injury patterns are:

Table 17.1 Classification of pelvic ring disruption (after Tile 1988)

Type A: stable		
	A1	Fractures of the pelvis not involving the pelvic ring
	A2	Stable, minimally displaced fractures of the pelvic ring
Type B: rotationally unstable, vertically stable		
	B1	Anteroposterior compression (open-book)
	B2	Lateral compression (ipsilateral)
	B3	Lateral compression (contralateral)
Type C: rotationally and vertically unstable (Malgaigne)		
	C1	Unilateral
	C2	Bilateral
	C3	Associated with acetabular fracture

- ipsilateral anterior and posterior injury (Fig. 17.3)
- contralateral (bucket handle) type (Fig. 17.4)

In the ipsilateral injury there may be fractures of the public rami or a locked symphysis anteriorly. In the contralateral injury the lateral compressive force is combined with a rotatory element and the anterior injury is combined with a posterior lesion on the opposite side.

Vertical shear

This fracture pattern was originally described by Malgaigne (1855) and consists of two vertical fractures, separating at one side of the pelvis and a middle fragment comprising the hip joint as shown in Fig. 17.5. The anterior lesion involves either both pubic rami or the pubic symphysis and is associated with massive disruption through the sacrum, ilium or the sacroiliac joint. This fracture is always grossly unstable in both rotational and vertical planes.

In summary, two important considerations affect the long-term results of these fractures:

- the degree of displacement and hence instability within the pelvic ring
- the associated injuries caused by the pelvic disruption, which may in themselves have predictable complication rates—these will be discussed later

The role of computerised tomographic (CT) scanning in the evaluation of major pelvic injuries has been described by Gill & Bucholz (1984) and Dalinka et al (1985). CT has an important role in the definition of the anatomy of the fracture.

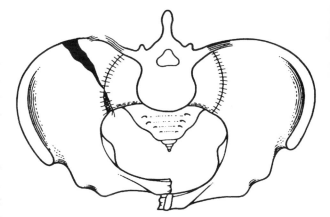

Fig. 17.3 Lateral compression injury: ipsilateral pattern.

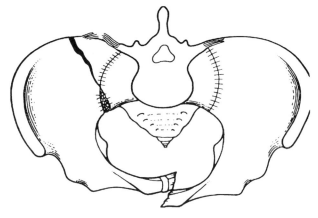

Fig. 17.4 Lateral compression injury: contralateral pattern.

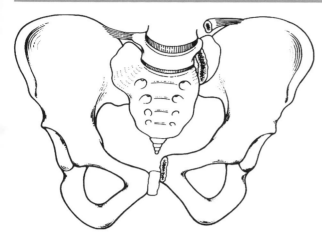

Fig. 17.5 The vertical shear pattern as described by Malgaigne (1855).

One further point concerns attitudes to the treatment of displaced pelvic fractures. Noland & Conwell (1930) reported that excellent functional results were frequent in cases in which a good anatomical position was not achieved. More recently, Watson Jones (1962) commented that excellent results were often found even when considerable displacement persisted. However, Letournel (1978) and Bucholz (1981) stated that the accuracy of reduction of major fracture dislocations of the hemipelvis appeared to be of central importance in the avoidance of late disability from these injuries. Certainly there is a trend at the present time, as with many other fractures, towards accurate reduction and stabilisation of pelvic fractures. In the assessment of sequelae of displaced fractures, the accuracy of reduction will be taken into account whenever possible.

Stable pelvic fractures

The surgeon is likely to be confronted either by a patient who has a clearly definable fracture pattern for which a prognosis is sought, or by a problem the future outlook of which is in question. Therefore the principal mechanisms of injury will be considered first, in this and the next two sections, followed by a discussion of specific complications.

Stable fractures of the pubic rami

The work of Gertzbein & Chenoweth (1980) demonstrated, using ^{99m}Tc methylene diphosphonate bone scans, that even in apparently isolated fractures of the pubic ramus there was disruption elsewhere in the pubic ring, usually in the acetabulum or sacroiliac regions. This probably explains the discomfort that patients with pubic

rami fractures experience in the hip and low back. This work shows that there is more to these simple, stable fractures than is at first apparent.

In 207 cases of 'isolated' pubic rami fractures reported by Peltier (1965), Dunn & Morris (1968) and Connolly & Hedberg (1969), only one long-term complication was reported—a non-union of two undisplaced pubic rami fractures. Connolly & Hedberg reported one urinary tract injury in their series of 82 unilateral pubic rami fractures, but the precise nature of the injury is not indicated. Levine & Crampton (1963), in a series which included 251 patients with pubic rami fractures, both stable and unstable, reported two cases of bladder rupture where only three pubic rami were fractured. Stress fractures of the pubic rami have been reported by Pavlov et al (1982) and Meurman (1980), and sporadically by other authors. Pavlov et al reported 12 cases, all of which occurred in the inferior pubic ramus near to the pubic symphysis. There were two complications, namely delayed union and refracture. Both of these problems occurred in patients who continued running despite pain and the fracture eventually healed after a period of rest.

Iliac wing fractures

In the reports of Peltier (1965), Dunn & Morris (1968) and Connolly & Hedberg (1969), there were 32 iliac wing fractures in a total of 497 pelvic fractures, giving an overall incidence of 6.5%. These fractures cause lower abdominal tenderness and rigidity, making exclusion of intra-abdominal injury difficult. There is no report of any significant long-term disability from this injury.

Summary

- Stable fractures and stress fractures of the pubic rami are rarely associated with long-term disability.
- Iliac wing fractures are not usually associated with long-term disability.

Rotationally stable/vertically unstable pelvic fractures

Anteroposterior compression fractures

The work of Peltier (1965), Dunn & Morris (1968) and Tile (1984) suggested an incidence of 18% for these injuries (90 of 497 pelvic fractures). This excludes avulsion injuries, acetabular fractures and pathological fractures (Figs 17.1 and 17.2).

Tile, in his series of 248 pelvic fractures, carried out the most careful and well-documented assessment of the results in the literature, and to a large extent we must be guided by these results. Tile's results were tabulated by a point system heavily weighted towards pain, with lesser scores for malunion, leg length discrepancy and non-union. Of 29 patients in Tile's series with anteroposterior compression injuries, 17 (59%) were free of pain and 11 (38%) had moderate pain, while one (3%) had severe pain. The mean follow-up was 45 months in these patients. The results were not broken down into types of symphyseal disruption or to identify isolated straddle fractures.

Tile (1984) pointed out that even in stage I injuries (i.e. less than 2.5 cm of separation of the symphysis pubis) there may be prolonged and significant pain and tenderness in the region of the pubic symphysis. Holdsworth (1945) reported that symphyseal pain often took up to 2 years to settle completely. Sarkin (1976) reported, at the South African Orthopaedic Association, 79 cases of symphyseal separation in black Africans. These patients were treated by 6 weeks of non-weight bearing. He found no permanent disability. Dunn & Morris (1968) described treatment of six cases in a pelvic sling. The patients were subsequently mobilised between 5 and 6 weeks from injury; two redisplaced, leading to persistent sacroiliac discomfort. Dunn & Morris also described 10 patients with straddle fractures who were treated conservatively; none of these patients suffered permanent disability.

Madsden et al (1983) reported a series of obstetric patients with a history of pelvic fracture. Of the three patients who developed problems, attributable to their pelvic injury during confinement, two were due to redisplacement of the pubic symphysis. This is an important consideration when preparing medico-legal reports on the prognosis of symphyseal disruptions in women of child-bearing age.

The differences in the reported results of anteroposterior compression injuries are difficult to explain. All the patients reported by Tile (1984) were involved in major high-energy injuries. The results in Tile's patients are comprehensive in that all patients were interviewed, examined and X-rayed at follow-up review. The incidence of post-injury pain in these patients has already been mentioned, and the overall incidence of satisfactory results was 21 of 29 (72%), with eight of 29 (28%) unsatisfactory results.

Lateral compression fractures

A lateral compression force causes marked inward rotation of the affected side of the pelvis (Figs 17.3 and 17.4). Many of these injuries leave the posterior ligaments intact and are vertically stable.

Tile's 1984 figures suggest that this is the most common type of pelvic injury mechanism. Other series fail to recog-

nise clearly and categorise this mechanism of injury and their figures are therefore difficult to interpret. Tile classified 183 (75%) of the pelvic fractures as lateral compression injuries. According to his rigorous criteria, 132 (72%) of these cases achieved a satisfactory result, while 51 (28%) had an unsatisfactory result. Tile looked specifically at pain following lateral compression injuries and found that 64% had no pain at all, 33% had moderate pain and 3% had severe pain.

Summary

- Anteroposterior compression injuries are associated with persisting moderate or severe pain in approximately 40% of patients. The overall incidence of unsatisfactory results is approximately 28%.
- Lateral compression injuries are associated with persisting moderate or severe pain in approximately 36% of patients. The overall incidence of unsatisfactory results is approximately 28%.

Rotationally and vertically unstable pelvic fractures (Malgaigne fractures)

The double vertical fractures have received much more attention in the literature than other types of unstable pelvic fracture. A study of the published reports reveals that some of these injuries are in fact severe anteroposterior or lateral compression injuries with associated major posterior disruption leading to vertical instability. However, the end-result in these circumstances is a rotationally and vertically unstable hemipelvic segment and the prognostic implications are the same.

The work of Noland & Conwell (1933), Peltier (1965) and Dunn & Morris (1968) suggested that the incidence of double vertical fractures was 8% in 374 pelvic fractures. Slatis & Huittenen (1972) stated that the incidence of vertical shear fractures was in the region of 20% from their own series and an extensive literature review, while Tile (1984) reported 34 cases in his series of 248 high-energy pelvic fractures—an incidence of 14%. The reason for this apparent disparity is that the report by Slatis & Huittenen included severe anteroposterior and lateral compression injuries with their double vertical fractures.

Slatis & Huittenen (1972) reported on 163 double vertical fractures, with a long-term follow-up on 65. When they considered patients of working age without major complicating injuries, 43% returned to work within 16 weeks, 74% within 24 weeks and 97% within 1 year of the injury.

Karaharju & Slatis (1978) described follow-up on 13 patients with double vertical fractures treated by external fixation using a trapezoid compression frame. The average time for return to work was 5–6 months. The longest period lost from work was 8 months. The authors felt that the incidence of low back pain and impaired gait was reduced by this method of treatment.

Slatis & Huittenen (1972) noted that recovery was more rapid where displacement was minimal; where displacement was present, recovery was related to the nature of the posterior injury. Symptoms resulting from dislocation of the sacroiliac joint took much longer to settle than fractures adjacent to the joint. Follow-up examination (1–7 years after injury) on 65 patients revealed an unexpectedly high incidence of late sequelae. Persistent dislocation of the hemipelvis secondary to unsatisfactory reduction gave rise to a limp, problems with walking and oblique inclination of the pelvis on sitting. Over half of these patients complained of chronic low back pain on the affected side in the region of the sacroiliac joint. There was no disabling pain in the pubic area even with wide separation of the symphysis or displaced pubic rami fractures.

Holdsworth (1945) had earlier reported similar findings in 50 patients with Malgaigne-type unstable fractures. Holdsworth reported a mean follow-up of 5 years and described a satisfactory result as the ability to return to pre-accident work or similar heavy work (in the case of women the ability to return to full household chores). He traced 42 cases and the results are shown in Table 17.2.

These results confirm that the nature of the posterior injury is important in determining the prognosis. Only 44% of patients with sacroiliac dislocations were able to return to heavy work, while 87% of those with fractures adjacent to the sacrum and ilium were able to do so. All patients in this series complained of pubic pain, but in each case it had disappeared 2 years after injury. Holdsworth (1945) appeared to be satisfied with the position achieved after conservative treatment with traction, and weight bearing was delayed for 12 weeks.

Lander (1984) confirmed that posterior disruption of the sacroiliac joint is associated with a poor prognosis. In his series of 31 sacroiliac disruptions treated conservatively, 15 were followed up for a mean period of 5.3 years. Thirteen (87%) complained of persistent low back pain,

three (20%) had to change their occupation, eight (53%) had difficulty with low or hard chairs and three (20%) had difficulty climbing stairs. He concluded that long-term disability follows traumatic sacroiliac disruption.

According to Langloh et al (1972), from a series of 24 double vertical fractures with posterior sacroiliac disruption, improvement may occur up to 12 months after injury and therefore a final prognosis should be deferred until this time.

Tile (1984) found that 14 (41%) of his 34 patients had a satisfactory result, while 20 (59%) had an unsatisfactory result. In terms of pain, 13 (38%) were pain-free while 15 (44%) experienced moderate pain and six (18%) suffered severe pain. Similar results were reported by Semba et al (1983), in a critical analysis of 30 patients with conservatively treated Malgaigne fractures followed for 2–12 years. They found that only 11 (37%) of the patients were symptom-free at follow-up.

Summary

- The most significant indicator of long-term disability is the nature of the posterior injury. Sacroiliac dislocations fare much worse than fractures of the sacrum or ilium.
- Symptoms may improve up to 12 months from injury and a final assessment should not be made before this time.
- Double vertical fractures are associated with persisting moderate or severe pain in approximately 62% of cases. The overall incidence of unsatisfactory results is 59%.

Specific complications

Tile (1984) analysed the factors resulting in unsatisfactory results in his patients. Of 104 such results, the most common factor was unacceptable pain, occurring in 69 (66%). Leg length discrepancy of over 2 cm accounted for nine unsatisfactory results. Permanent nerve damage accounted for 12 unsatisfactory results and urethral symptoms for six. These factors, together with the influence of pelvic fracture on subsequent pregnancy, will be considered in more detail.

Table 17.2 End-results in 42 double vertical fractures (adapted from Holdsworth 1945)

Fracture or dislocation of the pubis with:	Total	Able to return to heavy work	Painful
Sacroiliac joint dislocation	27	12	15
Fracture of the sacrum or ilium adjacent to joint	15	13	2

Neurological complications

Failinger & McGarity (1992) pointed out that neurological injuries were the most 'frequently overlooked' in patients with pelvic fractures. The most comprehensive reviews of the subject were provided by Patterson & Morton (1961) and Huittenen & Slatis (1971). The incidence of neurological complications is unclear. Patterson & Morton found the overall incidence to be 1.2% in a series of 809 pelvic fractures, while Huittenen & Slatis felt that the incidence was 10–12%. Huittenen & Slatis found a much higher incidence in double vertical fractures with 31 of 68 (46%) showing signs of nerve damage. In all cases with neurological injury in both series there was a significant posterior injury, either a fractured sacrum or sacroiliac dislocation.

Patterson & Morton (1961) considered the final results in 10 patients with neurological injury. Six were assessed as good. Since final disability was minimal and their original heavy occupation was resumed. Of the four others, one had persisting incontinence of urine as a result of neurological injury, while the others had poor results. Considering the neurological lesion in isolation, in no patient (even those where the final disability was minimal) did it recover fully. In this series the mean follow-up was 18 months.

Huittenen & Slatis (1971) found that the neurological signs affected all nerve roots from L4 to S5, with L5 and S1 being most commonly involved. Of the 31 cases with evidence of nerve injury 22 had motor signs and 26 had sensory signs; 17 had both motor and sensory signs. The follow-up was 1–5 years and even in those followed up for 5 years the authors found that the nerve lesion had not fully recovered.

Failinger & McGarity (1992) reported that neurological injuries were often missed at the time of the initial assessment and sometimes came to light when the patient failed to progress during rehabilitation. They concluded that 'the overall prognosis of a neurological injury in a patient who has a pelvic fracture is variable and depends on the degree and level of the nerve root involvement. Limited recovery has been reported in most series with frequent persistence of neuralgia and motor, sensory or reflex deficits'.

Summary

- Neurological injuries occur more commonly when there is dislocation of the sacroiliac joint or fracture of the sacrum.
- The prognosis following neurological injury is poor; in no case did the neurological lesion recover completely.

Urological injury and impotence

The urological injuries directly associated with pelvic fracture are rupture of the bladder and rupture of the urethra. Urethral rupture is by far the most serious of these injuries because of the high incidence of serious complications, namely stricture, incontinence and impotence.

The incidence of haematuria following pelvic fractures was 33% based on 623 cases reported by Noland & Conwell (1933), Flaherty et al (1968) and Slatis & Huittenen (1972). The incidence of significant bladder or urethral injury was much less, as shown in Table 17.3. The overall incidence of significant urological injury following pelvic fracture is in the region of 10–15% (Failinger & McGarity 1992).

Table 17.3 The reported incidence of urological injuries in 1158 patients

Reference	Pelvic fractures	Urological injury		
		Bladder ruptures	Urethral ruptures	Bladder and urethral ruptures
Noland & Conwell (1930)	125	22	9	
Levine & Crampton (1963)	425	8	5	1
Peltier (1965)	138	14	4	
Dunn & Morris (1968)	111	8	3	
Slatis & Huittenen (1972)	163	9	4	3
Colapinto (1980)	196	17	10	
Total	1158	78 (6.7%)	35 (3%)	4 (0.3%)

Colapinto (1980) observed in his series of 196 patients that all the urethral ruptures occurred in men. There were 96 female patients in this series, some with severe pelvic fractures, but none sustained a urethral rupture.

Froman & Stein (1967) believed that it was difficult to correlate fracture patterns with urological injury because of the complex forces involved. However, Kaiser & Farrow (1965), Flaherty et al (1968) and, more recently, Mitchell (1984) pointed out that straddle fractures cause over 50% of urethral injuries, while the rest are associated with various patterns of instability.

The incidence of urethral stricture is difficult to predict with any accuracy, because it depends upon precise knowledge of the original injury and on the subsequent management of the injury. Controversy still exists among urologists over the place of early surgery and the role of conservative management in the treatment of urethral ruptures.

However, if the urethra has been completely disrupted, an attempt should be made to re-establish its continuity by formal surgical exploration (Heyes et al 1983, Patterson et al 1983).

Kaiser & Farrow (1965) reported a careful follow-up of 22 cases of rupture of the bladder or urethra caused by pelvic fracture, with a minimum follow-up of 4 years. Of the six patients with a ruptured bladder who survived, the only long-term complication was a bladder calculus which was removed, leading to an uneventful recovery and a transient perineal fistula. These authors treated their urethral ruptures by a modified conservative method of realignment and approximation of the divided urethra, suprapubic catheterisation of the bladder and drainage of the prevesical space. Of the eight cases who survived, seven had complete recovery with no sequelae. One patient developed a fistula and a stricture. Mitchell (1984) pointed out that the outlook for patients with urethral strictures is better today with the use of the optical urethrotome.

The incidence of incontinence following urethral injury is unknown. Incontinence can also be caused by damage to the S2, S3 outflow at the sacral foraminae. Morehouse & MacKinnon (1969) believed that the statistics on incontinence were inadequate, but of 10 patients referred to them for urethroplasty for urethral stricture, seven were incontinent.

Impotence is a source of considerable personal embarrassment to the male patient and also, according to Mitchell (1984), is 'the most severe disability in the eyes of the Court'. Recently, more attention has been paid to this problem in the orthopaedic and urological journals. The incidence of impotence following a pelvic fracture is related to:

- the severity of the urethral injury
- the nature of the pelvic fracture
- the age of the patient

The severity of the urethral injury

King (1975) reported impotence in 13 of 31 cases with urethral injury (43%) and three of 59 cases without urethral injury (5%). King defined impotence as the inability to produce an erection, failure to achieve orgasm, failure to ejaculate and retrograde ejaculation. Similar observations were made by Chambers & Balfour (1963), who followed up 31 patients with pelvic fracture and urological injury; eight of the 17 (47%) with partial or complete rupture of the posterior urethra were permanently impotent. Mark et al (1995) found 57 of 92 patients to have permanent impotence following a pelvic fracture urethral injury.

A very important medico-legal consideration is the incidence and timing of the return of potency. Gibson (1970), in a report of 35 patients with a fractured pelvis with urethral rupture, identified 13 cases of permanent impotence (35%) and eight cases (22%) in which potency returned up to 19 months after injury. A similar experience was reported by Chambers & Balfour (1963): seven of their 31 cases reported loss of potency for 4 months to 4 years, with a mean of 19 months. These findings are summarised in Table 17.4. The figures from King's paper are not included, as duration of follow-up was not specified.

Table 17.4 Incidence of permanent and temporary impotence following urethral injury

Reference	Urethral injury (n)	Permanent impotence (n)	Temporary impotence (n)
Chambers & Balfour (1963)	17	8	7
Gibson (1970)	35	13	8
Mark et al (1995)	92	57	—
Total	144	78 (54%)	15 (28%)

The nature of the pelvic fracture

King (1975) noted that fracture patterns were broadly similar in potent and impotent patients. The major difference was the presence of disruptions of the pubic symphysis in five of the 16 (31%) impotent men, compared with similar disruptions in only 15 of 90 (17%) potent men. Mark et al (1995) found that bilateral pubic rami fractures were associated with a high incidence of impotence. They felt that impotence was due to disruption of the cavernosal nerves lateral to the prostatomembranous urethra behind the symphysis pubis.

The age of the patient

Mitchell (1984) reported that in his series of 23 patients, of those under the age of 30 all but one recovered normal potency; but of those over the age of 30, less than 50% recovered a normal, full and sustained erection.

Summary

- Significant urological injury occurs in approximately 10% of unstable pelvic fractures.
- Permanent impotence occurs in approximately 54% of patients with posterior urethral injury and unstable pelvic fracture.
- Final prognosis on impotence should be withheld for at least 2 years in patients with posterior urethral injury and unstable pelvic fracture, as potency may return in up to 28%.
- Impotence may occur in 5% of patients with unstable pelvic fractures and no urethral injury.

Non-union and delayed union

There are only three reports in the literature concerning non-union of pelvic fractures. Hundley (1966) described 20 cases of symptomatic non-union in 141 pelvic fractures. Pennal & Messiah (1980) reported on 32 cases of established non-union and 10 cases of delayed union in pelvic fractures. Tile (1984) described eight cases of non-union in his series of 248 pelvic fractures. These figures suggest that the incidence of non-union lies between 3 and 14%. Tile pointed out that non-union was more common in double vertical fractures and this was supported by analysis of the figures of both Hundley (1966) and Pennal & Messiah (1980). These showed that 56% of the non- and delayed unions occurred in double vertical fractures, as shown in Table 17.5.

In Pennal & Messiah's 1980 series the average time at diagnosis of delayed union or non-union was 9 months from the time of injury and the most common presenting symptoms were pain and a limp. Of their 42 patients, 18 underwent operation, which consisted of bone grafting and stabilisation in 14, onlay graft in two and excision of bone fragment in two. Their final results are shown in Table 17.6.

Summary

- Non-union and delayed union occur most commonly in double vertical fractures. The overall incidence is 3–14%.
- The best results in terms of functional outcome occurred in patients treated with bone grafting and stabilisation for their non-unions.

Malunion

Tile (1984) considered that minor degrees of malunion causing leg length inequality of less than 1 cm were common after major pelvic disruption. He believed that a smaller number of patients were left with significant malunions with leg length discrepancy of over 2 cm or with major rotational deformities of the pelvis. He quoted an overall incidence of 5%. Malunion is not always associated with pain.

Effect on subsequent pregnancy

When young women sustain unstable pelvic fractures, there are important medico-legal implications of the effect

Table 17.5 The incidence of non-union and delayed union in rotationally and vertically unstable fractures

Reference	Total number of unstable fractures	Total number of non-union and delayed unions	Number of non-unions in rotationally and vertically unstable fractures
Hundley (1966)	141	20	18
Pennal & Messiah (1980)	?	42	17
Total		62	35 (56%)

Table 17.6 The final disability assessment in non-union and delayed union of pelvic fractures (from Pennal & Messiah 1980)

Result	Group	
	Operative	Non-operative
Returned to pre-injury occupation	11	5
Returned to sedentary occupation	7	10
Permanently totally disabled	0	7
Permanently disabled by 50%	0	2
Total	18	24

of the fracture on future confinement. Watson Jones (1962) reported that problems with pregnancy were uncommon, and that even major deformities of the pelvic inlet were not incompatible with natural childbirth. Noland & Conwell (1933) reported one patient out of 44 women who required caesarean section because of impairment of the pelvic outlet.

Madsden et al (1983) have followed up 34 females with pelvic fractures through pregnancy. Ten of the patients had increased or recurrent pain throughout pregnancy; 27 had uncomplicated vaginal deliveries, including 13 patients with displaced pelvic fragments. Of the seven patients with complications, in only three cases could the complications be attributed to the previous pelvic fracture. Two developed re-disruption of the pubic symphysis and one underwent caesarean section because vaginal delivery was felt to be too dangerous.

Summary

- Some 9% of patients (three of 34) suffered complications of childbirth as a result of their pelvic fracture.
- In all, 29% of patients (10 of 34) suffered increased or recurrent pelvic pain during pregnancy.

Other groups

Sacral and coccygeal fractures

Isolated sacral fractures are uncommon. Sacral fractures usually occur as part of a more complex pelvic disruption. Fountain et al (1977) found six isolated sacral fractures in a group of 184 patients admitted with pelvic fractures—an incidence of 3%. All of the fractures involved S1, S2 or S3. All patients had evidence of urinary retention or a decrease in anal tone, or both. Five of the six failed to

improve and underwent sacral laminectomy and decompression. All of these patients improved over a 4–6 month period and no long-term disability was recorded.

It is generally felt that isolated sacral fractures cause no long-term problems; however, Foy (1988) reported on 16 cases with a mean 5.5 year follow-up. Two of these patients required excision of ununited low transverse sacral fractures. Of the remaining 14, only six (36%) were symptom-free; seven (50%) complained of mild or moderately severe pain (sacrodynia) at the site of their fracture and one (7%) complained of severe pain related to the site of the fracture. Two (14%) had evidence of persistent neurological dysfunction. In a report by Hazlett (1980), out of 50 cases of sacral fracture only one case of malunion was reported.

Coccygeal pain may be a source of persistent morbidity. There is often a history of trauma to the sacrococcygeal region. Torok (1974) reported that trauma was responsible in over 70% of the patients. Pyper (1957) reported a history of trauma to the coccyx in 14 of 28 cases (50%). In this group there was evidence of coccygeal fracture in only one case. All of the cases in Pyper's series underwent coccygectomy and 89% showed either marked improvement or complete relief of symptoms. Unfortunately, no study has followed up a group of patients with post-traumatic coccygeal pain to assess the risk of a painful disabling coccydynia.

Summary

- Isolated sacral fractures may give rise to long-term symptoms, particularly pain at the site of the fracture (sacrodynia). This occurred in 57% of 14 patients in one small series.
- The subject of coccydynia and its relationship to trauma remains unclear.

Pelvic fractures in children

The most comprehensive study of this subject was reported by Torode & Zieg (1985). Their specific aim was to determine the incidence of bony complications in children with pelvic fractures, and to formulate a classification bearing some relationship to the final outcome. They described 141 children with ages ranging from 2–17 years. Eleven of their patients died (a mortality rate of 8%), leaving 130 patients available for clinical review. They found the Pennal classification difficult to apply to children and suggested an alternative which essentially differentiated between stable and unstable injuries.

Torode & Zieg recognised an increased incidence of iliac wing fractures in children when compared to adults, there being 18 cases in their series (an incidence of 13%, compared to the incidence of 6.5% reported in adults earlier in this chapter). One patient with an iliac wing fracture also sustained a urethral injury. The authors noted that in the long term, iliac wing fractures—even those associated with injury to the iliac apophysis—did not cause any significant functional problems. Two patients appeared to have delayed ossification of the iliac apophysis, but at follow-up 2 years after the injury there was no significant difference between the two sides.

In their stable group of fractures (68 cases) Torode & Zieg (1985) identified two cases of delayed union of pubic rami fractures (incidence 3%). These fractures subsequently healed 1 year after injury. They noted that, in general, even displaced pubic rami fractures and gross displacement of the pubic symphysis were associated with good healing and no long-term symptoms. The better prognosis for symphyseal disruptions in children was explained in terms of the separation of the bone/cartilage interface and avulsion of a sleeve of periosteum, while in adults there is disruption of the fibrocartilaginous symphysis. Therefore, in the child, healing involves filling in with bone derived from the cartilaginous growth plate and periosteum. Torode & Zieg reported one urethral injury and one bladder injury in this group.

In the children with unstable pelvic fractures (40 patients) there were 13 bony complications (an incidence of 32%). These included eight cases of non-union of the pubic rami, three of premature closure of the triradiate cartilage, malunion of an acetabular fracture and one closure of the sacroiliac joint. There were five urethral injuries and three bladder ruptures in this group. It was not possible to correlate the results following operative and non-operative treatment as only three of the 40 patients underwent operative stabilisation.

Macdonald (1980) reported similar results to Torode & Zieg in a series of 15 displaced pelvic fractures in children.

Follow-up ranged from 6–24 years. Five of the 15 patients (33%) had residual symptoms and significant radiological changes.

Torode & Zieg (1985) reported seven urethral injuries (an incidence of 6%). Mitchell (1984) pointed out that it was particularly difficult to give a prognosis on the future fertility of a boy who sustained a fractured pelvis and a ruptured urethra, there being no long-term follow-up studies to assess potency and fertility in adult life following these injuries. Kelalis et al (1976) described seven boys with urethral rupture who were subsequently all potent; four of the patients had married and three had fathered children.

More recently, Schwarz et al (1998) reviewed 17 patients under the age of 12 with unstable pelvic ring fractures treated non-operatively. They were followed up for 2–25 years. The subjective long-term result depended on the presence or absence of low back pain. This correlated strongly with pelvic asymmetry. They concluded 'healing of an unstable pelvic fracture in malposition with asymmetry causes poor result and must be prevented'.

Summary

- Unstable pelvic fractures in children are associated with a 30–40% incidence of bony complications.
- Pelvic fractures in children are associated with a 6% incidence of urethral injury. The long-term prognosis is unclear, but the work of Mitchell (1984) and Kelalis et al (1987) revealed an optimistic outlook when considering a small number of patients.

References

Bucholz R W 1981 The pathological anatomy of Malgaigne fracture dislocation of the pelvis. Journal of Bone and Joint Surgery 63A: 100–404

Chambers H L, Balfour J 1963 The incidence of impotence following pelvic fractures with associated urinary tract injury. Journal of Urology 89: 702–703

Colapinto V 1980 Trauma to the pelvis; urethral injury. Clinical Orthopaedics 151: 46–55

Connolly W B, Hedberg E A 1969 Observations on fractures of the pelvis. Journal of Trauma 9: 104–111

Dalinka K D, Arger P, Coleman B 1985 CT in pelvic trauma. Orthopedic Clinics of North America 16: 471–480

Dunn A W, Morris H D 1968 Fractures and dislocations of the pelvis. Journal of Bone and Joint Surgery 50A: 1639–1648

Failinger M S, McGarity P L J 1992 Unstable fractures of the pelvic ring. Journal of Bone and Joint Surgery 74A: 781–791

Flaherty J J, Kelley R, Burnett B et al 1968 Relationship of pelvic bone fracture patterns to injuries of the urethra and bladder. Journal of Urology 99: 297–300

Fountain S S, Hamilton R D, Jameson R M 1977 Transverse fractures of the sacrum: a report of 6 cases. Journal of Bone and Joint Surgery 59A: 486–489

Foy M A 1988 Morbidity following isolated fractures of the sacrum. Injury 19: 379–380

Froman C, Stein A 1967 Complicated crushing injuries of the pelvis. Journal of Bone and Joint Surgery 49B: 24–32

Gertzbein S D, Chenoweth D R 1980 Occult injuries of the pelvic ring. Clinical Orthopaedics 151: 202–207

Gibson G R 1970 Impotence following fractured pelvis and ruptured urethra. British Journal of Urology 42: 86–88

Gill K, Bucholz R W 1984 The role of computerised tomographic scanning in the evaluation of major pelvic fractures. Journal of Bone and Joint Surgery 66A: 34–39

Goodwin M A 1959 Myositis ossificans in the region of the hip joint. British Journal of Surgery 46: 547

Hazlett J W 1980 Fractures of the sacrum. Journal of Bone and Joint Surgery 62B: 130–131

Heyes E E, Sandler C M, Corriere J N 1983 Management of the ruptured bladder secondary to blunt abdominal trauma. Journal of Urology 129: 946

Holdsworth F W 1945 Dislocation and fracture-dislocation of the pelvis. Journal of Bone and Joint Surgery 30B: 461–466

Huittenen V M, Slatis P 1971 Nerve injury in double vertical pelvic fractures. Acta Chirurgica Scandinavica 138: 571–575

Hundley J M 1966 Ununited unstable fractures of the pelvis. Journal of Bone and Joint Surgery 48A: 1025

Kaiser T F, Farrow F C 1965 Injury of the bladder and prostatomembranous urethra associated with fracture of the bony pelvis. Surgery, Gynecology and Obstetrics 120: 99–112

Karaharju E, Slatis P 1978 External fixation of double vertical pelvic fractures with a trapezoid compression frame. Injury 10: 142–145

Kelalis P P, King L R, Belman A B 1976 Clinical paediatric urology. W B Saunders, Philadelphia

King J 1975 Impotence after fractures of the pelvis. Journal of Bone and Joint Surgery 57A: 1107–1109

Lander R O 1984 Sacro-iliac injuries. Journal of Bone and Joint Surgery 66B: 611

Langloh N D, Johnson E W, Jackson C B 1972 Traumatic sacroiliac disruptions. Journal of Trauma 12: 931–953

Letournel E 1978 Pelvic fractures: annotation. Injury 10: 145–148

Levine J I, Crampton R S 1963 Major abdominal injuries associated with pelvic fractures. Surgery, Gynecology and Obstetrics 116: 223–226

Macdonald G A 1980 Pelvic disruptions in children. Clinical Orthopaedics 151: 130–134

Madsden L V, Jensen J, Christenson S T 1983 Parturition and pelvic fracture: a follow up of 34 obstetric patients with a history of pelvic fracture. Acta Obstetrica Gynaecologica Scandinavica 62(6): 617–620

Malgaigne J F 1855 Double vertical fractures of the pelvis. Reproduced and translated in Clinical Orthopaedics 151: 8–11, 1980

Mark S D, Keane T E, Vandemark R M, Webster G D 1995 Impotence following pelvic fracture urethral injury: Incidence, aetiology and management. British Journal of Urology 75(1): 62–64

Meurman K O A 1980 Stress fractures of the pubic arch in military recruits. British Journal of Radiology 53: 521–524

Mitchell J P 1984 Urinary tract trauma. John Wright, Bristol

Morehouse D D, MacKinnon K J 1969 Urological injuries associated with pelvic fractures. Journal of Trauma 9: 479–494

Noland L, Conwell H E 1930 Acute fractures of the pelvis. Treatment and results in 125 cases. Journal of the American Medical Association 94: 174–179

Noland L, Conwell H E 1933 Fractures of the pelvis: a summary of treatment and results attained in 185 cases. Surgery, Gynecology and Obstetrics 56: 522–525

Patterson D E, Barrett D M, Myers R P, Deweerd J H, Hall B B, Benson R C 1983 Primary management of urethral injuries. Journal of Urology 29: 573

Patterson F P, Morton K S 1961 Neurologic complications of fractures and dislocations of the pelvis. Surgery, Gynecology and Obstetrics 112: 702–706

Pavlov H, Nelson T L, Warren R F, Torg J S, Burstein A H 1982 Stress fractures of the pubic ramus. Journal of Bone and Joint Surgery 64A: 1020

Peltier L F 1965 Complications associated with fractures of the pelvis. Journal of Bone and Joint Surgery 47A: 1060–1069

Pennal G F, Messiah K A 1980 Non-union and delayed union of fractures of the pelvis. Clinical Orthopaedics 151: 124–129

Pennal G F, Sutherland G O 1961 Fractures of the pelvis. Motion picture in the American Academy of Orthopedic Surgeons film library

Pennal G F, Tile M, Waddell J P, Garside H 1980 Pelvic disruption; assessment and classification. Clinical Orthopaedics 151: 12–21

Pyper J B 1957 Excision of the coccyx for coccydynia: a study of 28 cases. Journal of Bone and Joint Surgery 39B: 733–737

Sarkin T L 1976 Injuries of the pelvis. Journal of Bone and Joint Surgery 58B: 396

Schwarz N, Posch E, Mayr J, Fishmeister F M, Schwarz A F, Ohner T 1998 Long term result of unstable pelvic ring fractures in children. Injury 29(6): 431–433

Semba R T, Yasukawa K, Gustilo R B 1983 Critical analysis of results of 53 Malgaigne fractures of the pelvis. Journal of Trauma 23: 535–537

Slatis P, Huittenen V-M 1972 Double vertical fractures of the pelvis: a report on 163 patients. Acta Chirurgica Scandinavica 138: 799–807

Tile M 1984 Fractures of the pelvis and acetabulum. Williams & Wilkins, Baltimore

Tile M 1988 Pelvic ring fractures: should they be fixed? Journal of Bone and Joint Surgery 70B: 1–2

Torode I, Zieg D 1985 Pelvic fractures in children. Journal of Pediatric Orthopaedics 5: 76–84

Torok G 1974 Coccygodynia. Journal of Bone and Joint Surgery 56B: 386

Watson Jones R 1962 Comment following presentation of a paper on pelvic fractures at a meeting of the British Orthopaedic Association 1961. Journal of Bone and Joint Surgery 44B: 216

The cervical spine
Gordon Bannister, John Hutchinson

Whiplash
Gordon Bannister

'Whiplash' is a loose term applied to any injury of the cervical spine other than an unequivocal fracture. Such physical pathology as has been defined includes disc disease (Jonsson et al 1994), facet arthritis (Barnsley et al 1995) and instability (James & Hooshmand 1965). 'Whiplash' correctly is a description of the mechanism of injury sustained in eight patients presented to the Western Orthopedic Association in San Francisco in 1928 by Harold Crowe. Other authors (Watson-Jones 1940, James & Hooshmand 1965) prefer the term 'cervical sprain'. Regardless of the name, the syndrome was recognised in the Edwin Smith Papyrus (Breasted 1930) and as 'spinal concussion' was described in a series of essays by Erichsen (1882) in the latter half of the 19th century, when the injury was designated 'railway spine'. Whiplash injuries are disproportionately represented in medicolegal practice. A relatively rare condition in the fracture clinic comprises 85% of all motor accident Personal Injury claims in the United Kingdom, 51% of the total injury cost for the insurance industry and 10% of premiums for motorists. The cost to the UK economy is approximately £3 billion. Some 300 000 people claim for whiplash injuries each year and the rate of increase is 5% per annum.

One in a 1000 of the population of Sweden are affected by whiplash injury (Bjornstig et al 1990), 5% of the Bristol population give an account of the injury (Gargan & Bannister 1997) and 1 in 40 American households are affected (Haines 1999).

Mechanism of injury
The acceleration to which the neck is subjected following a rear-end collision of 5 mph is of the order of 5G. By contrast, dropping heavily into a chair produces accelerations of between 6 and 9G in the horizontal and vertical planes. While there is an epidemic of whiplash injuries from Road Traffic accidents, only one has ever been recorded following a dodgem injury. Using human volunteers, McConnell et al (1993) found that three out of four doctors subjected to rear-end collisions of 4.5 mph reported pain the following day. Five of Castro et al's patients (1999) reported pain that settled after a week following collisions of between 6 and 7 mph. West et al's patients (1993) were reluctant to

take more than 7.3 mph and Mertz & Patrick's (1971) more than 8.2 mph. Most rear-end collisions are at around 15 mph and 10 mph is sufficient to cause a neck injury, there being little additional risk up to 30 mph. At lower speeds, there may be no vehicle damage.

Symptoms
The commonest symptoms are neck pain, occipital headache, shoulder and interscapular pain, thoracolumbar pain and upper limb paraesthesia with single figure percentages of other disorders (Table 18.1). In the majority of patients, onset is within 48 hours but the majority of upper limb pain and weakness presents later and between a quarter and a third of patients develop occipital headache, interscapular pain, thoracolumbar pain and upper limb paraesthesia after that time.

Hildingsson & Toolanen (1990) recorded that 59% of patients experienced symptoms on the day of the injury and 89% within three days, Deans et al (1987) found that 50% of neck pain presented after the initial A&E attendance and Maimaris et al (1988) 37% within an hour, 87% within a day and 13% later.

Back pain (Table 18.2)
Many reports omit lower back pain and this is almost certainly because of selective recording of data. Thus, when Gargan & Bannister (1990) reviewed Norris & Watt's 1983 series, a significant proportion described back pain dating from the time of the injury that was not recorded in the initial series. Thoracolumbar back pain appears to affect approximately a third of patients with whiplash injuries.

Physical signs
Although Norris & Watt (1983) recorded neurological deficit in 10 of their 63 patients and Maimaris et al (1988) in 16% of their series, Hohl (1974) found them in only 3% and Hildingsson & Toolanen (1990) in 4%. In practice, physical signs are difficult. Point tenderness is rarely recorded, although reputed to be consistent. Neck stiffness is potentially attractive but intra- and inter-observer error with a goniometer is 10° and range of movement can be restricted by painful inhibition. Painful inhibition, likewise, can produce muscle weakness and suppress reflexes.

Table 18.1 Acute symptoms (after Schutt & Dohan 1968, Hohl 1974, Wiley et al 1986, Hildingsson & Toolanen 1990, Gargan & Bannister 1994)

Symptom	%
Neck pain	87
Neck stiffness	65
Occipital headache	62
Shoulder and interscapular pain	49
Thoracolumbar back pain	46
Upper limb paraesthesia	22
Dysphagia	7
Visual disturbance	6
Tinnitus	4
Vertigo	2

Table 18.2 Back pain

Authors	Year	Total	Numbers
Gay & Abbott	1953	50	15
Hohl	1974	146	51
Balla	1980	300	60
Wiley et al	1986	192	115
Maimaris et al	1988	102	17
Gargan & Bannister	1990	43	18
Radanov et al	1991	78	26
Gargan & Bannister	1994	50	16
Total		961	318 (33%)

Severity of symptoms

The literature on whiplash injury rarely defines severity of symptoms. Most series record recovery or persisting complaints and a smaller proportion note those patients who are unable to work or are severely affected. In an attempt to improve reporting, the Quebec task force (Spitzer et al 1995) (Table 18.3) produced a classification which has not been validated, mixes symptoms and signs and does not measure functional disability. This classification has limited value in medico-legal reporting. Of greater value are the validated Gargan & Bannister classification (Table 18.4), and better still the Vernon & Mior neck disability index (Table 18.5) that allows the percentage score to be recorded and compared on subsequent examinations.

Apart from using different criteria to measure disability, series vary in the point of recruitment to study. Thus only 54% of patients presenting to Gotten (1956) in Neurosurgical Practice in Tennessee recovered, compared with 73% presenting to A&E departments in Belfast (Deans et al 1987, McKinney 1989) and Liverpool (Pennie & Agambar 1990). By contrast with all of these, 10% of Balla's 1982 series were severely disabled and not working, these being workmen's compensation cases reviewed two years after injury.

Recovery

Using only competent studies recruiting from A&E departments with 100% retrieval and at least 6 months' follow-up, it would appear that 55% of patients are absolutely pain-free after whiplash injury, 22% have

Table 18.3 Quebec task force classification of whiplash-associated disorders (Spitzer et al 1995)

Grade	Clinical presentation
0	No complaint about the neck
	No physical signs
I	Complaint of neck pain, stiffness and tenderness only
	No physical signs
II	Neck symptoms
	Decreased range of movement
	Point tenderness
III	Neck symptoms
	Decreased or absent reflexes, weakness and sensory deficit

Table 18.4 Gargan and Bannister scale (after Gargan & Bannister 1990)

Group	Symptoms
A	Symptom-free
B	Symptoms not interfering with occupation or leisure
C	Symptoms restricting occupation or leisure with or without frequent intermittent use of analgesia, orthotics or physical therapy
D	Loss of occupation, continuous use of analgesics, orthotics, repeated medical consultations

Table 18.5 Vernon and Mior's neck disability index (Vernon & Mior 1991). The questionnaire has been designed to give the doctor information as to how your neck pain has affected your abillity to manage in everyday life. Please answer every section and mark in each section only the ONE box which applies to you. We realize you may consider that two of the statements in any one section relate to you, but please just mark the box which most closely describes your problem.

Section 1 - Pain Intensity
- I have no pain at the moment
- The pain is very mild at the moment
- The pain is moderate at the moment
- The pain is fairly severe at the moment
- The pain is very severe at the moment
- The pain is the worst imaginable at the moment

Section 2 - Personal Care (Washing, Dressing etc.)
- I can look after myself normally without causing extra pain
- I can look after myself normally but it causes extra pain
- It is painful to look after myself and I am slow and careful
- I need some help but manage most of my personal care
- I need help every day in most aspects of self care
- I do not get dressed. I wash with difficulty and stay in bed

Section 3 - Lifting
- I can lift heavy weights without extra pain
- I can lift heavy weights but it gives extra pain
- Pain prevents me from lifting heavy weights off the floor, but I can manage if they are conveniently positioned, for example on a table.
- Pain prevents me from lifting heavy weights, but I can manage light to medium weights if they are conveniently positioned
- I can lift very light weights
- I cannot lift or carry anything at all

Section 4 - Reading
- I can read as much as I want to with no pain in my neck
- I can read as much as I want to with slight pain in my neck
- I can read as much as I want with moderate pain in my neck
- I can't read as much as I want because of moderate pain in my neck
- I can hardly read at all because of severe pain in my neck
- I cannot read at all

Section 5 - Headaches
- I have no headaches at all
- I have slight headaches which come in-frequently
- I have moderate headaches which come in-frequently
- I have moderate headaches which come frequently
- I have severe headaches which come frequently
- I have headaches almost all the time

Section 6 - Concentration
- I can concentrate fully when I want to with no difficulty
- I can concentrate fully when I want to with slight difficulty
- I have a fair degree of difficulty in concentrating when I want to
- I have a lot of difficulty in concentrating when I want to
- I have a great deal of difficulty in concentrating when I want to
- I cannot concentrate at all

Section 7 - Work
- I can do as much work as I want to
- I can only do my usual work, but no more
- I can do most of my usual work, but no more
- I cannot do my usual work
- I can hardly do any work at all
- I can't do any work at all

Section 8 - Driving
- I can drive my car without any neck pain
- I can drive my car as long as I want with slight pain in my neck
- I can drive my car as long as I want with moderate pain in my neck
- I can't drive my car as long as I want because of moderate pain in my neck
- I can hardly drive at all because of severe pain in my neck.
- I can't drive my car at all

Section 9 - Sleeping
- I have no trouble sleeping
- My sleep is slightly disturbed (less than 1hr sleepless)
- My sleep is mildly disturbed (1-2hrs sleepless)
- My sleep is moderately distrubed (2-3hrs sleepless)
- My sleep is greatly disturbed (3-5hrs sleepless)
- My sleep is completely disturbed (5-7hrs sleepless)

Section 10 - Recreation
- I am able to engage in all my recreation activities with no neck pain at all
- I am able to engage in all my recreation activities with some pain in my neck
- I am able to engage in most, but not all of my usual recreation activities because of pain in my neck
- I am able to engage in a few of my usual recreation activities because of pain in my neck
- I can hardly do any recreation activities because of pain in my neck
- I can't do any recreation activities at all

Table 18.6 Prognosis of whiplash injury using Gargan and Bannister grade (see Table 18.4)

Reference	Total	A	B	C	D
Hodgson & Grundy 1989	40	10	14	9	7
Pennie & Agambar 1990	130	111	14	3	2
Hildingsson & Toolanen 1990	93	39	13	27	14
Ryan et al 1994	29	10	17	1	1
Gargan & Bannister 1994	50	19	15	15	1
Total	342 (100%)	189 (55%)	73 (22%)	55 (16%)	25 (7%)

nuisance level discomfort, 16% have intrusive discomfort and 7% are disabled (Table 18.6). These figures are consistent with the only long-term prospective study recruiting at A&E departments (Murray, Pitcher & Galasko 1993). After between 2 and 3 years, Murray et al noted that 28% of patients with whiplash injuries had problems with sport, 16% with mobility, driving, hobbies and sleep, and 15% with washing, bathing and haircare (Table 18.7).

Signs

Hohl (1975), observed that 'physical findings after soft tissue neck injury are seldom commensurate with the severity of symptoms experienced'. Physical findings can change at different times within the same patient in the course of a day or working week (Hirsch et al 1988). Neck stiffness is associated with pain (Mealy et al 1986) and disruption of work and leisure activities (Watkinson et al 1991).

The surgeon seeking hard neurological signs will be disappointed in whiplash injury. Norris & Watt (1983) recorded neurological deficit in 10 of their 63 patients; 10 had altered sensation and six weakness. One patient had a diminished biceps jerk. Maimaris et al (1988) found neu-

rological signs in 21% of the 67 patients they examined, the population being heavily skewed towards symptomatic patients. The difficulty with neurological signs in whiplash is that sensory deficit rarely conforms to dermatomes, and power and reflexes can both be inhibited by pain (Gargan et al 1997).

Rate of recovery

Murray et al's prospective study over 4 years noted that symptoms plateaued after between 24 and 30 months, as did their severity (Table 18.8). The Bristol series originally reported by Norris & Watt (1983), and subsequently reviewed by Gargan & Bannister, recollected no change after 2 years, and in Leicester (Maimaris et al 1998) there was little change after 3 months. Gargan & Bannister (1994) prospectively reviewed 50 patients after 3, 12 and 24 months (Table 18.9). 93% of patients who were symptom-free and 86% of patients who were symptomatic after three months remained so after two years. After between 1 week and 3 months (Table 18.10) the majority of initial dysphagia, upper limb paraesthesia and interscapular

Table 18.7 Residual disability 2–3 years after whiplash (after Murray, Pitcher & Galasko 1993)

Activity	Problems %
Sport	28
Mobility/driving	16.5
Hobbies	16
Sleep	16
Washing/bathing/hair	15
Exercise	13
Housework	10
Dressing	8
Anxiety disrupting activity	5

Table 18.8 Rate of recovery (after Murray, Pitcher & Galasko 1993)

Time (months)	Symptom-free	Number of residual symptoms
0	3	4.09
6	29	2.09
12	46	1.54
18	54	1.32
24	56	1.26
30	59	1.2
36	60	1.18
42	60	1.15
48	60	1.16

Table 18.9 Prediction of prognosis after whiplash injury after 2 years (after Gargan & Bannister 1994)

Grade % after 3 months	A	B	C	D
A	93	3		
B	20	55	25	
C	7	20	73	
D			50	50
Grade % after 1 year	**A**	**B**	**C**	**D**
A	69	23	8	
B		70	30	
C	8	15	77	
D				100

Table 18.10 Resolution and later onset of symptoms between 1 week and 3 months (after Gargan & Bannister 1994)

Symptom	Resolution %	Later onset %	Persistent after 3 months %
Neck pain	24	6	77
Occipital headache	50	25	57
Interscapular pain	57	25	50
Thoracolumbar pain	38	33	71
Upper limb pain	50	75	80
Upper limb paraesthesia	60	25	47
Upper limb weakness	33	60	83
Dysphagia	88	0	13

pain had settled, but further upper limb pain and weakness had developed in a significant proportion of patients. Neck, thoracolumbar and upper limb pain and weakness tended to be persistent after 3 months.

Factors associated with outcome

The longer symptoms persist following whiplash injury, the less likely patients are to recover. A report prepared after 2 years is likely to be definitive, unless intervention of proven benefit is anticipated at that time. If a report has to be prepared before 2 years, factors associated with a poorer outcome may usefully be taken into account.

Awareness

Ryan et al (1994), in a series of 29 cases, noted that car occupants who were aware of an impending impact were 15 times less likely to have prolonged symptoms than those taken by surprise.

Pain distribution

Squires et al (1996) recorded pain maps and noted that patients with discomfort localised solely to the neck were eight times less likely to have prolonged symptoms than those whose pain radiated to the trapezii, interscapular region and shoulders.

Previous whiplash injury (Table 18.11)

Khan et al (2000) reviewed 79 patients who had suffered two whiplash injuries, of whom 84% reported increased symptomatology after the second impact. 97% who had been symptom-free before a second whiplash injury reported persisting discomfort, while over 30% of those who were left with symptoms after their original whiplash injury had disabling pain after a second. Seventy-three percent of the population had intrusive or disabling pain and overall the risk of deterioration increased by a factor of 5.

Table 18.11 Symptoms after second whiplash % (Khan et al 2000) Symptoms After second whiplash. Gargan & Bannister Grading (Table 18.4).

Original symptoms %		A	B	C	D
A	47	3	43	46	8
B	39	0	13	58	29
C	13	0	0	70	30
D	1	0	0	0	100
Total:			25	53	20

Pre-existing cervical spondylosis

Maimaris et al (1988) noted that 51% of patients who had pre-existing cervical spondylosis before whiplash injury were symptomatic long term, compared with 12% of necks that were radiologically normal. Likewise, they noted that 12% of patients who demonstrated a kyphosis were symptomatic, compared with 3% of those who did not. These two variables increased the risk of long-term symptoms by a factor of 4.

Abnormal neurology

Maimaris et al (1988) noted prolonged symptoms in 33% of patients who had abnormal neurology on presentation to the A&E department, compared with 10% of those who did not. Abnormal neurology thus increased the risk of long-term symptoms by a factor of 3.

Position in vehicle front or rear

Front seat passengers have a 2.8 fold greater risk of persisting symptoms than those in the rear (Allen et al 1985, Deans et al 1987, Otremski et al 1989).

Direction of impact

McNab (1964) associated a poorer outcome with rear-end collision and this was quantified further by Olney & Marsden (1986), Deans et al (1987) and the Quebec task force (Spitzer et al 1995). The risk of symptoms from a rear-end, rather than front or side, collision appears to be increased by a factor of 1.7.

Timing of onset and severity of pain

Deans et al (1987) noted long-term symptoms in 40% of patients who described these immediately on attendance at the A&E department and in 17% of those whose symptoms developed later. Thus, early onset of symptoms increases the risk of prolonged discomfort by a factor of 2.4. Hohl (1974) recorded significantly worse results in patients who had sufficient pain to require hospital admission and Radanov et al (1991) found that prolonged morbidity was associated with the severity of initial discomfort.

Age

Hohl (1974) noted that patients over the age of 50 fared less well following whiplash injury, an observation repeated by Nygren (1984) and Deans et al (1987). Patients over the age of 50 have an increased risk of 1.5 of long-term symptoms following whiplash injury.

Summary

■ Duration of symptoms is the most accurate prognostic indicator after whiplash.
■ Lack of awareness of impending impact, severe initial pain, widespread distribution of symptoms, previous whiplash injury, pre-existing cervical spondylosis, neurological symptoms and signs, front seat passengers, rear-end collisions and advancing age are all associated with a less favourable prognosis.
■ Neurological signs are rare, are associated with a poorer prognosis but their absence does not preclude this.
■ The severity of rear-end collision required to injure the neck may be insufficient to cause vehicle damage.

Employment

Murray, Pitcher & Galasko (1993) recorded a mean loss of 81 working days after whiplash in patients who were employed. Gozzard et al (2001) examined 717 medico-legal reports, noting that time off work was associated with severity of symptoms, manual employment, neurological signs or symptoms, and in women a psychological history. Gargan & Bannister (Table 18.4) Group A patients took 1 day off work, compared with 336 days in Group D. Manual workers took 14 days off, compared with 7 in clerical. Those with neurological symptoms and signs took 40% more time off work and females with a psychological history twice as much sickness absence. Seven percent of patients did not work again. All were in Gargan & Bannister Groups C and D. Thirteen percent of heavy manual, 9% of light manual and 5% of clerical workers did not resume employment after whiplash injury. Neurological signs and symptoms were twice as common in this group and again females with a psychological history were two and a half times more likely to remain off work indefinitely.

Summary

- On average patients who have sustained a whiplash injury lose 81 days from work.
- Time off work is increased according to severity of symptoms, relates to the manual nature of the Claimant's employment, is prolonged when there are neurological signs and symptoms and in women who have a history of psychological disease.
- 7% of patients claiming compensation after whiplash injury do not work again including 13% of heavy manual, 9.5% of light manual and 5% of clerical workers.

Imaging

The paucity of physical signs has encouraged radiological investigations in a quest for an objective indicator of disability. These involve plain X-rays, scintigraphy and magnetic resonance imaging (MRI).

Plain X-rays

Although Hohl (1974) noted sharp reversal of the cervical lordosis presaged disc degeneration at the level involved some 5 years later, and kyphosis is associated with a poorer outcome (Maimaris et al 1989), although other angular deformities seem benign (Miles et al 1988).

Case-control studies (Friedenberg & Miller 1963) demonstrate that cervical spondylosis at C5/6 and C6/7 respectively carry a 60% and 30% increase in risk of constitutional neck pain. However, only Maimaris et al (1988) have recorded more persistent symptoms in patients with degenerative changes, the observation being unsupported by Hohl & Hopp (1978), Balla (1980) and Hildingsson & Toolanen (1990).

Scintigraphy

Hildingsson et al (1989) noted normal scintographic findings and 31 of 35 acute soft tissue injuries of the cervical spine. Plain radiography demonstrated spondylitic changes in the remaining four. There was no correlation with outcome.

Magnetic resonance imaging

Davis et al (1991) compared T2 weighted MRI scans, nine patients injured in rear-end collisions and five with direct facial or anterior cranial trauma. Four of the nine patients who had been involved in rear-end collisions had pre-existing cervical spondylosis and three of these demonstrated disc herniation. Two of the patients with disc herniation also exhibited injuries to the anterior longitudinal ligament, fractures of the end plate, the anterior disc, and one patient

increased activity in the inter-spinous ligament. The study took place in a major trauma centre and it is likely that injuries were of higher violence than that normally caused in whiplash injury. The authors' observations were not confirmed in four patients described by Maimaris (1989), but similar pathology was recorded by Jonsson et al (1994).

Repeated radiological assessment

Jonsson et al (1994) investigated 24 patients with persisting symptoms by flexion and extension views and contrast-enhanced MRI scans. Ten of the 19 patients who had developed upper limb pain within days of the accident had Grade 3 or 4 cervical disc protrusions that correlated with the neurological signs. No patient with pain radiating to the upper limbs had abnormal flexion and extension views but five patients with central neck pain did and the two of these treated surgically had excellent results. Instability was defined as 3.5 mm of sagittal plane translation or 11° of angulation. Fresh injuries were found in all patients explored and the MRI scan underestimated the severity of disc injury in that lateral protrusions on MRI scan were found to be sequestrations when surgically explored.

Summary

- Plain X-rays are of little value and scintigraphy is unhelpful.
- Flexion–extension views may be helpful in localised neck pain and MRI scanning in upper limb radiation.

Natural history of neck pain

The medical expert is often asked to estimate the risk of neck pain, whether the accident has increased its speed of onset (acceleration), made inevitable constitutional neck pain worse (aggravation) and the potential effect of pre-existing degenerative change.

It would require a longitudinal study with regular X-rays over a 40 year period to give an accurate response to such requests and no such study exists. However, guidance can be obtained from cross-sectional studies. In the United Kingdom, the prevalence of neck pain in Belfast (Deans et al 1987) was 7% and in Bristol 8% (Hamer et al 1992). Neither of these studies specified the severity of pain. Lawrence (1969) recorded a history of neck pain and X-rayed over 3000 patients in Leigh, Wensleydale, Watford and the Rhonda. Symptomatically, pain was recorded as having occurred at any time in the past (pain at any time), being currently present (pain now) and time off work was noted. The definitions of radiological degeneration were Grade 1 (slight anterior wear of vertebral lip), Grade 2 (anterior osteophytes), Grade 3 (anterior

Table 18.12 Neck pain and disability % (Lawrence 1969)

Male

Radiological grade →	0–1				2				3–4			
Pain & disability →	Pain any time	Pain now	Off 1/52 +	Off >3/12	Pain any time	Pain now	Off 1/52 +	Off >3/12	Pain any time	Pain now	Off 1/52	Off >3/12
Age ↓												
15–24	19	2	1	1	33	0	0	0	0	0	0	0
24–34	32	4	5	1	26	5	5	0	100	0	0	0
35–44	35	6	4	1	30	6	4	2	34	8	12	4
45–54	42	8	3	0.5	40	13	5	2	45	16	12	2
55–64	40	12	7	3	34	9	3	1	38	10	4	4
65+	22	9	0	0	50	21	4	0	57	17	10	3

Female

Age ↓	Pain any time	Pain now	Off 1/52 +	Off >3/12	Pain any time	Pain now	Off 1/52 +	Off >3/12	Pain any time	Pain now	Off 1/52	Off >3/12
15–24	19	1	1	0.5	0	0	0	0	0	0	0	0
25–34	30	4	2	0	100	50	0	0	100	0	0	0
35–44	46	11	7	3	46	11	3	3	71	7	14	0
45–54	52	16	6	0.7	61	14	8	1	64	15	11	0
55–64	48	18	4	2	44	18	8	2	50	20	10	1
65+	57	12	10	7	60	13	7	5	61	13	7	2

osteophytes and narrowing of the disc) and Grade 4 (anterior osteophytes, disc narrowing and sclerosis of the vertebral plates). The risk of these symptoms in the male and female population is presented in Table 18.12. More advanced Grade 3 and 4 arthritis appears to have a greater effect on symptoms in patients under the age of 45 (Table 18.12), which is the population affected by whiplash injuries, rather more than those 45 years and over (Tables 18.13 & 18.14). Both advanced arthritis and increasing age increase symptoms of neck pain by between one and a half and two times.

Friedenberg et al (1960) followed 100 patients presenting with neck pain, radiating to the upper limb, noting that definite trauma preceded this in 25%, that 8% recovered, 60% improved, 17% remained unchanged and 15% deteriorated with time.

Gore et al reviewed 205 patients 10 years after initial consultation in orthopaedic practice. One hundred and twenty-one had been injured, of whom 76 had been involved in a Road Traffic accident. Ten years later 43% were pain-free, pain had decreased in 79% but 32% were left with moderate or severe discomfort. Neither injury nor litigation correlated with a poorer outcome but severity of initial symptoms did.

Friendenberg & Miller (1963) noted that twice as many patients with degenerative changes at C5/6 were symptomatic as those without and 50% more at C6/7. There was no significant difference between symptomatic and asymptomatic patients at other levels.

Treatment

Experts are often asked to opine on the merits of interventions to improve the outcome of whiplash injury and the contributory negligence of Claimants who decline treatment.

Cervical collars

Soft cervical collars are often prescribed, but there is little evidence to support their use. Four randomised prospective controlled trials failed to show benefit, compared with Maitland's manipulations (Mealy et al 1986), physiotherapy (Pennie & Agambar (1991), physiotherapy and self-mobilisation (McKinney 1989) or return to work and self-mobilisation (Borchgrevink et al 1998). If any immobilisation is to be used at all, a Philadelphia brace worn for 4 weeks (Guromoorthy et al 1999) gives significantly greater relief than an exercise programme.

Non-steroidal anti-inflammatories

A 14-day course of non-steroidal anti-inflammatory (NSAI) medication is significantly better than none at all in affording short-term relief (Gunzburg & Spalski 1998).

Physical Therapy

General physiotherapy seems no better than self-help (McKinney 1989, Borchgrevink et al 1998) but Maitland's manipulations are better than a soft cervical collar. In an observational study, chiropractic improves 93% of patients (Woodward et al 1996).

Table 18.13 Symptoms under 45 years in both sexes (%)

Symptoms	Radiological grades		
	0–1	2	3–4
Pain at any time	30	20	63
Pain now	5	4	9
Off work 1 week +	3	2	12
Off work 3 months +	1	2	2

Table 18.14 Symptoms over 44 years in both sexes (%)

Symptoms	Radiological changes		
	0–1	2	3–4
Pain at any time	46	46	51
Pain now	13	14	15
Off work 1 week +	5	6.3	8.5
Off work 3 months +	2	2	2

Pain clinic interventions

Sterile water injections into myofascial trigger points relieve pain better than saline (Byrn et al 1993). Radiofrequency neurotomy, particularly of the C5/6 facet joint after temporary improvement has been demonstrated by local anaesthetic, relieves symptoms in 75% of patients for a median of 8 months (Lord et al 1996).

Cervical fusion

Cervical fusion (Table 18.15) has been carried out either for disc protrusion and radiculopathy or instability. It is significant that the best results have been reported in large series published in the 1960s, but of the more recent literature only Jonsson et al (1994) have enjoyed general success. Comparing Jonsson's series with Algers' (1993), it is interesting to note that although both were carried out in the same country at the same time Jonsson operated within a year of injury, whereas Algers' patients waited a mean of 7 years and many had developed psychological disturbance. By contrast, Jonsson's approach was repeatedly to examine patients who had not recovered within 6 weeks, carry out flexion and extension views and contrast-enhanced MRI scans, and operate only on those whose symptoms and signs correlated closely with the radiological findings.

Bio-social factors

The difficulty in identifying organic pathology in whiplash injury has fostered the view that the condition is non-organic. The non-organic component may be psychological or bio-social.

Psychological response

In the earliest reports of whiplash injury, Gay & Abbott (1953) opined that 52% of their population demonstrated psycho-neurotic response and Gotten (1956) 85%. Anxiety was recorded in 5.3% of the Manchester series after 4 years (Murray et al 1993) and in 41% of the Bristol sample after 15 years (Squires et al 1996). Radanov et al (1991), in a non-consecutive population, found cognitive defects, some of which persisted after a year and could not be explained on the basis of pre-accident psycho-social factors. Mayou et al (1993) found depressive and post-traumatic symptoms in 18% of whiplash patients 3 months after injury and in 12% after 1 year, the depressive symptoms being associated with pre-accident psychiatric disorders. Using the General Health Questionnaire (Goldberg 1978), Gargan et al (1997) found comparable levels of psychological distress within the first week following whiplash injury, regardless of long-term outcome, but abnormal psychological scores in 81% of those with intrusive or worse symptoms after 3 months and 69% after 2 years.

Cultural response

In 1982, Balla compared a series of 300 patients, first reported in 1980, from South Australia, with 20 in Singapore. In Singapore, indigenous populations virtually never complained of disability, which was only ever reported by ex-patriot Europeans. This study is highly anecdotal. The South Australian patients were industrial rehabilitation cases reviewed after 2 years.

In 1986 Mills & Horne compared a year of Road Traffic accidents in New Zealand with those from Victoria, Australia. Population size and the numbers of cars were comparable, but in Victoria rear-end collisions were three and a half times as common, 10 times as many patients claimed compensation and five times as many were off work for more than 2 months. In New Zealand there was

Table 18.15 Cervical fusion after whiplash				
Author	**Year**	**Asymptomatic**	**Symptomatic**	**Severely symptomatic**
Gay & Abbott	1953	1	0	0
Gotten	1956	0	2	0
DePalma & Subin	1965	73	117	63
Janes & Hooshmand	1965	49	33	5
Hohl	1974	1	1	1
Wiley et al	1986	0	8	7
Hamer et al	1992	1	12	9
Algers et al	1993	0	11	9
Jonsson et al	1994	8	2	0
Total		134 (32%)	186 (45%)	94 (23%)

a 'no fault' compensation system, whereas in Australia an adversarial system operated. In 1987 (Awerbuch 1992), legislation was introduced in Victoria, requiring patients to report all whiplash injuries to the police and pay the first Australian 317 dollars of medical expenses. Claims fell by 68%. This suggests that the condition is substantially medicolegal, but Gibson et al (1999) recorded that 10% of Australians who had sustained whiplash injuries continued to have chronic neck pain after the 1987 legislation.

Schrader et al (1996) compared car occupants involved in motor vehicles accidents reported to the police in Lithuania with controls and found little difference in neck pain. This and the subsequent study from the same group (Obelieniene et al 1999), which used neighbours as controls, measures rear-end collision and not whiplash injury. As only 15% of patients involved in a rear-end collision ever develop neck pain (Freeman 1997), 94% of the accident victims would have had to have developed symptoms for the study to have reached statistical significance (Freeman & Croft 1996). Scrutiny of the data, rather than the conclusions, indicates that neck pain was one and a half times as frequent in the rear-end collision group than the control population and the discriminating power of the study was further blunted by the 33% prevalence of neck pain in the control group.

Legal influences

Claimants and all involved with the legal process have financial incentives in whiplash injury. A proportion of Claimants are fraudulent and there is an incentive for others involved in the legal process to maximise their gains. Claims to one leading insurance company occur three times more frequently in Manchester than the rest of the United Kingdom (Bachelor 2000). Insurance companies rely on solicitors to process claims but solicitors can earn fees only if Clients have sustained a personal injury. There is, therefore, incentive for solicitors to seek injury in Clients who would not otherwise pursue a legal case.

The Canadian province of Saskatchewan (Cassidy et al) changed from an adversarial to no-fault system with no payment for pain and suffering but generous replacement of medical costs and loss of income. Whiplash claims fell by 28% and there was a 54% decrease in the time to a settlement. Involvement of lawyers delayed settlement.

The concept that whiplash symptoms settle after litigation relies on anecdote, published in the 1960s, that is unsupported by more recent and robust literature.

'Accident neurosis' was proposed by Miller in 1961 in relation to minor head injuries and Harold Crowe in 1966 defined whiplash as 'any strain of the cervical spine that

does not resolve until all litigation is concluded'. There is no evidence from the ensuing literature that this is the case. Macnab (1964), Balla & Moraitis (1970), Hohl (1974), Norris & Watt (1983), Maimaris et al (1988), Ettlin et al (1992), Parmar & Raymakers (1993) Robinson & Cassar-Pullicino (1993) all found no difference in symptoms after conclusion of litigation, after whiplash, and Mendelson (1988) recorded a similar outcome from a wide variety of injuries. DePalma & Subin (1965) noted that 37% of litigants and 25% of non-litigants derived relief from cervical fusion.

Maimaris et al (1988) noted that symptoms were more common in patients pursuing litigation and Gargan & Bannister (1990) that litigation was most prolonged in patients whose symptoms were the most severe, whose settlements were the highest and therefore probably most keenly contested.

Summary

- Neck pain increases with age and in Grades 3 and 4 cervical disc degeneration in patients under the age of 45.
- Self mobilisation is better treatment than physiotherapy or soft cervical collars.
- A third of patients following cervical fusion are substantially relieved of pain and a quarter remain disabled. The results of cervical fusion are better if carried out in under 1 year than after 7.
- A significant proportion of patients with whiplash injuries develop a somatopsychic response as a reaction to the injury.
- Litigation influences the proportion of whiplash victims who claim but its conclusion is not accompanied by remission of symptoms.

■ References

Algers G, Pettersson K, Hildingsson C, Toolanen G 1993 Surgery for chronic symptoms after whiplash injury. Acta Orthopaedica Scandinavica 64 6: 654–656

Allen M J, Barnes M R, Bodiwalagg G G 1985 The effect of seat belt legislation on injuries sustained by car occupants. Injury 16: 471–476

Awerbuch M S 1992 Whiplash in Australia: Illness or injury. Medical Journal of Australia 157: 193–196

Bachelor M 2000 The cost of whiplash. Read at Whiplash 2000, Bath, England: May 16–18 2000

Balla J I 1980 The late whiplash syndrome. Australian and New Zealand Journal of Surgery 50: 610–614

Balla J I 1982 The late whiplash syndrome: A study of an illness in Australia and Singapore. Culture, Medicine and Psychiatry 6: 191–210

Balla J I, Moraitis S 1970 Knights in armour. A follow up study of injuries after legal settlement. Medical Journal of Australia: 355–361

Barnsley L, Lord S M, Wallis B J, Bogduk N 1995 The prevelance of chronic cervical zygapophyseal joint pain after whiplash. Spine 20 1: 20–26

Bjornstig U, Hildingsson C, Toolanen G 1990 Soft-tissue injury of the neck in a hospital based material. Scandinavian Journal of Social Medicine 18: 263–267

Borchgrevink G E, Kaasa A, McDonagh D, Stiles T C, Haraldseth O, Lereim I 1998 Acute treatment of whiplash neck strain injuries. A randomised trial of treatment during the first 14 days after a car accident. Spine 23 1: 25–31

Breasted J H 1930 The Edwin Smith Papyrus, Chicago, Vol. P452, Case 30. University of Chicago Press

Byrn C, Olsson I, Falkheden L, Lindh M, Hosterey U, Fogelberg M, Linder L E, Bunketorp O 1993 Subcutaneous sterile water injections for chronic neck and shoulder pain following whiplash injuries. Lancet 341: 449–452

Cassidy J D, Carroll L J, Cote P, Lemstram M, Berlund A, Nygren A 2000 Effect of eliminating compensation for pain and suffering on the outcome of insurance claims for whiplash injury. New England Journal of Medicine 342 16: 1179–1185

Castro W H M, Becke M, Schilgen M, Meyer S, Weber M, Peuker C, Wortler K 1999 Whiplash associated disorders in low speed rear impacts—fact or fiction? Whiplash Associated Disorders: World Congress '99, 8–11 Feb., Vancouver

Crowe H D 1928 Whiplash injuries of the cervical spine in proceedings of the section of insurance negligence and compensation law. American Bar Association, Chicago, pp. 176–184

Davis S J, Teresi L M, Bradley W G, Ziemba M A, Bloze A E 1991 Cervical spine hyperextension injuries MR findings Radiology 180: 245–251

Deans G T, Magalliard J N, Kerr M, Rutherford W H 1987 Neck sprain—a major cause of disability following car accidents. Injury 18: 10–12

DePalma A F, Subin D K 1965 Study of the cervical syndrome. Clinical Orthopaedics. 38: 135–142

Erichsen J E 1882 On concussion of the spine: nervous shock and other obscure injuries of the nervous system in their clinical and medicolegal aspects. Longmans, Green and Co., London

Ettlin T M, Kischka U, Reichmann S, Radii E W, Heim S, A'Wengen D, Benson D F 1992 Cerebral symptoms after whiplash injury of the neck: A prospective clinical and neuro psychological study of whiplash injury. Journal of Neurology, Neurosurgery and Psychiatry 55: 943–948

Freeman M D 1997 The epidemiology of late whiplash. PhD Dissertation, Oregon State University

Freeman M D, Croft A C 1996 Late whiplash syndrome. Lancet 348: 125

Friedenberg Z B, Broder M A, Edeiken J E, Spencer H N 1960 Degenerative disk disease of the cervical spine. Clinical and roentgenographic study. JAMA 174 4: 375–380

Friedenberg Z B, Miller W T 1963 Degenerative disk disease of the cervical spine. A comparative study of asymptomatic and symptomatic patients. Journal of Bone and Joint Surgery 45A: 1171–1178

Gargan M F, Bannister G C 1990 Long-term prognosis of soft-tissue injuries of the neck. Journal of Bone and Joint Surgery 72B: 901–903

Gargan M F, Bannister G C 1994 The rate of recovery following soft tissue injury of the neck. European Spine Journal 3: 162–164

Gargan M F, Bannister G C 1997 The comparative effects of whiplash injuries. Journal of Orthopaedic Medicine 19: 15–17

Gargan M F, Bannister G C, Main C, Hollis S 1997 The behavioural response to whiplash injury. Journal of Bone and Joint Surgery 79: 523–526

Gay J R, Abbott K M 1952 Common whiplash injuries of the neck. JAMA 152 18: 1698–1704

Gibson T, Bogduk N, Macpherson J, McIntosh A 1999 The accident characteristics of whiplash associated chronic neck pain. Whiplash Associated Disorders: World Congress '99, 8–11 Feb., Vancouver

Goldberg D 1978 Manual of the General Health Questionnaire. Nelson Publishing Company, Darville House, 2 Oxford Road East, Window SL4 1DF, Berks

Gore D R, Sepic S B, Gardner G M, Murray M D 1987 Neck pain: A long term follow-up of 205 patients. Spine 12 1: 1–5

Gotten N 1956 Survey of 100 cases of whiplash injury after settlement of litigation. JAMA 162 9: 865–867

Gozzard C, Bannister G C, Langkamer V G, Kahn S, Gargan M F 2001 Factors affecting employment after whiplash injury. Journal of Bone and Joint Surgery B: in press

Gunzberg R, Spalski M, Soeur M, Bauherz G, Michel M 1999 Efficacy of NSAID (tenoxicam) in the acute phase of whiplash. Whiplash Associated Disorders: World Congress '99, 8–9 Feb., Vancouver

Guromoorthy D, Twomey L, Batalin W J 1999 A prospective study of acute whiplash injury and its clinical management. Whiplash Associated Disorders: World Congress '99, 8–9 Feb., Vancouver

Haines F 1993 Automobile insurance—trends in neck soft-tissue injury claims. Whiplash Associated Disorders: World Congress '99, 8–11 Feb., Vancouver

Hamer A J, Gargan M F, Bannister G C, Nelson R J 1993 Whiplash injury and surgically treated cervical disc disease. Injury 8: 549–550

Hildingsson C, Heitala S-O, Toolanen G 1989 Scintigraphic findings in acute whiplash injury of the cervical spine. Injury 20: 265–266

Hildingsson C, Toolanen G 1990 Outcome after soft-tissue injury of the cervical spine. A prospective study of 93 car-accident victims. Acta Orthopaedica Scandinavica 61: 357–359

Hirsch S A, Hirsch P J, Hiramoto H, Weiss A 1988 Whiplash syndrome. Fact or fiction? Orthopaedic Clinics of North America 19 4: 791–795

Hodgson S P, Grundy M 1989 Whiplash injuries: Their long-term prognosis and its relationship to compensation. Neuro-orthopaedics 7: 88–91

Hohl M 1974 Soft-tissue injuries of the neck in automobile accidents. Factors influencing prognosis. Journal of Bone and Joint Surgery 56A: 1675–1681

Hohl M 1975 Soft tissue injuries of the neck. Clinical Orthopaedics 109: 42–49

Hohl M, Hopp E 1978 Soft tissue injuries of the neck II. Factors influencing prognosis. Orthopaedic Transactions 2: 29

Janes J M, Hooshmand H 1965 Severe extension-flexion injuries of the cervical spine. Mayo Clinical Proceedings 40(5): 353–369

Jonsson H, Cesarini K, Sahlstedt B, Rauschning W 1994 Findings and outcome in whiplash type neck distortions. Spine 19(24): 2733–2743

Khan S, Bannister G, Gargan M, Asopa V, Edwards A 2000 Prognosis following a second whiplash injury. Injury 31: 249–251

Lawrence J S 1969 Disc degeneration. Its frequency and relationship to symptoms. Annals of Rheumatic Disorders 28: 121–137

Lord S M, Barnsley L, Wallis B J, McDonald G J, Bogduk N 1996 Percutaneous radiofrequency neurotomy for chronic cervical zygoapophyseal joint pain. New England Journal of Medicine 335 23: 1721–1726

Maimaris C 1989 Neck sprains after car accidents. British Medical Journal 299: 123

Maimaris C, Barnes M R, Allen M J 1988 'Whiplash injuries' of the neck: A retrospective study. Injury 19 5: 393–396

Mayou R, Bryant B, Duthie R 1993 Psychiatric consequences of road traffic accidents. British Medical Journal 307: 647–651

McConnell W E, Howard R P, Buzman H H et al 1993 Analysis of human test subject kinematic responses to low velocity rear end impacts. Society of Automatic Engineering, Technical Paper No. 930889

McKinney L A 1989 Early mobilisation and outcome in acute sprains of the neck. British Medical Journal 299: 1006–1008

Macnab I 1964 Accelaration injuries of the cervical spine. Journal of Bone and Joint Surgery 46a: 1797–1799

Mealy K, Brennan H, Fenelon G C 1986 Early mobilisation of acute whiplash injuries. British Medical Journal 292: 656–657

Mendelson G 1998 Psychiatric aspects of personal injury claims. Charles C. Thomas, Springfield, Illinois

Mertz H J, Patrick L M 1971 Strength and response of the human neck. Society of Automotive Engineering, Technical Paper No. 710855

Miles K A, Maimaris C, Finlay D, Barnes M R 1988 The incidence and prognostic significance of radiological abnormalities in soft tissue injuries to the cervical spine. Skeletal Radiology 493–496

Miller H 1961 Accident neurosis. British Medical Journal 2: 992–998

Mills H, Horne G 1986 Whiplash—manmade disease? New Zealand Medical Journal 99: 373–374

Murray P A, Pitcher M, Galasko C S B 1993 The cost of long term disability from road traffic accidents four year study—final report. Transport Research Laboratory. Project Report 45. HMSO (ISBN 0968–4093)

Norris S H, Watt I 1983 The prognosis of neck injuries resulting from rear-end vehicle collisions. Journal of Bone and Joint Surgery 65B: 608–611

Nygren A 1984 Injuries to car occupants—some aspects of the interior safety of cars Acta Otolaryngology (suppl) 395

Obelieniene D, Schrader H, Bovim G, Miseviciene I, Trond S 1999 Pain after whiplash: A prospective controlled inception cohort study. Journal of Neurology, Neurosurgery and Psychiatry 66: 279–283

Olney D B, Marsden A K 1986 The effect of head restraints and seat belts on the incidence of neck injury in car accidents. Injury 17: 365–367

O'Neill B, Haddon W, Kelley A B, Sorenson W W. 1972 Automobile head restraints—frequency of neck injury claims in relation to the presence of head restraints. American Journal of Public Health 62: 399–406

Otremski I, Marsh J L, Wilde B R, McLardy-Smith P D, Newman R J 1989 Soft tissue cervical spinal injuries in motor vehicle accidents. Injury 20: 349–355

Parmar H, Raymakers R 1993 Neck injuries from rear impact road traffic accidents: Prognosis in persons seeking compensation. Injury 24(2): 75–78

Pennie B H, Agambar L J 1990 Whiplash injuries. A trial of early management. Journal of Bone and Joint Surgery 72B: 277–279

Radanov B P, Di Stefano G, Schindrig A, Ballinari P 1991 Role of psychosocial stress in recovery from common whiplash. Lancet 338: 712–714

Robinson D D, Cassar-Pullicino V N 1993 Acute neck sprain after road traffic accident. A long term clinical and radiological review. Injury 24(2): 79–82

Ryan G A, Taylor G W, Moore V M, Dolinis J 1994 Neck strain in car occupants: Injury status after 6 months and crash related factors. Injury 25 8: 533–537

Schrader M, Obelieniene D, Bovim G, Surkiene D, Mickeviene D, Miseviciene I, Sand T 1996 Natural evolution of late whiplash syndrome outside the medicolegal context. Lancet 347: 1207–1211

Spitzer W O, S'kovron M L, Salmi L R, Cassidy J D, Duranceau J, Suissa S, Zeiss E 1995 Scientific monograph of the Quebec task force on whiplash-associated disorders. Spine 20(85): 1–73

Squires B, Gargan M F, Bannister G C 1996 Soft tissue injuries of the cervical spine. 15 year follow up. Journal of Bone and Joint Surgery 788 6: 955–957

Vernon M, Mior S 1991 The neck disability index: A study of reliability and validity. Journal of Manipulative Physiotherapy and Therapeutics 14: 409–475

Watkinson A, Gargan M F, Bannister G C 1991 Prognostic factors in soft tissue injuries of the cervical spine. Injury 22: 307–309

Watson-Jones R 1940 Fractures and other bone and joint injuries. Williams and Wilkins Company, Baltimore, p. 723

West D M, Gough J P, Harper G T K 1993 Low speed rear-end collision testing using human subjects. Accident Reconstruction Journal 5: 22–26

Wiley A M, Lloyd G J, Evans S G, Stewart B M 1986 Musculoskeletal sequelae of whiplash. Advocates Quarterly 7: 65–73

Woodward M N, Cook J C H, Gargan M F, Bannister G C 1996 Chiropractic treatment of chronic whiplash injuries Injury 27 9: 643–645

Cervical spine injuries
John Hutchinson

Introduction

Modern management of trauma, such as Advanced Trauma and Life Support (ATLS) based systems in appropriate receiving hospitals, has increased the survivability of spinal trauma. The development of spinal injury as a speciality has prolonged the life expectancy of quadriplegic and paraplegic patients. Widespread access to CT, MRI and radioisotope imaging has increased the detection rate of spinal injuries. Nevertheless, there is a relative paucity of studies on the outcome of cervical spine fractures. This part of the chapter draws together published series to give an idea of outcome, but in many cases 'first principles' are required to arrive at a prognosis.

Imaging

Cervical spine injuries are missed in 3 to 25% of patients, and one-third of these cases develop neurological sequelae (Chapman & Anderson 1997).

X-rays

The standard series of X-rays in neck trauma are a lateral (occiput to C7-T1), open mouth and anteroposterior views. These are between 33 and 85% sensitive in detecting fractures (Chan et al 1980; Clark et al 1988; Davis et al 1993; Enderson et al 1990; Streitweiser et al 1983). The lateral view allows assessment of the retropharyngeal tissue.

MRI

This evaluates the neural elements, the intervertebral disc, the anterior and posterior longitudinal ligaments, the ligamentum flavum and the interspinous ligaments. Blood, oedema and occult fractures are all demonstrated. In a single sagittal acquisition, the alignment of the cervical spine is assessed. Multiple fractures are common in cervical trauma, making MRI a useful screening tool.

CT

Excellent in detailing the anatomy of a fracture, assessing the mechanism of injury and planning surgery; it is widely used in North America as a screening tool for cervical trauma in the Emergency Room (Chapman & Anderson 1997).

Dynamic radiology

This is useful where there is neck pain, normal radiographs, no neuropathy and the patient has free movement of the cervical spine. The flexion-extension views should be with active, not passive, movement. There is some controversy attached to their use in most other circumstances.

Stability

The presence of a bony or ligamentous injury requires stability to be assessed. Confusion arises from the use of the term 'spinal instability' which is used interchangeably with the term 'segmental instability' as a possible aetiology of low back pain. For this reason the term 'unstable fracture' is used to avoid misunderstanding. An unstable fracture is one which will displace under physiological load. White & Panjabi (1990) expanded this definition in the spinal context to *'a loss of the ability under physiological loads to maintain relationships between vertebrae in such a way that there is neither damage nor subsequent irritation to the spinal cord or nerve roots and there is no development of incapacitating deformity or pain due to structural changes'*.

The signs of a possibly unstable fracture are:

- Increased retropharyngeal soft tissue interval: 3 mm at C3: 8–10 mm below C4
- Compression fractures (present if there is more than 3 mm loss of anterior height when compared with the posterior vertebral body)
- Avulsion fractures near the insertion of spinal ligaments
- Disc space widening of 1.5 times or more compared to adjacent levels (White et al 1976)

The signs of a probably unstable fracture are:

- Angulation of more than 11° between adjacent vertebral bodies (White & Punjabi 1990)
- More than 3.5 mm translation of the vertebral body
- Increased interspinous distance
- Facet joint malalignment
- Spinous process malalignment on the AP view
- Lateral tilting of the vertebral body on the AP view

Bohlman & Anderson (1992) documented that the torn posterior ligament complex in flexion injuries may not heal even after prolonged rigid immobilisation. Soft tissue injuries treated conservatively thus have a risk of late instability, or failure under relatively small load.

Pharmacological treatment and the timing of surgery

There is considerable debate regarding the optimal acute treatment of spinal cord injuries.

Many surgeons do not carry out early decompression because of increased perioperative complications and worsening neurological status (Sonntag & Francis 1995; Rosenfeld et al 1998). Much of the evidence for this is based upon studies published before 1990. A prospective randomised study by Vacarro et al (1997) showed no difference in neurological outcome between patients operated on early and late. Other clinical studies have suggested some benefit of surgery within 24 hours, but have not elucidated a more accurate timeframe (Bracken et al 1990; Levi et al 1991).

Although not demonstrated by any human study, there is a certain time period (probably less than 2–3 hours) in which surgical decompression may benefit neural recovery (Carlson et al 1997). Some major spinal centres aim to decompress cervical trauma with neurological deficit as soon as possible after admission.

Early surgical stabilisation (within 24 hours) may decrease the length of acute hospital stay (Campagnolo et al 1997).

Injury to the spinal cord results in the release of neurotoxic and inflammatory mediators which cause further damage (Bracken et al 1990; Delamarter et al 1995; Salzman & Betz 1996). Many pharmacological agents are being investigated with a view to modifying this secondary damage, and high dose methylprednisolone is widely given in the acute treatment of cord injury (Bracken et al 1990; Bracken et al 1997). It is the authors' opinion that the case for giving high dose steroids in acute spinal injury is unproven.

Other agents are being evaluated with a view to promoting neural recovery (Vaccaro & Singh 2000).

Classification of cervical injuries

An ideal classification of cervical injuries would reflect progressive osteoligamentous injury as well as neurological damage. To date no such classification exists. The AO classifications of spine fractures are complex but comprehensive. In the medico-legal context a description of the bony and soft tissue injuries, along with a proposed mechanism of injury, is suggested.

It is important that standard terms are used to describe injuries, allowing comparison of treatments and facilitating prognosis.

The American Spinal Injury Society's (ASIA) functional and neurological classification should be used in all cases (ASIA 1992). Cord lesions are named as the last useful (antigravity) level, and are classified as intact, complete or incomplete. Sacral sparing indicates an incomplete lesion. Anterior, posterior, central and Brown-Séquard cord injuries are described. Function is classified using a modification of Frankel's grades. Individual muscle function should be described with the Medical Research Council's scoring system (Table 18.16).

Cervical injuries are arbitrarily divided into lesions above C2–3 where there is atypical anatomy, and sub-axial injuries, which have a more heterogeneous pattern. Allen

Table 18.16 Muscle grading chart

Grade	Muscle action
0 = zero	Total paralysis
1 = trace	Visible or palpable contraction
2 = poor	Active movement, gravity eliminated
3 = fair	Active movement against gravity
4 = good	Active movement against resistance
5 = normal	Active movement against full resistance

Frankel grade

Grade	Function
A	Complete neurological injury
B	Preserved sensation distal to level of injury
C	Preserved motor non-functional
D	Preserved motor functional
E	Preserved sensation, normal power

et al (1982) have suggested a complex but comprehensive classification for sub-axial injuries (Fig. 18.1). This is of help in surmising the mechanism of injury.

Atlanto-occipital dislocations

These are high-energy injuries which are usually fatal. The survival chance is less than 1% (Bucholz & Burkhead 1979). The vast majority of these injuries described in the literature are associated with a head injury and/or a spinal cord injury. An apparent increase in incidence probably reflects improved emergency medical care. There is often a delay in diagnosis, reflecting the difficulties in assessing images. There are many radiological measurements to aid diagnosis, including Powers Ratio (Fig. 18.2). (AO:BC) is the most commonly used. MRI is the best means of diagnosing the injury.

Atlantocervical dislocation is sometimes associated with an avulsion fracture of the dens or occipital condyles. Traylenis et al (1986) described anterior, vertical and posterior patterns, depending on the position of the condyles in relation to the atlas (types I–III respectively). Types I and III can be reduced with gentle traction. A trial of halo-vest immobilisation, followed by flexion-extension X-rays, is reasonable, but most of these injuries will require operative stabilisation.

Atlanto-occipital dislocations biomechanically require fusion from the occiput to the axis, but clinical series suggest a lower level of fusion is most often performed

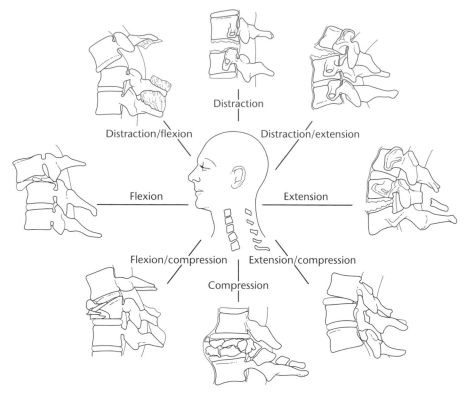

Fig. 18.1 Classification of sub-axial injuries (From Allen & Fergusson 1982, with permission).

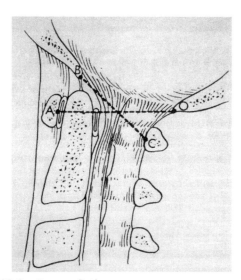

Fig. 18.2 Powers Ratio.

because of coexisting injuries (Eismont & Bohlman 1978; Montane et al 1991).

The results depend on the severity of injury and the emergency and early hospital treatment. Some improvement in neurological status has been recorded (Eismont & Bohlman 1978; Montane et al 1991).

Most patients will have a fusion of the upper two motion segments at least.

The motion available at the occipitocervical junction is 21° extension, 3° flexion, 7° rotation and 5° lateral bending (Werne 1957; Panjabi et al 1988). The atlanto-axial joint accounts for 50% of cervical rotation (Penning & Wilmink 1987).

Several series have reported 100% fusion rates following instrumented occipito-cervical fusion, with no loss of reduction (Roy-Camille et al 1989; Sasso et al 1994; Smith & Anderson 1994).

Occipital condyle fractures

Again this is a rare injury, but 21st century medicine will see an increase in diagnosis and survivability. Anderson & Montesano (1988) described and categorised these injuries (Fig. 18.3):

I: an impaction of the condyle occurring as a result of axial loading.

II: condyle fractures associated with basilar skull fractures; caused by a direct blow.

III: occur with rotation or lateral bending, and are caused by avulsion of the condyle by the alar ligament.

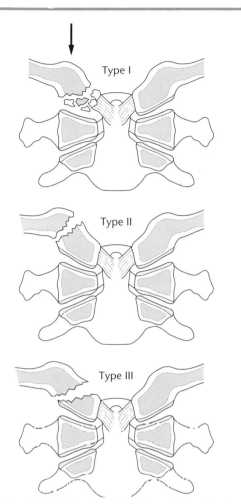

Fig. 18.3 Occipital condyle fractures (from Anderson & Montesano 1988; with permission).

Patients present with base of skull pain and often with clinically obvious rotational deformities.

If the tectorial membrane, or contralateral alar ligaments are damaged, there is considerable craniocervical instability.

Often, detection is possible by MRI, but exact diagnosis is dependent on CT.

Types I and II are relatively stable injuries and can be treated in a rigid cervical collar for 6–8 weeks. The treatment of type III cases depends on the degree of ligamentous injury. Halo immobilisation for 12 weeks or occipitocervical fusion is indicated.

Roy-Camille (1995) reviewed 30 cases published between 1978 and 1994. The long-term result of type I and II injuries appeared satisfactory. The author would suggest that the variety of instability and neural injury within type III fractures requires them to be regarded as a heterogeneous group. The outcome will depend on the degree of damage, the treatment given, and the quality of healing which occurs.

Fracture of the atlas

This was first described by Sir Astley Cooper in 1822, with a 46 further cases described before Geoffrey Jefferson's eponymous description of 1920.

Full understanding of these fractures requires a knowledge of the ligamentous and bony anatomy, and an appreciation of the embryology and anomalies.

The classification of injuries of C1 has evolved slowly. Five types of fracture have been demonstrated clinically (Fig. 18.4).

The fact that few series (Levine 1983; Highland & Salciccioli 1985; Ersmark and Kalen 1987; Segal et al 1987; Lee et al 1998) have reported large numbers of atlas fractures, coupled with the high incidence of concominant cervical spine injuries, makes logical conclusions about specific injuries hard to arrive at. These series also reflect a diversity of treatment regimes, the choice of which again is often determined by the associated injuries.

Stable injuries do well in rigid cervical collars (Lee et al 1998).

A combined displacement of the lateral masses of more than 6.9 mm implies a transverse ligament rupture (Spence et al 1970).

The critical feature of these injuries, however, is that the transverse ligament fails under tension with axial loading. The remainder of the upper cervical ligaments are normally intact. Fielding et al (1974) has demonstrated that selective rupture of the transverse ligament results in minimal instability at C1–2. Prophylactic fusion may be warranted in adults, where there is unlikely to be ligamentous healing and further trauma may be catastrophic. Where there is significant displacement (7–10 mm total) of the lateral masses, non-union is common (Segal et al 1987), and incongruity of the joints can become an important factor. In these fractures the bony elements can be reduced with traction, but this position is often lost in a halo-jacket. Trans-articular C1–2 screws can be used to allow mobilisation rather than a period of traction in bed.

For patients with posterior arch fractures, the expected result is a union with minimal to no symptoms (Levine 1998). Any residual symptoms are most commonly related to concomitant injuries.

Where there is an associated traumatic spondylolisthesis of C2 (both are hyperextension injuries), there may be late degeneration of the C2–3 facet joint. This joint is probably damaged at the time of injury.

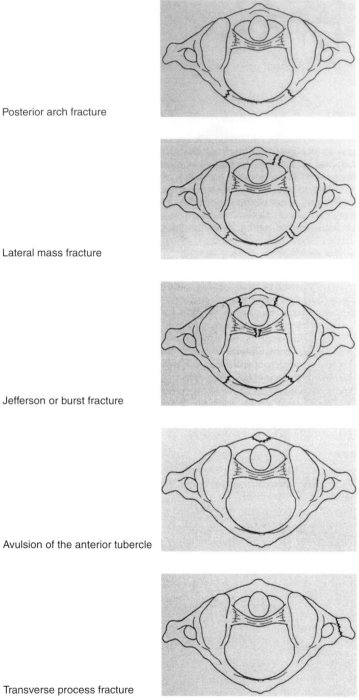

Posterior arch fracture

Lateral mass fracture

Jefferson or burst fracture

Avulsion of the anterior tubercle

Transverse process fracture

Fig. 18.4 Classification of fractures of the atlas.

Patients with minimally displaced Jefferson and lateral mass fractures, treated in a halo, usually progress to union with less than 2 mm further displacement. Dynamic radiography shows no late instability in these patients (Levine 1998).

Where there is greater displacement stability still appears to be ubiquitous; however the non-union rate is 17% and is related to the degree of displacement (Levine 1983). Levine & Edwards (1991) reported that 80% of these patients having some residual neck pain.

Late neurological complications have been reported (Levine 1998). Cranial nerve lesions and greater occipital nerve damage have been described (Zielinski et al 1982).

Although it is not well documented, incongruency of the occipito-atlantal and atlanto-axial joints will lead to degenerative changes, unilaterally or symmetrically, with consequent arthropathy.

Twelve percent of atlanto-axial injuries, treated operatively and non-operatively, will produce chronic pain (Ersmark & Kalen 1987).

Odontoid fractures

Odontoid fractures constitute 18% of cervical spine fractures and dislocations. This figure is much higher in young children because of large head-to-body mass ratio. The elderly suffer osteoporotic fractures with a relatively high incidence.

Unsatisfactory alignment and non-union may result in pain and progressive neuropathy (Crockard et al 1993; Carlson et al 1998).

Anderson & D'Olonzo (1974) reported on 60 patients and described three levels of fracture (Fig. 18.5). This classification gives a prognosis for fracture union (Apuzzo et al 1978; Hadley et al 1988; Clark 1991).

Type I fractures occur cephalad to the transverse ligament and represent avulsion fractures. They are often 'incidental' fractures, but can be associated with craniocervical instability. Treatment usually comprises radiological exclusion of significant instability, and a collar for symptomatic treatment.

They are often excluded from clinical series. Anderson & D'Olonzo (1974) reported two type I fractures which healed without problem. Even if there is a non-union it is usually asymptomatic (Carlson et al 1998).

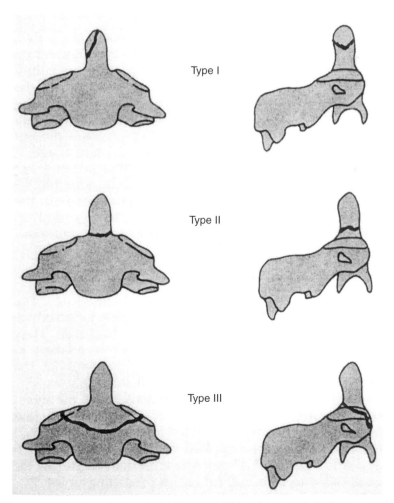

Type I

Type II

Type III

Fig. 18.5   Odontoid fractures (from Anderson & D'Olonzo 1974, with permission).

Type II fractures occur at the base of the dens. Reported non-union rates vary from 11% (Hadley et al 1985; Lind et al 1987) to 100% (Maiman & Larsen 1982).

Factors of proven significance in non-union are (Carlson et al 1998):

- Displacement (translation or angulation)
- Ability to achieve or maintain a reduction
- Age
- Delayed diagnosis or treatment

Factors of probable significance are:

- Comminution (Hadley & Browner 1988)
- Distraction (Ryan & Taylor 1982)

The Cervical Spine Research Society's multi-centre study found a non-union rate of 32%. Displacement of 5 mm and angulation of 10° or more are associated with non-union or malunion.

Primary operative stabilisation (either anterior or posterior) is recommended where there is:

- Displacement of 5 mm or more
- Angulation of 10° or more
- Comminution
- Coronal oblique fractures
- Polytrauma
- A patient who will not tolerate orthoses
- Concomitant C1 fractures
- Pathological fractures
- Irreducible C1–2 fractures.

Type III fractures are through the body of C-2. Union is reported as between 87 and 100% (Clark & White 1985; Hadley et al 1985). Poorer results are associated with cervical orthoses rather than halo-vests.

Twelve percent of atlanto-axial injuries, treated operatively and non-operatively, will produce chronic pain (Ersmark & Kalen 1987).

Transverse ligament rupture

The transverse ligament is part of the cruciform ligament, and is the strongest part of the occipito-cervical hinge.

The maximum normal atlanto-dens interval (ADI) is 3 mm in the adult and 5 mm in children (Fielding et al 1974). Any ADI over 5 mm puts the cord at risk.

In normal patients the maximum anterior translation of C1 on C2 is 4.0 mm in children and 2.5 mm in adults (Jackson 1950).

MRI can demonstrate both mid-substance rupture and lateral bony avulsion.

This injury is often fatal, but many case-reports exist. There is a high association with head-injury. Clinical reports suggest a common mechanism, with an impact to the occiput, usually with associated local injuries, causing hyperflexion. Traumatic rupture has been reported in children.

Treatment consists of surgical stabilisation, as the remaining ligamentous structures are not strong enough to resist similar trauma. Transarticular C1–2 screws are the treatment of choice. Jeanneret & Magerl (1992) showed a solid arthrodesis in 12 of 12 patients.

Other fusion techniques probably have a higher rate of non-union.

Traumatic spondylolisthesis of the axis (hangman's fracture)

This was described in judicial hangings by the Rev. S. Houghton in 1866, who calculated the fall in feet required to produce fracture by dividing 1260 by the prisoner's weight in pounds.

Levine and Edwards' 1985 classification has been modified by Levine (1998) to include five fracture types (Figs 18.6 to 18.10).

A Type I injury has a fracture through the pars of C2 just posterior to the junction of body and pedicle. There is less than 3 mm displacement, little or no angulation, and the fracture is almost vertical. This pattern results from a hyperextension and axial load.

A Type IA or 'atypical' injury has essentially no angulation or displacement. The fracture line runs obliquely through the body on one side, and through the neural arch or foramen transversaium on the other. This fracture is not

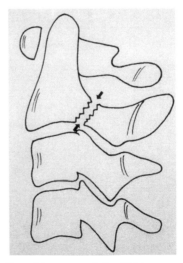

Fig. 18.6   Type I hangman's fracture.

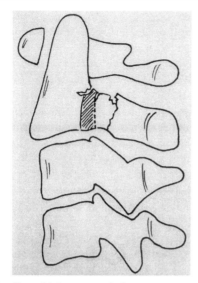

Fig. 18.7   Type IA hangman's fracture.

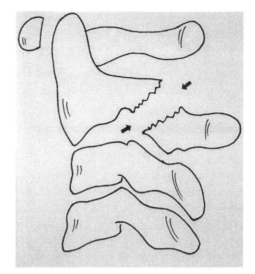

Fig. 18.9   Type IIA hangman's fracture.

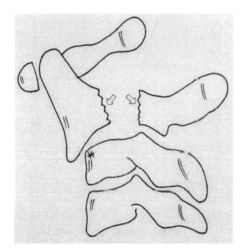

Fig. 18.8   Type II hangman's fracture.

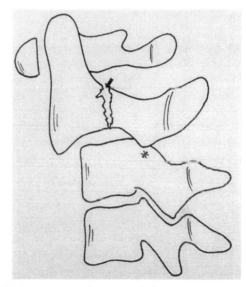

Fig. 18.10   Type III hangman's fracture.

readily apparent on lateral X-ray, but should be suspected if there is malalignment of the anterior C2–3 bodies, apparent lengthening of the body, and normal alignment of the posterior C2–3 bodies.

Type II fractures have more than 3 mm translation and variable angulation. There is usually a compression of the anterosuperior body of C3. The mechanism is a hyperextension fracturing the pars, followed by flexion disrupting the posterior longitudinal ligament and disc. The anterior longitudinal ligament is intact, allowing reduction with traction. It is essential to differentiate these injuries from type IIA fractures.

Type IIA injury is the result of failure of the neural arch under tension as a result of flexion. The fracture is much more horizontal than the extension injuries. C2 hinges on the anterior annulus of the C2–3 disc, giving angulation with little translation at the fracture. The anterior longitudinal ligament can rupture.

If traction is applied there can be dramatic vertical displacement.

Type III fracture is a combination of a Type I injury with facet joint disruption.

Francis et al (1981) showed a 6.5% incidence of neurological injury in C2 traumatic spondylolisthesis.

Treatment and prognosis

Type I and IA fractures can be treated in an orthosis.

A Type II injury with moderate displacement can be managed in a halo-vest. Wider displacement requires reduction, prolonged traction or operative fixation. IIA fractures are flexion-distraction injuries, and are reduced with extension and axial compression. A halo-vest is applied for up to 12 weeks.

Type III injuries usually require open reduction and internal fixation.

Operative stabilisation can be with anterior C2–3 fixation or posterior C2 pedicle screws.

Type I injuries have 98% union and few long-term problems (Levine 1998). These injuries are often associated with posterior atlas fractures or dens fractures. As previously noted, approximately 10 to 30% of patients with these injuries will have degeneration of the C2–3 facet joint as a result of axial loading at the time of injury (Hadley et al 1985). These patients complain of local pain, which is often exacerbated during cold weather. Late arthrodesis is indicated.

Type IA have been reported with neurological injury. The union rate is probably over 98% with few long-term problems.

Type II injuries again are often associated with other injuries, but few patients have neurological deficits as a result of this fracture. Displacement of more than 5 mm often leads to non-union at the fracture site. Seventy percent of these patients will develop an anterior ankylosis at C2–3. Symptomatic non-union is unusual, but is probably more common in lower-grade injuries with less damage to the disc and anterior portion of C2 (Levine 1998).

Coric & Kelly (1996) reviewed 39 hangman's fractures with less than 6 mm displacement. None had significant disability or neurological sequelae at follow-up. Poorly reduced type II fractures will have local kyphosis, which is often symptomatic. There may also be loss of extension.

Patients with high quadriplegia as a result of type III fractures have a poor prognosis. The long-term symptomatic results of C2–3 fusion are excellent (Levine 1998).

Twelve percent of atlanto-axial injuries, treated operatively and non-operatively, will produce chronic pain (Ersmark & Kalen 1987).

Cervical burst fractures

Burst fractures are different from compression and teardrop fractures. They are caused by axial load with varying degrees of flexion causing comminuted body fractures with varying canal occlusion. There may be failure of the posterior vertebral arch.

Treatment depends on assessment of stability and the wish to decompress the spinal cord. Both of these are controversial topics (Benz et al 1998). A wide variety of con-servative and operative options may be appropriate depending on the patients' needs and the surgeon's experience.

Cervical fractures treated in a halo-vest have a 90 to 95% union rate (Lind et al 1988; Murphy et al 1990).

There is a high incidence of neurological damage (Marar 1972; Bohlman & Anderson 1992). Surgical decompression has been shown to improve outcome. Anderson & Bohlman (1992) showed a 63% neurological improvement with decompression an average of 15 months after complete neurological injury. Earlier surgery tended to show better results. The same authors reported the results of decompression in 58 patients with incomplete injuries. If surgery was within 12 months 81% had good (gained one or more root level), or excellent (became independently mobile) results. After 12 months only 50% had good or excellent results (Anderson & Bohlman 1992).

Fusion of more than one motion segment, anterior procedures, lower (C5—T1) segment fusions, Frankel A-C grades and hyperflexion injuries are all associated with late adjacent level degeneration (Capen et al 1985; Goffin & Van Loon 1995). Symptoms, however, do not directly correlate with radiological changes.

Pain and degenerative changes are associated with kyphosis of 20° or more (Jenkins et al 1994).

Flexion teardrop fractures

These are high-energy flexion-compression injuries. The antero-inferior border of the vertebra fractures (giving the characteristic appearance), and the posterior fragment retropulses into the canal (Fig. 18.11). There can be disruption of all or most of the soft tissues, including disc and ligaments, at the level of the fracture.

There is a neurological injury dependent on the degree of canal compromise of between 25 and 91% (Allen et al 1982). Operative treatment is aimed at obtaining good spinal alignment, decompressing the spinal canal and allowing early mobilisation.

If there is no significant ligamentous or posterior element injury then non-operative management can be considered.

Hyperxtension teardrop injuries

These are avulsion fractures with Sharpeys fibres from the annulus pulling off a small fragment of bone. Most commonly occurring at C2, they tend to be stable injuries (Levine & Lutz 1992), but can be associated with posterior element injury.

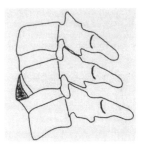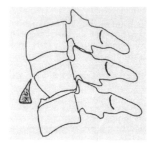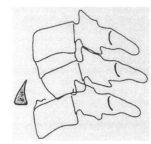

Fig. 18.11 Teardrop fractures: progressive severity.

Central cord syndrome has been described by Monroe et al (1986) but neurological injury tends to be rare (Levine & Lutz 1992).

The vast majority of these injuries progress uneventfully to asymptomatic bony or fibrous union.

Sub-axial facet joint dislocations and fractures

The majority of these injuries are flexion-distractions, with rotation possibly causing fracture of the articular process. Extension-compression may cause a fracture separation of the articular mass. The injury occurs most often at the C5–6 or C6–7 levels. Injuries include facet subluxation, perched facets, dislocated facets and fracture of one or both articular processes. These injuries can be unilateral or bilateral. Unilateral facet joint ligamentous injuries are the most common. Unilateral facet fractures and dislocations have similar degrees of translation and rotation: 4 mm and 5–7°. The facet dislocation is associated with much more soft tissue disruption, especially of the posterolateral portion of the disc. Bilateral facet dislocations produce as much as 50% translation of the vertebral body.

Delayed diagnoses of unilateral facet injuries have been widely reported.

Roy-Camille et al (1988) found that 24% of patients with unilateral dislocations had cord symptoms, and 68% had radicular symptoms. In the same paper he describes 66 patients with facet fractures who had radiculopathy, but none with myelopathy. Rorabeck et al's 1987 series of 26 patients with unilateral injury included 11 with root injury and three with cord injury.

Treatment aims to restore cervical alignment and decompress the neural elements. Reduction can be with serial traction, closed or open manipulation. Ligamentous injuries are best treated with operative stabilisation, which can be anterior or posterior via a variety of techniques.

Considerable controversy surrounds the indications for MRI in facet injuries of the cervical spine (Doran et al 1993). Worsening neurology as a result of disc retropulsion with reduction of dislocation has been described (Arena et al 1988; Tribus 1994). Discal abnormalities on MRI are present in 60% of cases, but disc retropulsion occurs in only 4% of cases, most of whom have severely displaced uni- or bi-facetal dislocation (Marshall 1987).

The loss of reduction in halo-vests has been described. This orthosis does not control rotation or 'snaking' in the mid-cervical spine (Perry 1972).

In Rorabeck et al's 1987 study, all patients with reduced dislocation had good outcomes, while seven out of 10 patients with untreated dislocation had disabling pain. Beyer & Cabanela (1991) reported 10 of 24 patients treated conservatively having long-term symptoms while one of 10 treated operatively had long-term pain.

Post-traumatic syringomyelia

While incidences of up to 50% in spinal cord injury have been reported, this probably represents primary lesions. The incidence of post-traumatic syringomyelia causing progressive neuropathy is thought to be between 0.3 and 2.3% of spinal cord injuries according to some authors (Rossier 1981; Williams 1981). However, a more recent prospective study of 449 spinal cord injury patients followed yearly for 6 years found that 6% developed a symptomatic syrinx (Schurch et al 1996).

■ References

Allen B L Jr, Ferguson R L, Lehman T R et al 1982 A mechanistic classification of closed, indirect fractures and dislocations of the cervical spine. Spine 7: 1–27

American Spinal Injury Association and International Medical Society of Paraplegia 1992 Standard for neurological and functional classification of spinal cord injury, revised. American Spinal Injury Association, Atlanta, GA

Anderson L D, D'Alonzo R T 1974 Fractures of the odontoid process of the axis. Journal of Bone and Joint Surgery (Am) 56: 1663

Anderson P A, Bohlman H H 1992 Anterior decompression and arthrodesis of the cervical spine: Long-term motor improvement. Part II—Improvement in complete traumatic quadriplegia. Journal of Bone and Joint Surgery (Am) 74: 683–692

Anderson P A, Montesano P X 1988 Morphology and treatment of occipital condyle fractures. Spine 13: 731–736

Apuzzo M L J, Heiden J S, Weiss M H et al 1978 Acute fractures of the odontoid process: An analysis of 45 cases. Journal of Neurosurgery 48: 85

Arena M J, Eismont F J, Green B A 1988 Intravertebral disc extrusion associated with cervical facet subluxation and dislocation. Journal of Bone and Joint Surgery (Am) 72: 43

Benz R, Abitbol J J, Ozanne S, Garfin S R 1998 Cervical burst fractures in *Spine Trauma*. Levine, Edmont, Garfin, Zigler. (eds) W B Saunders

Beyer C A, Cabanela M E 1991 Unilateral facet dislocations and fracture-dislocations of the cervical spine: a review. Orthopaedics 15(3): 311

Bohlman H H 1972 Pathology and current treatment concepts of cervical spine injuries. Instructional Course Lecture 21: 108–115

Bohlman H H 1979 Acute fractures and dislocations of the cervical spine. Journal of Bone and Joint Surgery (Am) 61: 1119–1142

Bohlman H H, Anderson P A 1992 Anterior decompression and arthrodesis of the cervical spine: Long-term motor improvement. Part I—Improvement in incomplete traumatic quadriplegia. Journal of Bone and Joint Surgery (Am) 74: 671–682

Bracken M B, Shepard M J, Collins W F, Holford T R, Young W, Baskin D S 1990 A randomised, controlled trial of methylprednisolone or naloxone in the treatment of acute spinal-cord injury. New England Journal of Medicine 322: 1405–1411

Bracken M B, Shepard M J, Holford T R, Leo-Summers L, Aldrich E F et al 1997 Administration of methylprednisolone for 24 or 48 hours or tirilazad mesylate for 24 or 48 hours in the treatment of acute spinal cord injury: results of the third National Acute Spinal Cord Injury Randomized Controlled Trial. National Acute Spinal Cord Injury Study. JAMA 277(20): 1597–1604

Bucholz R W, Burkhead W Z 1979 The pathological anatomy of fatal atlanto-occipital dislocations. Journal of Bone and Joint Surgery 61(A): 248–249

Campagnolo D L, Esquieres R E, Kopacz K J 1997 Effect of the timing of stabilization on length of stay and medical complications following spinal cord injury. Journal of spinal Cord Medicine 20(3): 331–334

Capen D A, Garland D E, Waters R L 1985 Surgical stabilization of the cervical spine. A comparison of anterior and posterior spine fusions. Clinical Orthopaedics 196: 229–237

Carlson G D, Minato Y, Okada A, Gorden C D, Warden K E, Barbeau J M et al 1997 Early time-dependent decompression for spinal cord injury: vascular mechanisms of recovery. Journal of Neurotrauma 14(12): 951–962

Carlson G D, Heller J G, Abitbol J J, Garfin S R 1998 Odontoid fractures in *Spine Trauma*. Levine, Edmont, Garfin, Zigler. (eds) W B Saunders

Chan R N W, Ainscow D, Sikorski J M 1980 Diagnostic failures in the multiply injured. Journal of Trauma 20: 684–687

Chapman J R, Anderson P A 1997 The Adult Spine: Principles and Practice. Frymoyer J W (ed) Lippincot-Raven, p 1245–1295

Clark C R 1991 Dens fractures. Seminal Spine Surgery 3: 39

Clark C R, Ingram C M, El Khoury G Y, Ehara S 1988 Radiographic evaluation of cervical spine injuries. Spine 13: 742–747

Clark C R, White A A 1985 Fractures of the dens. Journal of Bone and Joint Surgery (Am) 67: 1340

Coric D, Kelly D L 1996 Treatment of traumatic spondylolisthesis of the axis with non-rigid immobilization: a review of 64 cases. Journal of Neurosurgery 85: 4, 550–554

Crockard H A, Heilman A E, Stevens J M 1993 Progressive myelopathy secondary to odontoid fractures: Clinical, surgical and radiological features. Journal of Neurosurgery 78: 579

Davis J W, Phreaner D L, Hoyt D B, Mackersie R C 1993 The etiology of missed cervical spine injuries. Journal of Trauma 34: 342–345

Delamarter R B, Sherman J, Carr J B 1995 Pathophysiology of spinal cord injury: recovery after immediate and delayed decompression. Journal of Bone and Joint Surgery 77A: 1042–1049

Doran S E, Papadopoulos S M, Ducker T B, Lillehei K O 1993 Magnetic resonance image documentation of coexistent traumatic locked facets and disc herniation. Journal of Neurosurgery 79: 341–345

Dunn E J, Blazer S 1987 Soft tissue injuries to the lower cervical spine. Instructional Course Lecture 36: 499–512

Eismont F J, Bohlman H H 1978 Posterior atlanto-occipital dislocation with fractures of the atlas and dens. Journal of Bone and Joint Surgery 60A: 397–399

Enderson B L, Reath D B, Meadors J, Dallas W, Deboo J B, Maull K I 1990 The tertiary trauma survey: a prospective study of missed injury. Journal of Trauma 30: 666–669

Ersmark H, Kalen R 1987 A follow-up study of 85 axis and 10 atlas fractures. Clinical Orthopaedics Rel Res 217: 257–260

Fielding J W, Cochran G V B, Lawsing J F et al 1974 Tears of the transverse ligament of the atlas: A clinical and biomechanical study. Journal of Bone and Joint Surgery (Am) 56: 1683–1691

Fielding J W, Hawkings R J 1977 Atlanto-axial rotatory fixation. Journal of Bone and Joint Surgery (Am) 59: 37

Fielding J W, Hawkins R J, Ratzan S A 1976 Spine fusion for atlantoaxial instability. Journal of Bone and Joint Surgery (Am) 58: 400

Francis W R, Fielding J W, Hawkins J R 1981 Traumatic spondylolisthesis of the axis. Journal of Bone and Joint Surgery 63: 311–318

Goffin J, Van Loon J et al 1995 Long-term results after anterior cervical spine fusion for fractures and/or dislocations of the cervical spine. Journal of Spinal Disorder 8: 500–508

Hadley M N, Browner C, Sonntag V K 1985 Axis fractures: A comprehensive review of management and treatment of 107 cases. Neurosurgery 17: 281

Hadley M N, Browner C M, Liu S S et al 1988 New subtype of acute odontoid fractures (type IIA). Neurosurgery 22: 67

Hadley M N, Dickman C A, Browner C M et al 1989 Acute axis fractures: A review of 229 cases. Journal of Neurosurgery 17: 642

Highland T R, Salciccioli G G 1985 Is immobilization adequate treatment of unstable burst fractures of the atlas? Clinical Orthopaedics 201: 196–200

Jackson H 1950 The diagnosis of minimal atlanto-axial subluxation. British Journal of Radiology 23: 672

Jeanneret B, Magerl F 1992 Primary posterior fusion of C1–2 in odontoid fusion: Indications, techniques and results of transarticular screw fixation. Journal of Spinal Disorder 5: 464–475

Jefferson G 1920 Fracture of the atlas vertebra. British Journal of Surgery 7: 407

Jenkins L A, Capen D A, Zigler J E, Nelson R W, Nagelberg S 1994 Cervical spine fusions for trauma. A long-term radiographic and clinical evaluation. Orthopaedic Review Supplement 13–19

Lee T T, Green B A, Petrin D R 1998 Treatment of stable burst fracture of the atlas (Jefferson fracture) with rigid cervical collar. Spine 23: 18, 1963–1967

Levi L, Wolf A, Rigamonti D et al 1991 Anterior decompression in cervical spine trauma: does the timing of surgery affect the outcome? Neurosurgery 29: 216–222

Levine A M 1983 Avulsion of the transverse ligament associated with fracture of the atlas. Orthopedics 6: 1467

Levine A M 1998 Fractures of the atlas in *Spine Trauma*. Levine, Edmont, Garfin, Zigler. (eds) W B Saunders

Levine A M 1998 Traumatic spondylolisthesis of the axis (Hangmans fracture) in *Spine Trauma*. Levine, Edmont, Garfin, Zigler (eds) W B Saunders

Levine A M, Edwards C C 1985 The management of traumatic spondylolisthesis of the axis. Journal of Bone and Joint Surgery (Am) 67: 217–226

Levine A M, Edwards C C 1991 Fractures of the atlas. Journal of Bone and Joint Surgery (Am) 73: 680–691

Levine A M, Lutz B 1992 Extension teardrop injuries of the cervical spine. Cervical Spine Research Society: Dec, abstract 49

Lind B, Nordwall A, Sihlbolm H 1987 Odontoid fractures treated with halo vest. Spine 12: 173

Lind B, Sihlbom H, Nordwall A 1988 Halo-vest treatment of unstable cervical spine injuries. Spine 13: 425–432

Locke G R, Gardner J I, van Epps E F 1966 Atlanto-dens interval in children: A survey based on 200 normal subjects. AJR 97: 135

Maiman D J, Larson D J 1982 Management of odontoid fractures. Neurosurgery 11: 471

Marar B 1972 The pattern of neurological damage as an aid to the diagnosis of mechanism in cervical spine injuries. Journal of Bone and Joint Surgery (Am) 56: 1648–1654

Marar B D, Balachandran N 1973 Non-traumatic atlanto-axial dislocation in children. Clinical Orthopaedic Rel Res 92: 220

Marshall L F, Knowlton S, Garfin S R 1987 Deterioration following spinal cord injury. Journal of Neurosurgery 66: 400–404

Monroe B E, Wagner L K, Harris J H 1986 Hyperextension dislocation of the cervical spine. AJR 146: 803–808

Montane I, Eismont F J, Green B A 1991 Traumatic atlanto-occipital dislocation. Spine 16: 112–116

Moore K R, Frank E H 1995 Traumatic atlantoaxial rotatory subluxation and subluxation. Spine 20: 1928–1930

Murphy K P et al 1990 Cervical fractures and spinal cord injury: Outcome of surgical and non-surgical management. Mayo Clinical Processes 65: 949–959

Ono K, Yonenobu K, Fuji T et al 1985 Atlantoaxial rotatory fixation: Radiographic study of its mechanism. Spine 10: 602

Panjabi M, Dvorak J, Duranceau J et al 1988 Three dimensional movements of the upper cervical spine. Spine 13: 726–730

Penning L, Wilmink J T 1987 Rotation of the cervical spine. A CT study in normal subjects. Spine 12: 732

Perry J 1972 The halo in spinal abnormalities. Orthopedic Clinics of North America 3: 69–80

Phillips W A, Hensinger R N 1989 The management of rotatory atlantoaxial subluxation in children. Journal of Bone and Joint Surgery (Am) 71: 664

Robertson P, Swan H 1992 Traumatic bilateral rotatory facet dislocation of the atlas on the axis. Spine 17: 1252–1254

Rorabeck C H, Rock M G, Hawkins R J 1987 Unilateral facet dislocation of the cervical spine: An analysis of results of treatment in 26 patients. Spine 12: 23–27

Rosenfeld J F, Vaccaro A R, Albert T J, Klein G R, Coiler J M 1998 The benefits of early decompression in cervical spinal cord injury. American Journal of Orthopaedics 1: 23–28

Rossier A B, Foo D, Shillito J et al 1981 Progressive late post-traumatic syringomyelia. Paraplegia 19: 96–97

Roy-Camille R, Mazel G, Edourard B 1988 Luxations et luxations-fractures. In: Roy-Camille R (ed) Rachis Cervical Inferieur: Sixiemes Journées D'Orthopedie de la Pitie. Paris, Masson, pp 93–103

Roy-Camille R, Saillant G, Mazel C 1989 Internal fixation of the unstable cervical spine by a posterior osteosynthesis with plates and screws. In: The cervical spine, 2nd edn. J B Lippincott, Philadelphia pp 390–403

Ryan M D, Taylor T K F 1982 Odontoid fractures. A rational approach to treatment. Journal of Bone and Joint Surgery 64: 416

Salzman S K, Betz R R 1996 Experimental treatment of spinal cord injuries. In: Betz R R (ed.) The child with a spinal cord injury. American Association of Orthopedic Surgeons: 63

Sasso R C, Jeanneret B, Fischer K, Magerl F 1994 Occipitocervical fusion with posterior plate and screw insertion. A long-term follow-up study. Spine 19: 2364–2368

Schurch B, Wichmann W, Rossier A B 1996 Post-traumatic syringomyelia (cystic myelopathy): A prospective study of 449 patients with spinal cord injury. Journal of Neuro Neurosurgical Psychiatry 60: 61–67

Segal L S, Grimm J O, Stauffer E S 1987 Non-union of fractures of the atlas. Journal of Bone and Joint Surgery (Am) 69: 1423–1434

Smith M D, Anderson P A 1994 Occipitocervical fusion. Technical Orthopaedics 9: 37–42

Sonntag V K H, Francis P M 1995 Patient selection and timing of surgery. In: Benzel E C, Tator C H (eds) Contemporary management of spinal cord injury. American Association of Neurological Surgeons, Park Ridge, Il: pp 97–108

Spence K F, Decker S, Sell K W 1970 Bursting atlantal fracture associated with rupture of the transverse ligament. Journal of Bone and Joint Surgery (Am) 52: 543–549

Streitwieser D, Knopp R, Wales L R, Williams J L and Tonnemacher K 1983 Accuracy of Standard Radiographic Views in Detecting Cervical Spine Fractures. Annals of Emergency Medicine 12: 538–542

Traylenis V C, Marano G D, Dunker R O, Kaufman H H 1986 Traumatic atlantooccipital dislocation: case report. Journal of Neurosurgery 65: 863–870

Tribus C B 1994 Cervical disc herniation in association with traumatic facet dislocation. Technical Orthopaedics 9: 5–7

Vaccaro A R, Singh K 2000 Pharmacological treatment and surgical timing for spinal cord injury. Contemporary Spine Surgery, Vol. 1:9: 55–62

Vacarro et al 1997 Neurologic outcome of early versus late surgery for cervical spinal cord injury. Spine 22(22): 2609–2613

Werne S 1957 Studies in spontaneous atlas dislocation. Acta Orthopaedica Scandinavica (suppl) 23: 1–150

White A A, Panjabi M 1987 Update on the evaluation of the lower cervical spine. Instructional Course Lecture, 36: 499–520

White A A, Panjabi M 1990 The problem of clinical instability in the human spine: A systematic approach. In: White A A et al (eds) Clinical biomechanics of the spine, 2nd edn. J B Lippincot, Philadelphia, pp 277–378

White A A, Southwick W O, Panjabi M M 1976 Clinical instability of the lower cervical spine. Spine 1: 15–27

Williams B, Terry A F, Jones H W F et al 1981 Syringomyelia as a sequel to traumatic paraplegia. Paraplegia 19: 67–80

Worzman G, Dewar F P 1968 Rotatory fixation of the atlantoaxial joint. Radiology 90: 479

Zielinski C J, Gunther S F, Deeb Z 1982 Cranial nerve palsies complicating Jefferson fracture. Journal of Bone and Joint Surgery (Am) 64: 1382–1384

The thoracic and lumbar spine

Jeremy C. T. Fairbank

■ Assessment of thoracic and lumbar spinal problems in patients in personal injury cases

Introduction

The clinician delivering a medical report on a patient with spinal symptoms following personal injury must rely principally on the patient's history, aided by all available medical records, especially those of the general practitioner, other legal reports and submissions and investigations. Examination is important, and may provide additional valuable information, but this is normally secondary to the history. On occasions, special investigations may be commissioned to supplement or confirm an opinion. This chapter is concerned with these aspects of medico-legal reporting.

Causation of back pain

Chronic pain is very common in community surveys, and back pain heads the list of more specific complaints (Elliott et al 1999, Health Department 1999). This leads to difficulties in dissecting out how much symptoms are attributable to a specific incident and how much is due to societal and degenerative factors.

It is important to appreciate, and when appropriate to emphasise in the report, that in many cases the true cause of back pain is not well understood, and is often unknown. Classification systems of back pain are discussed elsewhere (Fairbank & Pynsent 1992) and are not appropriate for the medico-legal environment. In the author's view, there is accumulating evidence that the intervertebral disc is involved in many cases of chronic back pain, although the mechanisms are not well understood. Intervertebral discs degenerate in all adults, and some adolescents. Often this process is asymptomatic, and the process of distinguishing symptomatic from asymptomatic discs is complex and idiosyncratic in different clinicians. There is experimental evidence from Fraser's group in Adelaide that disc degeneration can be precipitated by trauma in sheep, and that this process occurs *gradually* over a period

after the insult (4–12 months in his sheep model; Osti et al 1990, Moore et al 1992). A recent report from Finland suggests very strongly that intervertebral disc degeneration is implicated in back pain in adolescents and young adults (Salminen et al 1999). Another study from the same country pointed to the early onset of low back pain (around the age of 15) in patients hospitalised with diagnoses related to lumbar disc disorders, including disc prolapse. This study does not record 'injury' as a factor.

The earlier observations by Park in Oswestry of the posterior annular tear (Park et al 1979) are also of importance. Axial injuries to the spine of young people (a 4-year-old was an exceptional example in the author's experience, although it did not present until the age of 16) can produce symptomatic annular tears which are difficult to diagnose, and symptoms may therefore be misinterpreted as psychosomatic. A post-mortem study has also linked annular tears with trauma (Osti et al 1992). Thus, in this author's view, high-velocity road traffic accidents and falls may also produce injuries to the annulus of the intervertebral disc. Such a lesion may become symptomatic gradually after the accident, but in most cases significant pain is present from the time of injury. Such pain may be masked by symptoms from other injuries. This may *not* be associated with intervertebral disc herniation, and therefore may *not* be visible in myelography or computed tomographic (CT) examinations. These injuries may be identified on high-quality magnetic resonance scans (MRI) or discography. Spondylolysis and spondylolisthesis are recognised sources of back symptoms diagnosed from plain radiographs. However, even the presence of these abnormalities can be misleading, and the pain can be arising from elsewhere in the lumbar spine. Both these findings may be asymptomatic. In general, other congenital anomalies of the lumbar spine are asymptomatic.

In the end, the clinician has to take a view on all the available evidence as to whether the spine symptoms are attributable to the injury or not. The younger the victim, the more likely is MR and discographic evidence to be attributable.

Pain following fractures

Significant long-term pain following spinal fractures was for a long time denied by advocates of the conservative management of these injuries. The publication from the

Perth group (Hardcastle et al 1987) has shown that this is not the case. This study suggested that a long fusion was probably deleterious to function in paraplegics. MRI scanning has demonstrated the frequency of disc injuries accompanying vertebral body fractures, and it is possible that these are important sources of chronic back pain. A recent, and important, multi-centre non-randomised trial of conservative v. operative treatment of burst fractures in 1019 patients has shown that wedging of greater than 30 is closely related to chronic pain (Gerzbein 1992). This study also suggests that effective surgery is better at reducing the incidence of pain in these fractures, and is probably more effective in improving neurological status than conservative care.

Litigation and illness behaviour

Litigation has long been recognised as an adverse feature in back pain patients (Krusen & Ford 1958, Hammonds et al 1978, Waddell et al 1979, Spengler et al 1980, Leavitt et al 1982, Carron et al 1985, Frymoyer et al 1985, Trief & Stein 1985, Vallfors 1985, Sternbach 1986, Hurme & Alaranta 1987, Jamison et al 1988, Kleinke & Spangler 1988, Greenough & Fraser 1989, Talo et al 1989, Burns et al 1995, Rainville et al 1997, Vaccaro et al 1997). This must be accepted as a fact of life, and the prognosis, even in the most clear-cut pathological circumstances, altered accordingly. All patients will exhibit some degree of illness behaviour. This may be magnified in certain personality types, in the presence of secondary gain, where doctors have failed to deliver a convincing diagnosis and where treatment has failed. This area has been a major preoccupation of Waddell's group (Waddell et al 1992). These patients are very difficult to assess, and it may be appropriate to use specialised questionnaires (Main et al 1992). In the medico-legal environment, it may be necessary to obtain a clinical psychologist's opinion on the patient's behaviour. In some circumstances, defendants have resorted to private detectives to monitor activities of daily living.

The well-known inappropriate physical signs should not be used in isolation. In a study that the author undertook on physical examination, these signs were very unreliable (McCombe et al 1989). In a Canadian study (Bradish et al 1988) it was shown that they did not predict outcome in a group of patients with chronic back pain receiving workman's compensation, although others have found them to be of predictive value (Dzioba & Doxey 1984). They should be reported, but interpretation must be cautions. Lancourt & Ketteelhut (1992) have identified other social factors that predict return to work following industrial injury, including the following: a history of workman's compensation; an Oswestry score over 55; adverse

family factors; employment for less than 6 months; financial difficulties; poor coping skills, etc. McIntosh et al (2000) prospectively observed 1752 workmen's compensation claimants for 1 year. Prolonged claims were associated with 1) working in the construction industry (about half the rate of those in other industries); 2) older age (also found in other studies); 3) lag from injury to treatment; 4) pain referred into the leg; and 5) three or more Waddell signs (which, incidently, were found in 9.4% of this sample). Reduced time receiving benefit was associated with 1) a less severe score on a disability scale (a modification of the Low Back Pain Outcome score (Greenough & Fraser 1992)); 2) intermittant pain; and 3) a previous episode of back pain (this finding conflicts with those of all other studies). This study suffers from the usual problems of selectivity, as it includes only patients seeking compensation and treatment through the channels of one particular back pain service. Even so, these factors explain only 25% of the varience, so there are many other unknown factors working here. Waddell & Main have emphasised that their signs should be used with great caution in an individual and have confirmed that their signs are unsuitable for use in a medico-legal environment (Main & Waddell 1998).

Pre-existing back problems

Great difficulties arise where there have been back symptoms or successful spinal surgery before the injury in question, or where there are obvious abnormalities on X-ray which predate the injury. Each case must be taken on its merits, and a careful history and examination of the available evidence made before an opinion is given. Lawyers frequently demand an opinion on the risk of the symptoms developing if the accident had not occurred. This question is often impossible to answer, as useful data are not available from the literature. An estimate is usually offered of the number of years that a particular injury has brought forward symptoms that might otherwise have occurred. It is important to remember that the incidence of back pain often diminishes in later years (Fairbank 1986, Health Department 1999). Kellgren & Lawrence's epidemiological work in the 1950s is an important source of the relationship of degenerative changes of the lumbar spine to back symptoms, although this study did not attempt to measure the severity of symptoms (Lawrence 1969). One good long-term study from Denmark put the relative risk of a history of back pain at 2.71 (95% Confidence Intervals (CI) 1.75–4.21). This study also finds a higher incidence of sickness absence in unskilled workers and in those with poor job satisfaction (Müller et al 1999). This supports the findings of the Boeing study where this was found to be much the strongest predictor of back pain in a working population (Bigos et al 1991).

Attempts have been made to link many environmental factors to back pain. Driving, smoking and exposure to vibration are the strongest of these factors in relation to disc prolapse (Kelsey et al 1984), and may be commented on where appropriate.

Low back pain is more common in heavy manual workers than others (Kelsey et al 1992). The occupations with the highest incidence are truck driver, material handling, nursing and nursing aids. These figures must be qualified by compensation factors and the difficulties of returning to heavy physical work with a degree of back pain which may be tolerable only in less physically demanding jobs.

Frequency and amount of lifting may be a factor over 11.3 kilograms, but there are conflicting findings in the literature (Kelsey et al 1992). Unexpected sudden maximal effort may also be associated with back pain. These points are all based on epidemiological findings, and individual cases must be interpreted on their own merits. Sedentary jobs may also have an increased incidence of back pain (Kelsey et al 1992).

Outcome measures

Recently, there has been increasing interest in defining outcome measures. There are different requirements in the fields of clinical research, clinical audit and medico-legal reporting. Outcome measures should be transferred from one requirement to another with great care. Medico-legal reports concern the circumstances of an individual, and so it should be made clear when interpreting from the general to the particular. Specific outcome measures have to be defined for an individual. For example, in a retired man whose main interest is golf, the capacity to play golf and the number of holes he can manage could be used as a principal outcome measure, while in a young labourer the principal outcome measure may be his working capacity. A woman's capacity to look after a young family or her ability to sit may be equally important. Other patients may be more concerned with walking or carrying capacity.

The Oswestry Disability Index (Fairbank et al 1980) and the Roland–Morris scale (Roland & Morris 1983) are two widely used condition-specific outcome measures. The author does not use these self-report scales in the medico-legal environment (Fairbank & Pynsent 2000) as their validity depends on statistical tests made on many patients. A single patient has to show large changes in the scale before any absolute improvement with time or treatment can be established. Absolute measures can give only general guidance as to severity of perceived symptoms (Roland & Fairbank 2000).

Assessment

The history of injury is of paramount importance. All histories are flawed and, ideally, should be corroborated by other evidence. The reliability of history-taking in this area has been investigated (Biering-Sorenson & Hilden 1984, Thomas et al 1989, Walsh & Coggan 1991), but these studies are difficult to apply to the individual medico-legal situation.

History of injury

A detailed history of the original injury must be taken from the patient. Records are not infrequently inaccurate or incomplete. A check list of relevant factors includes:

- The mechanism of injury, an indication of the violence involved (degree of damage to vehicle, height fallen, estimated speed, weight lifted, whether another party let go, etc.).
- Whether this was an abnormal or normal working practice.
- Which part of the body struck the ground first (with corroborating evidence of other injuries) should be ascertained.
- The nature of the work or working practices may be relevant, including training in lifting and handling.

The timing of the onset of symptoms is important. Back pain may be noticed some time after the injury, particularly in association with other fractures, head, chest or abdominal injuries. In general, a 2 week delay in the onset of symptoms following a high-energy injury is acceptable, and this period might be prolonged in the case of head injury or enforced recumbancy. This view is a matter of opinion, and hard to justify one way or another from the literature. Herniated discs can occur in association with injury (again a matter of opinion, and the exception rather than the rule) and back pain may precede the onset of root symptoms by hours, days, weeks or even months. Causation may be difficult to establish, but the back pain should start very soon after the injury. In normal clinical practice, herniated discs start with an insidious onset of back pain, and clear-cut trauma is not often implicated.

Management

The time of arrival of the patient in hospital (or, where appropriate, the timing of his first medical consultation) should be noted. Where ambulance records are available, the timing of first call, etc., should also be noted. Details of the subsequent medical management, investigations, conservative and operative procedures should be recorded.

The patient's subsequent course, noting hospital and other attendances, return to work, interference with social life, hobbies and other leisure activities should be noted, as these details may give an indication of disability.

Present symptoms

These provide the main basis for developing a prognosis. In the author's view, they should not be assessed until at least a year following the injury in question, however. If surgery has been carried out, the final assessment should be made at least a year after the intervention. Referred journals require a 2–5 year follow-up, but this ideal has to be seen in the light of the legal and financial demands for settlement.

Pain pattern

This is helpful in distinguishing referred pain from root pain. Back pain is normally experienced at or below the level of the lesion, either in the midline or to one side. In a small study (Fairbank 1982), the author found pain from definite sites of pathology (tumours or fractures) to be referred about two segments distally in the thoracic and upper lumbar spine. In the low lumbar spine, pain may be referred into the buttocks, posterior thighs and sometimes, when severe, into the calves. This phenomenon was first described by Kellgren (Kellgren 1938, 1939, 1941, 1977) and was later called sclerodermal pain. Sufferers of this type of referred pain often report more distal radiation when their symptoms are worse (what the author has come to call 'thermometer' pain). This pain is frequently confused with root pain. The term 'sciatica' is to be abhorred as it has never received an accepted medical definition, and in many doctors' minds is equivalent to root pain. Patients and doctors alike have difficulty in distinguishing the 'leg' from the 'thigh', and 'all the way down the leg' may or may not include the foot.

Root pain is usually in a dermatomal distribution. The upper lumbar roots (L2 and L3, and sometimes L4) refer to the anterior thigh. Sclerodermal pain from these levels may refer to the groin and genitalia (McCall et al 1979). S1 root pain tends to be felt in the sole or lateral side of the foot, while L5 is felt on the dorsomedial aspect of the foot or toes. The symptoms of neurogenic claudication are often difficult for the patient to localise precisely.

Patients with chronic back pain may exhibit total spinal or whole body pain, and many will also display features of pain behaviour. This can occur with clear-cut pathology, but is often seen where all treatment has failed, and no pain source can be identified. It is best shown by a self-reported pain pattern (Ransford et al 1976), which in

some reports has been found to be a predictor of poor outcome of treatment (most recently in spinal fusion for spondylolisthesis (Möller and Hedlund 2000)).

Pain severity

This is difficult, but not impossible, to measure. A full discussion of the issue was presented by Jadad (1993). However, it is difficult to interpret in medico-legal reports. A pain diary may be of some value.

Current disabilities

These concern activities of daily living, working ability, time taken off work, interference with leisure activities, sports, hobbies, etc., and the use of walking aids, wheelchairs, etc. Again, formal measures of disability such as the Oswestry index (Fairbank et al 1980, Baker et al 1989, Fairbank & Pynsent 2000) can be used, but are difficult to interpret in isolation (Lancourt & Ketteelhut 1992).

Exacerbating and relieving factors

These can be useful in distinguishing root pain from referred pain. Root pain is generally but not always exacerbated by walking. An important group of back pain patients have their symptoms exacerbated by sitting and relieved by activity. Chronic back pain is usually activity related, but patients cannot usually define a walking distance, unlike those with neurogenic claudication. Claudicants relieve their pain by sitting, squatting or stooping, and have to wait 5–20 minutes before they can carry on. This is in contrast to vascular claudicants, who usually have to wait for only a minute or two. Neurogenic claudicants cannot 'walk through' their symptoms, and they describe a wide variety of these, ranging from heaviness to non-dermatomal pain, and, on occasion, they may have symptoms such as bladder fullness and penile erection. Classically, these patients can ride a bicycle without symptoms (Dong & Porter 1989). Night pain can be associated with acute disc herniations, although this is also an indicator of spinal tumours or infection.

Bladder/bowel/sexual disabilities

These should be recorded in those individuals with cauda equina symptoms and chronic low back pain. The orthopaedic expert should be careful in keeping within his/her expertise in interpreting the significance of these symptoms.

Record of abilities/disabilities

In these days of covert video surveillance, it is important to document the subject's reported walking and carrying capacity, and what his normal day-to-day activities are. Clearly, it is easier to throw doubt on an individual's case if he or she is seen to do something that he or she has reported that they 'never' do. However, if he/she reports 'sometimes' or 'good and bad days', then video evidence of a capacity on a single occasion is less impressive. It is worth recording the frequency of reported incapacity in this event.

Examination
General considerations

The examination starts on the first sight of the patient. Inconsistencies between his or her behaviour and reported disability are noted. The shape of the spine is normally reported descriptively, but special techniques, such as photography or ISIS, can be used. Direct measurements from plain radiographs can also be presented.

Neurological signs should be reported individually but, on occasion, the Frankel score is of value (Frankel et al 1969), although it must be clearly explained to lawyers. Bladder function is not included here, and must be defined separately, or be referred to experts.

Waddell's group has published a paper on the assessment of physical impairment in patients with chronic low back pain, and produced a score in terms of total flexion, total extension, average lateral flexion, average straight leg raise and spinal tenderness, with a clear description of how these tests were applied. However, this is difficult to apply to the individual, with the usual problems of arguing from the general to the particular. One test described in this paper, which is not generally used, but which may be applicable in medico-legal examinations, is the bilateral straight leg raise. This involves asking the supine patient to raise both legs six inches off the couch, and to hold this position for 5 seconds. The examiner is not permitted to count the seconds out loud, and the calves must be clear of support for a positive result (Waddell et al 1992).

Look

Skin blemishes, injury scars and surgical scars should be described and measured. Unsightly lumps and bumps relating to the injury should be recorded, and leg length discrepancies and limb circumferences noted. The latter are useful in confirming loss of function, disuse or neurological damage. Grip strength can be assessed with a commercial device or a rolled-up sphygmomanometer cuff. Lower limb muscle strength can be assessed using the MRC scale. Always compare the affected with the unaffected side.

Feel

Look for tenderness, particularly over the spine. This was surprisingly reliable in the midline in the author's study (McCombe et al 1989). Waddell has confirmed these findings, and gives a clear description of this technique (Waddell et al 1992).

Movement

Range of movement is important in the assessment of spinal pain, but is not always easy to measure. Waddell's advice concerning 'warm-up' (Waddell et al 1992), which encourages patients to carry out the manoeuvre several times before a measurement is taken, is highly recommended. Modified Schrober tape measurements (MacVae & Wright 1969) or goniometer measures can be used (Ohlen et al 1989, Waddell et al 1992), as can descriptive measures in percentages, or the distance that the fingertips reach down the lower limbs. McCombe found the tape measure method to be reliable (McCombe et al 1989). Another technique is the flexicurve method (Burton 1986), which can also be applied to the cervical spine.

Straight leg raise (SLR)

This is an important test in clinical practice. However, it does vary day to day, and there is no absolutely agreed method of performing the test. In the medico-legal environment this may mean that apparently discordant observations reflect badly on the patient.

The author's preferred method is to lie the patient supine and flat. The symptomatic side is examined first. The hip and knee are passively flexed to their full extent. The hip joint may be rotated at this stage if it is thought to be symptomatic. The knee is extended gently until straight, allowing the hip joint to extend as symptoms and mobility permit. This angle is the straight leg raise. Other tension signs may be elicited at this stage if required. The manoeuvre is then repeated on the other side. It should be done with care in patients with considerable nerve root irritability, whom it may otherwise hurt. This method is less familiar to the 'professional patient', so that, in the author's view, a more reliable measurement is obtained. If the patient can sit up on the couch with knees extended, this should be recorded. This is not quite the same as a unilateral SLR, but is equivalent to raising both legs at once. It allows the pelvis to rotate so that the tension on the sciatic nerve and lumbar roots is diminished compared with a unilateral SLR. Nevertheless, a patient who does not permit an SLR but can sit up on a couch should be considered to be behaving inappropriately.

Neurological examination

This should be undertaken in all cases, and either reported as normal, or the abnormalities specified.

Investigations
Plain X-ray

This is an essential part of the assessment of the back pain patient. However, its limitations should be clearly appreciated. There is a wealth of asymptomatic abnormality to be found on X-rays of the lumbar spine, some of which has been alluded to above. Not infrequently, films can be found of the offending part taken before the accident for other reasons, and these can also be of value, both in detecting changes that might be consequent on the accident, and in providing a check on the patient's history. All relevant dates and findings should be included in the medical report. The most important feature of plain X-rays is that they are rather less 'operator dependent' than more complex investigations.

Contrast studies

The myelogram is rapidly becoming an historical investigation, although it is generally accepted as the 'gold standard' on which more modern investigations are validated. It is still sometimes used in combination with CT, particularly in neurosurgical departments. It may be of value in the assessment of post-surgical complications (Montaldi et al 1988). It is not an appropriate test to commission for medico-legal reasons where more modern techniques are available.

CT scans

Computed tomography is of great value in the assessment of fractures and vertebral canal dimensions and, rarely, where other bone pathology is indicated. It cannot easily be extended to the whole spine without massive exposure to radiation, or by making the cuts so thick as to be diagnostically useless. CT will demonstrate herniated discs nicely, but is misleading in the assessment of the failed surgical patient (Montaldi et al 1988). It can be used in conjunction with myelography. There is a high incidence of abnormal findings in the asymptomatic spine (Weisel et al 1984). Spiral (or helical) CT is an evolution of the same technology, giving better quality imaging.

MRI scans

The introduction of magnetic resonance imaging has transformed the investigation of the spine. It is a very sophisticated technique, and is both machine and operator dependent. The early machines produced indifferent pictures by modern standards, but even the best machine will produce poor quality images in the hands of an inexperienced operator. As in all investigations of the spine, there is a plethora of asymptomatic abnormality (Powell et al 1986, Boden et al 1990). Where there is abnormality, it has to be interpreted against the background of the clinical problem, and the radiologist should be familiar with this. There is much sub-specialisation in radiology, as in other fields of medicine, and reports should be accepted only on the basis of the repute of the signature.

There are some useful applications of MRI in the field of medico-legal work. In some cases the medical expert should advise that an MRI scan be obtained, and insist that it is done by the appropriate radiologist. The principal indications are for the investigation of neck and low back pain following road traffic accidents. Not all whiplash patients require MRI, but it is of value in young patients where a disc injury is suspected. These injuries have been identified on post-mortem examinations in the neck (Taylor & Twomey 1990, Davis et al 1991, Jonsson et al 1991).

Provocative radiography

This term was coined by the late Bill Park of Oswestry, who became skilled at inserting needles into various structures in the spine (especially intervertebral discs and facet joints). Injection of contrast may provoke no pain, new pain or the patient's own pain, which should be relieved by local anaesthetic, the contrast and local anaesthetic together forming a sort of 'Koch's postulates' to localise pain. Such a technique is most commonly used in discography, nerve root blocks and facet blocks; it is rarely, if ever, indicated for medico-legal purposes, and should only be used on clinical grounds if surgery is being considered.

Outcome measures in chronic back pain

As discussed above, these should be designed for the individual; general outcome measures should be avoided, unless they are being used to monitor progress between one consultation and the next.

Other 'objective' measures of back pain

A number of machines designed to measure isometric back strength have been developed in North America over the past decade. All are expensive. It is claimed that one application of these machines is 'objectively' to measure back performance. In the author's view, these claims should be treated with considerable scepticism, and the devices should be considered as research tools. A useful study from British Columbia (Cooke et al 1992) concludes that 'lumbar dynamometry should be regarded as an indicator of the level of performance at the time of testing, more as a psycho-physiological test than as a valid measure of true physical capacity'. In other words, it measures the patient's perception of his performance, and is therefore subjective. Furthermore, the authors conclude that these devices still require further validation for the measurement of back strength in well-motivated volunteers. These machines have been used as an outcome measure by Szpalski et al (1990) and for monitoring progress (Gomez et al 1991, Cooke et al 1992).

Frequently asked questions

Note that the answers to questions for an individual is a matter of opinion, and only rarely are there data available designed to answer this type of question. The opinions are based on epidemiological data. This means arguing from the general to the particular.

What is the risk of an individual developing back pain?

In the South Manchester prospective survey of 2715 adults with no history of back pain, 34% of males and 37% of females reported a new episode of back pain in the following year (Croft et al 1999). 'Poor general health' was the best predictor of back pain (Relative Risk (RR) 1.5; 95% CI 0.8–2.7). Obesity did not predict pain in men, but did in women (RR 1.4; 95% CI 1.0–2.0). Height was not found to be a predictor of back pain. In this study, other aspects of daily living, such as fitness, smoking and watching TV, were not predictors for back pain. Do-it-yourself in males was a weak predictor. This is in contrast to previous studies that have shown physical fitness to be a strong preventer of back pain (Leino 1993, Videman et al 1995, Harreby et al 1997).

What proportion of individuals recover after an episode of back pain? (all these data reviewed by Andersson 1999)

60–70% by 6 weeks
80–90% by 12 weeks
Slow and uncertain >12 weeks
Diagnosis 'back pain', 60% better by 10 days
Diagnosis 'sciatica', 40% better by 10 days
What is lifetime incidence? 49–69%
What is point prevalence of back pain? 12–30%
What is period prevalence of back pain? 25–42%

Return to work

Off work injury 3.6 months
On work injury 14.9 months
Disability >6 months—only 50% return to work
Disability >2 years—virtually 0% return to work

Is this individual more likely to develop back pain if he/she. . .

Has a history of low back pain

There is strong evidence for this from many studies. The relative risk is 2.71 (95% CI 1.75–4.21) from a Danish study (Müller et al 1999).

. . .Smokes

Yes (Kelsey et al 1984, Deyo & Bass 1989, Ducker 1992, Ernst 1993, Müller et al 1999, Scott et al 1999)
No (Croft et al 1999)

. . .drinks alcohol

No available evidence

. . .is overweight (high body mass index)

The literature contains conflicting information. A careful review found only 32% of studies in favour, but the overall conclusion is inconclusive (Leboeuf-Yde 2000).

. . .takes no exercise

Evidence unclear (Croft et al 1999, Müller et al 1999)

Is too tall

Evidence unclear (Croft et al 1999)

What is the risk of an individual with disc degeneration developing chronic back pain?

Limited evidence. A cross-sectional study using radiographs is the only one that this author knows of which relates symptoms to radiological disc degeneration (Kellgren & Lawrence 1958). The incidence of 'MR disc degeneration' is likely to be much higher. Boos et al followed 46 individuals for 5 years with MR evidence of disc hemiations. 41% developed back pain which, suggests that disc degeneration has limited predictive power for back pain. None developed serious back pain.

How probable is this disc herniation caused by an injury?

No available evidence.

Having had a previous disc herniation, how likely is this individual to have another?

An estimate is a 10% chance of recurrence in 10 years at the same or a different level, regardless of whether or not the individual has surgery. This is interpreted from Weber's data (Weber 1983).

The re-operation rate following lumbar surgery is 9.5% in Ontario in a 4 year follow-up of all patients operated on in the province (Hu et al 1997), and 7.5% of microdiscectomy patients followed up for 4.5 years in a Japanese study (Hirabayashi et al 1993).

How likely is this individual with chronic back pain to return to work?

In a prospective study observing 1752 workmen's compensation claimants for 1 year (McIntosh et al 2000), prolonged claims were associated with 1) working in the construction industry (about half the rate of those in other industries); 2) older age (also found in other studies); 3) lag from injury to treatment; 4) pain referred into the leg; and 5) three or more Waddell signs (which, incidently, were found in 9.4% of this sample). Reduced time receiving benefit was associated with 1) a less severe score on a disability scale (a modification of the Low Back Pain Outcome score (Greenough & Fraser 1992)); 2) intermittent pain; and 3) a previous episode of back pain (this finding conflicts with those of all other studies). This study suffers from the usual problems of selectivity, as it includes only patients seeking compensation and treatment through the channels of one particular back pain service. Even so, these factors explain only 25% of the variance, so there are many other unknown factors working here.

Is there any place for rehabilitation in managing patients with chronic low back pain?

Yes. The evidence is somewhat conflicting, but a recent study is strongly in favour.

This paper carries many references to previous work (Vendrig et al 2000).

References

Andersson G 1999 Epidemiological features of chronic low-back pain. Lancet 354: 581–585

Baker D, Pynsent P, Fairbank J 1989 The Oswestry Disability Index revisited. In: Roland M, Jenner J (eds) Back pain: New approaches to rehabilitation and education. Manchester University Press, Manchester, pp 174–186

Biering-Sorenson F, Hilden J 1984 Reproducability of the history of low back trouble. Spine 9: 280–286

Bigos S, Battie M, Spengler D et al 1991 A prospective study of work perceptions and psychosocial factors affecting the report of back injury. Spine 16: 1–6

Boden S, McCowin P, Davis D et al 1990 Abnormal magnetic-resonance scans of the cervical spine in asymptomatic subjects. A prospective investigation. Journal of Bone and Joint Surgery America 72: 1178–1184

Boos N, Semmer N, Effering A et al 2000 Natural history of individuals with asymptomatic disk abnormalities in magnetic resonance imaging: predictions of low back pain-related medical consultation and work incapacity. Spine 25: 1484–1492

Bradish C, Lloyd G, Aldam C et al 1988 Do non-organic signs help to predict the return of activity of patients with low-back pain? Spine 13: 556–560

Burns J, Sherman M, Devine J, Mahoney N, Pawl R 1995 Association between workers' compensation and outcome following multi-disciplinary treatment for chronic pain: Role of mediators and moderators. Clinical Journal of Pain 11: 94–102

Burton A 1986 Regional lumbar sagittal mobility; measurement by flexicurve. Clinical Biomechanics 1: 20–26

Carron H, DeGood D, Tait R 1985 A comparison of low back pain patients in the United States and New Zealand: Psychosocial and economic factors affecting severity of disability. Pain 21: 77–89

Cooke C, Menard M, Beach G, Locke S, Hirsch G 1992 Serial lumbar dynamometry in low back pain. Spine 17: 653–662

Croft P, Papageorgiou A, Thomas E, Macfarlane G, Silman A 1999 Short-term physical risk factors for new episodes of low back pain: Prospective evidence from the South Manchester back pain study. Spine 24: 1556–1561

Davis S, Tensi L, Bradley W 1991 Cervical spine hyperextension injuries: MR findings. Radiology 180: 245–251

Deyo R A, Bass J E 1989 Lifestyle and low back pain: the influence of smoking and obesity. Spine 14: 501–506

Dong G, Porter R 1989 Walking and cycling tests in neurogenic and intermittent claudication. Spine 14: 965–969

Ducker T B 1992 Cigarette smoking and the prevalence of spinal procedures. Journal of Spinal Disorder 5: 135–136

Dzioba R, Doxey N 1984 A prospective into the orthopaedic and pschological predictors of outcome of first lumbar surgery following industrial injury. Spine 9: 614–623

Elliott A, Smith B, Penny K, Smith W, Chambers W 1999 The epidemiology of chronic pain in the community. Lancet 354: 1248–1252

Ernst E 1993 Smoking: a cause of back trouble? British Journal of Rheumatology 32: 239–242

Fairbank J 1982 The anatomical sources of low back pain, with particular reference to the intervertebral apophyseal joints. MD, Cambridge

Fairbank J 1986 Incidence of back pain in Britain. In: Hukins D, Mulholland R (eds) Back pain: Methods for clinical investigation and treatment. Manchester University Press, Manchester, pp 1–12

Fairbank J, Couper J, Davies J, O'Brien J 1980 The Oswestry low back pain questionnaire. Physiotherapy 66: 271–273

Fairbank J, Pynsent P 1992 Syndromes of low back pain and their classification. In: Miv J (ed.) Lumbar spine and back pain, 4th ed. Churchill Livingstone, Edinburgh, pp 273–290

Fairbank J, Pynsent P 2000 The Oswestry Disability Index. Spine 25: 2940–2953

Frankel H, Hancock D, Hyslop G 1969 The value of postural reduction in the initial management of closed injuries of the spine with paraplegia and tetraplegia. Paraplegia 7: 179–192

Frymoyer J, Rosen J, Clements J, Pope M 1985 Psychological factors in low back pain disability. Clinical Orthopaedics 195: 178–184

Gerzbein S 1992 Scoliosis Research Society: Multicenter spine fracture study. Spine 17: 528–540

Gomez T, Beach G, Cooke C, Hrudey W, Goyert P 1991 Normative database for trunk range of motion, velocity and endurance with the Isostation B-200 dynamometer. Spine 16: 15–21

Greenough C, Fraser R 1989 The effects of compensation on recovery from low back injury. Spine 14: 947–955

Greenough C, Fraser R 1992 Assessment of outcome in patients with low back pain. Spine 17: 36–41

Hammonds W, Brena S, Unikel I 1978 Compensation for work-related injuries and rehabilitation of patients with chronic pain. Southern Medical Journal 71: 664–666

Hardcastle P, Bedbrook G, Curtis K 1987 Long-term results of conservative and operative management in complete paraplegics with spinal cord injuries between T10 and L2 with respect to function. Clinical Orthopaedic Relative Responses 224: 88–96

Harreby M, Hesselsøe G, Kjer J, Neergaard K 1997 Low back pain and physical exercise in leisure-time in 38-year-old men and women: a 25-year prospective cohort study of 640 school children. European Spine Journal 6: 181–186

Health Department 1999 The prevelence of back pain in Great Britain in 1998. Stationary Office, London, p 18

Hirabayashi S, Kumano K, Ogawa Y, Aota Y, Maehiro S 1993 Microdiscectomy and second operation for lumbar disc herniation. Spine 18: 2206–2211

Hu R, Jaglal S, Axcell T, Anderson G 1997 A population-based study of reoperations after back surgery. Spine 22: 2265–2270

Hurme M, Alaranta H 1987 Factors predicting the result of surgery of lumbar intervertebral disc herniation. Spine 12: 933–938

Jadad H 1993 The measurement of pain. In: Pynsent P, Fairbank J, Carr A (eds). Outcome measures in orthopaedics. Butterworth-Heinemann, Oxford

Jamison R, Matt D, Parris W 1988 Effects of time-limited versus unlimited compensation on pain behavior and treatment outcome in low back pain patients. Journal of Psychosomatic Responses 32: 277–283

Jonsson H, Bring G, Rauchning W, Sahlstedt B 1991 Hidden cervical spine injuries in traffic accident victims with skull fractures. Journal of Spinal Disorders 4: 251–263

Kellgren J 1938 Observations on referred pain arising from muscle. Clinical Science 3: 175–190

Kellgren J 1941 Sciatica. Lancet 1: 561–564

Kellgren J 1977 The anatomical source of back pain. Rheumatology Rehabilitation 16: 3–12

Kellgren J, Lawrence J 1958 Osteo-arthrosis and disc degeneration in an urban population. Annals of Rheumatological Discovery 17: 388–397

Kellgren J H 1939 On the distribution of pain arising from deep somatic structures with charges of segmental pain areas. Clinical Science 4: 35–46

Kelsey J, Githens P, O'Conner T 1984 Acute prolapsed intervertebral disc: an epidemiological study with special reference to driving automobiles and cigarette smoking. Spine 9: 608–613

Kelsey J, Mundt D, Golden A 1992 Epidemiology of low back pain. In: Jayson M (ed.) The lumbar spine and back pain. Churchill Livingstone, Edinburgh, pp 537–549

Kleinke C, Spangler A 1988 Predicting treatment outcome of chronic back pain patients in a multidisciplinary pain clinic: Methodological issues and treatment implications. Pain 33: 41–48

Krusen E, Ford D 1958 Compensation factor in low back injuries. JAMA 166: 1128–1133

Lancourt J, Ketteelhut M 1992 Predicting return to work for lower back pain receiving worker's compensation. Spine 17: 629–640

Lawrence J 1969 Disc degeneration: its frequency and relationship to symptoms. Annals of Rheumatic Diseases 28: 121–138

Leavitt F, Garron D, McNeill T, Whisler W 1982 Organic status, psychological disturbance and pain report characteristics in low back pain patients on compensation. Spine 7: 398–402

Leboeuf-Yde C 2000 Body weight and low back pain: A systematic literature review of 56 journal articles reporting on 65 epidemiologic studies. Spine 25: 226–237

Leino P 1993 Spine 18: 863–871

MacVae I, Wright V 1969 Measurement of back movement. Annals of Rheumatic Diseases 28: 584–589

Main C, Waddell G 1998 Spine update. Behavioral responses to examination: a reappraisal of the interpretation 'nonorganic signs'. Spine 23: 2367–2371

Main C J, Wood P L R, Hollis S, Spanswick C C, Waddell G 1992 The distress and risk assessment method: A simple patient classification to identify distress and evaluate the risk of poor outcome. Spine 17: 42–52

McCombe P, Fairbank J, Cockersole B, Pynsent P 1989 Reproducibility of physical signs in low back pain. Spine 14: 908–918

McIntosh G, Frank J, Hogg-Johnson S, Bombardier C, Hall H 2000 Prognostic factors for time receiving workers' compensation benefits in a cohort of patients with low back pain. Spine 25: 147–157

Möller H, Hedlund R 2000 Surgery versus conservative treatment in adult isthmic spondylolisthesis. A prospective randomized study Part 1. Spine

Montaldi S, Fankhauser H, Schnyder P, de Tribolet N 1988 Computed tomography of the postoperative intervertebral disc and lumbar spinal canal: investigation of twenty five patients after successful operation for lumbar disc herniation. Neurosurgery 22: 1014–1022

Moore R, Osti O, Vernon-Roberts B, Fraser R 1992 Changes in endplate vascularity after an outer anulus tear in the sheep. Spine 17: 874–878

Müller C, Monrad T, Biering-Sørensen F et al 1999 The influence of previous low back trouble, general health, and working conditions on future sick-listing because of low back trouble: a 15-year follow-up study of risk indicators for self-reported sick-listing because of low back trouble. Spine 24: 1562–1570

Ohlen G, Spangfort E, Tingvall C 1989 The measurement of spinal sagittal configuration and mobility with Debrunner's kyphometer. Spine 14: 580–583

Osti O, Vernon-Roberts B, Fraser R 1990 Anulus tears and intervertebral disc degeneration. Spine 15: 762–767

Osti O, Vernon-Roberts B, Moore R, Fraser R 1992 Annular tears and disc degeneration in the lumbar spine. Journal of Bone and Joint Surgery 74B: 678–682

Park W, McCall I, O'Brien J, Webb J 1979 Fissuring of the posterior annulus fibrosus in the lumbar spine. British Journal of Radiology 52: 382–387

Powell M, Wilson M, Szypryt P, Symonds E, Worthington B 1986 Prevelence of lumbar disc degeneration observed by magnetic resonance in symptomless women. Lancet ii: 1366–1367

Rainville J, Sobel J, Hartigan C, Wright A 1997 The effect of compensation involvement on the reporting of pain and disability by patients referred for rehabilitation of chronic low back pain. Spine 22: 2016–2024

Ransford A O, Cairns D, Mooney V 1976 The pain drawing as an aid to the psychological evaluation of patients with low back pain. Spine 1: 127–134

Roland M, Morris R 1983 A study of the natural history of low back pain. Part 1: Development of a reliable and sensitive measure of disability in low-back pain. Spine 8: 141–144

Roland M, Fairbank J 2000 The Roland–Morris disability questionnaire and the oswestry disability questionnaire. Spine 25: 3115–3124

Salminen J, Erkintalo M, Pentti J, Oksanen A, Kormano M 1999 Recurrent low back pain and early disc degeneration in the young. Spine 24: 1316–1321

Scott S, Goldberg M, Mayo N, Stock S, Poitras B 1999 The association between cigarette smoking and back pain in adults. Spine 24: 1090–1098

Spengler D, Freeman C, Westbrook R, Miller J 1980 Low back pain after multiple lumbar spine procedures: Failure of initial selection. Spine 5: 356–360

Sternbach R 1986 Survey of pain in the United States: The Nuprin pain report. Clinical Journal of Pain 2: 49–53

Szpalski M, Poty S, Hayez J, Debaize J 1990 Objective assessment of trunk function in patients with acute low back pain treated with Tenoxicam. Neuro Orthopaedics 1: 41–47

Talo S, Hendler N, Brodie J 1989 Effects of active and completed litigation on treatment results: Workers' compensation patients compared with other litigation patients. Journal of Occult Medicine 31: 265–269

Taylor J, Twomey L 1990 Disc injuries in cervical trauma. Lancet 336: 1318

Thomas A, Fairbank J, Pynsent P, Baker D 1989 A computer interview for patients with back pain—a validation study. Spine 14: 844–846

Trief P, Stein N 1985 Pending litigation and rehabilitation outcome of chronic back pain. Archives of Physical and Medical Rehabilitation 66: 95–99

Vaccaro A, Ring D, Scuderi G, Cohen D, Garfin S 1997 Predictors of outcome in patients with chronic back pain and low-grade spondylolisthesis. Spine 22: 2030–2034

Vallfors B 1985 Acute, subacute and chronic low back pain: Clinical symptoms, absenteeism, and working environment. Scandinavian Journal of Rehabilitative Medicine 11 (suppl) 1–98

Vendrig A, van Akkerveeken P, McWhorter K 2000 Results of a multimodal treatment program for patients with chronic symptoms after a whiplash injury of the neck. Spine 25: 238–244

Videman T, Sarna S, Battie M et al 1995 The long-term effects of physical loading and exercise lifestyles on back-related symptoms, disability and spinal pathology among men. Spine 20: 699–709

Waddell G, Kummel E, Lotto W et al 1979 Failed lumbar disc surgery and repeat surgery after industrial injuries. Journal of Bone and Joint Surgery America 61: 201–207

Waddell G, Somerville D, Henderson I, Newton M 1992 Objective clinical examination of physical impairment in chronic low back pain. Spine 17: 617–628

Walsh K, Coggan D 1991 Reproducibility of histories of low back pain obtained by self administered questionnaire. Spine 16: 1075–1077

Weber H 1983 Lumbar disc herniation: a controlled, prospective study with ten years of observation. Spine 8: 131–140

Weisel S, Tsourmas N, Feffer H C C, Patronas N 1984 A study of computer-assisted tomography: I. The incidence of positive CAT scans in an asymptomatic group of patients. Spine 9: 549–951

Chapter 20

Thoracolumbar spine fractures

Guy Selmon and Michael A. Foy

Introduction

The management of injuries of the thoracic and lumbar spine is changing. Historically, most injuries have been treated non-operatively, but more fractures are now being treated surgically. However, the majority of these fractures are amenable to conservative treatment.

The thoracolumbar junction is the commonest site for fractures. This is due to the fact that, unlike the cervical and lumbar areas, the thoracic spine is relatively rigid due to the ribs. Therefore the cervicothoracic and thoracolumbar junctions represent transition zones between mobile and restricted segments. Injuries are concentrated in these areas (White & Punjabi 1990). Fortunately there are important anatomical characteristics at the thoracolumbar junction that allow greater recovery from neurological deficits compared to elsewhere in the spine.

Motor vehicle accidents are the most frequent cause (45%) of injuries to the vertebral column, followed by falls (20%) sports (15%) and acts of violence (15%). In patients over the age of 75 years falls account for 60% of spinal fractures. Males are injured four times more frequently than females (Rockwood et al 1996). Gertzbein (1992) reported the distribution of fractures as follows: spinal cord level (T1–T10) 16%, conus medullaris level (T11–L1) 52% and cauda equina level (L2–L5) 32%.

It should be noted that there is a reported incidence of between 6 and 17% for non-continuous spinal injuries in patients with documented spinal fractures. An awareness of this and a full examination are therefore essential in each case. Comprehensive imaging of the whole spine should be undertaken if an injury is found.

The majority of patients with fractures of the thoracolumbar spine are neurologically intact but 15 to 20% do sustain neurological injury. The management of these patients requires a multidisciplinary approach and this is usually best achieved at a specialist centre. It is recommended that the preparation of reports for these patients is performed by spinal injury specialists (see Chapter 22). However, orthopaedic surgeons may be asked to prepare reports on more specific aspects of a case, such as the patient's initial management in the A&E department, and may be asked to give a prognosis for neurologically intact patients as regards pain and deformity.

Classification

An ideal classification for spinal fractures should be simple but complete, take account of mechanism of injury, assist in deciding treatment and give an idea of prognosis.

Currently, there is no universally accepted classification system for thoracolumbar injuries. Nicoll (1949) was one of the first to describe these types of injuries and pointed out that they generally had stable or unstable patterns. Holdsworth (1963, 1970) modified and expanded Nicoll's classification and from this all subsequent classification schemes have been based. He classified these fractures into five groups according to the mechanism of injury. This classification was developed using a two-column concept and did not take into account the possibility of an unstable burst fracture.

Denis (1983) developed a three-column concept. The anterior column contains the anterior longitudinal ligament, the anterior half of the vertebral body and the anterior part of the annulus fibrosus. The middle column contains the posterior longitudinal ligament, the posterior half of the vertebral body and the posterior part of the annulus fibrosus. The posterior column contains the neural arch, the ligamentum flavum, the facet joints and the interspinous ligaments. He noted that each column may fail individually or in combination although in practice isolated middle column failure is not encountered. They may fail as a result of four basic mechanisms of injury: compression, distraction, rotation and shear. From this, four major types of thoracolumbar injuries can be described:

1. Compression (48%)
2. Burst (14%)
3. Seat belt type (5%)
4. Fracture–dislocation (16%)

The numbers in brackets are the incidences for each type found by Denis in his study of over 400 thoracolumbar fractures. Denis also described a fifth group of minor injuries which includes transverse process fractures (14%) and fractures of the articular processes (1%), spinous processes (2%) and pars intra-articularis (1%).

The AO group (Magerl et al 1994) have introduced another classification based on the pathomorphological characteristics of the injuries. The simple 3–3–3 grid of the AO group is used. There are three types, A, B and C, and each of these have three subgroups. There are three subgroups within these groups. Type A (vertebral body compression) concentrates on injury patterns of the vertebral body. Type B injuries (anterior and posterior element injuries with distraction) are characterised by transverse disruption either anteriorly or posteriorly. Type C injuries (anterior and posterior element injuries with rotation) describe injury patterns resulting from axial torque. The final classification was devised as a result of more than 10 years of work and a review of over 1400 consecutive thoracolumbar injuries. This classification reverts to the two-column concept as popularised by Holdsworth. The classification is undoubtedly useful for research purposes and is slowly gaining popularity in everyday clinical use. To date, however, there are few, if any, publications using this classification to describe results.

The majority of the recent literature still uses Denis' classification, although this may change as the AO classification takes over. For the purposes of this chapter the papers reviewed continue to classify the injuries into major (compression, distraction and fracture–dislocation) and minor (pars and transverse process fractures).

Anatomical considerations

Injuries in the thoracic spine may have inherent stability due to the ribs and the sternum; bracing may be all that is required. In children with complete neurological injuries at thoracic level or of the thoracolumbar junction stabilisation is required to prevent late kyphotic deformity.

The transition zone of the thoracolumbar junction is also associated with an increase in disc size, a lordosis and a reorientation of the facet joints. This junction also marks the emergence of the nerve roots in the cauda equina. These roots have significant healing potential. This is due partly to the relative increase in canal space and partly to the increased vascularity in this area of the spine. It is possible to have some recovery from complete lesions as well as having greater potential for recovery from partial lesions.

In the lumbar spine, compression fractures tend to have more stability as a result of the size of the vertebral bodies and the strength of the surrounding muscles. Lower down the lumbar spine, as the weight bearing line passes posterior to the vertebral bodies, fractures tend to be more stable still. At the L5–S1 level significant forces may be required to cause disruption and these injuries may be less stable.

Finally, many authors have noted that there is no direct correlation between the severity of neurological deficit and the degree of spinal canal compromise due to retropulsed bone and disc fragments.

Outcome following thoracolumbar fractures

The long-term prognosis of patients who have suffered thoracolumbar injuries is related to the level and severity of the initial bony/ligamentous injury and the efficacy of the chosen treatment in avoiding symptomatic, late sequelae. The work of Davis (1929) and Watson Jones (1931) recorded the outcome of thoracolumbar injuries to be excellent. The latter postulated that poor results were due to inadequate reduction and subsequent deformity.

However, Nicoll (1949) published his results on a series of 152 miners with thoracolumbar injuries. Outcome in this series was much less satisfactory.

Fifty-eight percent complained of persistent pain, which was thought to be of two types: 40% had pain at the fracture site while 60% complained of pain in the low back irrespective of the location of the fracture. (Table 20.1)

Table 20.1 The effect of fracture type on outcome Nicoll (1949)

Fracture type	Fracture Distribution		Outcome		Site of Pain	
	Total number of cases	%	Number with pain	% of total with pain	Pain at site of fracture (%)	Low back pain (%)
Anterior wedge fracture	88	58	58	66	28	72
Lateral wedge fracture	21	14	15	71	93	7
Fracture dislocation	29	19	7	24	43	57
Neural arch fracture	14	9	9	64	33	67
Overall	152	100	89	58	40	60

Nicoll found little correlation between the anatomical result and outcome. Of the 50 patients with 'perfect functional results', 48% had residual deformity.

Compression fractures

Compression fractures occur as a result of axial loading combined with either flexion or lateral bending. There is failure of the anterior column. Depending on the direction of the axial force either the common anterior wedge compression fracture results or the less common lateral wedge fracture. The middle column remains intact and these fractures are usually stable and not associated with neurological deficit. Some authors believe these fractures occur as a result of low-energy injuries in incompetent bone. In younger patients involved in high-energy injuries these fractures are rare and other major fracture types should be suspected. True compression injuries can be treated with short-term bed rest and appropriate analgesia. Bracing can be helpful, although it may be cumbersome in the elderly.

Although wedge and burst fractures are two distinct fracture types, many reviews consider them together. The following section covers compression fractures as a whole and there is then a review of burst fractures.

One of the largest studies published on conservative treatment of thoracic and lumbar injuries remains the work done by Aglietti et al (1984). They reviewed 275 patients who formed two groups: those who were neurologically intact and those who had associated neurological deficit. The groups were reviewed separately. All fractures were treated conservatively.

Neurologically intact patients

Two hundred and twenty-two patients were available for review in this group; 66% were male and nearly half of the group were employed in heavy manual labour. Fractures were classified according to morphology and presumed direction of disruptive force, i.e. wedge, compression (there were three subtypes in this group), flexion–rotation, extension, shear and distraction. Ninety-seven percent of fractures were wedge or compression types. The exact

method of early treatment varied between different clinicians. There was attempted reduction using a hyperextension brace in 93 patients. This was worn for about 2 months. The remainder were treated in plaster jackets and mobilised according to their symptoms. Average follow-up was 9 years; 33% had no pain but 8.5% were restricted at work by their pain; 82% returned to their previous jobs at an average of 6 months post injury, 15% had changed jobs and 3% had become chronic invalids. The authors also noted that in patients with possible gain associated with their injury, there were significant differences in outcome, as seen in Table 20.2.

No significant correlation was established between residual kyphosis and pain. There was no significant difference in clinical or functional parameters between single and multiple fracture levels. Overall about 60% of patients with stable vertebral body fractures achieved excellent or good results as judged by persistence of pain. Eighty percent of patients were able to return to their previous occupations. There were no significant differences found in the outcomes between males involved in light and heavy manual work. No difference was found when looking at wedge or burst fracture separately. Spontaneous fusion had no influence on the long-term outcome. There was an increased incidence of spondylotic changes noted radiologically in compression fractures, although this could not be correlated with the presence or absence of pain.

The authors also looked at fracture reduction, residual kyphosis, single v. multiple fractures and various other possible prognostic indicators but were unable to identify any factors in the early stages which could be used for longer-term prognosis. None of their patients required late surgery. Their findings matched those of Nicoll some 30 years previously.

Neurologically impaired patients

Although over 150 patients with thoracolumbar injury and paraplegia were treated at the unit only 53 were available for review. Thirty-one had died within 2 months of injury and this highlights the severity of these types of injury and associated injuries. Three-quarters of the patients had

Table 20.2

Hospital classification	Return to previous occupation	Change of occupation	Chronic invalid	No back pain	Back pain—mild work interference
Public	95%	3%	1%	47.5%	21%
Worker's compensation	70%	23%	5%	20.7%	41.5%
	p=0.0	p=0.0001	n.s.	p=0.0002	p=0.0002

complete lesions on admission; 40% were at T12 and L1. The bony lesion involved was not restricted to compression fractures and therefore comparison is difficult. However, some conclusions on the conservative treatment of these injuries can be drawn from their results. The problems arising from the neurological lesion are more important than those arising from the bony lesion. Utmost care must be taken to avoid all complications from the moment the patient enters hospital. Consideration should be given to early stabilisation of these fractures to enable early rehabilitation.

Review of combined series of compression/burst fractures

Muckle et al (1984) reviewed 42 patients who had sustained stable 'crush' fractures between T12 and L4. None had sustained neurological deficit. Average follow-up was 9 years. There was a combination of both compression fractures and burst fractures (17%). All the patients had been treated conservatively with bed rest and lumbar supports. Fifty-five percent had occasional backache but had returned to their previous occupation. However, 62% of all patients had discomfort at L4/5 and L5/S1. Patients with burst fractures, multiple fractures and fractures at L3 or L4 seemed to be more likely to develop persistent symptoms.

Hazel et al (1988) studied 25 patients with stable compression fractures for an average of nine years. Twenty patients had single level fractures. No patients had neurological deficits and compaction of the fracture was less than 50% in all cases. The patients' average age was 37 years. Treatment involved several modalities including bed rest, analgesia, physiotherapy and braces.

Nineteen patients had no or occasional back pain with no limitation of activity. One patient developed chronic, disabling back pain. He had a history of drug abuse. The remainder needed modification of activity due to more frequent pain. Twenty-one returned to their previous jobs and only one did not return to any employment. Of the patients with persisting symptoms, half had been suffering from back pain prior to the accident. Increased radiological compression (of more than 10%) had occurred over time in seven patients. In six of these, the increase was evident 1–4 months post injury. No correlation was found between signs and symptoms at follow-up and the degree of initial compression of the fracture.

Singer (1995) studied the long-term functional prognosis of a group of British Army personnel with thoracolumbar vertebral fractures without neurological deficit. There were 69 males and four females. Mean follow-up was 64 months (range 6–120). Ninety percent, had sustained simple compression fractures as judged by using biplanar radiographs. The remaining 10% had sustained failure of the middle column, resulting in burst fractures. Severity of the fracture was assessed by measuring the ratio between the anterior and posterior vertebral heights for compression fractures. For burst fractures, the ratio was calculated using the anterior (or posterior if more affected) height of the fractured vertebra and that of the one above. Twenty-six percent were 'minor', 64% 'moderate' and 10% 'severe'. Thirty-one percent of fractures occurred in the thoracic area, 47% at the thoracolumbar junction and 22% in the lumbar area.

Eighty-three percent were treated with bed rest and mobilisation (without bracing) as pain allowed; 14% were fitted with thoracolumbar–sacral orthoses and the remainder (3%) underwent surgical reduction and posterior stabilisation using Harrington rods. Functional outcome was assessed using the patient's medical employment status category. This is a grading of a soldier's ability to perform arduous and physically demanding military tasks.

The results according to fracture type are seen in Table 20.3. The difference is statistically insignificant (P=0.5). There is also a trend towards poorer outcome with increasing severity of fracture but this is also insignificant. Neither the number of vertebrae fractured nor the method of treatment had any statistically significant effect on outcome. It can be seen that up to three-quarters of patients with stable thoracolumbar injuries will achieve an excellent functional outcome. However, the group studied were predominantly fit, young, motivated males who had non-compensatable injuries. Possible bias in the outcome may be introduced as a result.

Summary

■ The outcome of these injuries is very variable; up to 60% of people with compression fractures may have residual symptoms.

Table 20.3

Fracture type (N)	OUTCOME (%)		
	Excellent	**Good**	**Fair/poor**
Wedge (66)	76	14	11
Burst (7)	57	29	14

- The majority of people return to their pre-injury occupations.
- Radiological evidence of degenerative change is more common following compression fractures but this does not seem to correlate to the presence or absence of pain.
- There do not appear to be any specific prognostic indicators associated with compression fractures.

Burst fractures

According to Denis, failure of the anterior and middle columns leads to burst fractures. These may be associated with retropulsed fragments of bone or disc material into the spinal canal and neurological deficits are thus more common in these injuries than in compression fractures. As mentioned previously, there is little direct correlation between the degree of spinal canal compromise and severity of neurological deficit.

While the management of compression fractures is generally accepted to be conservative, much more controversy exists as to the appropriate management of burst fractures. This is mainly due to the fact that there is no universally accepted definition of the unstable burst fracture. There is also debate as to whether bony fragments should be removed from the spinal canal. Limb et al (1995) proposed that in a neurologically stable patient, with or without a partial cord lesion, spinal decompression is not required simply on the basis of canal compromise. They argue that neurological damage occurs at the time of the injury and is not due to impingement seen radiologically after the event. It has also been observed that retropulsed fragments will remodel with time.

Shen & Shen (1999) reviewed the outcome of neurologically intact patients with thoracolumbar junction burst fractures at a single level. They excluded fractures with an initial angle of kyphosis of more than 35° but included patients who had evidence of posterior column damage. Thirty-eight patients were followed up for an average of 4 years. The majority were mobilised as pain allowed from day one without bracing. Thirty-two patients reported minimal or no pain and 76% were able to return to work at the same level. No neurological deterioration was found. The average kyphosis angle increased from 20° to 24°. Two patients went on to require surgery for persistent back and buttock pain respectively.

Chow et al (1996) retrospectively reviewed 24 patients with 'unstable' burst fractures but excluded patients with evidence of posterior column fracture. Average follow-up was nearly 3 years. Their patients were managed with a short period of bed rest followed by mobilisation in an extension brace. Nineteen out of 24 patients had minimal or no pain. Two patients went on to require surgery for persistent back pain. Eighteen returned to work, 13 to a similar job to that which they held prior to their accident.

Mumford et al (1993) undertook another retrospective review of outcome of the conservatively managed thoracolumbar burst fracture. All the 41 patients were neurologically intact. They were treated with a period of bed rest and log-rolling for a mean duration of 4 weeks. They were then mobilised in a thoracolumbar–sacral orthosis. No patients required late surgery. Fifteen percent were unable to work following injury but 63% were able to return to a similar job to that which they held previously.

Weinstein et al (1988) retrospectively reviewed 41 patients with thoracolumbar burst fractures which were treated conservatively. Average follow-up was over 20 years and this represents the longest follow-up of this type of injury in the literature. Seventy-eight percent were neurologically intact at the time of injury. All were treated conservatively. At follow-up only 10% reported no pain, the majority having minimal to mild back pain. Nearly 90% had been able to return to their pre-injury occupation. There had been no neurological deterioration in any of the patients. Two patients had required surgery for conditions related to their injuries. One had required anterior and posterior fusion at T10–L3 for significant back pain and kyphosis. The other had anterior decompression and fusion for proven canal stenosis. The authors' suggestions were that neurologically compromised patients should probably be treated surgically whereas those who were neurologically intact should probably be treated non-operatively.

The largest study on the functional outcome of low lumbar burst fractures to date was carried out by Seybold et al (1999). They concentrated on fractures between L3 and L5, pointing out that these three vertebrae form the main lumbar lordosis. Axial compression forces in these vertebrae tends to put them into further lordosis as opposed to kyphosis. Forty patients were followed up for an average of 45 months; 24 (57%) were neurologically intact at presentation, 20 were treated with initial bed rest and mobilisation in an orthosis; of these, two required later surgery for symptoms and signs of claudication. The remainder underwent surgery. Sixteen out of 18 patients with neurological deficit underwent surgery and this typifies most surgeons' approach to this injury. The functional outcome of operatively treated patients was not significantly different from those treated conservatively. Over 40% of patients who underwent an operation required further surgery, such as for removal of metal implants, even with modern instrumentation. In this group of fractures neither progressive kyphosis nor vertebral collapse occurred.

McEvoy & Bradford (1985) retrospectively reviewed 53 patients who had sustained burst fractures of the thoracic and lumbar spine. Average follow-up was more than 3 years. Thirty-eight patients had some neurological deficit, while 31 underwent early surgery, including laminectomy, posterolateral decompression, posterior spinal fusion usually with Harrington rods and anterior spinal fusion. Of the 22 patients initially treated conservatively, six went on to require surgery.

Neurological improvement was seen in 68% of the group treated with surgery. However, back pain was more common in the surgical group but disability less common. Poor functional outcome was less common in the surgical group. Little increase in deformity was seen in either group.

This paper and another by An et al (1991) confirm that back pain is more common in patients who have had long segment instrumentations or fusions. Back pain was also more common in people who had lost their lumbar lordosis. The authors suggest that long fusion with distraction instrumentation should be avoided in the low lumbar spine to reduce the possibility of long-term back pain. Short rigid fixation is likely to be more beneficial.

A recent review from the Leeds burst fracture study group also included an extensive meta-analysis concerning outcomes following burst fractures (Boerger, Limb, Dickson 2000). They emphasised that neurological damage occurred at the time of the injury and there was *no* evidence that decompression of the neural elements (either direct or by ligamentotaxis) improved outcome. In fact, because of the complications associated with surgical intervention there was evidence that surgically treated patients fared worse, although this was not statistically significant. They emphasised that as burst fractures are not inherently unstable they do not fall into the category of a fracture dislocation requiring prompt surgical stabilisation. They also emphasised that painful post-traumatic kyphosis occurs in less than 10% of all cases and cannot be used as a justification for surgical stabilisation.

Summary

- Neurological deterioration in initially neurologically intact patients is rare.
- There appears to be no correlation between initial radiographic severity of injury or residual deformity following conservative treatment with symptoms at follow-up.
- Conservative treatment of burst fractures in neurologically intact patients is unlikely to lead to neurological deterioration or progressive deformity.

- The majority of patients who have a burst fracture of the thoracolumbar spine have good or fair results whether treated operatively or not.
- Many patients with evidence of posterior column injury (although not facet fracture or dislocation) can be treated conservatively.
- Pain appears less of a problem following short segment fusions.
- There is no evidence that surgical decompression with stabilisation improves neurological function or reduces painful post-traumatic kyphosis.

Seat-belt type/flexion–distraction injuries

These injuries constitute several types of fractures which have similar but not identical bony and ligamentous configurations.

Denis (1983), in his classification, described a seat-belt type injury occurring with failure of both the posterior and middle columns as a result of flexion around the hinge of the anterior column. Other flexion–distraction injuries occur when there is compressive failure of the anterior column around the hinge of the middle column with the posterior column failing in tension. Many management principles are the same for both type of injury. The originally described Chance fracture was purely a bony injury. It consists of a horizontal fracture extending through the spinous process, the pedicles and exiting through the superior part of the vertebral body. There are also purely ligamentous flexion–distraction injuries which may be harder to pick up on plain radiographs. They are all as a result of forced flexion with or without distraction. The main risks with all these injuries is progressive kyphosis, deformity and pain.

Injuries associated with the use of seat-belts are usually restricted to the lumbar spine, although T12 fractures are sometimes encountered. A characteristic bruising or abrasion is often seen as a result of trauma associated with the use of seat-belts ('seat-belt sign'). Abdominal injury is a common association and should be excluded early. In some series, there is a delay in diagnosis of an intra-abdominal injury for over 24 hours in over 50% of the cases.

The incidence of this type of injury is between 5 and 15% of all thoracolumbar spinal injuries. In their review of the topic, Triantafyllou & Gertzbein (1992) remind us that intervertebral disc injury is common. Over 85% of their series of 40 were treated surgically. Monosegmental fixation appears to achieve satisfactory results without jeopardising other segments of the spine.

Anderson et al (1991) reviewed 20 consecutive flexion–distraction injuries at their unit. They classified the injuries as bony Chance fractures, ligamentous Chance injuries and flexion–distraction injuries. Their average age was 21 years and all except one had been involved in road traffic accidents. Fourteen patients were neurologically intact, three had incomplete lesions, one had sensory disturbance in the legs only and one had a complete neurological lesion. Thirteen required laparotomies for intra-abdominal pathology. Treatment was decided on according to the exact injury. Bony Chance-type injuries with no neurological deficit and less than 10° of kyphosis were treated in extension bracing for 3–6 months. Ligamentous injuries were treated with Harrington rods or interspinous wiring. Flexion–distraction injuries were treated with Harrington rods. Accordingly, seven patients were treated non-operatively. Follow-up was short (average 12.4 months). All the partial neurological deficits recovered fully following surgery. The complete paraplegic patient was unchanged following surgery. Kyphosis was measured radiologically on admission and at follow-up. The average change in angle was significantly more in the surgically treated group. Those who were treated non-operatively had more back pain than the surgically treated group although this was not statistically significant. The authors advocated operative treatment for those with kyphosis of more than 15°, ligamentous injuries, neurological deficits or those who are multiply injured.

Summary

- These injuries usually occur in the lumbar region, although the 12th thoracic vertebra can be affected.
- Associated intra-abdominal injuries are common and should be excluded early.
- Surgical treatment is usually undertaken acutely to prevent late deformity and restore normal anatomy.
- Patients should be fully investigated early with both CT and MRI scans to delineate the exact pathology.

Fracture–dislocations

These injuries are characterised by complete three-column ligamentous disruption from a combination of tension, hyperflexion, rotation or shear. The bony columns fail and subluxation or dislocation results. In Denis' series in 1983 these injuries had an incidence of 16%. They are highly unstable and are usually associated with neurological deficit. They are likely to progress to a kyphotic or translational deformity.

They can also be associated with severe intra-abdominal pathology and this should be excluded early. Denis divided these injuries into several subtypes: flexion–rotation, shear and flexion–distraction. The assessment of the patient with a spinal injury is considered more fully in Chapter 22.

Minor vertebral fractures

These fractures form their own group together with the other four main fracture types described by Denis. They include isolated fractures of the transverse processes, fractures of the spinous processes, fractures of the pars interarticularis and fractures of the facet joints. For all these injuries it is important to establish that there are no other associated spinal fractures which may produce an unstable spinal injury. They are rare and outcome is poorly documented. One of the more well known of these injuries is the 'Clay Shoveler's Fracture'. This is a fracture of the spinous process of the lower cervical or upper thoracic vertebrae. In isolation these fractures can be treated conservatively. However, they may be caused by flexion–distraction injuries, in which case the treatment is likely to be operative stabilisation. Acute fracture of the pars is extremely rare.

Transverse process fractures

One of the few reviews in the literature that has been carried out on transverse process fractures was by Aglietti et al in their large spinal series in 1984. They were able to review 21 patients who had isolated lumbar transverse process fractures at an average follow-up of 13 years. Fifteen of the patients had fractures at multiple levels. Most of the fractures were at the L2 and L3 levels. The majority were in heavy manual workers. Fifty-two percent were symptom free or suffered only minimal pain. Two were severely restricted at work but 90% had returned to their previous employment. There was a 10% non-union rate although it is not clear if these were symptomatic. Reis & Keret (1985) pointed out that an isolated fracture of the fifth lumbar transverse process may be suggestive of a significant pelvic injury such as a lateral compression fracture–dislocation.

Specific complications of thoracolumbar fractures

When initial treatment of thoracolumbar fractures is not successful, instability may persist and result in deformity, pain and increased neural deficit. Fractures that are thought to be stable initially may also cause subsequent problems under a period of physiological loading.

Deformity

Kyphosis is the most common post-traumatic deformity encountered. It may be associated with increasing neurological deficit and is therefore also the most potentially serious. There is a definite association between isolated laminectomy and the development of kyphosis and this single procedure should be avoided in the trauma setting. Many factors contribute to the development of deformity including the age of the patient, the type and stability of the original injury and its early management. The amount of kyphosis tolerated will vary according to the level of the deformity and the lifestyle of the patient. Mechanical sequelae of kyphosis include pain, abnormal flexion and extension and difficulty sitting.

Many surgeons use 30° of kyphosis as a cut off to performing surgery in the acute stages of a fracture. Retropulsed fragments in the spinal canal may make the individual much less tolerant of kyphotic deformity even with remodelling of the spinal canal. Kyphosis is much less well tolerated in the lumbar spine due to the limited potential for sagittal compensation.

The decision to operate on post-traumatic kyphosis will depend on many factors. Indications to operate include the development of a new neurological deficit or progression of an old one. Unremitting pain and cosmesis are also important factors.

Post-traumatic scoliosis is much less common and the indications to intervene are the same as for the kyphotic deformities.

Flatback deformity

Kyphotic deformity of the lumbar spine was originally described in scoliotic patients who had been treated with distraction instrumentation. It is now a well recognised complication of the surgical treatment of lumbar spine fractures. It is caused by over distraction of the lumbar spine during instrumentation, producing a loss of the lumbar lordosis. Patients develop a stooped posture, pain and fatigue secondary to this kyphosis. Treatment consists of avoiding over distraction in the first place! Established flatback deformity can be treated surgically, although this often has to be extensive.

Pain

Pain following thoracolumbar trauma is common. While for most people this will not interfere significantly with their lives, up to 20% become disabled by it. The incidence of pain is the same in groups that are treated operatively or non-operatively. Pain may be related to deformity and in these cases the exact origin of the pain may be elusive. It may be due to a combination of bony and soft tissue problems. Patients can develop subtle instability without deformity, for example with posterior ligamentous injuries. These injuries may be apparent only on flexion–extension views or on MRI scanning.

Whether there is deformity or not, patients may develop pain as a result of neural compression. Intervertebral discs may have been injured at the time but become symptomatic only at a later date. These patients require thorough investigation with a full history and examination. Treatment will depend on the perceived cause of the pain. However, in the medico-legal context, the question of attributability of a low back problem to a specific injury is difficult when one considers that 70 to 80% of westernised populations experience back pain anyway.

Neurological deficit

Patients can develop new neurological deficits for several reasons. Progressive kyphotic deformity, incomplete resorption of fragments within the spinal canal, secondary degenerative changes and post-traumatic syringomyelia can all cause symptoms related to neural compression. Depending on the degree of disability, surgical intervention may be considered.

Spondylolysis and spondylolisthesis

Spondylolysis is the term used to describe a defect in the pars intra-articularis without vertebral slippage. When one vertebra slips forward on another a spondylolisthesis is present. The prevalence of spondylolisthesis is about 5%. It is equally common in men and women. The isthmic type seems to result from a stress fracture that occurs in children with a genetic predisposition to the lesion. It is never seen at birth and it is not seen in chronically bedridden people. Some workers believe that the pars is thinner and less resistant to shear forces in children than in adults. However, up to 50% of Eskimos are reported to have the condition compared to 6 or 7% of white males. This supports the theory that there is a genetic predisposition to spondylolisthesis. Dickson (1998) gives an excellent account of current opinion on this topic.

Friedrickson et al (1984) prospectively studied 500 unselected children for over 20 years. They found that the incidence of spondylolysis with or without spondylolisthesis is 4.4% at the age of six years compared to 6% in adulthood. Slipping may increase up to age of 16 but this happens rarely. Most patients with a spondylolysis, with or without a sponylolisthesis, do not have pain. They also found that spina bifida occulta occurs more frequently in patients with a pars defect.

People with spondylolistheses do have a higher frequency of chronic low back pain than the general population, although many slips are asymptomatic. It has been found that in the 25–45 year age group there is a statistically higher incidence of degenerative disc disease in patients with spondylolistheses. However, it remains an enigma as to why symptoms often develop in adulthood if the lesion has been present for many years. Trauma is sometimes associated with the onset of symptoms but this is very variable. Post injury X-rays often show no change when compared to pre-injury films. Patients with spondylolistheses can also present with radicular pain. The cause for this is often easier to determine.

Younger patients with a spondylolisthesis may also develop a scoliosis which may be of three types: sciatic, olisthetic or idiopathic. The sciatic variety is due to muscle spasm and usually resolves with relief of symptoms. The olisthetic variety results from asymmetrical slipping of the vertebra and usually resolves after treatment of the slip. Idiopathic scoliosis and spondylolisthesis found simultaneously should be treated as separate problems.

Classification

The classification that is currently favoured by the International Society for the Study of the Lumbar Spine is that proposed by Wiltse et al (1976). Five categories are recognised:

1. **Dysplastic**, where there is congenital dysplasia or even aplasia of the posterior facet joints of the L5/S1 levels.
2. **Isthmic**, where the underlying lesion is in the pars interarticularis. It is generally felt now that separation of the pars occurs as a result of a fatigue fracture. Acute fractures of the pars have been described but are very rare.
3. **Degenerative**, where there is degenerative incompetence of the posterior facet joints. This type is most common at the L4/5 level. It hardly ever occurs before the age of 50 years.
4. **Traumatic**. Acute fracture in the area of the bony hook other than in the pars interarticularis.
5. **Pathological**. Lesions such as tumours and Paget's disease usually affect the whole motion segment and not just the pars.

Approximately 50% of spondylolistheses are of the isthmic type, 25% are degenerative and 21% are dysplastic.

From a medico-legal standpoint, it has already been mentioned that patients with a spondylolisthesis often attribute the onset of symptoms to an injury. It is also well documented that acute fractures of the pars are extremely rare. Hilibrand et al (1995) published results on five cases of acute fracture of the pars presenting with acute spondylolisthesis following trauma. Four of the patients were under the age of 20 years. They had all been involved in

some form of trauma (road traffic accidents in four cases). The L5/S1 level was involved in four of the cases. The spondylolisthesis was Grade 1 in four of the cases. Four out of five patients were treated conservatively initally, with bedrest and a thoracolumbar orthosis. The fifth, who had a Grade 1 slip, was treated with short-segment instrumentation and fusion within 48 hours of injury. Of the four treated conservatively, three required surgical procedures subsequently for progressive neurological deficits and symptomatic progression of the slip.

Floman et al (1991) reported on the effect of axial skeleton trauma on pre-existing lumbar spondylolisthesis. The aim was to document the stability of the pre-existing lumbosacral slip in patients who had sustained burst fractures of the lumbar spine. In a 10 year period five such cases were encountered. Two of the patients had a history of back pain with known spondylolistheses. In the other three, the slip was confirmed as being old with the help of a negative bone scan as well as radiographic and operative findings. All the cases were Grade 1 L5/S1 slips. Although this was only a small series the authors concluded that Grade 1 spondylolistheses have no less ability to absorb vertical compression forces than normal adjacent tissue. They also suggested that, if the slip was found to be old, and the new fracture was being treated surgically, the slip should not be included in the fusion.

They highlighted the point that acute spondylolytic spondylolistheses are rare and that in the face of major trauma the slip should be dated with a bone scan. A negative bone scan together with radiographic findings of a smooth, well rounded pars defect indicates that the slip is old and not related to any recent trauma.

The prognosis of symptomatic spondylolisthesis is poorly documented. Most children's symptoms can be controlled with restriction of sporting activities and other conservative measures. Risk of further slippage at the L5/S1 level is very rare and occurs only in the first few years if ever. This is particularly so with slips that are less than 30%. Increased risk of slippage occurs more in girls and particularly between the ages of nine and 15 years. Radiologically, patients with dysplastic slips and more than 50% slips are more at risk of further slippage. Surgery is usually performed for slips of more than 50% and in children with symptomatic slips who have failed conservative treatment. Success rates for the myriad of surgical procedures that exist vary widely, although the younger the patient, the better the results.

Summary

- An inherited predisposition to spondylolisthesis is common.

- The commonest type is the isthmic variety which is usually a result of repetitive stresses or a fatigue fracture through the pars interarticularis.
- Spondylolisthesis is often asymptomatic.
- Acute pars fractures are very rare and in cases of trauma and spondylolisthesis the slip is hardly ever new.
- A bone scan is helpful in dating the slip, together with plain radiographs.

References

Aglietti P, Di Muria G V, Taylor T K F et al 1984 Conservative treatment of thoracic and lumbar vertebral fractures. Italian Journal of Orthopaedic Traumatology 9 (suppl) 83–105

An H S, Vaccaro A, Cottler J M, Lin S 1991 Low lumbar burst fractures: comparison among body cast, Harrington rod, Luque rod and Steffee plate. Spine 16 (suppl) S441–S444

Anderson P A, Henley M B, Rivara F P, Maier R V 1991 Flexion distraction and Chance injuries to the thoracolumbar spine. Journal of Orthopaedic Trauma 5, 2: 153–160

Boerger T O, Limb D, Dickson R A 2000 Does 'Canal Clearance' affect neurological outcome after thoracolumbar burst fractures? Review Article. Journal of Bone and Joint Surgery 82B (No. 54): 629–635

Chow G H, Nelson B J, Gebhard J S et al 1996 Functional outcome of thoracolumbar burst fractures managed with hyperextension casting or bracing and early mobilisation. Spine 21(18): 2170–2175

Denis F 1983 The three-column spine and its significance in the classification of acute thoracolumbar injuries. Spine 8: 817–831

Dickson R A 1998 Spondylolisthesis. Current Orthopaedics 12(4): 273–282

Floman Y, Margulies J Y, Nyska M, Chisin R, Libergall M 1991 Effect of major axial skeleton trauma on preexisting lumbosacral spondylolisthesis. Journal of Spinal Disorders 4(3): 353–358

Fredrickson B E, Baker D, McHolick W J, Yuan H A, Lubicky J P 1984 The natural history of spondylolysis and spondylolisthesis. Journal of Bone and Joint Surgery 66A: 699–708

Frymoyer J W, Ducker T B, Hadler N M, Kostuik J P, Weinstein J N, Whitecloud III T S 1997 The adult spine, 2nd ed. Lippincott-Raven, Philadelphia

Gertzbein S D 1992 Scoliosis Research Society: multicenter spine fracture study. Spine 17: 528–540

Hazel W A, Jones R A, Morrey B F, Stauffer R N 1988 Vertebral fractures without neurological deficit. Journal of Bone and Joint Surgery 70A: 1319–1321

Hilibrand A S, Urquhart A G, Graziano G P, Hensinger R N 1995 Acute spondylolytic spondylolisthesis. Journal of Bone and Joint Surgery 77A: 190–195

Holdsworth F 1963 Fractures, dislocations and fracture–dislocations of the spine. Journal of Bone and Joint Surgery 45B: 6–20

Holdsworth F 1970 Fractures, dislocations and fracture–dislocations of the spine. Journal of Bone and Joint Surgery 52A: 1534–1551

Limb D, Shaw D L, Dickson R A 1995 Neurological injury in thoracolumbar burst fractures. Journal of Bone and Joint Surgery 77B: 774–777

Magerl F, Aebi M, Gertzbein S D, Harms J, Nazarian S 1994 A comprehensive classification of thoracic and lumbar fractures. European Spine Journal 3: 184–201

McEvoy R D, Bradford D S 1985 The management of burst fractures of the thoracic and lumbar spine. Spine 10(7): 631–637

Muckle D S, Fansa M, Bruce R J 1984 Long-term prognosis of stable lumbar fracture in young adults. Journal of Bone and Joint Surgery 66B: 285

Mumford J, Weinstein J N, Spratt K F, Goel V K 1993 Thoracolumbar burst fractures—the clinical efficacy and outcome of nonoperative management. Spine 18(8): 955–970

Nicoll E A 1949 Fractures of the dorso-lumbar spine. Journal of Bone and Joint Surgery 31B: 376–394

Reis N D, Keret D 1985 Fracture of the transverse process of the fifth lumbar vertebra. Injury 16(6): 421–423

Rockwood C A, Green D P, Bucholz R W, Heckman J D 1996 Fractures in adults, 4th ed. Lippincott-Raven Publishers, Philadelphia

Seybold E A, Sweeney C A, Fredrickson B E, Warhold L G, Bernini P M 1999 Functional outcome of low lumbar burst fractures. Spine 24(20): 2154–2161

Shen W J, Shen Y 1999 Non-surgical treatment of three-column thoracolumbar junction burst fractures without neurological deficit. Spine 24(4): 412–415

Singer B R 1995 The functional prognosis of thoracolumbar vertebrae fractures without neurological deficit: a long-term follow-up study of British Army personnel. Injury 26(8): 519–521

Terry Canale S 1998 Campbell's operative orthopaedics, 9th ed C V Mosby, St Louis

Triantafyllou S J, Gertzbein S D 1992 Flexion distraction injuries of the thoracolumbar spine: A review. Orthopedics 15, 3: 357–364

Watson Jones R 1931 Manipulative reduction of crush fractures of the spine. British Medical Journal 1: 300–303

Weinstein J N, Collalto P, Lehmann T R 1988 Thoracolumbar 'burst' fractures treated conservatively: A long-term follow-up. Spine 13(1): 33–38

White A A, Punjabi M 1990 Clinical biomechanics of the spine, 2nd ed. J B Lippincott, Philadelphia

Wiltse L L, Newman P H, Macnab I 1976 Classification of spondylolysis and spondylolisthesis. Clinical Orthopaedics and Related Research 117: 23–29

Chapter 21

Traumatic spinal cord injuries

John R. Silver

Introduction

Traumatic spinal cord injuries have been known for thousands of years. The first account was given by the ancient Egyptians: they recognised that the patients invariably died within a few days of injury and felt that it was a condition not to be treated. This high mortality continued throughout ancient times, the middle ages and until comparatively recent times. During the First World War, when the practice of medicine was well developed, virtually all of the patients with spinal injuries died from pressure sores and ascending urinary tract infection within weeks of injury. It was only with the advent of the Second World War and the setting up of spinal centres, in which the patients were all congregated together with all aspects of their treatment supervised by one doctor, combined with better bladder management and understanding of the importance of regular turning, that paraplegic patients began to survive the initial injury and leave hospital.

Initially, the speciality was developed in the UK in Emergency Medical Service Hospitals. A series of spinal units were set up but these were not very satisfactory until Sir Ludwig Guttmann showed how the treatment should be carried out. From the outset civilian patients were treated but with the advent of the National Health Service a comprehensive service was developed.

During the past 50 years, centres have been set up throughout the world. Initially, the patients were treated by a variety of doctors (neurosurgeons, orthopaedic surgeons, neurologists and urologists), but with the increasing development of skills and services, spinal injuries is now recognised as a speciality in its own right. There are now consultants in spinal injuries in the UK who devote themselves exclusively to the management of patients with spinal cord injuries, and who have an appropriate higher training accreditation which is recognised by the Royal Colleges of Physicians and Surgeons.

Patients with spinal injuries are now being resuscitated in intensive care units and transferred within hours—by helicopter or ambulance—to an appropriate spinal injury centre. As a result of this rapid transfer, the better understanding of the management of patients and the evolution of treatment, the immediate mortality has been reduced.

In the early years, although paraplegic patients were leaving hospital, the initial mortality among tetraplegic patients was 100%. Even by 1968 one in three complete tetraplegics died (Silver & Gibbon 1968), but as a result of improved methods of treatment, oral anticoagulants and chest management, the mortality rate is now about 2%—although patients are surviving with severe disability.

Now patients on ventilators are being kept alive, but this carries a high morbidity and mortality. They are returning to their families but need an enormous amount of care and support. Efforts are being made to discontinue the ventilator by electronically pacing the diaphragm. This has a better prognosis but there is still a high mortality. Of 19 ventilator patients studied by Professor Carter over a period from 1968 to 1992 only seven were alive (that is 37%). By contrast, of the 23 patients who were electrophrenically paced, there were eight males and six females living (Carter 1993).

The long-term problems of returning the patient to society and finding suitable work and housing to enable the patient to lead an independent, integrated existence still remain. It is accepted that patients should survive, and so the major problem of returning them to society and finding suitable work requires an understanding of their needs and the ability and wherewithal to make suitable provisions for them. Clearly, someone who is confined to a wheelchair will be unable to use stairs or resume work as a roofer or a jockey, but with suitable treatment, retraining, provision of care and adaptations to housing, a useful, happy, productive life is possible. With suitable electronic aids, patients who have function only in their mouths can work again. This is a major challenge.

Head and spinal injuries are among the most expensive cases in terms of compensation: a straightforward paraplegic with full liability can expect to receive £1 million, a tetraplegic £1.8 million and the ventilator–dependent patient in excess of £4 million. This money is largely given to compensate for loss of earnings and to pay for the amount of care required to allow the person to live in society. With ventilator cases, building a suite of rooms for the carers may be considered: in effect, a small intensive care unit in the house.

Consequently, determination of the natural history of the condition, complications, the ability to return to work with appropriate retraining, the development and subsequent treatment (or prevention) of complications and the prognosis largely govern the amount of compensation allocated.

Guidelines governing compensation

There are five aspects:

- Loss incurred directly as a result of the accident, damage to clothes, travelling to hospital by the family, damage to car and loss of earnings.
- Pain and suffering.
- The present condition.
- What the future holds—the prognosis and natural history of the condition.
- The question of the future of the NHS and the balance between private care and the support that can be expected from the state and whether it has to be paid for.

Direct loss

The doctor is not going to be concerned with the loss—that is easily computed by the patient's legal advisers. He will be asked to sign a certificate that the patient was confined to hospital and was unable to follow his normal occupation.

Pain and suffering

There is a difference here between UK and USA practices. In the UK one cannot evaluate and make a distinction between pains: how can the pain of blindness be compared with the pain of a mother who has lost a child? As such, under the UK legal system an arbitrary sum is allocated for this and the doctor will not be asked to advise, this being more of a philosophical and moral question. However, there are tables of figures which act as guidelines which can be consulted.

The present condition and future outlook

The question that the doctor is concerned with is the patient's condition at the moment. He should also assess how it will be in the future: whether it will improve, in which case the damages will be reduced, or deteriorate, so that greater damages will accrue when greater care is necessary.

Satisfactory settlement of the case is a major factor in returning patients to society. Little research has been done in this area, but the following studies, from general accident cases, show that the reports very often do not pro-duce the required information on which the lawyers can base a reasonable settlement.

In a study of 818 settled claims, Cornes (1987) found that in most cases the effects of the injury, the treatment and the recovery were adequately dealt with, but in the majority of cases information about the patient's social situation was inadequate and may have had an adverse effect on the assessment of compensation requirements. The median time from accident to settlement was 29 months.

Cornes & Aitken (1992) followed this up and found that the speciality receiving the most frequent requests for the provision of reports was orthopaedic surgery. They studied files from insurance companies on 203 patients, which contained 602 reports, the majority of which were given by consultants. Of the 602 reports, 368 had been given by consultants and 255 by orthopaedic surgeons. They found striking omissions in the possibilities of rehabilitation. In only 24 of the 203 cases was onward referral for rehabilitation made, and these made no specific reference as to what needed doing. Medical history was not recorded. The authors were critical of opinions based on subjective 'rules of thumb'.

Lee & Aitken (1984) found that orthopaedic surgeons predicted only 48% of the surgical and psychosocial problems that occurred after surgery. This indicated the importance of repeated assessment at intervals in order to overcome the inaccuracy of prediction.

The future of the National Health Service

In the old days the NHS was always available for care, emergency or routine, but now with budgeting there is an increasing tendency to budget for private care within these claims.

A certain amount of the medical care may have to be paid for privately, such as Baclofen pumps to deal with spasticity. Some of the statutory allowances may have to be paid back and come off the claim. Incredible as it is to believe, a patient who stays in hospital would have had to pay for food at home, so this is deducted from his claim.

The content of the report

In common with other cases, the consultant who is treating the patient is in the best position to give the report on the patient's behalf, because he knows the patient and the future treatment that is planned and he has an understanding of the various sequelae and consequences of spinal injuries. When there is doubt about the extent of the knowledge of the doctor treating the patient, other opinions may be requested on the patient's behalf. For example, if a patient with a spinal injury has sustained a fractured wrist as part of his initial injury, then the risks of arthritis or stiffness or the need for osteotomy should be assessed by an orthopaedic surgeon and a report requested.

It should be remembered that the limbs are not being used in a normal manner. The upper limbs in a paraplegic will be used for transferring, throwing greater strains on the shoulder, and the problem of standing in the paralysed person may have to be considered.

After a spinal cord injury, fractures complicate rehabilitation in up to 6% of cases with a median time of onset of 9 years after the injury. This is due to osteoporosis due to disuse. Initially these fractures were confined to the lower limbs but now that tetraplegics are living independently using their arms for transferring, they are occurring in the upper limbs.

If the patient has difficulty in emptying his bladder, with recurrent urinary tract infection, then the views of a urological surgeon on the efficacy of bladder surgery may have to be requested.

Settlement of these cases involves such large sums of money that the insurance company or the solicitors for the other party will require their own expert to see the patient to assess whether the reports and the views expressed are acceptable.

There is now an increasing number of rehabilitation reports from specialists in housing, equipment for the disabled, employment, nursing, physiotherapy, occupational therapy, sexuality and fertility, psychiatric, psychological assessment with psychometric testing, counselling and driving. There are maybe 30 000–40 000 people who make a significant portion of their income from being an expert and thousands more who are occasionally in Court (The Observer 8.11.98).

These reports are very time-consuming, and consultants may not have the time and/or access to other professional resources to undertake more formal assessments of residual function, working conditions and the labour market (Cornes & Aitken 1992).

It is necessary for the Court to know not only how the patient is now, but whether the disability will increase or the need for care will alter in the future. This will depend on an accurate examination and history of the injury. Previous medical conditions, such as alcoholism, heavy smoking, drug addiction or suicide attempts, are unlikely to be improved by spinal injury and will have an adverse effect upon future management. It is necessary to consider the housing situation and care arrangements, the effect of the injury upon the patient's physical state and how it has altered from normal.

The following points may be discussed, assessed and analysed: family history; who is currently treating the patient; which specialists or alternative practitioners the patient is currently attending (physiotherapists, chiropracters, aromatherapists, reflexologists); how they are being funded (privately or on the NHS); are they doing the patient any good; is further treatment contemplated; motor power; ambulation; the need for a wheelchair; the preservation of sensation; head injury; the presence of pressure sores; the presence or absence of spasms; the type and nature of the pain; bowel and bladder management; sexual function; future and present housing needs; the patient's method of transport; the need for physiotherapy; occupational therapy; previous employment; the possibilities of obtaining work; independence; the need for care; how that care is to be provided; implications upon the family and upon the children; the self-esteem of the patient; time spent in bed with illness; the patient's mental state; counselling; change in lifestyle; the ability to take holidays; how this is to be achieved (specialised hotels and carers to accompany the patient); immediate and remote risks; what future treatment is contemplated; what the patient considers would improve his life; the patient's attitude to disability; the need for special equipment; and life expectancy.

Clearly, to discuss all these things in detail would involve writing a textbook on spinal injuries, but certain points have to be emphasised.

General examination

It is advisable that the patient is examined within 6 months of the Court hearing. The practice of going to Court with stale reports–some, 3–4 years old—is to be deplored, as the patient's condition can deteriorate rapidly. When the doctor is called to substantiate his opinions it is embarrassing to be confronted with a patient covered with pressure sores which have developed since the time of the last examination. The wife or the carers may have left and the patient may have changed his housing or his home. Unless the best information is available, such points can only be brought out in Court to the patient's and the doctor's detriment.

The practice of submitting reports based on the study of case notes is also to be deplored, since it relies on the accuracy of examination by another doctor who may be inexperienced. Frequently, errors are copied from one set of notes to another and from one report to another.

Some orthopaedic surgeons routinely do not see new patients at any stage, the care being allocated to junior doctors (Lourie 1998); in other clinics, particularly for those with back pain, patients are being seen by physio-therapists who can order X-rays, but in 41% of cases they do not ensure that they are checked by a radiologist (Weatherley & Hourigan 1998). It is necessary to disentangle from handwritten notes who is responsible for decision-making and treatment at any given stage of the patient's career.

Medical reports written from case notes do not take account of the social impact of an injury. A whiplash injury in a keen or professional sports person can be devastating, while a similar injury will not be as incapacitating for a person working in a sedentary job.

It is desirable to see the patient at home so that adaptations can be inspected, their suitability commented on and further changes requested. A paraplegic patient may be totally dependent in his own housing before modification as he cannot get into the toilet or bathroom, having to be bed bathed by the carers, whereas if he is in modified accommodation he ought to be independent for these activities. It may be possible to interview the carers and tell-tale signs such as empty drink and drug bottles and tensions within the family noted.

It is advisable to have discussions with a member of the family, because they are going to be responsible for looking after the patient; their whole attitude will govern the course of successful rehabilitation and future care. The medical examination can be a very frightening and exhausting business for the patient, and one which will certainly require special transport and care arrangements for the rest of the family.

The demeanour of the patient has to be carefully studied. Osler (see Bean 1950) has drawn attention to the patient who comes with a piece of paper and a list of complaints—'la maladie du petit papier', as indicative of neurasthenia—and Miller (1961) has pointed out that in cases of anxiety neurosis the patient is almost invariably accompanied by a carer who prompts and answers many questions, while the patient, with a resigned air, finds it all too fatiguing.

Difficulty in attending the appointment and numerous phone calls from the patient or family can all be significant. It is striking that so many of the patients are ex-directory. A large number are unable to give all the information and have to write a voluminous letter, or phone in, because they are unable to express themselves adequately at the examination.

The patient may feel that he has revealed too much or has fallen out with the examining doctor and this may be followed up some weeks or months later by a letter of complaint about the method of performing the examination or the content. Patients frequently do not understand the questions that are being asked.

Although not always feasible, it is desirable that female patients have a chaperone when seen by the examining doctor, since complaints, by consensus within the medical profession, are increasing.

Patients with organic illness, irrespective of who the medical expert is appearing for, are only too happy to attend for examination because they welcome an audience and hope someone will be able to help them. The fact that patients make excuses and do not turn up is an important prognostic feature indicating either that they may have something to hide or that they do not take the examination seriously. At the very least, they have scant regard for the time of the professional person who has arranged to see them.

Documentation

These cases are complicated. Numerous reports are required on housing, equipment for the disabled, nursing care and employment and occupational therapy by case managers and psychologists; occasionally, reports by private detectives are accompanied by a video.

All the previous X-rays and medical records should be obtained by the solicitor. The notes should be paginated and indexed by a special reader before being submitted to the examining doctor, who should not be reluctant to charge for the time spent studying them. Patients who deny any injury to their back prior to the accident complained of, will, when confronted with a 15 year history—predating the accident—of back pain, admissions to hospital and investigations, blandly say that they had forgotten or did not think you would have the information available or that it mattered. This does not go down well in Court, either for the patient or the doctor's own expertise.

When you see the patient it is inevitable that the documentation will not be complete. You can either wait months or years until the documents all arrive, in which case you will have forgotten what you thought, or submit a preliminary report which is subject to correction when the full documentation arrives. If the examining doctor finds that the documentation does not tally with what the patient tells him then it has to be recorded because his report is for the Court.

The reports have to be formatted in a special way to meet the Court's requirements, with pre-Trial disclosure. They have to be in order and carefully submitted, and the consultant or the secretary may not have the time to devote to this.

The outcome of the Court hearing may be the most important aspect of the patient's successful return to society.

Physical examination

The problem of general examination is a very difficult one, since the majority of patients do not expect to have to undergo a general examination: if they have a whiplash injury of the neck they do not expect to have their cardiovascular system examined. This seems to be in keeping with Cornes & Aitken's findings (1992), in which only 13% of examining doctors carried out a general examination.

It is a difficult and controversial area, since a woman with back pain may well have secondary deposits from a carcinoma of the breast.

It is necessary to be able to perform an accurate and comprehensive examination of the nervous system, which normally requires the doctor to have done a neurological house job and preferably a registrar job in neurology, since, almost without exception, the following features—which could affect the prognosis—are ignored even by specialists.

Head injury

It is almost impossible to fracture the cervical spine without sustaining a head injury. Fifty percent of admissions to a spinal unit are cervical spine injuries causing tetraplegia, and the presence of head injury with spinal injury is frequently overlooked. The patient's rehabilitation can be impaired because of difficulty in concentrating, aggression, forgetfulness and impairment of intellect. This has to be taken into account and amplified by psychiatric, psychological and psychometric assessments, MRI and CT scans, reports from previous employers and the GP, and interviews with the spouse.

Rehabilitation is a learning process and if a patient has a severe head injury and cannot learn or adapt to his spinal injury, however mild, then rehabilitation is virtually impossible.

Specialist rehabilitation with a head injury costs £900–2000 a week, depending on the needs of the patient.

Motor power

The patient should be examined. Unfortunately, one is often confronted with reports submitted only from study of the notes or, if the patient has been seen at home, he may not have been examined at all, or may have been examined in a wheelchair. It may seem self-evident, but motor power cannot be evaluated unless a patient is undressed; the shoulder muscles and the posterior muscles are almost invariably ignored. In cauda equina lesions the glutei and soleus muscles are frequently not examined, being on the posterior aspect, and their paralysis is ignored, as the patient has not been turned on his side.

Reflexes

For aesthetic reasons, a vital reflex, the anal reflex, is usually omitted. This is a most important indicator of bladder function and a predictor of the return of bladder activity.

Sensation

The sensory examination may well be carried out in a perfunctory manner only. The ascent of sensory loss in post-traumatic syringomyelia is frequently missed and sensory sparing, which may well be around the anus in cauda equina lesions, is again frequently missed and the sacral segments are not examined, for aesthetic reasons.

Unfortunately, cauda equina lesions, where a patient is incontinent and impotent, are frequently missed and these patients, because they are seen to be walking about, receive scant sympathy.

Examination of the spine

Note should be taken of laminectomy scars, kyphosis and deformity, and a series of tests carried out to determine whether pain is organic or non-organic (Waddell 1991).

Pressure sores

Unless the patient is examined and all dressings removed, the presence of pressure sores might be missed, since the patient may be ashamed or unwilling to disclose these sores.

The presence of a pressure sore, which can lead to amyloid disease and septicaemia, is again understated and not appreciated.

Bladder

In the past, life expectancy was entirely governed by the function of the urinary tract and for this reason we will elaborate on the subject. There are two aspects, the social problem and the effect on life expectancy. In females, it is impossible to fit a satisfactory appliance and almost invariably paraplegic women are incontinent of urine, having to change their clothes several times a day. This is extremely embarrassing socially, and yet women will make light of it and not complain unless specifically asked. If they have a permanent indwelling catheter, it is going to lead to dilatation of the urethra, requiring a urinary diversion. However, the development of the sacral anterior nerve-root stimulator has changed this prognosis. This implant does require neurosurgical intervention, though. The implants are expensive and the necessity and cost of such treatment, which is not available under the NHS, should be discussed. In contrast, males can have a satisfactory device, but the presence of a collecting device and leg bag is embarrassing and hinders sexual activity.

In both sexes, the presence of defective emptying leads to ascent of infection to involve the kidneys, which can shorten the patient's life expectancy due to stones, scarring, pyelonephritis and amyloid disease. Evaluation of these matters is clearly a subject for the specialists—the urological surgeon and renal physician—and requires extensive investigation in the form of X-rays, ultrasound tests, urine cultures, clearance studies and blood estimation.

The bladder should be evaluated neurophysiologically by pressure studies, ultrasound and urodynamics, as this will enable an opinion to be given as to whether a sacral nerve-root stimulator could be used. These are clearly matters for 'ultra'-specialists in neurosurgery and urology, but they do change the patient's outlook and can transform his life from one of dribbling incontinence to independence.

Sexual function

This aspect is almost totally ignored, yet when one considers what a dominant factor it is, it should obviously be discussed in full and not purely in mechanical terms. Female patients may be able to have children, but will need extra care in looking after them: the effect of pregnancy upon a tetraplegic patient is a specialist subject, as the patient may develop severe infections and autonomic dysreflexia. Although female patients may be fertile, they may well have a total loss of appreciation and—due to anaesthesia, spasms and incontinence—the sexual act may be impossible or totally distasteful: sexuality should be distinguished from fertility. Marriage prospects are reduced. In contrast, male patients may well be infertile but may be able to achieve intercourse. Skilled advice is needed to evaluate this loss.

The previous pessimistic views on fertility in males have had to be revised because of the pioneering work of Steptoe and Edwards at Bourn Hall and of Professor Brindley. Fertility can be achieved in a small but significant number of patients who were previously dismissed as being infertile. This is a very sensitive subject, which should be evaluated by expert practitioners. It is costly and a course of treatment from a specialised centre can give up to a 20% chance of success (Table 21.1). It involves both psychological and physical assessment of both partners.

Social and psychological problems

These problems are vast and cannot be adequately dealt with in a text of this size. Housing is a major problem in everyone's lives. Although the population in this country has remained static, people no longer live at home until they get married and therefore they need small units.

Table 21.1 Typical cost of fertility treatment in November 1998

Initial consultation	£120.00
IVF treatment	£2200.00
+ female drugs	£1000.00
+ electro-ejaculation	£650.00
Freezing an embryo	£250.00
HIV & hepatitis screening	£160.00
Licensing fee for establishment	£40.00

Large houses are broken up into flats. People may have had a satisfactory flat before injury, but it is totally unsuitable when they are paralysed in a wheelchair. Early provision of suitably modified or purpose-built accommodation is a major factor in trying to return any patient to society. This may well be available in a compensation case by means of an interim payment and can transform the rehabilitation programme. The Courts accept that the patient should have proper housing, paid for privately, and this cannot be provided by the state. The kind of problems involved in organising rehousing are illustrated in Table 21.2. Clearly, the patient requires ground floor accommodation suitable for a wheelchair, or adequate lifts, and this is an area in which specialist reports by architects should be obtained. The doctor may well be asked to comment on the suitability of adaptations, and to discuss any omissions.

The details of the housing are not the province of the medical expert but the principles are that the patient is not entitled to better himself—he should be living in the same state as he was before or anticipated but he is entitled to the housing suitable to his disability. He is entitled to an adapted toilet, a bathroom suitable for a wheelchair, and rooms for carers and a guest.

Care

Some paraplegic patients can be completely independent, but while they require no care it is not desirable for them to live on their own. It may take them a long time to get their clothes on and equipment together, which might preclude them from going to work, so it is desirable that they have some assistance. On the other hand, high tetraplegics, with C4 transections, require total care and cannot be left on their own for more than a short period. There are tetraplegic patients with C6 lesions living on their own who can do their own transfers. Fifty percent of admissions at spinal injury centres are tetraplegics.

There are difficult ethical and moral questions here. Some patients have carers living in the house who turn the

Table 21.2 Details of the main processes involved in the adaptations required for disabled persons (from Cardiff City Council, with permission)

Adaptation for disabled costing over £250 and requiring County Architect's involvement

DETAILS OF PROPOSED MAIN PROCESSES

Social Services	1	Receive request for adaptation.
	2	Contact tenant and assess problem.
	3	Inform tenant of time of visit.
	4	Property visited by occupational therapist.
	5	Assessment of need.
	6	Request Engineer for site visit.
Social Services and Engineers	7	Visit site. Decide to inform authority.
Social Services	8	Inform Architects by telephone.
Social Services and Architects	9	Make joint visit.
Social Services	10	Confirm adaptation to Architects and Housing.
Architects and Housing	11	Receive confirmation of adaptation.
Architects	12	Prepare scheme.
	13	Submit drawing and estimate to Social Services and Housing, and drawings to Building Control, and if necessary Planning.
Social Services, Building Control and Planning	14	Receive details from Architects.
	15	Receive Building Register's approval and planning permission.
Social Services	16	Visit tenant. Fill in grant form. Inform Housing that plans meet requirements and enclose completed grant form.
Housing	17	Receive grant form. Send to grant section with copies of plans and schedules, recommendations from Social Services and certificate of future occupation and estimate.
Grants	18	Receive grant application and process.
Housing	19	Inform area office to visit property, assess work and report to HQ.
	20	Instruct Architects to prepare documents and seek tenders.
Architects	21	Prepare documents and seek tenders.
Housing	22	Inform Social Services of intention to seek authorisation from Chairman or Committee.
Social Services and Housing	23	Seek Housing Chairman and Director of Social Services authorisation or report to respective committees.
	24	Confirm contributions.
Grants	25	Send list of approvals to Social Services and Housing and approval to tenant.
Social Services and Housing	26	Receive list of approvals.
Architects	27	Inform Housing of tender figures.
Housing	28	Receive tender figures.
	29	Write to Architects to proceed with work and issue works order.
Architects	30	Receive instructions, get works order signed. Agree any increases. Start on site.
	31	Inform Housing of any additions or variations.
Housing	32	Receive details of any changes.
Architects	33	At practical completion. Inform departments concerned by standard letter.
Social Services, Housing and Grants	34	Receive letter from Architects.
Architects	35	At final completion. Inform departments concerned by standard letter.
Social Services, Housing and Grants	36	Receive letter from Architects.

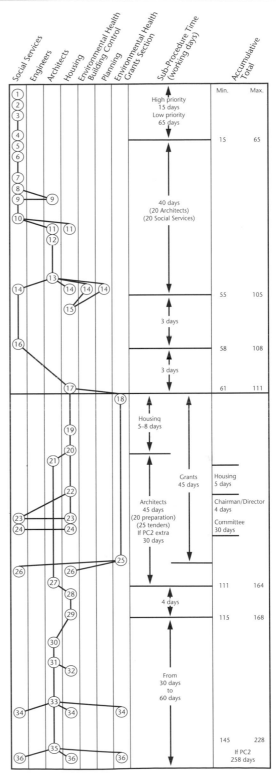

patients throughout the night. Other patients, who are working and require just one turn at night, appear at the clinic and say that they have a carer coming in to turn them who steps across their wife in the double bed and state quite blandly that they have been instructed by their solicitors to get the carer to come in so that they can increase the size of their claim.

Physiotherapy

It is reasonable for patients to have passive movements which can be carried out by the carers and perhaps a session a month with a physiotherapist to check whether they are getting contractures. It is not reasonable for them to be attending for physiotherapy on a private basis three times a week. A good guide to the right balance is the amount of physiotherapy they are receiving currently prior to settlement of the claim.

Counselling

Again, it is suggested that patients should be counselled/psychologically managed on a monthly or weekly basis. Again frequency could be determined by their counselling regime prior to the settlement of the case. It has to be recognised that although counselling can do good it can also do harm and may not be in the patient's best interests (Effective Health Care Bulletin 1997).

Wheelchairs

A vast number of wheelchairs can be claimed (up to six). If the patient has never tried out any of these wheelchairs, it seems unreasonable that the insurance company should pay for them.

Who provides the care, and how is it to be provided?

This is a complex issue. There are nursing agencies, the family, children, neighbours, district nurses, twilight schemes and local authorities. It has been suggested that a manager should be employed to coordinate all of these agencies.

In general, after the Second World War patients with spinal injuries were accommodated in hostels, rather like large boarding schools, where they could live with a certain amount of support and go out to work. Things have now moved on and people expect to live as normal members of society. It has been assumed, in the past, that the family would provide care on discharge from hospital, but this is not necessarily the best solution; in fact, surveys have shown that it is probably the worst. What is required is advice from social workers, interviews with the family and accurate assessment of how much care is needed to look after the patient at home. It is important to evaluate between carers, the trained and nurses. It costs £17 000 per

nurse per year for an 8 hour day, but if 24 hour care is necessary this will involve costs of £40 000 per year. Some lifts and transfers involving heavy patients are much better carried out by two people; in fact, in hospitals nurses are advised against single-handed lifts. The Courts accept that it is the patient's right to live independently in society and that carers have to be provided. How this is to be achieved is a matter for specialist discussions with the nursing agencies. Ventilator-dependent patients require round the clock nursing.

It is the patient's present state that can be dealt with by examination. However, the questions that the doctor is most often asked are: 'What is going to happen to the patient in the future?' 'How long is the patient going to live and what complications are likely to develop?' Again, this is an enormous subject but, clearly, if the patient is going to die from pressure sores within days of the Court hearing then a great deal of money will be spent by the insurance company, not for the patient, but for the benefit of his dependants. On the other hand, if the amount of money required to look after a patient is underestimated, then the patient is confronted with a situation in which he may run out of money while still requiring care. The present situation is unsatisfactory.

Notwithstanding the previous strictures, many patients are looked after by their families. While the family are strong and young they can do this, but as they age, the carer's health deteriorates, and the patient puts on weight and becomes less mobile, and the family becomes less capable. At this stage the patient may well develop pressure sores and require a great deal more care. Thus, evaluation has to be made of the carer's health and future arrangements and at what stage more help will be needed (Thiyagaragan & Silver 1984). The doctor may well be asked at what stage the patient will become totally disabled and when help will be needed. A much more sensitive issue is whether a carer is going to leave or in the case of a marriage what are the possibilities of it not continuing. Bearing in mind that the divorce rate in the UK is 40%, this is something that has to be considered. While in some cases the development of paraplegia can be an ennobling and bonding experience, this is not universally so.

The legal profession has been discussing this, and looking at the development of a structured compensation scheme whereby money is paid out according to the patient's needs. Structured settlements are ideally suited to the problem but they need careful evaluation of the likelihood of the patient developing syringomyelia or being confined to bed or wheelchair, so that the Barristers can decide how much money has to be paid now and how much has to be paid into Court for later developments.

Further problems have been raised on the question of contingency fees. The Legal Aid Scheme has now virtually been abolished and suggestions have been made that doctors can participate on a conditional or contingency fee basis. Doctors cannot participate on a conditional/contingency fee basis as they lose their independence. Doctors cannot participate on a contingency fee basis because they are required to sign a declaration at the end of every report as follows: 'I confirm that I have not entered into any arrangement where the amount or payment of my fees is in any way dependent on the outcome of the case.'

Prognosis

While it is difficult enough to evaluate the patient's present condition, to predict the natural history or the various complications would require not one textbook of spinal injuries but many. The nature of the complications that can affect the patient in the future, which the doctor will be asked about in his report, are listed below.

Chest complications

Because of the paralysis of the intercostal muscles, tetraplegic patients are liable to develop pneumonia and die suddenly.

Urinary tract infections

Acute ascending urinary tract infections used to kill patients rapidly after injury. These have been largely eliminated in the acute stage, but are still liable to occur. Later on, the development of stones, amyloid disease, chronic pyelonephritis and hypertension are all recognised complications that can lead to premature death of the patient, although their course can be modified by treatment.

Pressure sores

Among spinal injury patients, pressure sores are the most common cause of re-admission to hospital. Untreated sores lead to septicaemia, penetration of bone, chronic ill health and amyloid disease. There are many causes apart from loss of sensation.

There is still great ignorance about the treatment and management of pressure sores. In general, you can put anything you like on a pressure sore apart from the patient, but this lesson is still not universally appreciated. There are various items of equipment, such as hoists, low air loss beds and turning beds, which can prevent pressure sores from occurring, but none will compensate for a well trained carer. Sores are a marker of the patient's care, and of the skill and devotion of the carer.

Cystic degeneration

The development of post-traumatic syringomyelia is ill-understood, but it does occur in a significant proportion of cases—as many as 20% of patients develop it. A post-traumatic cyst may give rise to ascent of sensory loss and progression of the paralysis, and 1% of patients require surgery. The treatment is still unsatisfactory and is currently being modified.

With the development of MRI scans, it is possible to diagnose cystic change and follow its progress (Figs 21.1 and 21.2). As yet, these scans are not universally available on all spinal injury services, but it is unwise to go to Court without having an MRI scan carried out and it is reasonable—at this stage of knowledge—to carry out MRI scans on paraplegic and tetraplegic patients at regular intervals to follow the patient's progress. These scans are expensive and it is often argued that they should be carried out no more than three-yearly or else be paid for privately. This is very difficult to justify, especially if the patient has never had an MRI before or it has not been carried out by the treating doctor.

Life expectancy

This is the subject most frequently addressed. It depends on the patient's present state, age, level and completeness of the lesion and the nature of the treatment that the patient is undergoing. Has the patient suffered, or is he

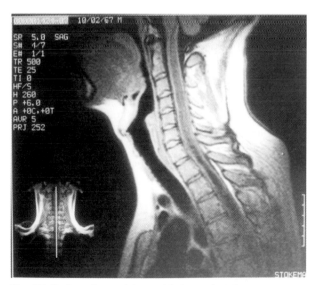

Fig. 21.1 A patient with a mid-thoracic injury, satisfactorily rehabilitated, developed ascent loss of sensation. MRI shows the features of a cyst of the spinal cord. A shunt was inserted and progress monitored by repeat MRIs since the treatment are not very satisfactory.

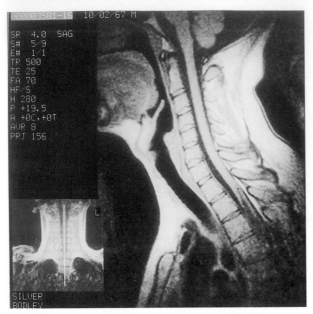

Fig. 21.2 The cyst appears to have collapsed, but either fresh cysts can form or the cyst can dilate.

likely to develop, complications? The most important of these have been mentioned, and they depend upon comparing the population of paraplegic patients with a matched normal population.

Life expectancy is an area of romance, guesswork and bargaining, and few accurate figures are available. In earlier times, all spinal injury patients died within a few weeks. Latterly it has been clear that patients are surviving for much longer. Few patients lived for many years after sustaining spinal injuries during the First World War. These patients invariably had non-interference with their bladders or were catheterised for only a short period, since life expectancy was then governed by the development of ascending urinary tract infections. Patients died of renal failure.

With improved methods of treatment, this rate of mortality was reduced. Until the Second World War, veterans with spinal injuries died rapidly of pressure sores. With better understanding of the development of sores, this risk has been reduced but is still a major cause of admission to hospital, and there is always a risk of the patient dying of sores and the late development of amyloid disease, or the development of respiratory failure in high tetraplegic patients as paralysis of the intercostal muscles enables secretions to accumulate and pneumonia to develop. There is an increased risk of suicide, cancer particularly of the bladder, and cystic degeneration. Patients are unable to exercise so there is an increased risk of coronary heart disease. It is well established that lack of exercise can

lead to a change in the lipid profile with a corresponding decrease in life expectancy (Bauman et al 1998).

Comprehensive studies have been carried out in Canada based on the whole population of spinal patients, showing that there is an increased mortality compared with the general population. From this, predictions have been made of the expectation of life in the future. However, these studies have been based on extrapolation of the mortality, rather than on actual survivals (Geisler et al 1983).

The only way in which mortality can be evaluated is by comprehensive assessment of all the patients passing through a spinal unit, correlating the causes of death with the level of the lesion, complications and bladder function, compared with a similar population in that country at the same time. This evaluation has now been carried out and shows a considerable improvement on the extrapolated figures from Canada but they are still not normal.

Despite the fact that accurate figures based on survival are available, many extraordinary statements have been made—patients with spinal cord injury being given longer life expectancy than a healthy man of a comparable age and patients on ventilators being said to have a normal life expectancy—so critical assessment of the figures produced is required with study of the references. Such phrases as 'everybody accepts' or 'it is universally accepted' are coded messages which the counsel and Judges will pick up meaning that one has absolutely no authority for this statement except one's own opinion and it also implies that anyone who disagrees with it is an aberrant thinker or has aberrant views.

This is an area of controversy. Does a patient who becomes tetraplegic at the age of 20 and has lived to the age of 40 years have the same life expectancy as a person who becomes tetraplegic at the age of 40? What can be said is that a tetraplegic has a worse life expectancy than a paraplegic, but a great deal depends on the care with which the patient looks after himself and how well he or she is motivated. It is fundamental to all life expectancy, irrespective of the disease, that any estimation must be made from the time of onset of the disease.

Up to this point we have dealt with the question of discussing the patient as he is and the natural history of the condition. However, there is a controversial and difficult situation when one is confronted with the patient and one feels that better or different treatment could change the prognosis. In general, one should report on the patient's current condition. However, it may well be that different treatment could bring about improvements and one might well recommend further treatment. Certainly, one should recommend further investigations to determine the nature of the condition.

A much more difficult area is when one is confronted with, perhaps, a straightforward road traffic accident where the patient has been negligently diagnosed or treated at the receiving hospital. This may well be an issue of litigation against the hospital, which will diminish the insurance company's liability. How this is dealt with is a matter of conscience for the doctor, but it is clearly an issue which has to be considered.

Who gives reports?

Who should give a report on a spinal injury case? The first point is that in general the number of reports that are asked for depends upon the cost of the case. Thus with a very minor injury (a sprained wrist), which may settle for under £1000, the insurance company will not necessarily go to the expense of obtaining a report by their own doctor and may be satisfied with a report from the GP. In cases of greater complexity, the hospital consultant treating the patient will be asked to report; but where cases are of the greatest complexity, with sums in excess of £4 million awarded, then reports will be requested from many specialists, particularly where there are contentious issues. In general, the Courts listen to and take account of the doctor who is treating the patient, because he is familiar with the patient's condition, has treated the patient from the outset and will have plans in mind as to what the treatment involves. He is responsible for the patient's care and, as such, the Judge will listen to him but he may not have the time or the conscience to submit the type of report that will obtain the most money. It is common that when reports have been submitted the insurance company will ask another doctor to go and see the patient. In spinal cases this is now almost invariably a spinal consultant—who will have an understanding of the natural history of the condition and the complications.

Other specialists may be called in to give reports—a urological surgeon on the bladder management, a neurosurgeon on the syringomyelia and a plastic surgeon on the pressure sore management.

An orthopaedic surgeon may well be requested to give a report on aspects such as the management of the initial fracture or of the spinal fracture, whether it needs fixation, whether it is unstable, whether arthritis is developing as a result of fractures in the upper limbs, the management of associated fractures, the management of complications such as contractures, tendon release and the natural history of osteoporosis in disused bones (Table 21.3). Reports may be required from a psychiatrist or psychologist to assess adjustment to injury or post-traumatic stress disorder. Litigation itself can add to the stress suffered by a patient.

Because of the way in which cases are treated in the UK, it may well be that the spinal patient will have been admitted in the first instance to an A&E department and then transferred to a spinal centre within days. An orthopaedic surgeon may be asked to produce a report on the patient's initial treatment and complications while in A&E or, at a later stage, when the patient has returned home, he may see the patient in a follow-up clinic and be asked to produce a report for the insurance company. It is of course up to the individual conscience and competence of any doctor to choose what he writes about, but such reports dealing with the more complicated aspects of spinal injury, such as post-traumatic syringomyelia, life expectancy and pressure sores, are best dealt with by the appropriate spinal, urological or neurosurgical consultant. It does happen that general reports from an orthopaedic

Table 21.3 Areas usually covered by an orthopaedic surgeon
The initial fractures and how they can affect the patient
The question of osteoprosis and stress fractures
Excessive use of the arms leading to osteoarthritis of the shoulders
The possibility of tendon transfers to improve the function of the upper limbs
Tenotomies to improve the function of the lower limbs
Specific surgery for the spine (usually the province of a spinal surgeon)
Brachial plexus (usually the province of a specialist in this field)
The problems of osteomyelitis secondary to pressure sores
The possibilities of calliper training

surgeon are submitted in the absence of these specialist reports and then, when the case is approaching hearing and is being evaluated, there is a great flurry of activity and only then are reports requested from the relevant experts. These are produced at great expense and lead to irritation on the part of the patient, who will already have been examined by innumerable consultants.

If a doctor writes a report he should be prepared to go to Court to substantiate the findings. It is essential that he examine the patient and see the previous medical records before giving the report. Once he has given a report it has to be recognised that this will be read by the patient, solicitors and Barristers for the patient, and by those for the other side, and will eventually go to Court. Once the report is submitted and signed, the patient may wish to make corrections. If there are errors of fact on the doctor's part these have to be checked against his notes, and then it is reasonable to make an alteration.

On the other hand, if the patient has clearly told the doctor something and now wants to alter it, this can be dealt with by:

- Leaving the report as it is
- Re-examining the patient
- Requesting the solicitor to produce a sworn affidavit from the patient and then appending it to the report

The fax machine and the internet have made the issuing of reports much more complicated. Solicitors are working to a time schedule and, as soon as the reports are received, faxes or e-mails come back with requests for alterations which cannot be made immediately and which demand further research. At this point, reports from the other side are received, together with a voluminous package of experts' reports—all of which need commenting on. Unfortunately, many are mere shopping lists for an idealised paralysed patient who bears no relation to the patient on whom the doctor is reporting. Lines of treatment may be proposed that the treating doctor has no intention of implementing, all to be paid for privately. The ostensible purpose of this is merely to inflate the claim.

The examining doctor may well be questioned in Court about these complicated reports, and it is important that he go through these other experts' reports with the patient to see if he has seen and will use the equipment requested, which the examining doctor has been asked to endorse, for example a Baclofen pump or a bladder stimulator. Not uncommonly, the patient may have never heard of the equipment or if it has been discussed with him he does not wish to use it.

The next stage is that the solicitor or Barrister may wish to manipulate the doctor's report in order to give the most favourable interpretation. While this may be tempting, it has to be recognised that it is the doctor's independent report. Barristers have been specifically instructed not to pressurise doctors to alter their reports, and it has to be recognised that doctors are the experts and that they are providing their reports for the benefit of the Courts. This is only too apparent when extraordinary extraneous statements coached in legalese creep into a medical report. It could be extremely unfortunate in Court if one's original notes are produced and found to be different to the report submitted. As all Judges have been Barristers prior to sitting, they are not entirely unfamiliar with this practice, and have given specific instructions that this is not to take place. Furthermore, any statements that one makes should be able to be substantiated not by rule of thumb or reference to authority but by reference to established, accepted practice. It is not sufficient to say that one knows some similarly misinformed doctor, akin to oneself, who practices some bizarre form of treatment.

The examining doctor may be asked to participate in a conference with other experts. This is perfectly reasonable if one is dealing with reasonable doctors but the rules are quite clear. The solicitor has to produce the questions that he wants answered. His expert may sit down with the other expert, but he does not have to agree. He can say whether a point is agreed or disagreed. Then the report is written and signed by both experts and is submitted to the other side. One's draft report is *not* to be submitted to the other side's solicitors for amending/manipulation.

When litigation crosses international boundaries, an examining doctor should make scrupulous efforts to adhere to the customs and practices of the country in which the case is being heard.

Having been mulled over by the solicitor and Barrister, the report may be returned to the examining doctor with closely written questions which demand the knowledge of a Nobel Prize winner, the judgement of Solomon and a good measure of 'economy with the truth'.

Armed with the final draft of one's report, one may be summoned to a case conference. This is designed to be intimidating. One's reports may have been gone through and discussed, amended, improved, dissected or otherwise mutilated. Ostensibly, the reason for this is to discuss the report with the doctor, but in practice it is to see how the doctor will stand up in Court against the Judge. The Barrister will act as 'devil's advocate'. The doctor may be sent away with innumerable requests for information. It is wisest for the doctor to ask for the minutes of the meeting to be sent to him so he can make any appropriate 'revisions', because after 2 hours of questioning he may be totally confused as to what he thought he said and what he actually did say. There may be as many as two Barristers, a Barrister-in-training, solicitors, articled clerks and an insurance company representative, and occasionally the patient may be present.

Alternatively, the report may not have been looked at at all as the Barrister who has been dealing with the case has been replaced at the last moment for various reasons, to the patient's detriment and then the examining doctor will have to explain to the counsel the difference between a paraplegic and a tetraplegic and what a pressure sore is.

Giving evidence in Court can be a very time-wasting exercise, involving sitting around for days in corridors. Many consultants cannot afford the time away from their clinical practice and decline to give reports. The problem is compounded by that fact that solicitors ask consultants to be available for up to a week to give evidence and then, at the last minute, postpone or cancel the case. These cases may well take place at Courts some distance from the consultant's practice and necessitate overnight stays: this is to be deplored and the reluctance of consultants to appear is understandable. This has given rise to a great deal of friction between the medical and legal professions with regard to cancellation fees, to such a degree that the matter has been dealt with in the High Court.

In an article in the British Medical Association News Review (1986) Judge Bingham stressed that each case for payment must be judged on its own merits, but he made it clear that there were limits on what could be demanded of witnesses in the name of public duty. In this case, the cancellation had been made only 24 hours before the hearing was due. It was unreasonable to expect that the witnesses would not lose income as a result, said the Judge. He added:

The Court is undoubtedly very much assisted by the expert evidence of medical and other witnesses at the peak of their professions. If such men are to respond to invitations to give expert evidence in Court and to keep time free for that purpose, it is right that they should not run the risk of a last minute cancellation which would leave them substantially out of pocket. It would, therefore, be very unfortunate if witnesses such as these were deterred from making their services available, and if the Court were dependent on the evidence of those who had no very pressing demands on their time.

The practice that is now accepted in the UK is as follows:

■ Cancellation of Court hearing with notice of 48 hours or less, full fee payable

■ Cancellation of Court hearing with notice of 48 hours to 1 week, half fee payable

Similar practices are followed in other countries.

Obviously, the size of the fee is a matter for negotiation, but if one gives a report it is essential that one settle one's terms to give the report, attend a case conference or to attend Court, whether the fee is to be met by the patient, the solicitor or a government agency, and whether one agrees to the fee being subject to taxation, prior to agreeing to appear in Court.

Suzanne Burn, Secretary, Civil Litigation Committee, The Law Society, at the 1998 Expert Witness Conference, pointed out that relations between doctors and solicitors were fragile and nearly all the complaints referred to fees (Burn 1998).

It is to be hoped that matters should improve with the implementation of the Civil Justice reforms because the intention is for fixed trial dates to be offered in many more cases and much earlier. In the larger claims the Courts will, in theory, be much more pro-active, organising case management conferences and pre-Trial reviews, and working with the parties and their legal representatives to narrow the issues and, if a case goes to Trial, to plan and timetable the Trial. If the pre-action protocols, new offers to settle and encouragement to use the ADR are at all successful, the last minute settlement should become less common.

Summary

■ Spinal injury cases are among the most expensive that come to court.

■ Many different disciplines are involved in the formulation of the final claim: orthopaedic surgeons, neurosurgeons, urological surgeons, psychologists, nurses and housing experts.

■ Physicians or surgeons should restrict themselves to the areas where they have specific expertise.

■ The orthopaedic surgeon should regard himself in this light. The purpose of this chapter has been to outline the complexities of spinal injury cases, and it should be understood that the orthopaedic surgeon's report would be considered as one among many before a large claim can be settled.

■ References

Bauman W A et al 1998 The effect of residual neurological deficit on serum lipoproteins in individuals with chronic spinal cord injury Spinal Cord 36: 13–17

Bean W B 1950 Osler's aphorisms. Henry Schuman, New York, p 136

British Medical Association News Review 1986 Doctors win fight over court fees (July)

Burn Suzanne 6.11.98 The 1998 Expert Witness Conference. Bond Solon Training

Carter R E 1993 Experience with ventilator dependent patients. Paraplegia 31: 150–153

Cornes P, Aitken R C B 1992 Medical reports on persons claiming compensation for personal injury. Journal of the Royal Society of Medicine 85: 329–333

Cornes P F 1987 Rehabilitation and return to work of personal injury claimants. Report, Rehabilitation Studies Unit, University of Edinburgh

Effective Health Care Bulletin 1997 Vol 3 No 3 ISSN: 0965–0288

Geisler W O, Jousse A T, Wynne-Jones M, Breithaupt D 1983 Survival in traumatic spinal cord injury. Paraplegia 21: 364–373

Lee R H, Aitken R C B 1984 Prediction of fracture patients' rehabilitation problems by orthopaedic surgeons. Health Bulletin 42: 174–186

Lourie J 1998 Delegation of orthopaedic workload. Annals of the Royal College of Surgeons Eng (Suppl) 80: 260–264

Miller H 1961 Accident neurosis. British Medical Journal 1: 919–997

The Observer 8.11.98 Woolf pounces on experts' fees

Silver J R, Gibbon N O K 1968 Prognosis in tetraplegia. British Medical Journal 4: 79–83

Thiayagarajan C, Silver J R 1984 Aetiology of pressure sores in patients with spinal cord injury. British Medical Journal 289: 1487–1490

Waddell G 1991 Low back disability—a syndrome of western civilisation. Neurosurgery Clinics of North America 2(4): 719–738

Weatherley C R, Hourigan P G 1998 Triage of back pain by physiotherapists in orthopaedic clinics. Journal of the Royal Society of Medicine 91: 377–379

Whiteneck G G, Charliefue S W et al 1991 Mortality, morbidity and psychosocial outcomes of a person's spinal cord injured more than 20 years ago. Paraplegia 30(9): 617–630

Chapter 22

Head injury

Bryan Jennett

■ Introduction

Considerable confusion often arises when doctors and lawyers discuss the consequences of head injury. There are several reasons for this. One is that, unlike injuries to other parts of the body where the severity of damage is usually maximum at the moment of injury, a relatively mild injury to the head can lead to serious complications. These may be temporarily life-threatening, yet if they are competently treated there may be complete recovery. But there is the possible paradox that severe permanent disability can be the outcome of an injury that initially was not serious because complications resulted in secondary brain damage.

Another problem is that while the most disabling sequelae are often the psychosocial rather than the physical, these may not be obvious when the patient is examined for a medico-legal report. Defining their nature and severity usually depends on skilled interpretation of accounts of the patient's behaviour by others. The opinion of a neuropsychologist and/or psychiatrist experienced in this particular field can be useful, and sometimes essential.

Yet another difficulty is the development of complications months or years after injury (e.g. epilepsy, meningitis), when the patient has already made a good recovery. There may then be arguments about establishing the causal relationship between previous injury and a long delayed complication.

Early complications

These can develop within the first few hours or days after injury and can cause secondary brain damage which far exceeds that sustained in the original accident.

Intracranial complications

These include swelling of the brain, infection and the development of haematoma. Such a blood clot may be either on the surface of the brain (extradural or subdural) or within its substance (intracerebral). Intracranial haematoma can pose a threat to life and rapid surgical intervention to remove the clot is then required. Even when this is done there is considerable early mortality and many survivors have persisting deficits or a high risk of developing late traumatic epilepsy, or both. The problem is that this serious complication, the commonest cause of

avoidable mortality and morbidity, frequently occurs after injuries that did not initially appear serious. Thus more than half the operated patients in one large series had talked after injury, some having been fully conscious and sent home from general hospitals—either from the A & E department or after being admitted for observation (Miller et al 1990). It is therefore important to identify which patients are at risk in order to ensure that they are kept under observation and have a CT scan. This complication is more common in adults than children, and in older than younger adults, in victims of falls than of road accidents, and in those with a linear skull fracture (see below). Guidelines for identifying which adult patients should be X-rayed, admitted, scanned or referred to a neurosurgeon to reduce risks from this complication were originally published in 1984 (Briggs et al 1984). These were then updated to include children and to take account of the greater availability of CT scanning in general hospitals (Bullock & Teasdale 1990; Teasdale et al 1990). A more recent version of these guidelines has now been published (Society of British Neurological Surgeons 1998).

Early traumatic epilepsy, defined as fits developing during the first week after injury, is more frequent in children, in whom it can occur after quite mild injury. Adults have early fits only when there has been substantial brain damage, as evidenced by depressed fracture, intracranial haematoma or post-traumatic amnesia. Repeated early fits or status epilepticus may cause secondary brain damage. The significance of early epilepsy for predicting late epilepsy is discussed later.

Extracranial complications

About a third of head injured patients also have major extracranial injuries and complications related to these can cause or aggravate secondary brain damage. Extracranial complications which combine to damage the brain include low blood pressure or shock, inadequate respiration and loss of blood due to haemorrhage. Their effect is to reduce the oxygen supply to the brain.

Secondary brain damage

In some cases it is obvious that secondary brain damage is dominant, in that the patient was clearly not severely affected soon after injury, but then developed intracranial or extracranial complications. In other cases it is a matter of conjecture how much of the eventual brain damage resulted from primary as distinct from secondary factors. A matter raised in some cases is the extent to which secondary complications might have been avoided and the secondary brain damage might have been less if medical management had been more appropriate. Where neurosurgical services are regionalised, as they are in Europe, delay in referral to a neurosurgeon can occur. Sometimes the delay is simply a function of distance, but more often it is because the risks of certain complications were underestimated or the early signs of their development were not recognised. Initial assessment and observation in the first few hours and days after injury are therefore concerned with discovering factors which increase the risk or likelihood of complications before they develop and instituting appropriate observation and investigation, and with detecting the early signs when these do develop so that timely treatment can be provided.

Attempts are sometimes made by lawyers defending those responsible for a head injury by accident or assault to argue that the injury that their client caused was not severe, and that the consequences flowed mainly from inadequate medical care. Such a defence is unlikely to be successful, however, because the chain of causation from the head injury to the complications is continuous—and the opportunity for suboptimal treatment and its consequences would not have occurred had the patient not suffered the original injury. Such allegations may also be the basis of a complaint against a hospital or health authority for making inadequate provision for care, or against individual doctors for having been negligent. Those asked to report on such cases should be cautious about stating with certainty that the outcome would definitely have been more favourable had the medical management been different.

Significance of skull fractures

It is brain damage that matters after head injury but damage to the scalp, the skull and the face bears witness to the head having been subjected to a certain degree of violence. Thousands of patients who attend A&E departments with lacerations or bruising of the face or scalp have sustained no brain damage. More than half of these mild injuries occur in children, many of them with scalp laceration. Unless a fracture of the skull vault or the base indicates the possibility that secondary intracranial complications may develop, these patients can usually be sent home without risk. Only 1 or 2% of those who attend A&E departments after head injury have a skull fracture.

Because severe brain damage can occur without a skull fracture, and a skull fracture can occur without brain damage or complications, there has been continuing controversy about the significance of discovering a fracture, and therefore about the indications for taking a skull X-ray (Jennett 1987, Lloyd 1998). A distinction must be made between a linear fracture of the vault of the skull, a compound depressed fracture of the vault of the skull and a fracture of the base of the skull. The latter two fractures indicate a breach in the integrity of the coverings of the brain and each is associated with a risk of intracranial infection. Their significance is therefore not in doubt.

Compound depressed fracture of the vault

A compound depressed fracture of the vault of the skull underlying a scalp laceration usually causes some local brain damage but unless the brain as a whole has been subjected to damage there will have been no loss of consciousness. At least a quarter of patients with compound depressed fractures are fully conscious when first seen, have had no alteration of consciousness and have no abnormal neurological signs. In a patient who is fully conscious it is easy to overlook a depressed fracture unless there is obvious penetration of the brain, as evidenced by brain and cerebrospinal fluid (CSF) coming out of the laceration. A compound injury is even more likely to be missed if the brain has been penetrated by a sharp object which has been withdrawn, leaving only a small puncture wound. Examples are when a child falls against a knitting needle or the axle of a toy wheel, or when an assault has been carried out at any age with a sharp instrument such as a screwdriver. If a scalp laceration or puncture wound overlying a penetrating injury wound is treated by simple suture without proper debridement there is a risk of meningitis or brain abscess.

Fracture of the base of the skull

Meningitis is also a risk after a fracture of the base of the skull involving the air sinuses or the middle ear cavity. This kind of injury is usually associated with some initial impairment of consciousness. Clinical clues to a basal fracture are the development of bilateral black eyes or bruising behind the ear several hours after the injury; or the leakage of blood and CSF from the nose or one or both of the ears. In the event of there also being facial injuries these sinister signs may easily be overlooked. Meningitis may be delayed for months or years after a fracture of the base of the skull. Some such patients have continuing CSF rhinorrhoea or otorrhoea, but when the leak is trivial or intermittent the fistula is often not recognised although the risk of meningitis remains. When meningitis first occurs after months or years its causative relationship to a preceding injury may not initially be recognised.

Linear fracture

A linear fracture of the skull does not in itself call for any immediate treatment. For this reason its detection has been considered to be unimportant by radiologists who are concerned about the large number of patients with mild injuries who are X-rayed in A&E departments. When such a fracture is associated with clinically severe head injury there is no call for an immediate X-ray because such patients will obviously be admitted and radiological examination (usually CT scanning) can be carried out from the ward. There may be no fracture of the skull in some serious (even fatal) head injuries where acceleration/deceleration forces have led to deep unconsciousness.

A linear fracture is of greatest importance in the patient who is walking and talking on arrival at the A&E department and who could safely be sent home if it were known that he did not have a skull fracture. In such mildly injured patients a skull fracture increases the likelihood of the development of an acute intracranial haematoma several hundred times (Teasdale et al 1990). This is a potentially lethal complication and its successful treatment depends on early recognition followed by expeditious surgery. It is therefore considered wise to admit patients at risk to hospital for observation rather than to risk their developing this complication at home, when some delay in appropriate management would be inevitable. That is the rationale for advising that a skull radiograph should be taken when a fracture is possible, rather than likely. Even so, only about half the head injuries coming to A&E departments in the UK have a skull X-ray, and that is quite appropriate because many of these are mildly injured children very unlikely to have a fracture or to develop complications. Apart from deciding which mild injuries should be kept under observation rather than sent home, a fracture is also important in patients who are confused because in these cases it also indicates an increased risk of intracranial haematoma. This is important when it comes to deciding when patients should have a CT scan and which should be transferred to a regional neurosurgical unit.

Apart from the small minority of patients who have a penetrating injury, evidence of brain damage depends largely on observed or reported alteration of consciousness, and much less often on the presence of focal neurological signs. All but 5% of head-injured patients are fully conscious by the time they arrive at the A&E department, although witnesses may testify to some of them having been briefly unconscious or dazed. The most direct evidence of this altered consciousness is whether the patient himself remembers the accident and events subsequent to it, such as roadside conversations or being transported to hospital. The presence of post-traumatic amnesia is the most reliable clue to minor brain damage, and a few minutes of amnesia may occur in patients whom witnesses reliably report never to have been unconscious.

Glasgow Coma Scale

If a patient is confused or in a coma then the extent and duration of this is usually recorded at the time by the Glasgow Coma Scale (Table 22.1; Teasdale & Jennett 1974). This also makes it possible to define coma more clearly and to distinguish it from other states of reduced consciousness or responsiveness. Coma is defined as not opening the eyes, not obeying commands and not uttering recognisable words. Many doctors, however, still use the word loosely and may qualify it as light or deep coma, although there are no agreed definitions for these terms. The advantages of using the Glasgow Coma Scale is that overall severity may be expressed by the total score on the scale. The scale was used to classify a large series of head injuries into three grades of severity (Table 22.2). The study showed that severe injuries are relatively infrequent and that many patients who developed haematomas, and those with poor outcomes, had been classified as mild or moderate on admission.

Another advantage of using this scale when observing the patient in the early hours or days after injury is that it enables any deterioration in conscious level to be rapidly recognised. Such a change is the earliest and most consistent sign that intracranial complications are developing—in particular an intracranial haematoma. For these reasons the use of the scale as a basis for observation is increasingly accepted as part of standard, good practice.

Post-traumatic amnesia

The best guide to the severity of brain damage that is available to the doctor who is called on months later to submit a legal report is the duration of the post-traumatic amnesia (Greenwood 1997). Its advantage is that it can be ascertained by asking the patient when he himself realised where he was. It is usually possible to distinguish this from what he was told by friends and relatives. The duration of the post-traumatic amnesia is always much longer than the time when witnesses report that he first woke or spoke. Only an approximate estimate of post-traumatic amnesia is needed in order to categorise the severity of injury according to this scale:

<5 minutes	very mild
5 minutes – 1 hour	mild
1–24 hours	moderate
1–13 days	severe
> 14 days	very severe

Table 22.1   Glasgow Coma Scale

Variable	Score
Eye-opening	E = 4
Spontaneous	3
To speech	4
To pain	1
Nil	1
Best motor response	
Obeys	M = 6
Localizes	5
Withdraws	4
Abnormal flexion	3
Extensor response	2
Nil	1
Verbal response	
Oriented	V = 5
Confused conversation	4
Inappropriate words	3
Incomprehensible sounds	2
Nil	1
Coma score (E+M+V) = 3–15	

Table 22.2   Distribution of severity of 1919 admissions (derived from Miller & Jones 1985)

Glasgow Coma Scale*	Severe, < 8 (%)	Moderate, 9–12 (%)	Mild, 13-15 (%)
All admissions	5	11	84
Computerised tomography scans	40	21	29
Intracranial haematoma	59	23	18
Hospital > 1 month	50	25	25
Vegetative or severe at 1 month	28	28	44

* On this 14-point scale, < 7,8–12, 13 or 14 – here adjusted for full scale.

In assessing severity it is important whenever possible to distinguish the severity of the initial injury to the skull and to the brain from the subsequent brain damage due to complications. An apparently mild injury may become serious because complications develop. An initially serious injury or a life-threatening complication may be followed by a good recovery, but that does not mean that the damage was not severe.

Sequelae of uncomplicated mild injuries

Most patients after head injury complain for a time of headache and dizziness, and sometimes of poor concentration and memory, and of fatigue and irritability. These symptoms comprise the post-concussional syndrome and because they commonly occur in patients who have had only a few minutes of post-traumatic amnesia, or none at all, it was once believed that they were psychological in origin, and not related to organic dysfunction of the brain. That has now been disproved, because for some 2–3 weeks after such a mild injury it can be shown that all patients have some impaired processing of information when formal psychological tests are carried out. There may also be disorders of the vestibular apparatus controlling balance, and an increased sensitivity to noise (hyperacusis). If these various subjective complaints are ignored by doctors, instead of the patient being reassured that they are likely to be temporary and are not evidence of serious damage, the symptoms may become a source of anxiety to the patient and this may make matters worse. These symptoms may be exaggerated or prolonged if the patient returns to work too soon, particularly if this involves paper work and intellectual effort. Normally these complaints do not persist for more than a month but there are a few patients who, for reasons that are often not obvious, continue to complain for months and a few who find it difficult to adjust to normal life again. This has been termed an accident neurosis and if this is suspected then a skilled psychiatric opinion should be obtained. In view of the clear organic background to these symptoms in the early stages, it is unwise to assume that the patient is malingering or exaggerating. The post-traumatic stress syndrome, related to recalling the frightening circumstances of the accident, is not a feature of patients with a significant head injury, as they are amnesic for these events.

Sequelae of more severe injuries
Glasgow Outcome Scale

The development of the Glasgow Outcome Scale (Jennett & Bond 1975) has made it easier to place brain-damaged patients into broad categories and to define the timescale of recovery. The scale refers to the patient's social capacity rather than to neurological deficits, and it does so on a simple scale of four for survivors (Table 22.3). A good recovery is recorded if the patient has either assumed all normal activities or is judged capable of doing so, although he may have some minor deficits. A moderate recovery describes a patient who has a clear-cut deficit— it may be a weakness in a limb, defective vision or hearing, or paralysis of one or more cranial nerves. However, the patient is fully independent, able to travel by public transport and capable of fending for himself. He may have returned to his own work but that does not mean that he is not to some extent disabled. It is important not

to regard failure to return to work as evidence of deficit, or return to work as evidence that there is no deficit.

Patients are classified as severely disabled if they are conscious but dependent, in the sense of requiring another person for some activity every day. That dependence can vary from being bedridden to needing help only with going out of doors or perhaps with some particular task during each day. Dependence is usually required because of a combination of physical defects, such as paralysis or loss of speech and mental disorder. Some patients who have no physical deficit may be wholly dependent because they are so seriously impaired mentally that they are unable to be left alone in the house or to fend for themselves. Usually mental deficits, including memory impairments, personality change and lack of motivation, are more disabling than physical deficits. Yet this mental deficit may not always be immediately obvious, and careful enquiry needs to be made of friends and relatives. If there is a marked mental deficit formal assessment by a psychologist and psychiatrist should be carried out in order to establish the nature and extent of the deficit. Although undue dependence on relatives sometimes develops so that patients are not making full use of their capabilities there is usually no doubt about a patient being dependent. There can, however, be differences of opinion about the exact degree of dependence for various activities.

Vegetative state

A patient in the vegetative state (Jennett & Plum 1972) has lost all function in the cerebral cortex. After head injury this is usually the result of severe initial diffuse axonal injury in the white matter of the cerebral hemispheres and brain stem. When this is the case the patient has almost always been deeply unconscious from the outset. There is often no skull fracture and a CT scan in the acute stage may show only small abnormalities, although these are of significance when interpreted by a skilled neuroradiologist. They include small haemorrhagic contusions in the corpus callosum and superior cerebellar peduncle and often some blood in the third ventricle. Occasionally, this condition

Table 22.3	Glasgow Outcome Scale (from Jennett & Bond 1975)
Outcome	**Patient's social capacity**
Dead	
Vegetative	Eyes open, not sentient
Severely disabled	Conscious but dependent
Moderately disabled	Independent but disabled
Good recovery	Normal activities

results from severe secondary hypoxic brain damage, especially when there has been an episode of cardiac arrest. Patients who die after several months in the vegetative state show marked cerebral atrophy with ventricular dilatation, and this can be shown in life on CT scans.

Patients in the vegetative state are awake but not aware. That is, they have long periods of eye-opening (with sleep–wake rhythm) but they show no signs of any psychologically meaningful responses. Because the brain stem is relatively intact they breathe on their own, can swallow and have a wide range of reflex activities, moving their spastic limbs in response to painful stimuli; they may briefly follow a visual stimulus or turn towards a loud noise. They never utter a word but can groan or cry out. These physiologically decerebrate patients are sometimes said to be in a permanent coma but that is a misleading term for someone whose eyes are open. They are of course quite different from patients who are brain dead, whose brain stem no longer functions and who are ventilator-dependent. They must also be distinguished from patients with a locked-in syndrome who are paralysed but fully conscious; this results from a brain stem stroke and very seldom results from head injury.

Although some patients recover consciousness after being vegetative for some months it is agreed that the vegetative state can be declared permanent 12 months after injury (Royal College of Physicians 1996). Provided that they are tube-fed and have basic nursing care these patients can live for many years and can attract very large sums in compensation, based on their care requirements as well as lost earning capacity. Many observers have described this as a state worse than death. There is now a consensus in several countries that no benefit comes from continuing treatment, and that this (including artificial nutrition and hydration) can be withdrawn (Jennett 1997). In the UK at present prior approval from the High Court is required before this is done, but this rule may be relaxed in future.

Neurophysical deficits

These are best classified as those affecting cranial nerves and vision, those affecting language function and those affecting the limbs. The commonest cranial nerve deficit is loss of sense of smell or anosmia. This frequently occurs with fractures of the base of the skull but it can also occur after a relatively mild concussion; it is usually a permanent deficit. It can be of considerable significance in certain jobs and it also deprives the patient of warning smells, such as fire or escaping gas. Apart from that there is the loss of pleasure because the aroma of food, which is part of the taste, is affected.

Visual symptoms may consist of a squint, double vision, loss of part of the visual field or even loss of all sight in one or both eyes.

Loss of hearing in one ear is quite common due to damage to the nerve to the inner ear associated with the fracture of the petrous temporal bone.

Facial paralysis is likewise due to a fracture of the base of the skull but is less common; it may be permanent although partial recovery is usual.

Disorder of language function most commonly affects the patient's ability to speak fluently even though he may be able to think of the words to say—so-called expressive dysphasia. More subtle forms involve the ability to read, to understand the spoken word or to write. This more commonly occurs with damage to the left side of the brain but in some left-handed persons it may result from damage to the right side. Damage to the controlling mechanisms of one or more of the limbs can result in hemiplegia, resembling a stroke, or to problems affecting one limb or all four. Some patients suffer severe ataxia and loss of balance as a result of damage in the cerebellum and brain stem. The frequency of these features after severe injury is shown in Tables 22.4 and 22.5 (Jennett et al 1981).

Mental dysfunction

This includes disorders of behaviour, changes in personality and impaired cognitive performance (Brooks 1984). There are many neuropsychological tests for measuring different aspects of cognition—attention, vigilance, memory, complex information processing, problem-solving and learning new tasks. It is such tests of performance rather than verbal IQ tests that show deficits after head injury. However, the scores of some patients are well within the normal range of the population as a whole, yet they may be performing well below their pre-traumatic levels as estimated from their educational or occupational attainments. The patterns of impairment can vary widely between patients with seemingly similarly severe brain damage. No doubt this is because of the widespread and varied nature of the lesions as well as of pre-traumatic psychosocial status. For example, alcoholism and social deviancy are more common among the head injured than in the population as a whole, and these can adversely affect recovery after severe injury.

Personality changes and altered behaviour are common in patients with definite cognitive deficits, but also in those whose test results show little abnormality. Again the patient may not seem beyond the range of normal, but may nonetheless be greatly changed according to his family. Reduced drive and depression are common and these combine to frustrate attempts at rehabilitation or

Table 22.4   Neurophysical sequelae at 6 months post injury (from Jennett et al 1981)

	All cases, *n*=150 (%)	After, intracranial haematoma, *n*=77 (%)	No intracranial haematoma, *n*=73 (%)
Any cerebral hemisphere dysfunction	65	62	67
Cranial nerve palsy			
All cases	37	38	36
As the only sign	13	10	15
Alaxia	9	4	14

Table 22.5   Sequelae of cerebral hemisphere damage at 6 months post injury (from Jennett et al 1981)

	All cases, *n*=150 (%)	After, intracranial haematoma, *n*=77 (%)	No intracranial haematoma, *n*=73 (%)
Hemiparesis			
All cases	49	56	62
As the only hemisphere sign	24	14	34
Dysphasia			
All cases	29	32	26
As the only sign	7	10	4
Hemiparesis and dysphasia	21	17	26
Hemianopia			
All cases	5	5	5
As the only sign	1	1	1
Epilepsy			
All cases	17	25	8
As the only sign	8	12	1

re-employment and may also result in lack of insight about his deficits. Lack of social restraint, tactlessness, irritability and impulsive behaviour characterise some patients. These behavioural problems and the stress and burden they cause to the family tend to get worse rather than better after the first few months and may last for years. This may be because the tolerance and optimism of the family during the early post-traumatic period are difficult to sustain as they realise that the changes are permanent.

Timescale of recovery

This is important for managing the patient medically, for advising him socially and for knowing when it is time to settle a legal case. Most substantial recovery occurs within the 6–12 months after injury. It is unusual for a person to move from one category on the Glasgow outcome scale to the next better one after 1 year. But that is not to deny that there may be considerable improvements within the categories of moderate or severe disability. Such recovery more often reflects adaptation or acceptance of disability rather than actual return of function. Even in the severest cases, it is therefore usually possible a year after injury to state with confidence that the patient is likely always to have a severe degree of disability and to be dependent, and this should usually be enough to consider the settlement of a case.

Sometimes false hopes of substantial later recovery are held out to the patient or his family but it is now generally recognised that careful assessment a year or 18 months after injury will usually enable a confident prognosis to be given. Questions are sometimes asked about the expectation of life of severely disabled survivors in order to calculate legal awards. There is little reduction in expectancy, which means that many patients face 40 years of disability because most are under 30 years of age when injured.

Post-traumatic epilepsy

This is the only common late complication, and it can develop in patients who have made a good recovery. About 5% of patients admitted to hospital after head injury develop later epilepsy (after the first week) but the incidence is very much higher after certain types of injury (Jennett 1995). When there has been an acute intracranial haematoma evacuated within 2 weeks of injury the risk is approximately 35% (higher for intradural than extradural clots). The risk is only around 20% in patients in whom a CT scan has shown a significant intracerebral haematoma, but who do not require surgery. The risk after depressed fracture ranges from less than 3% to more than 60% according to various combinations of four factors—post-traumatic amnesia of greater than 24 hours, tearing of the dura, focal signs and early epilepsy. In patients without intracranial haematoma or depressed fracture the risk of epilepsy is low unless there has been an early fit. In that event the risk is approximately 25% and this applies whether post-traumatic amnesia is more or less than 24 hours. More than half the patients developing late epilepsy have their first fit in the first year after injury, and the risk steadily diminishes as the year pass without a fit occurring.

Once a late fit does occur, the tendency for fits to recur continues and this has serious implications for the patient, particularly in limiting eligibility to drive. Patients who have suffered a high-risk type of injury will normally not be eligible to drive a private car for a year after injury; those whose job depends on driving heavy goods vehicles or public service vehicles may find themselves debarred for longer (Taylor 1995). Unfortunately prophylactic anticonvulsant drugs have little effect on the incidence of traumatic epilepsy.

Summary

- The best guide to the severity of brain damage available to the doctor called upon to submit a medico-legal report months after head injury is the duration of the post-traumatic amnesia.
- Whether a head injury has initially been mild or severe, many sequelae are possible. The relationships between the sequelae, the severity of the injury, the complications and the management are often complex.
- The commonest cranial nerve deficit following severe head injury is anosmia. It occurs particularly after basal skull fracture.
- The most substantial recovery after severe head injury occurs within 12 months of injury. A confident prognosis can usually be given 12–18 months after injury, although some improvement may still occur.
- About 5% of patients admitted to hospital with head injuries develop late epilepsy (after the first week), but after certain injuries the rate is much higher.

■ References

Briggs M, Clark P, Crockard A et al 1984 Guidelines for the initial management of head injury in adults. British Medical Journal 288: 983–985

Brooks D N 1984 Psychological, social and family consequences of closed head injury. Oxford University Press, Oxford

Bullock R, Teasdale G 1990 Head injuries (in ABC of major trauma). British Medical Journal 300: 1515–1518 and 1576–1579

Greenwood R 1997 Value of recording duration of post-traumatic amnesia. Lancet 349: 1041

Jennett B 1995 Epilepsy after head injury and intracranial surgery. In: Hopkins A, Shorvon S, Cascino G (eds) Epilepsy, 2nd ed. Chapman and Hall, London, pp 401–416

Jennett B 1997 A quarter of a century of the vegetative state: an international perspective. Journal of Head Trauma Rehabilitation 12: 1–12

Jennett B, Bond M 1975 Assessment of outcome after severe brain damage. Lancet I: 480–484

Jennett B, Plum F 1972 Persistent vegetative state after brain damage. Lancet I: 734–737

Jennet B, Snoek J, Bond M R et al 1981 Disability after severe head injury; observations on the use of the Glasgow outcome scale. Journal of Neurology, Neurosurgery and Psychiatry 44: 285–293

Lloyd D H 1998 Skull radiographs and children with blunt head injury. British Journal of Surgery 85: 590–581

Miller J D, Jones P A 1985 The work of a regional head injury service. Lancet I: 1141–1144

Miller J D, Murray L S, Teasdale G M 1990 Development of a traumatic intracranial haematoma after minor head injury. Neurosurgery 27: 669–673

Royal College of Physicians Working Group 1996 The permanent vegetative state. Journal of the Royal College of Physicians London 30: 119–221

Society of British Neurological Surgeons 1998 Guidelines for the initial management of head injuries. British Journal of Neurosurgery 12: 349–352

Taylor J F (ed.) 1995 Medical aspects of fitness to drive: a guide for medical practitioners, 5th ed. The Medical Commission on Accident Prevention, London

Teasdale G, Jennett B 1974 Assessment of coma and impaired consciousness; a practical scale. Lancet ii: 81–84

Teasdale G, Murray G, Anderson E et al 1989 Risks of an acute intracranial haematoma in children and adults: implications for managing head injuries. British Medical Journal 300: 363–367

Further Reading

Goldrein I, de Haas M, Frenkel J (eds) 2000 PI Major Claims Handling — cost-effective case management. Butterworths, London

Jennet B, Lindsay K 1994 Introduction to neurosurgery, 5th ed. Heinemann, London

Jennett B, Teasdale G 1981 Management of head injuries. F A Davis, Philadelphia

Reilly P, Bullock R (eds) 1997 Head injury. Chapman & Hall, London

Teasdale G 1995 Head injury. Journal of Neurology, Neurosurgery and Psychiatry 58: 526–539

Section 5

Miscellaneous topics

Repetitive strain injury

Campbell Semple

Introduction

This chapter differs significantly from the rest of this volume, in a number of ways:

- We are not dealing with an 'injury' in the accepted sense of trauma to the body at a specific point in time.
- Many patients with a claim for repetitive strain injury (RSI) do not in fact have any conventional diagnosable condition in the upper limb.
- The concept of RSI is novel, vague and lacks any precise definition.
- Most of this volume deals with the *results* of treatment of various injuries and fractures: this chapter concentrates on *causation* of various possible diagnoses affecting the upper limb.
- There is little debate on the causation or definition of a fractured scaphoid, or dislocated hip, by contrast, in this area of industrial upper limb litigation it is fundamental that clear statements and definitions of diagnostic categories are made, and supported by good quality medical papers, reviews and statistics, where such exist.

History of RSI epidemics

Problems of aching and painful arms and hands, associated with industry and manual labour, have been known of—and written about—for many years (Rammazini 1713, transl. 1940), and phrases such as 'washerwoman's wrist', 'potter's arm' and 'chicken plucker's wrist' are well known in parts of the country where such occupations are established; indeed, this is a source of initial confusion, as many people in the Potteries (Staffordshire, UK) for example, who complain of painful wrists, may indeed be pottery workers, but this does not necessarily mean that their complaints are *caused* by their pottery work, as they may simply reflect the high proportion of potters in that general population. There have been very few worthwhile comparative studies of upper limb problems in industry, with equivalent figures from the non-industrialised population, and most useful studies have come from Scandinavia (Allander 1974, Kuorinka & Kostinen 1979, Luopajarvi et al 1979, Waris 1980, Viikari-Juntura 1984, Kivi 1984, Roto & Kivi 1984, Dimberg 1987).

In Japan in the 1970s a large number of cases of upper limb complaints were recorded in Nippon Telephone & Telegraph (Maeda 1977, Hocking 1987) and the general term of 'occupational cervico-brachial disorder' was used to cover them.

A similar but larger epidemic occurred in Australia in the 1980s, and this has been well documented by, for example, Brooks (1986), Hadler (1986), Lucire (1986), Cleland (1987), Ferguson (1987) and Hocking (1987). It was during this epidemic that the concept of repetitive strain injury was raised, and certainly the phrase, and its RSI acronym, has a persuasive ring to it, and has been much used in the Australian, and now UK, media. In the USA the phrase 'cumulative trauma disorder' is used: unfortunately, these acronyms have taken root firmly in the media, and it is not an easy task to persuade newspaper editors and TV reporters, many doctors, and most of all patients, that this condition may well not exist (see Definitions below).

During the Australian epidemic it should be appreciated that much high profile media advertising, such as evening TV adverts in immigrant languages, kept the concept of possible industrial injuries, and their associated legal claims, well in the forefront of popular thought, and similar attitudes have been prevalent in many countries over the past decade.

In the UK we are in the midst of our own RSI epidemic (Waldron 1987), and a further epidemic is occurring in the USA where cumulative trauma disorder (CTD) is the preferred descriptor. It is important to appreciate that the definitions and descriptions in this chapter relate mainly to the UK, and there are significantly different ground rules and social security regulations in the USA, Australia and Japan which affect the manner in which these epidemics may rise and fall in each country.

In the UK the Department of Social Security (DSS) has defined a number of Prescribed Industrial Diseases, on the basis of which an employee may receive compensation from the government if he has been exposed to a harmful environment, and suffered a disease as a consequence (see below under Definitions for details). The amount of compensation is not great, and there is a strong and increasing tendency for employees to bring a Civil Negligence Claim against their employer, in effect accusing the employer of being negligent in allowing the circumstances to arise, or continue, in which the Plaintiff suffered his condition. The damages possible in such civil tort cases are considerable and there is much activity among insurance companies (for the defendants) and trades unions (for Plaintiffs) in trying to have the RSI concept justified or refuted.

It is worth emphasising that the DSS and the Health & Safety Executive (HSE) in their literature do not define RSI, and indeed reject the term, but generally refer to specific and generally accepted diagnostic categories. RSI as a clear diagnostic label has not formed the basis of any successful High Court claim in the UK, although some lower Courts have accepted the RSI label.

The medical/legal debate

In many ways it is frustrating that what is essentially a medical problem (whether or not RSI exists, how it can be defined, and what causes it) is being fought out in Courts of law, which are very imperfect forums for this exercise, particularly with an emotive background of media interest and speculation, not to mention the financial implications (Hadler 1984a,b, 1985, 1986).

It is worth being aware of recent legal Judgements in relation to RSI, and it is also important to appreciate that a Judge's decision in any particular case does not establish or refute a medical matter or diagnosis for the future; many of the legal cases over the past decade or two have revolved around points of law, which is no doubt proper in a Court of law. However, this chapter is viewing the matter from the medical point of view, and clarification of the medical debate in this area should be through good quality medical scientific research, epidemiology and logical analysis.

Pepall v. Thorn EMI [1985]

Nine women won modest damages, relating to a variety of diagnoses in the arm and hand claimed to be the result of electronic assembly work. This case is often used as a precedent for the employers' duty to warn employees of the danger of developing *tenosynovitis* in the workplace.

McSherry v. British Telecom [1992]

Two women, both data processors, won damages on the basis that their *cervical spondylosis* and *tennis elbow*, respectively, had been caused or contributed to by inadequate seating or other office furniture. This judgement carried implications for a large group of potential British Telecom claimants.

Mountenay and others v. Bernard Matthews [1993]

Six plaintiffs in a poultry processing plant won damages, and three lost their claims, on the basis of varied upper limb diagnoses having been caused or aggravated by their work. The damages awarded were relatively modest, and have enabled numerous further claims to be settled out of Court. The Judge awarded one claimant damages on the basis of her experiencing more than ordinary pain, albeit she had not suffered any recognisable injury; this point has been legally disputed by the Judge in *Moran* v. *South Wales Argus, vide infra*.

Mughal v. Reuters [1993] (HC)

This claimant (using a keyboard) claimed specifically to be suffering from RSI, rather than a more conventional diagnosis.

His claim was rejected in the High Court, on the basis that RSI did not exist as a recognised medical diagnosis, but also because the workplace was considered satisfactory and had not caused any injury to the plaintiff.

Moran v. South Wales Argus [1994] (HC)

This second High Court judgement has also firmly rejected the concept of non-specific RSI in a keyboard worker; in the course of this case the chapter on repetitive work in Hunter's Diseases of Occupations, 8th edition (1993), was comprehensively criticised, and most of the scientific references therein were shown to be inappropriate or misleading. This chapter has now been rewritten and avoids mention of RSI, preferring to discuss *upper limb pain*. The Judge also rejected the concept suggested in *Mountenay* (above) that compensable pain might exist without a definable injury or disease process.

Amosu et al v. Financial Times [July 1998] (HC)

A group of financial journalists failed in their claim that they had suffered either RSI or other significant injury or disease process as a consequence of their journalistic/keyboard activities.

Pickford v. ICI

The arguments in this case revolved around the diagnosis of writer's cramp. The Court at first instance rejected the claim, and the Court of Appeal overturned that Judgement, but on further Appeal the House of Lords restored the original Judgement. Much of the legal argument related to the relevance of psychological causation to the diagnosis of writer's cramp, or muscle dystonia, which is, strictly speaking, within the definition of PD A4, but few other PI cases have been argued on this basis.

Alexander et al v. Midland Bank [1998]

Five claimants argued that their intense work for the Midland Bank on keyboard numerating had led to pains and problems in their upper limbs. The Judge accepted that they had suffered from fibromyalgia, and that this condition was caused by their work, and awarded them damages. The Appeal Court rejected a further defendants' claim and the Claimants were successful.

Comment It is worth noting that the matter of diagnosis, in a strictly medical fashion, has moved and varied around these various cases, and indeed among the many unquoted cases. It is important for any student, be he medical or legal, to appreciate that this entire subject of 'RSI', as a definition or diagnosis, remains an extremely fluid and unfocussed debate.

UK law at present
Prescribed Diseases

It is important to understand these categories where they relate to the upper limb as many claims start off as PD (Prescribed Disease) claims, and then tend to develop into EL (Employer's Liability) claims, where the ground rules are very different.

PD A4 Cramp of the hand or forearm (writer's cramp)

This disease concept arose in the early years of last century, but it has rarely been used as the basis of a negligence action in recent times; it is not easy to understand the precise pathology in this condition, and current neurology would class it as a muscle dystonia, and perhaps it is a variant of what would now be classed as a (psychological) stress disorder. Writer's cramp was a significant element of the recent Appeal Court Judgement in the *Pickford* case (*vide supra*).

PD A5 Beat hand/A7 Beat elbow

This is essentially subcutaneous cellulitis over the elbows, but may occasionally occur in the hand. Such cellulitis originally occurred in underground miners crawling on their hands and knees in low coal seams, but it is now a rare condition. It may still occur from time to time in the knees of carpet layers. This diagnosis has very rarely, if ever, been invoked in Personal Injury claims in the past 30 years.

PD A8 Tenosynovitis

MS10 (1977) and Notes on the Diagnosis of Occupational Diseases (Greenfield 1985) imply inflammation of synovial sheaths of finger extensor tendons, and quote Thompson & Plewes (1951), which is indeed a good description of an outbreak of tenosynovitis in a UK factory. By definition, PD A8 cannot exist in an anatomical situation where there is no synovial sheath, e.g. around the elbow; indeed, peritendinitis crepitans (Thompson & Plewes 1951) occurs outwith the wrist tendon sheaths, and the syndrome has more recently been termed 'crossover syndrome' (Wood & Linscheid 1973, Williams 1977). Recently, a new edition of Guidance Notes from the DSS (1991) has included trigger finger and thumb and de Quervain syndrome under PD A8, but this argument runs directly contrary to the conclusions of the BOA study group on the subject (BOA 1990).

From time to time the DSS produces Guidance Notes on the Diagnosis of these various PDs, and the interested student should be aware of these diagnostic criteria, while being aware that they are rarely clear–cut, and considerable uncertainty and overlap exists among these various disease entities.

The MS10 pamphlet, published in 1977 by the HSE, describes tenosynovitis as the second most common (prescribed) industrial disease in the UK, occurring in many factory situations. Semple (1986) has criticised the basis for this statement, which is based on unreliable statistics.

In 1990, the HSE published a further pamphlet, entitled Work Related Upper Limb Disorders, with the intention of clarifying some of the ambiguities in MS10 (1977), but it is doubtful if this has been achieved.

PD A11 Episodic blanching (vibration white finger)

This condition was prescribed as an Industrial Disease in 1985, to cover the small vessel circulation problems induced by long exposure to chain saws, grinding and fettling equipment, and the like. It is essentially a separate matter from RSI, and will not be considered further here, but good reviews do exist (see Griffin 1987, Raffle 1987).

PD A12 Carpal tunnel syndrome (CTS)

This PD prescription relates to CTS *only* as a consequence of the prolonged use of vibrating tools or equipment.

Trade union and consumer group advice

Numerous pamphlets and guidance notes have been issued for the education and information of the general and working public. Their quality varies, and certainly, from a medical point of view, some information is simply wrong, or significantly misleading. Tackling Teno (GMB Union 1986) is a pamphlet written in popular style, and to a suggestible reader implies that many common upper limb conditions are caused by working practices; it is important to appreciate that many Claimants are familiar with such publications, but may not realise that much of their contained material is, to say the least, contentious.

Definitions

There has been no definition of RSI in any reputable medical paper or textbook, with the exception of Hunter's

Diseases of Occupations (Hunter 1987, 1993, 7th and 8th editions) (and even that is a loose description of symptoms rather than a clear definition), and, more importantly, the term RSI has been roundly condemned by numerous authoritative bodies, such as the Royal Australasian College of Physicians (1986) and the British Orthopaedic Association (1990). The review by four senior British hand specialists (Barton et al 1992) points out that the three descriptors, *repetition*, *strain* and *injury*, are all inappropriate, and that the phrase/acronym should not be used; also, that much unnecessary debate and confusion between doctors, specialists, lawyers, and most of all patients, would be avoided if RSI was rejected as a diagnostic entity (Barton 1989).

The concept of RSI originated in Australia, and descriptions of the 'syndrome' can be found in Browne et al (1984), McDermott (1986) and Thompson et al (1987). In the UK, the chapter in Hunter's Diseases of Occupations (Hunter 1987, 7th edition) has been much quoted—and criticised—in Court. Any orthopaedic/ rheumatology/ hand surgery expert who is considering a Court appearance as an expert witness in such cases would be well advised to consider the RSI chapter in Hunter carefully; much of this chapter is inaccurate, and in particular the quoted references in relation to 'etiology' are confused and do not support the statements in the text: these inaccuracies are compounded in the later chapter written by Hazleman (1993, 8th edition). The most recent edition, the 9th, of Hunter has been completely rewritten by different authors, and they avoid the RSI concept, referring simply to 'chronic upper limb pain'.

A variant of the RSI concept is the 'overuse syndrome', described by Fry (1986a), again in Australia, but there have been no independent supporting articles (see Fry 1986b, Dennett & Fry 1988) and a number of critical comments on Fry's concept (Semple et al 1988).

The proponents of RSI/overuse argue that a pathological condition can occur in the upper limb from excessive use, this condition being separate from the recognised syndromes such as carpal tunnel syndrome (CTS), tennis elbow, tenosynovitis, and so on. If a professional medical expert witness wishes to argue that RSI exists, then he must be prepared to go to Court armed with the necessary evidence to support his case. Some speculative theories on the possible pathological basis for this 'condition' may be found in Fry (1986), Smythe (1988) and Cohen et al (1992).

A recent paper by Greening & Lynne (1998) has been used by proponents of the RSI concept as implying a proven connection with white collar work, but a careful reading of the paper will show that it is no more than a hypothesis.

Outwith the strictly medical field there have been numerous ergonomic papers which imply that various medical conditions may be caused, or aggravated, by faulty or inadequate seating, furniture or working environments, including pace of working, rates of repetitive work and the like. Any medical man approaching Court on this subject would do well to familiarise himself with some of the relevant papers, such as those by Wallace & Buckle (1987), Armstrong et al (1982), Armstrong (1986) and Silverstein et al (1986). One of the considerable difficulties in this overall debate is that the ergonomists tend to be analysing working practices in terms of *complaints*, rather than in terms of specific *disease* or *injury* as a consequence of a particular industrial process.

It has been suggested (*Mughal* v. *Reuters* (High Court) [1993], Prosser J.) that holding the wrist/hand in a particular position while typing/word processing has caused a pathological condition in the arm or hand, but there is no reliable evidence that tenosynovitis, or any other diagnosable condition, has resulted from such activity in an otherwise fit, healthy, individual trained for such work. Many ergonomists have argued that variations in seat height, or other aspects of the office position, may lead to RSI or other more specific pathologies in the arm or hand, but there is little hard evidence of such a relationship.

Causation

While tenosynovitis (PD A8) is an accepted industrial disease (by the DSS and the HSE), numerous claims are now being brought on the basis that other conditions are caused by industrial working practices, and it is worth analysing the evidence for and against these claims.

Much debate, both in and out of Court, has occurred on this point (Barton 1989), and the medical expert must make up his mind clearly here, after assessing the relevant literature.

Because of the general debate on the matter of causation of various upper limb diagnoses, the Industrial Injuries Advisory Council asked the British Orthopaedic Association for their views on whether any further diseases or diagnoses should be 'prescribed', beyond the current A4, A5, A7 and A8. The subcommittee appointed by the BOA, consisting of four senior hand surgeons, produced a full report on the matter, and concluded that there was no convincing evidence that any further diseases should be so prescribed; they also firmly rejected the concept of RSI as a diagnostic concept (Barton et al 1992). This is an important review, which has been much quoted in Courts, and should be the starting point for any medical expert considering a possible work-related upper limb complaint.

In the absence of a specific traumatic episode, there are a number of common constitutional conditions which can lead to aches and pains in the upper limb.

Cervical spondylosis

Essentially, this is naturally occurring osteoarthritic degeneration of the skeleton, but it may be aggravated by specific injury. It is a widely diagnosed condition in patients in their middle years and beyond, and represents the natural ageing process of the human skeleton, more marked in some patients than others. It may be attributed to trauma, such as a whiplash injury in a road traffic accident, or similar situations in which a forceful extreme of movement can be demonstrated, associated with appropriate X-ray changes. In most cases, however, cervical spondylosis is simply a variant of the ageing process, with attendant aches and pains in the neck, and referred root pains in the arms and hands. There is no scientific or statistical evidence to show that cervical spondylosis is any more common in patients in any particular trade or job of work than in other patients of comparable age or sex (Lawrence 1969, Murray-Leslie & Wright 1976).

Rotator cuff/shoulder capsulitis

The shoulder joint has only rarely been implicated (by lawyers) under the concept of RSI, and indeed it is difficult to find any reliable research or studies relating shoulder problems to specific working practices, manipulations or forces. The shoulder joint and its immediate soft tissue anatomy (the rotator cuff) is certainly well recognised as being prone to degenerative change, and also to tears which may be a consequence of *specific* trauma. Diagnostic confusion also occurs when trying to separate aches and pains in the shoulder region from nerve root symptoms emanating from the (degenerate) cervical spine. The BOA study (1990) considered there was no good evidence of work-related causation, although the authors felt more studies would be welcome.

Epicondylitis: tennis elbow (lateral) and golfer's elbow (medial)

These are common presenting conditions in the general population, that is those working and those not working in manual occupations, in general practitioner surgeries, and orthopaedic and rheumatological clinics (Coonrad & Hooper 1973, Allander 1974, Hamilton 1986), and indeed on this basis, that is that they occur commonly in the general population, they have been repeatedly rejected as possible PDs by the Industrial Injuries Advisory Council, for there is

no evidence that they are any more common in arduous or manual occupations than in sedentary work (Hamilton 1986, DSS 1991, Barton et al 1992). The terms 'tennis elbow' and 'golfer's elbow' are both very poor descriptors.

A number of studies have shown epicondylitis to be particularly common in the 35–55 age range, and more common in women than men. Kurppa et al (1979b) claim that a literature review of industrially related musculoskeletal conditions is almost entirely anecdotal, but subsequent studies from Scandinavia have suggested an increased incidence of epicondylitis among workers in heavier occupations, e.g. meat-cutters (Roto & Kivi 1984). However, Dimberg (1987) implies that the incidence among blue collar patients is of similar incidence to that among white collar patients, the former group simply tending to complain more than the latter.

Tenosynovitis

The definitions of this condition have formed the basis for much legal argument in the past decade. It is important to appreciate the various ways in which 'tenosynovitis' may be used as a diagnosis.

Tenosynovitis is unfortunately used commonly, and quite inaccurately, to describe a patient with an otherwise unexplained ache or pain in the arm or hand. This term should *not* be used unless there is clear evidence on clinical examination of swelling crepitus and pain along the anatomical line of a tendon at the level of the wrist where it has a tendon sheath. If no such physical signs are evident, it may be that no clear diagnosis can be made, and the problem should be labelled as an 'aching forearm' or a 'painful wrist', or by a similar non-specific term.

Acute tenosynovitis of finger/wrist extensors, usually with crepitus, following arduous or unaccustomed exertion, has been well described by Williams (1977) and Thompson & Plewes (1951), who suggested the name 'peritendinitis crepitans'; more recently, the concept of intersection syndrome (Grundberg & Reagan 1985) has been used to describe the anatomical site where the thumb extensor tendons cross over the wrist extensors.

Industrial tenosynovitis (PD A8) is defined in MS10 (1977) and Guidance Notes (1991). It involves synovial tendon sheaths, and occurs after a period of arduous or unaccustomed work. It settles rapidly with rest (Greenfield 1985).

Numerous other types of tenosynovitis, or tenovaginitis stenosans, occur commonly in the general population, particularly triggering of thumb and finger tendons, and de Quervain's syndrome (essentially triggering of the thumb extensor tendons), and there is no evidence that they are any more common in any particular working population than in those who are not doing manual work. There is also no evidence that these triggering conditions are a consequence of an inflammatory condition in the tendons or their sheaths, except in the rheumatoid arthritic situation (BOA 1990, Kurppa et al 1979a, Barton et al 1992).

De Quervain's syndrome is a stenosing or triggering condition affecting the thumb extensor tendons in the first dorsal compartment of the wrist. It occurs commonly in the general population and is only rarely related to manual work (Clarke M 1998). De Quervain's syndrome is often misdiagnosed; it should be remembered that there are numerous causes for pain/tenderness on the radial aspect of the wrist, such as C5/6 root irritation, scaphoid pathology, crossover syndrome/peritendinitis crepitans, or osteoarthritis of thumb carpometacarpal (CMC) joint, and de Quervain should not be diagnosed unless there is clear and precise tenderness over the first dorsal compartment, together with evidence of thumb extensor tendon difficulties such as catching or nodularity. Finkelstein's test may be helpful, but is often positive in the other conditions mentioned above. The BOA study (1990) considered that the majority of de Quervain problems were not caused by work, but felt that a case for work causation might occasionally be made (Evans 1987, Barton et al 1992).

Carpal tunnel syndrome (CTS)

This common condition is often quoted, apocryphally, as being due to repeated movement or exertion of the fingers, but there is no statistical evidence to support this contention. The General Practice Morbidity Statistics (1983) described CTS as occurring in 0.5% of women from 45–64 years of age, per annum. Nathan et al (1988) and Fuchs et al (1991) show that age and sex are the only determining factors in this condition, and that manual activity or occupation is not a relevant factor. More recently, Burke (1997) have underlined this point in their analysis of CTS in the English Midlands, where occupation was unrelated to the occurrence of the condition. The BOA group (1990) and Barton et al (1992) also considered CTS and firmly stated that it should not be considered as a possible PD. Hadler (1989) contains an excellent review of arguments for and against CTS as an Industrial Disease, and agrees with Barton. The study by Greening & Lynne (1998) suggests some connections between keyboard work and peripheral neuropathy, but this is no more than a hesitant hypothesis.

Dupuytren's contracture

Many manual workers are prone to attribute the flexion deformities of their fingers to their employment; there is no evidence to support this concept, however, and much

evidence to show that the condition is an inherited trait, unaffected by particular forms of occupation. Heuston (1987) discusses the possible industrial aetiology of Dupuytren's contracture, and convincingly shows the condition to be of constitutional/genetic origin, with no detectable causation from hard or repetitive manual work. Heuston points out that a patient with a strong diathesis (predisposition) is more likely to develop significant contracture after a traumatic incident in the hand, e.g. a fracture, than a person without the diathesis (Heuston 1987).

Ganglions

Ganglions are generally considered to be benign synovial cysts, most commonly arising on the dorsal aspect of the scapholunate joint, on the back of the wrist. There is no statistical evidence to show any likely correlation with work. Most orthopaedic/hand surgeons are familiar with wrist ganglions presenting in teenage girls, often before they have reached employable age (BOA 1990).

Osteoarthritis of the base of the thumb

Osteoarthritis in the joints at the base of the thumb is common, and is generally part of the ageing process in the musculoskeletal system, existing in 33% of postmenopausal women (radiologically), one-third of whom had painful symptoms (Armstrong et al 1994). A previous injury, such as a Bennett's fracture, may increse the risk of degenerative joint disease, but there is no good evidence that any particular form of work or manual labour predisposes an otherwise healthy adult to such changes. Various joints may be involved in such degenerative changes, but the commonest are the carpometacarpal joint, and the joint between the scaphoid, trapezium and trapezoid bones (the STT joint). Hadler et al (1978) in a careful study, showed that the anatomical locus, but not the incidence, of distal IPJ osteoarthritis in the finger may be influenced by long-term manual activity.

Summary

- 0.5% of women aged 45–64 years develop CTS per annum.
- 10% of the general population have pain in an upper limb per annum.
- The RSI/overuse diagnosis is unsupported and undefined in law or medicine.
- There is a 3–10% incidence of tennis elbow, unrelated to occupation.
- Beware of Hunter's Diseases of Occupation.
- Dupuytren's contracture is not due to manual work.
- de Quervain's syndrome and trigger finger/thumb are contentious.

- 'Tenosynovitis' is a highly suspect diagnosis, especially by GPs and A&E departments.
- Extensor tenosynovitis (properly diagnosed) is a Prescribed Industrial Disease (A8).
- Thumb, carpometacarpal joint and STT osteoarthritis is common, and part of the natural ageing process.

Examination, report and opinion
History taking and examination

Taking a medical history following a fractured femur in a road traffic accident (RTA) is generally a simple matter of excluding any significant previous medical problems. In RSI cases the matter is likely to be much more indistinct, regarding both the timescale and the origin of symptoms. Most adults experience aches and pains in their upper limbs from time to time (Lawrence 1969, Hadler 1989) and it may be difficult, and occasionally impossible, to separate a sequence of mild complaints from the emergence of more significant problems, leading to the symptoms in question under a legal claim. It is important to be aware of the importance which the law, solicitors and Barristers will attach to the date of the commencement of symptoms, and the examining expert's notes on this point need to be precise, or at least as precise as the patient's history will allow. GP or works medical records may well offer clues as to initial symptoms.

Similarly, note must be taken of the progress of the complaint: did it reach a peak and then subside? Did it commence slowly and then reach a plateau? Did it occur suddenly on one particular morning? Has it continued to worsen with time? Has it improved or worsened after various treatment modalities? All such aspects of the patient's problem need to be noted and analysed.

It is perhaps worth noting here that it is the natural and expected course of any *injury* or *physical insult* to the limb to improve with the passage of time, if not to normality, at least to a plateau of healing. Situations in which the symptoms continue at a steady level, or indeed worsen, imply the presence of other factors, such as unsuspected infection, or other underlying disease or psychological factors.

It should be possible to obtain a clear description of the work which the Plaintiff was doing at the time the alleged problems arose; it may well be that the work was extreme or unreasonable, either in general, or for that particular person (e.g. he was too small or light for the job, or had not been properly trained for it). By all means record the Claimant's description of the forces involved, the pressure of work, rest breaks etc. but bear in mind that the Claimant often has a somewhat exaggerated view of the matter, and it is frequently the case that the actual weights involved, or the hours worked, are less than appear from an initial interview.

Summary

- Establish the time scale: dates of starting and finishing work, and reasons for finishing.
- Pre-exposure morbidity: were there other rheumatic problems?
- Exact description of work: was it arduous or unaccustomed?
- Initial diagnosis from history (GP and hospital records).
- The clinician's own findings, analysis and current diagnosis.
- Relate the current diagnosis to original work: is there a thread of causation?
- The presence of other diagnoses, unrelated to work exposure.
- The presence of other factors, such as psychology or neurosis.
- The prognosis, including working capacity.

■ References

Allander E 1974 Prevalence, incidence and remission rates of some common rheumatic diseases or syndromes. Scandinavian Journal of Rheumatology 3: 145–153

Armstrong A I, Hunter J G, Davis T R C 1994 The prevalence of degenerative arthritis in the base of the thumb in post-menopausal women. Journal of Hand Surgery 3B: 340–341

Armstrong T J 1986 Ergonomics and cumulative trauma disorders. Hand Clinics 2: 553–565

Armstrong T J, Foulke J, Joseph B, Goldstein S 1982 Investigation of cumulative trauma disorders in a poultry processing plant. American Industrial Hygiene Association Journal 43(2): 103–116

Barton N J 1989 Repetitive strain disorder. British Medical Journal 299: 405–406

Barton N J, Hooper G, Noble J, Steel W M 1992 Occupational causes of disorders in the upper limb. British Medical Journal 304: 309–311

Bell D S 1989 'Repetition strain injury': an iatrogenic epidemic of simulated injury. The Medical Journal of Australia 151: 280–284

British Orthopaedic Association 1990 Working party report

Brooks P 1986 Occupational pain syndromes. Medical Journal of Australia 144: 170–171

Browne C D, Nolan B M, Faithfull D K 1984 Occupational repetition strain injuries. Guidelines for diagnosis and management. Medical Journal of Australia 140: 329–332

Burke F 1997 Median nerve compression syndrome at the wrist. In: Hunter J (ed.) Tendon and nerve surgery in the hand. Mosby, London, pp 145–148

Clarke M et al 1998 The histopathology of de Quervain's disease. Journal of Hand Surgery 23B: 732–734

Cleland L G 1987 'RSI': a model of social iatrogenesis. Medical Journal of Australia 147: 236–239

Cohen M L, Arroyo J F, Champion D G, Browne C D 1992 In search of refractory cervicobrachial pain syndrome. Medical Journal of Australia 156: 432–436

Coonrad R W, Hooper W R 1973 Tennis elbow: its course, natural history, conservative and surgical management. Journal of Bone and Joint Surgery 55A: 1177–1182

Dennett X Fry H J H 1988 Overuse syndrome: a muscle biopsy study. Lancet 905–908

Department of Health and Social Security (DHSS) 1972 Traumatic inflammation of the tendons of the hand or forearm or of the associated tendon sheaths. PD34. DHSS Notes on the Diagnosis of Occupational Diseases, p 38

Department of Social Security (DSS) 1991 Notes on the diagnosis of prescribed diseases. HMSO

Dimberg L 1987 The prevalence and causation of tennis elbow (lateral humeral epicondylitis) in a population of workers in an engineering industry. Ergonomics 30(3): 573–579

Evans G 1987 Tenosynovitis in industry: menace or misnomer? British Medical Journal 294: 1569–1570

Ferguson D 1984 The 'new' industrial epidemic. Medical Journal of Australia, 140(6) 318–319

Ferguson D A 1987 'RSI': Putting the epidemic to rest. Medical Journal of Australia 147: 213–214

Fry H J 1986a Overuse syndrome, alias tenosynovitis/tendinitis: the terminological hoax. Plastic and Reconstructive Surgery 78(3): 414–417

Fry H J H 1986b Physical signs in the hand and wrist seen in the overuse injury syndrome of the upper limb. Australian and New Zealand Journal of Surgery 56: 47–49

Fuchs P C, Nathan P A, Myers L D 1991 Synovial histology in carpal tunnel syndrome. Journal of Hand Surgery 16A: 753–758

GMB Union 1986 Tackling teno: a GMB guide to upper limb disorders

Golding D N 1985 Tennis and golfer's elbow. Arthritis & Rheumatism Council, p 2

Greenfield P R 1985 Notes on the diagnosis of occupational diseases. Department of Health & Social Security Pamphlet

Greening J, Lynne B (1998) Vibration sense in the upper limb in patients with repetitive strain injury and a group of at risk office workers. International Archives of Occupational Environmental Health 71: 29–34

Griffin M J 1987 Assessing the hazards of whole-body and hand-arm vibration. Recent Advances in Occupational Health 3: 191–202

Grundberg A B, Reagan D S 1985 Pathologic anatomy of the forearm: intersection syndrome. Journal of Hand Surgery 10A: 299–302

Hadler N M 1978 Hand structure and function in an industrial setting: influence of 3 patterns of stereotyped repetitive usage. Arthritis and Rheumatism 21(2): 210–220

Hadler N M 1984a Medical management of regional musculoskeletal diseases. Grune & Stratton

Hadler N M 1984b Occupational illness: the issue of causality. Journal of Occupational Medicine 26: 587–593

Hadler N M 1985 Illness in the workplace: the challenge of musculoskeletal symptoms. Journal of Hand Surgery 10A: 451–456

Hadler N M 1986 Industrial rheumatology: the Australian and New Zealand experiences with arm pain and backache in the workplace. Medical Journal of Australia 144: 191–195

Hadler N M 1989 The roles of work and of working in disorders of the upper extremity. Bailliere's Clinical Rheumatology 3: 121–141

Hadler N M 1990 Cumulative trauma disorders: an iatrogenic concept. Journal of Occupational Medicine 32: 38–41 (editorial)

Hamilton P G 1986 The prevalence of humeral epicondylitis: a survey in general practice. Journal of the Royal College of General Practitioners 36: 464–465

Hazleman B L 1993 Repeated movements and repeated trauma. In: Hunter's diseases of occupations, 8th ed, pp 515–530

Health & Safety Executive 1977 Beat conditions, tenosynovitis. Guidance Note MS10

Health & Safety Executive 1990 Work related upper limb disorders—a guide to prevention. Pamphlet

Hocking B 1987 Epidemiological aspects of 'repetition strain injury' in Telecom Australia. Medical Journal of Australia 147: 218–222

Hooper G 1990 Cystic swellings. In: Tumours of the wrist and hand. Churchill Livingstone, Edinburgh

Hueston J T 1987 Dupuytren's contracture and occupation. Journal of Hand Surgery 12A: 657–658

Hunter D 1987 Repeated movements and repeated trauma. In: Hunter's diseases of occupations, 7th ed, pp 620–633

Industrial Injuries Advisory Council 1992 Work related upper limb disorders. HMSO, London

Ippolito E, Postachini F, Scola E, Belocci M, De Martino C 1985 De Quervain's disease: an ultrastructural study. International Orthopaedics 9: 41–47

Ireland D C R 1988 Psychological and physical aspects of occupational arm pain. Journal of Hand Surgery 13B: 5–10

Kivi P 1984 Rheumatic disorders of the upper limbs associated with repetitive occupational tasks in Finland in 1975–1979. Scandinavian Journal of Rheumatology 13: 101–107

Kuorinka I, Koskinen P 1979 Occupational rheumatic diseases and upper limb strain in manual jobs in a light mechanical industry. Scandinavian Journal of Work Environment and Health 5: 39–47

Kurppa K, Waris P, Rokleanen P 1979a Peritendinitis and tenosynovitis. Scandinavian Journal of Work Environment and Health 5: 19–24

Kurppa K, Waris P, Rokkanen P 1979b Tennis elbow: lateral elbow pain syndrome. Scandinavian Journal of Work Environment and Health 5: 15–18

Lawrence J S 1969 Disc degeneration—its frequency and relationship to symptoms. Annals of the Rheumatic Diseases 28: 121–138

Lucire Y 1986 Neurosis in the workplace. Medical Journal of Australia 145: 323–327

Luopajarvi T et al 1979 Prevalence of tenosynovitis and other injuries of the upper extremities in repetitive work. Scandinavian Journal of Work Environment and Health 5: 48–55

Maeda K 1977 Occupational cervicobrachial disorder and its causative factors. Journal of Human Ergology 6: 193–202

McDermott F T 1986 Repetition strain injury: a review of current understanding. Medical Journal of Australia 144: 196–200

Medical Editors 1985 Carpal tunnel syndrome (reports on rheumatic diseases). Arthritis & Rheumatism Council, p 2

Murray-Leslie C F, Wright V 1976 Carpal tunnel syndrome, humeral epicondylitis, and the cervical spine: a study of clinical and dimensional relations. British Medical Journal 1: 1439–1442

Nathan P A, Keniston R C, Myers K D, Meadows K D 1992 Longitudinal study of median nerve sensory conduction in industry: relationship to age, gender, hand dominance, occupational hand use, and clinical diagnosis. Journal of Hand Surgery 17A: 850–857

Nathan P A, Meadows K D, Doyle L S 1988 Occupation as a risk factor for impaired sensory conduction of the median nerve at the carpal tunnel. Journal of Hand Surgery 13B: 167–170

Nelson J, Howard M D 1937 Peritendinitis crepitans (a muscle-effort syndrome). Journal of Bone and Joint Surgery 2: 442–459

Porter K M 1989 Neck sprains after car accidents. British Medical Journal 298: 973–974

Raffle 1987 Vibration. In: Hunter's diseases of occupations, 7th edn, pp 460–471

Ramazzini B 1940 De morbis artificium (translated by W C Wright). University of Chicago Press, Chicago (first published in 1713)

Roto P, Kivi P 1984 Prevalence of epicondylitis and tenosynovitis among meatcutters. Scandinavian Journal of Work Environment and Health 10: 203–205

Royal Australasian College of Physicians 1986 College wants name 'RSI' changed. Statement by the Royal Australasian College of Physicians

Semple J C 1986 Tenosynovitis—editorial. Journal of Hand Surgery 11B: 155–156

Semple J C 1991 Tenosynovitis, repetitive strain injury, cumulative trauma disorder, and overuse syndrome, et cetera. Journal of Bone and Joint Surgery 73B: 536–538

Semple J C, Behan P O, Behan W M, Brooks P, Hocking B, Littlejohn G, Miller M 1988 Overuse syndrome. Lancet 1464–1466 (collection of letters)

Silverstein B A, Fine L J, Armstrong T J 1986 Hand/wrist cumulative trauma disorders in industry. British Journal of Industrial Medicine 43: 779–784

Smythe H 1988 The 'repetitive strain injury syndrome' is referred pain from the neck. Journal of Rheumatology 15: 1604–1608

Thompson A R, Plewes L W 1951 Peritendinitis crepitans and simple tenosynovitis: a clinical study of 544 cases in industry. British Journal of Industrial Medicine 8: 150–157

Thompson D, Rawlings A J, Harrington J M 1987 Repetition strain injuries. Recent Advances in Occupational Health 3: 75–89

Viikari-Juntura E 1984 Tenosynovitis, peritendinitis, and the tennis elbow syndrome. Scandinavian Journal of Work Environment and Health 10: 443–449

Waldron H A 1987 Anyone for teno? British Journal of Industrial Medicine 44: 793–794 (editorial)

Wallace M, Buckle P 1987 Ergonomic aspects of neck and upper limb disorders. International Reviews of Ergonomics 1: 173–200

Waris P 1980 Occupational cervicobrachial syndromes: a review. Scandinavian Journal of Work Environment and Health 6: 3–14

Welch R 1973 The measurement of physiological predisposition to tenosynovitis. Ergonomics 16: 665–668

Williams J G P 1977 Surgical management of traumatic non-infective tenosynovitis of the wrist extensors. Journal of Bone and Joint Surgery 59B: 408–410

Wood H A, Linscheid R L 1973 Abductor pollicis longus bursitis. Clinical Orthopaedics and Related Research 93: 293–296

Chapter 24

Soft tissue injuries, including burns

Orla Austin and Simon Kay

Introduction

The plastic surgeon has a key role to play in both the acute and the long-term management of patients with soft tissue injuries. The input required depends on the nature and severity of the wound. The aim of management in dealing with any soft tissue injury is to heal the wound as quickly as possible and at the same time achieve the best functional and cosmetic outcome. To do this, a reconstructive ladder is employed to plan the type of closure, ranging from primary closure to tissue transfer, either locally from the area surrounding the injury, or from a distant site (Fig. 24.1). This chapter discusses various aspects of wound management together with the treatment of burns injury. It also briefly considers the provision of skin cover for the injured upper and lower extremity.

Primary closure

Wounds can be closed primarily where there is little or no skin loss. The most important aspect of wound closure is the precise approximation of the skin edges without undue tension. This ensures healing with minimal scarring. Care should be taken to remove the skin sutures or staples at the appropriate time in order to

avoid ugly cross-hatching or suture marks surrounding the scar.

Skin grafts: definition and terminology

A skin graft is an auto-transplant of skin, one site to another, without an intact blood supply and without the blood supply being restored surgically. It is dependent on neovascularisation from the recipient bed for survival.

Split-thickness skin grafts (SSG) contain epidermis and some dermis, and are described as thick, medium or thin depending on the thickness of the included dermis. Since the sweat glands, sebaceous glands and hair follicles lie deep in the dermis, SSGs do not grow hair and often remain dry and scaly due to the lack of glandular elements. Split-thickness skin grafts are insensate and provide poor cosmesis, especially on the face. Being thinner than ordinary skin, they are readily traumatised. Because of trauma within the dermis, they inevitably undergo contraction and can distort surrounding structures or cause joint contractures.

A skin graft may be taken with either a skin graft knife or a power dermatome. Before the introduction of dermatomes, all skin grafts were harvested with hand-held knives, such as the Humby knife. Since the advent of power dermatomes, the hand-held knife is used less frequently as a power dermatome allows better and more consistent control of the length, width and depth of the skin graft. The skin graft may be harvested under local or general anaesthetic.

SSGs can be used as sheet grafts or meshed grafts. A meshed graft allows the passage of exudate from the wound, permits the graft to lie in close contact over an irregular surface and can be stretched to a size greater than the original (such as 1.5:1 or 3:1), depending on the meshing board used. Meshed skin covers a larger area, contours easily and adapts to fit an irregular bed, allows any exudate to drain freely and provides increased edges from which re-epithelialisation occurs. However, it also has several disadvantages: it leaves much of the wound to heal by secondary intention, potentially resulting in wound contracture, and gives an unsightly 'string vest' appearance.

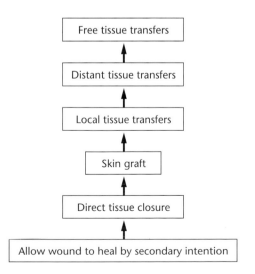

Fig. 24.1   Reconstructive ladder for wound closure.

Full-thickness skin grafts (FTSGs) contain epidermis, dermis and skin appendages and so provide improved cosmesis, and they resist wound contraction better than SSGs, possibly because the dermis is not destroyed. They can grow hair and are self-moisturising but, in common with SSGs, they remain poorly sensate for practical purposes.

Skin grafts are used for replacing missing skin when the recipient bed is capable of angiogenesis and so is judged to have potential for developing granulation tissue. The word 'take' as applied to skin grafts implies neovascularisation and physical adherence of the graft to the wound.

Skin grafts are contraindicated in circumstances in which angiogenesis is poor or absent, e.g. an avascular wound bed such as exposed cortical bone, bare tendon, bare cartilage and exposed prostheses following radiation damage. They are also contraindicated is cases of purulent discharge, infection with streptococci group A bacteria, and if there is a need for future surgery through the graft.

All skin autografts have a donor site. Donor defects for FTSGs need to be closed surgically, leaving a linear scar. They are generally harvested from an area where the skin is thin, and the scar can be hidden, such as the postauricular area, supraclavicular fossa and groin.

SSG donor sites heal spontaneously from epithelial remnants. The time for the healing of donor site varies from 10–14 days, depending predominantly on the thickness of the harvested graft in proportion to the skin thickness at the site, postoperative wound infection, the age and general condition of the patient, and the nature of the dressings used. SSG donor sites are painful until healed; they will almost always leave a scar, varying from an area of altered pigmentation to a lumpy, hypertrophic area, depending on the thickness of the graft taken, the healing process, the site from which harvested and the presence of postoperative infection. The donor site should therefore be chosen with care, using an area that is cosmetically acceptable such as the upper thigh or lateral buttock.

Skin grafts: outcome

Crusting and scaling of SSGs are to be expected and usually require application of agents such as Nivea, E45 or lanolin. Skin grafts change colour as they heal. Those from the abdomen, buttocks and thighs ultimately appear yellow, while FTSGs on the face look redder than the surrounding skin for up to 12 months. Skin grafts always shrink as the graft/wound interface contracts. FTSGs tend to contract less, whereas SSGs contract the most; the thinner the graft, the greater is the contraction. This secondary contraction can distort normal features and interfere with normal movement if a SSG crosses a joint. Thin grafts applied on periosteum can be unstable and, being thin and insensate, are more prone to trauma and subsequent chronic breakdown. It is important to remember that the junction of a skin graft with surrounding normal skin is a scar and will behave like one—with the potential for hypertrophy, atrophy or contraction.

Donor sites for SSGs also show scaling and crusting with diminished excretion of sweat and sebaceous glands initially, but usually recover within 3 months. The pattern of hair growth can be disturbed. Recovery of sensibility is normal. Formation of small cysts or milia is common, but diminishes with time. Pigmentary changes are unpredictable, but can be very significant in people with pigmented skin. Like all wounds, there are significant colour changes with time. The early erythematous appearance gradually lightens over 12–24 months. Exposure to sun in the early stages can worsen the erythema and alter the pigmentation.

FTSG doner sites appear as linear scars and can undergo hypertrophy, remain narrow or stretch.

Skin grafts: reporting

The graft *and* the donor site should be reported upon. The following features should be recorded.

The graft

- Type
- Dimensions
- Site
- Method of harvest
- Aesthetics—sheet or meshed; colour; scaliness; hair growth; ulceration
- Contour
- Sensation, dysaesthesia
- Junctional scar
- Effect on surrounding structures
- Effect on joint position and function
- Symptoms

SSG donor site

- Site
- Time for healing
- Dimensions
- Aesthetics—colour and contour
- Whether or not easily concealed
- Symptoms

Full-thickness donor site

- Site
- Dimensions
- Aesthetics—colour and contour, scar width
- Whether or not easily concealed
- Effect on surrounding structures
- Symptoms

Skin grafts: results

In an ideal situation grafts should achieve 100% take. Most skin graft failures are due to problems with the recipient site rather than technical errors in harvesting the graft. Flowers (1970) identified the two commonest causes of graft failure as haematoma and infection. Other reasons include excess pressure (>30 mmHg), and inappropriate bed, shearing motion in the graft/bed interface and fluid collections.

SSG donor sites should heal within 2–3 weeks without granulation tissue. The presence of granulations implies a full-thickness loss of graft, either at the time of harvest or later, following infection. Similarly, a donor site showing a hypertrophic scar implies deep injury. Pruritus can be a problem in a recent donor site.

Skin flaps: definition and terminology

A skin flap is a unit of skin and subcutaneous tissue (Hodges 1986) which maintains its connection with the body during all stages of transfer or has the vascular connection restored immediately following transfer by means of microvascular anastomosis. As a flap carries its own blood supply it is not dependent for its survival on the vascularity or angioneogenic potential of the recipient bed. This is the fundamental difference between a graft and a flap.

The defect to be closed is termed the 'primary defect', while the defect subsequent to raising a flap is the donor or 'secondary defect'. The secondary defect can be closed directly or with a skin graft or another flap.

Flaps can be described geometrically (rhomboid, bilobed, Z-plasty etc.), geographically (local, regional or distant), on the pattern of transfer (rotation, advancement, transposition or microsurgical) and, most importantly, on the basis of the vascular supply. If a flap contains an anatomically recognised artery and vein, the flap is an axial pattern flap (McGregor & Morgan 1963) and can be made thinner and longer than flaps without a specific identifiable vascular pedicle but instead relying on the random pattern of skin blood supply.

Tissues other than skin can be transferred as flaps (bone flaps, muscle flaps and fascial flaps) and flaps can be composed of more than one tissue (myocutaneous flaps, fasciocutaneous flaps etc.). Fasciocutaneous flaps contain the deep fascia in addition to the overlying skin and subcutaneous tissues for the purpose of including the muscular plexus that runs with the fascia (Ponten 1981). Myocutaneous flaps contain skin, fascia and muscle and provide a good, reliable blood supply together with bulk for dead space closure.

A flap rather than a skin graft is indicated to restore surface in an avascular wound, to restore volume, to reconstruct complex structures and to provide lost function. A flap is also indicated when the need is for thick pliable skin, or where it is necessary to re-operate through the wound at a later date to repair underlying structures. The advantages are healing by primary intention, maintenance of skin appendage function, meeting of complex needs in one operation, better aesthetics, obliteration of dead space and the possibility of maintaining sensation. The disadvantage is the creation of an additional wound (the secondary defect) with its own morbidity and aesthetic burden. Flap reconstruction is technically demanding and can be time-consuming. Flaps can suffer partial or total necrosis and invasive procedures may be necessary for the monitoring of flaps and patients. At the recipient site (the primary defect) volume mismatch can make the flap bulky, requiring revision surgery. The junction of the flap with the surrounding tissues can be the site of neuromata; flaps—especially free cutaneous flaps—can be insensate; and regional and distant flaps may show significant mismatch in aesthetic appearance at the recipient site.

Skin flaps: reporting

All flaps have a donor site that also has to be considered.

Flap

- Symptoms
- Site
- Flap constituents—skin, fascia, fat, muscle, bone
- Dimensions
- Shape
- Aesthetics—colour, contour, hair growth
- Marginal scarring
- Sensation
- Ulceration

Donor site

- Symptoms
- Site
- Method of closure
- Aesthetic appearance
- Scarring
- Neurological deficit
- Functional/musculoskeletal deficit (in the case of myocutaneous flaps)
- Whether or not easily concealed

Skin flaps: results

A flap can be described as unsuccessful if it fails to achieve the purpose for which it was raised. Conversely, even if a flap does not survive in its entirety but serves the reconstructive purpose, then it should be deemed successful. Flaps fail for a number of reasons which may be technical (design error, tension, poor blood supply, anatomical incongruity or infection) or due to patient factors (smoking, obesity, age, site, polycythaemia, non-compliance with after-care).

■ Skin cover in the lower limb

Reconstructive options for the provision of skin cover in the lower extremity range from simple skin grafts to complex microsurgical transfers of composite tissues. The spectrum of lower extremity trauma extends from simple pretibial lacerations to traumatic amputations. The particular technique chosen should be safe, and provide the best functional and aesthetic reconstruction with a high success rate, the least morbidity and the shortest rehabilitation. Special requirements in the lower extremity are stability over bone, durability on weight-bearing surfaces, ability to obliterate bony cavities, suppleness over joints and the capacity to withstand the dependent position. Sensibility is desirable but not essential (Rautio 1991).

Injuries

Pre-tibial flap lacerations

These lacerations are characterised by undermining of a flap of tissue and these flaps have a high incidence of necrosis, particularly if sutured back to their original site. Common predisposing factors are infirmity, old age, imbalance, visual problems and steroids. There is a lack of agreement about the best way of treating these common injuries. Opinions differ about the role and the timing of surgery, the use of skin graft or of the defatted flap, postoperative mobilisation, the management of the skin graft donor site

and the role of DVT prophylaxis. Skin grafts have success rates of greater than 85%, and the main problem in these patients is the postoperative social rehabilitation.

Compound fractures

Treatment protocols for the management of severe lower extremity injuries involving skeleton and soft tissue disruption have now been used for a couple of decades (Byrd et al 1981). Godina (1986) pioneered the concept of emergency microvascular flaps in the management of complex lower extremity trauma, and demonstrated an infection rate of 1.5% when the wounds were closed within 24–72 hours. Ninkovic classified the timing of treatment and showed that surgery does not need to be performed on the day of injury. Arnez et al (1999) proposed a new scoring system for predicting the outcome in severe lower limb injury. The practice of combined assessment by plastic and orthopaedic surgeons, radical debridement of bone and soft tissue either serially or primarily, stabilisation of fractures and either primary or delayed primary flap cover have decreased the incidence of infection and subsequent morbidity (Godina 1986, Yaremchuk et al 1987). The two most important determinants of outcome of these severe injuries are the mechanism of injury and the adequacy of debridement (Walton & Rothkopf 1991). Joint guidelines for the optimal management of open tibial fractures were published by the British Orthopaedic Association and the British Association of Plastic Surgeons in 1997.

Compound tibial fractures

These can be classified in a variety of ways. The two commonly used systems are those described by Byrd et al (1985) and the Gustilo et al classification (1984; see below), the latter a modification of the earlier Gustilo classification of 1976 and particularly useful in discussing skin reconstruction:

- Type I—an open fracture with a cutaneous wound <1 cm.
- Type II—an open fracture with a cutaneous wound >1 cm without extensive soft tissue damage.
- Type IIIA—high-energy trauma irrespective of the size of the wound. There is adequate soft tissue coverage of the fractured bone, despite extensive soft tissue lacerations or flaps. Gustilo et al (1984) reported an infection rate of 4% and no amputations.
- Type IIIB—there is an extensive soft tissue injury with loss of tissue, accompanied by periosteal stripping and bone exposure. These wounds are usually associated with massive contamination. With conventional management, a very high proportion, 52% (Gustilo et al 1984), of these patients develop infections. Sixteen per-

cent eventually require amputations. With aggressive treatment, salvage rates of 93% and chronic infection rates of 6.9% have been recorded (Francel et al 1992). Three year follow-up results from the USA in patients with Gustilo IIIB fractures who had successful free tissue transfer within 15 days of injury reveal a major complication rate of 3.6%, successful limb salvage in 93%, good aesthetic results in 80% and patient satisfaction in 96%. However, 66% of patients exhibit decreased ankle motion, 44% have swelling and oedema requiring elastic support and activity modification, and 50% occasionally require an assistance device for ambulation. The long-term employment rate was 28% and no patient returned to work after 2 years of unemployment. In contrast, 68% of amputees after lower extremity trauma over the same period returned to work within 2 years (Francel et al 1992).

■ Type IIIC—these are open fractures associated with arterial injury requiring repair. The infection rate for these injuries is 42%, and 42% of patients have amputations (Gustilo et al 1984). Primary amputation should be considered. However, salvage rates of 70% have been reported with early revascularisation and soft tissue reconstruction (Russell et al 1991).

The shortcoming of the Gustilo classification is that it does not adequately describe severe injuries that do not include fractures (Francel et al 1992).

Choice of flaps

Flaps used for soft tissue defects of the lower limb may be mobilised from either a local or a distant (free) source. The choice depends on the site or level of injury, the type of injury sustained and the tissue type that needs to be replaced. Frequently used flaps are the gastrocnemius muscle flap for upper third tibial defects, and the fasciocutaneous flap or tibialis anterior muscle or soleus muscle flap for middle third tibial defects. Lower third tibial defects require microvascular free tissue transfers as there is a paucity of local tissues to be used as flaps. Latissimus dorsi muscle with or without overlying skin and the rectus abdominis muscles are the two frequently used free flaps in the lower extremity.

Foot injuries

As the characteristics of sole skin cannot be duplicated by any other tissue, the requirements in this area are unique and are ideally provided by tissue from the sole itself. The reconstructive method and flap chosen should be able to withstand weight bearing, the forces of shear between bone and soft tissue, and ideally be sensate. The flap should not be bulky, to avoid interference with footwear.

SSGs can be used to cover shallow defects. Long-term morbidity includes hyperkeratosis and junctional scar instability and hypersensitivity.

Controversy exists about the choice of flaps for covering the sole—whether myocutaneous, muscle with skin graft or fasciocutaneous. The use of innervated flaps in preference to others is not supported by clinical series (Francel et al 1992). The proximal plantar area and the weight-bearing heel can be covered either by local flaps, by the island instep fasciocutaneous flap or by the flexor digitorum brevis muscle flap with skin graft (Saltz et al 1991). The non-weight-bearing heel, achilles tendon and the malleoli can be covered with fasciocutaneous flaps (Francel et al 1992) or muscle flaps, using the extensor digitorum brevis muscle from the dorsum of the foot. Large defects will require microvascular tissue transfer, the exact choice being determined by local wound characteristics. For small lesions of the forefoot, local flaps or flaps from discarded toes can be used. Large defects would necessitate the use of microvascular free tissue transfer. Skin grafts play a major role in covering wounds over the dorsum of the foot. Large defects with bone or joint exposure are treated most commonly with microvascular muscle transfer. Rehabilitation is quicker for patients with foot injuries compared to leg injuries, as weight bearing can be commenced early in the absence of bony injury. The average time to full weight bearing was 106 days (range 90–280 days) in one series (Francel et al 1992).

Severe degloving injuries

These should be managed by conservative serial debridement and expanded meshed grafting unless specific indications for flap cover are found.

Skin cover in the lower limb: reporting

In addition to reporting on the flap or graft, as before, the following should be recorded:

■ pre- and post-injury employment
■ pre- and post-injury ambulation status
■ pre- and post-injury gait
■ aesthetic appearance
■ use of footwear

Skin cover in the lower limb: results

See the general comments above.

Re-employment is the end-result of successful rehabilitation. Less than 30% of patients with severe tibial fractures return to work, while the return-to-work rate is 78% in patients with foot reconstructions (Francel 1992).

Scars

Scars are sometimes viewed as incidental and unremarkable in comparison to the surgery that has dictated them, but to the patient they may be the only permanent evidence of their trauma and, quite apart from their disfiguring qualities, they may assume a psychological significance out of apparent proportion to their appearance. Rather than simply stating the presence of a scar, the reporting surgeon should describe the quality of the scar and have an understanding of scar maturation, so that he may give a confident prognosis as to the likely appearance and timing of the final blemish.

Scar: natural history

Scars go through phases of development, the length and timing of which may vary with the site on the body and from age to age in the same individual. After uncomplicated wound closure the site of injury appears as a fine line within skin, but as the proliferative or fibroblastic phase of wound healing progresses the vascularity increases and more collagen is deposited, making the scar appear red, firm, raised and pruritic. Most scars are at their worst between 2 weeks and 2 months after injury (Parsons 1977). Scars show improvement in appearance once the wound enters the stage of maturation characterised by collagen homoeostasis (Madden & Peacock 1971). The end-point of maturation may take from 4–24 months (Parsons 1977) and is complete when the scar is soft, pliable and has lost the increased vascularity. Scar revision should await scar maturation (Parsons 1977) unless there is a threat to function.

Scar: factors affecting results

First and foremost, an ideal scar should not interfere with function; and secondly, it should be aesthetically acceptable. Scars become noticeable when they interrupt the homogenous flow of tissue planes because of differences in colour, contour and texture, e.g. hyperpigmented, depressed or elevated scars.

Factors that have an effect on the final appearance of scars can be considered in terms of patient factors, wound factors and technical factors. Patient factors such as the genetic background, the racial characteristics of the individual, age, nutritional status, drug therapy and so on are outside the control of the surgeon, but can interfere with the normal processes of scar maturation.

Wound factors

The final appearance of a scar is more influenced by the method of injury than by the method of suture (Parsons 1977). Confused or infected wounds, traumatic tattooing, improper orientation against relaxed skin tension lines and across flexor joint surfaces, closure under tension, bevelling of edges and tangentially raised skin flaps are predictors of an ultimately poor result. Trapdoor scars result from scar contraction around areas of skin surrounded on three sides by scar tissue, and are very difficult to revise.

The site of a scar has a profound influence on its outcome, and patients will often point to a near-perfect appendicectomy scar and compare it critically with a scar on the volar forearm or the knee. Sites on the body which are particularly prone to the formation of thick scars are the pre-sternal, pre-clavicular and shoulder regions. Scars on the back seldom remain hairline and tend to stretch with time. On the limbs, the volar forearm and the knee are well known sites for poor scars. Broadening of a scar is related to its initial lumpiness.

Technical factors

Crikelair (1960) summarised the fundamentals of surgical techniques to minimise scarring. The most important is placement of the incision, which should follow tension lines and avoid longitudinal incisions across flexor surfaces. Differences among suture materials are negligible, although technical factors of suture placement and timing of suture removal do affect the final scar (Parsons 1977). Suture marks can be avoided by using subcuticular sutures, while scar stretching can be minimised by avoiding tension in closure and by using subcuticular sutures which provide prolonged dermal support (Chantarask & Milner 1989, Elliot & Mahaffey 1989). Ninety percent of scar stretching is seen within the first 6 months (Sommerlad & Creasey 1978).

Hypertrophic and keloid scars

Optimum healing produces a fine-line scar that compromises neither function nor appearance. Hypertrophic and keloid scars are abnormal scars and cannot be differentiated histologically (Grabb 1967), but may be differentiated by their clinical behaviour (Brown & Pierce 1986).

Hypertrophic scars appear to be a self-limiting type of overhealing following injury (Niessen et al 1999). They contain excess collagen that remains within the confines of the original wound, are found in all areas of the body, and predominantly in young people, and follow a natural history of growth followed by a spontaneous decrease in volume (Peacock et al 1970). Keloids are pseudotumours of collagen (Rohrich & Spicer 1986) or benign tumours that extend beyond the boundary of the original wound (Grabb 1967), and—in contrast to hypertrophic scars—tend to persist.

Keloids also display a significant familial predilection and are more common in Afro-Caribbeans than in

Caucasians by a ratio of 3.5:1 to 15:1 (Brown & Pierce 1986). They may occur at any age, but very young children and older adults are rarely affected.

No universally effective method of treatment of keloids is available. Surgical excision is followed by 100% recurrence (Rohrich & Spicer 1986), and adjuvant treatment is essential to reduce this. Surgical excision followed by intra-operative and postoperative corticosteroid injections, pressure therapy or radiation (brachytherapy) have been used in the past, with variable results (Darzi et al 1992, Tang 1992). More recently, interferon has shown some benefits in reducing scarring.

Hypertrophic scars may resolve spontaneously over a period of between 9 months and 2 years, or in response to local pressure (Larson et al 1974), but the pressure needs to be maintained constantly for 6–9 months. Early release may be followed by relapse (Kisher et al 1975, Brent 1978). Intralesional steroids are also effective (Ketchum et al 1974), and hypertrophic scars have been shown to respond to silicone gel application (Quinn 1987).

Surgery for hypertrophic scars is often successful when the scar lies against an optimal direction and the revision procedure reorients the scar. However, it is imperative to warn patients undergoing scar revision surgery that the new scar will go through the same cycle of worsening before improving, and that hypertrophy may recur.

Scars: reporting

Despite the problems of cutaneous scarring, there is a paucity of objective clinical scales for evaluation and reporting scar appearance. Beausang et al (1998) suggested a visual analogue scale incorporating scar colour, contour, texture and distortion. Other authors have suggested the use of a pneumanometer (Spann 1996).

Scar analysis should include the following:

- location
- orientation
- dimensions
- thickness, colour, shape
- associated symptoms
- behaviour over preceding months/years
- local distortions, contour defects, shadows
- interference with function
- previous treatment
- tenderness
- aetiology

Burns: treatment

It is estimated that more than 100 000 burn victims are treated in A&E departments in the UK every year. The extent of their injuries range from minor burns with no permanent sequelae to major disfiguring and life-threatening burns.

The cardinal determinants of burn mortality have traditionally been burn area and age (Bull 1971). Other factors shown to be of statistical significance in predicting mortality are full-thickness burn area, bronchopulmonary disease, pO_2, carboxyhaemaglobin and airway oedema associated with inhalation injury (Zawacki et al 1979). Higher than expected death rates have been reported in obese patients (Purdue et al 1990) and those with other injuries who have been burnt in motor vehicle accidents (Purdue et al 1985).

The extent of body surface area that has been burnt also determines the need for intravenous resuscitation. Children with burns >10% of body surface area and adults with burns >15% need to be resuscitated.

The primary determinant of long-term appearance and function is burn depth, which may be characterised in degrees or descriptively. Simple erythema (1st degree burn) heals without sequelae. In superficial burns there is a partial thickness injury (2nd degree) to the skin, which heals spontaneously from surviving epithelial remnants without significant scarring within 2–3 weeks. Deep dermal burns (2nd degree) involve the deeper (reticular) layers of the dermis and may take longer to heal, and there may be more scarring than in the case of the superficial burn. Deep burns (3rd degree) involve the full thickness of the skin and sometimes deeper structures (4th degree) as well. These burns almost always need surgery in the form of debridement and appropriate reconstruction. Despite currently available technology, clinical observation remains the standard for burn depth diagnosis (Heimbach et al 1992).

Burns showing simple erythema and superficial burns are best managed conservatively. Burns diagnosed to be full thickness should be debrided and appropriately reconstructed as soon as medically safe, usually within 2–5 days. Early excision and grafting are widely accepted because of the low morbidity rate (Settle 1996). No firm guidelines can be set about the correct management of deep dermal burns. Conservative treatment with surgery for those failing to heal at the end of 2–3 weeks, or early debridement and skin grafting within 2–5 days, is acceptable. The advantage of the latter is a shorter hospital stay but an increased requirement of blood transfusion. In a randomised controlled study, Engrav et al (1983) were unable to show any significant difference in function between the two treatment approaches, and at best a marginal difference in appearance in the long term.

Burns: outcome

Blisters appear on healed burns, grafted burns or on donor sites. They can be seen between 2–6 weeks, diminish with time but may continue for months. Dryness can be a problem for 6–8 weeks until natural lubricants return (Warden 1987). Dermatitis, either allergic or irritant, is common. Avoidance of sunlight is recommended for 6 months to avoid sunburn and permanent hyperpigmentation (Warden 1987). Itching of healing burns can be troublesome and the pathogenesis is ill understood. Hypertrophic scarring and contractures are common after burns which have taken longer than 3 weeks to heal. Neoplastic change in unstable burn scars is a long-term problem. The problems associated with both skin grafting and donor sites are similar to those mentioned previously.

Burns: reporting

History

- The time and place of the incident
- The cause of the burn
- The extent and depth of the burn
- Activity at the time of the burn
- Other injuries or illnesses
- Smoke inhalation
- Any use of alcohol or drugs
- First aid measures and time interval before initiation of treatment
- Casualty treatment
- Definitive treatment—resuscitation, wound management
- Time for wound healing
- Surgery—timing
    —use of skin graft, artificial skin (Integra), skin flaps etc.
- Effects on growth (in children)
- Psychological consequences
- The extent of the burn

Examination

- Aesthetic appearance
- Functional consequences
- Symptoms such as itching, discomfort, tightness or dryness
- The need for further treatment
- The overall degree of disability
- Rehabilitation needs
- Psychological assessment

- Texture, contour, colour, hair growth
- Sensation, sweating and areas of breakdown
- Comment on any grafts, flaps, donor sites or scars

Gunshot wounds

Gunshot wounds are occurring with increasing frequency in the UK. There is a trend in modern warfare to cause maiming rather than death. The type and severity of injury are dependent on the type and velocity of the weapon used and the distance from which it was fired.

Injuries may be classified as high or low velocity. The higher the velocity of the missile, the greater the area of damage around the missile track. Low velocity injuries such as those caused by a pistol travel at a rate of less than 1100 feet per second, leading to a direct effect on tissues by laceration and crushing within the narrow confines of the missile track. High velocity injuries are caused by weapons such as rifles and cause more extensive injuries with more extensive tissue destruction beyond the missile tract. The entrance and exit wounds do not indicate the considerable damage that may have occurred to the deeper structures.

Reconstruction of gunshot wounds depends on the extent of the injury and the nature of the structures injured. Initial treatment consists of resuscitation, thorough wound lavage and debridement of devitalised tissues, reconstruction of vital structures and appropriate skin and soft tissue reconstruction. It must be noted that it is not necessary to remove all pellets from a shotgun injury.

Reporting on gunshot wounds incorporates all previous points on scars, grafts and flaps together with functional outcome and capacity to return to work. A recognised scoring system called PULHHEEMS or the Army Fitness Score (Ministry of Defence 1987) can be employed to aid assessment of functional outcome, although it is more useful within an army setting (Matthews 1994).

Nail Bed

The fingernails have a multiplicity of functions as well as contributing to the cosmesis of the hand. In addition to scratching, they protect the dorsal surface of the finger, allow tiny objects to be grasped, contribute to thermoregulation and enhance tactile sensitivity, by providing counter-support of the pulp.

Nail injuries: treatment

The most common nail/nail bed injury is in the long finger (Zook 1981). Nail injuries can be classified as simple or complex, i.e. with or without tissue loss or fractures (Magalon & Zalta 1991). Primary treatment provides the best opportunity for preventing late morbidity. Such treatment should be carried out following the principles of hand surgery, including the judicious use of a tourniquet, magnification, atraumatic technique, fine instruments and absorbable sutures for the nail bed. Nail bed lacerations should be meticulously repaired and subungual haematomas drained. The nail fold should be maintained and the nail plate should be adequately supported. Missing segments of the nail bed should be replaced with toe nail bed partial-thickness grafts or toe nail and bed microvascular transfers. Associated fractures of the distal phalanx are usually uncomplicated.

If the injury is severe or the treatment is inadequate, deformities of the nail plate such as splitting, and abnormal curvature such as claw nails, are common. The nail might lose adhesion to the bed and keratin cysts can occur. Painful nail spikes can be troublesome.

Nail injuries: reporting

- The condition of the nail plate
- The condition of the nail bed
- The condition of the nail bed support
- Adherence of the nail to the bed
- Any associated symptoms
- Aesthetic deformity
- Cold intolerance

■ Skin cover in the upper limb

A basic principle in reconstructive hand surgery is that lost skin should be replaced with tissue that most closely resembles it. Other factors that need to be taken into consideration in choosing appropriate skin cover in the upper limb include pliability, bulk, sensibility. aesthetic appearance, hair growth, interference with hand elevation and physiotherapy. General factors are the site and nature of the wound, donor site morbidity, the patient's condition, age and sex, smoking (Gilbert & Brockman 1991), the patient's wishes and the surgeon's technical ability.

As anywhere else in the body, the choice lies between grafts and flaps of different types, or even combinations, and varies with the site of the defect, i.e. dorsum of the hand, volar surface of the hand or other sites in the upper limb.

The aim should be to provide the best reconstruction (functional and aesthetic) with the least morbidity and in the shortest period of time.

Dorsum of the hand

The requirement is for thin and pliable skin to permit full flexion.

Dorsum of the hand: skin grafts

In suitable conditions SSGs should be obtained from distant sites such as the thigh (large area) or local sites such as the arm and volar forearm. The dorsal forearm should not be used, as the donor site is difficult to conceal. The disadvantage of a volar forearm donor site is the 60% incidence of hypopigmentation (Xavier & Lamb 1974).

Dorsum of the hand: flap cover

In the event that flap cover is indicated, thin supple skin can be obtained as local flaps in the case of small defects. Larger areas require distant flaps transferred with or without microsurgical anastomoses. The flap of choice is the radial forearm flap because it is thin and because its arc of rotation allows coverage of the entire dorsum without difficulty. Other flaps used include the free lateral arm flap or a posterior interosseous septocutaneous flap. Although they are relatively thin, the fasciocutaneous flaps described above can still be bulky. Transferring fascia as a flap and covering it with a SSG provides the thinnest reconstruction. Examples include a microsurgical fascial flap obtained from the lateral arm or from the scalp (temporoparietal fascia), or transferred conventionally from the volar forearm (radial forearm fascial flap) or the dorsal forearm (posterior interosseous flap).

Volar surface

The need is for thick glabrous skin which can resist contraction and continue to grow (in children). It is also important that the skin has sweat glands to enhance the friction needed in gripping.

Volar surface (palm): skin grafts

Healing by secondary intention may be acceptable for distal defects in the absence of other injuries, using the McCash (1964) open palm technique.

Although FTSGs are preferable in the palm, for larger areas of skin loss, SSGs may be used, at least initially. Several useful donor sites have been described. The most common is the groin, as abundant skin is available with an easily concealed scar. However, the colour match is often imperfect and the cosmetic result marred by hair growth. Small areas can be harvested from the hypothenar eminence (Schenk & Cheema 1984), the wrist crease, the volar forearm and so on. Thick SSGs can be obtained from the instep of the foot (Namba et al 1977) as plantar skin makes an ideal substitute for palmar skin. Donor site hypertrophy can occur in 25% of patients (Nakamura et al 1984).

Volar skin (palm): flaps

Durability, resistance to contraction, return of sensation and potential for growth are best provided by local flaps or regional flaps, from the dorsum of the proximal phalanges or, for larger areas, from distant sites such as the lateral arm, using microsurgical techniques or the radial forearm flap.

Volar skin (fingers and thumbs)

The choice between conservative treatment, skin grafts, flap cover or terminalisation is dependent on a variety of factors, such as the extent and severity of injury and the patient's needs.

SSGs are adequate in most instances. Local flaps have the major advantage of replacing like with like, and the practical benefit of being in the same anaesthetic field. Significant pulp losses in the thumb can be replaced using microvascular pulp transfer from the great toe (Buncke & Rose 1979). It is also important to maintain the first web space in order to achieve maximal hand function and a variety of flaps may be used for this including the posterior interosseous flap or the dorsal foot flap.

Arm

The requirements for skin cover are much less specialised than in the hand, and the principles applicable at other sites are applicable here, too. A number of local options are available, depending on the site and size of the defect, including the latissimus dorsi and scapular flaps which may be rotated on their vascular pedicle. The latissimus dorsi muscle flap may also be used as a functional transfer for the reconstruction of biceps or triceps.

Skin cover upper limb: reporting

Apart from the general details of the flap/graft (recipient and donor sites), additional information as given below should be recorded:

- Hand function
- Sensation
- Social hand usage
- Cosmesis
- Hand use for leisure and occupational activities
- Reflex sympathetic dystrophy
- Cold intolerance
- Return to employment—original or alternative profession
- Time for return to employment

■ References

Arnez Z M, Tyler M P H, Khan U 1999 Describing severe limb trauma. British Journal of Plastic Surgery 52: 280–285

Beausang E, Floyd H, Dunn K W, Orton C I, Ferguson M W J 1998 A new quantitative scale for clinical scar assessment. Plastic and Reconstructive Surgery 102: 1954–1961

Brent B 1978 The role of pressure therapy in management of ear lobe keloids: preliminary report of a controlled study. Annals of Plastic Surgery 1: 579

British Orthopaedic Association and British Association of Plastic Surgeons 1997 The Management of Open Tibial Fractures

Brown L A, Pierce H E 1986 Keloids: scar revision. Journal of Dermatology, Surgery and Oncology 12: 51–56

Bull J 1971 Revised analysis of mortality due to burns. Lancet ii: 1133–1134

Buncke H J, Rose E H 1979 Free toe-to-finger tip neurovascular flaps. Plastic and Reconstructive Surgery 63: 607–612

Byrd H S, Cierny G III, Tebetts J B 1981 The management of open tibial fractures with associated soft tissue loss: external pin fixation with early flap coverage. Plastic and Reconstructive Surgery 68: 73

Byrd H S, Spicer T E, Cierney G 1985 Management of open tibial fractures. Plastic and Reconstructive Surgery 76: 719

Chantarask N D, Milner R H 1989 A comparison of scar quality in wounds closed under tension with PGA (Dexon) and polydioxanone (PDS). British Journal of Plastic Surgery 42: 687–691

Crikelair G F 1960 Surgical approach to facial scarring. Journal of the Medical Association of America 172: 140

Darzi M A, Chowdri N A, Kaul S K, Khan M 1992 Evaluation of various methods of treating keloids and hypertrophic scars: a 10 year follow up study. British Journal of Plastic Surgery 45: 374–379

Elliot D, Mahaffey P J 1989 The stretched scar: the benefit of prolonged dermal support. British Journal of Plastic Surgery 42: 74–78

Engrav L H, Heimbach D M, Reus J L 1983 Early excision and grafting vs non-operative treatment of burns of indeterminant depth: a randomised prospective study. Journal of Trauma 23: 1001–1004

Flowers R 1970 Unexpected postoperative problems in skin grafting. Surgical Clinics of North America 50: 439

Francel T J 1992 Clinics in Plastic Surgery 19: 871–879

Francel T J, Vander Kolk C A, Hoopes J E, Manson P N, Yaremchuk M J 1992 Microvascular soft-tissue transplantation for reconstruction of acute open tibial fractures: timing of coverage and long-term functional results. Plastic and Reconstructive Surgery 89: 478–487

Gilbert A, Brockman R 1991 Flap coverage for the upper extremity. In: Meyer V E, Black M J M (eds) Microsurgical procedures. Hand and upper limb series. Churchill Livingstone, Edinburgh, pp 132–150

Godina M 1986 Early microsurgical reconstruction of complex trauma of the extremities. Plastic and Reconstructive Surgery 78: 285

Grabb W C 1967 Keloid and hypertrophic scars. University of Michigan Medical Journal 33: 38

Gustilo R B, Mendoza R M, William D N 1984 Problems in the management of type III (severe) open fractures: a new classification of type III open fractures. Journal of Trauma 24: 742

Heimbach D, Engrav L, Grube B, Marvin J 1992 Burn depth: a review. World Journal of Surgery 16: 10–15

Hodges P L 1986 Principles of flaps. Selected Readings in Plastic Surgery 4(3): 1–19

Ketchum L D, Cohen I K, Masters F W 1974 Hypertrophic scars and keloids: a collective review. Plastic and Reconstructive Surgery 53: 140

Kisher C W, Shetlar M R, Shetlar C L 1975 Alteration of hypertrophic scars induced by mechanical pressure. Archives of Dermatology 111: 60

Larson D L, Abston S, Willis B 1974 Contracture and scar formation in the burn patient. Clinics in Plastic Surgery 1: 653

Magalon G, Zalta R 1991 Primary and secondary care of nail injuries. In: Foucher G (ed.) Fingertip and nail bed injuries. Hand

and upper limb series. Churchill Livingstone, Edinburgh, pp 103–113

Matthews S J E 1994 Missile and gunshot wounds. In: Outcome measures in Trauma. Butterworth-Heinemann Ltd

McCash C R 1964 The open palm technique in Dupuytren's contracture. British Journal of Plastic Surgery 17: 271–280

McGregor I A, Morgan G 1963 Axial and random pattern flaps. British Journal of Plastic Surgery 26: 202

Monafo W W, Bessey P Q 1992 Benefits and limitations of burn wound excision. World Journal of Surgery 16: 37–42

Nakamura K, Namba K, Tsuchida H 1984 A retrospective study of thick split thickness plantar skin grafts to resurface the palm. Annals of Plastic Surgery 12: 508

Namba K, Tsuchida H, Nakamura K 1977 Split-skin grafts from the hairless area for resurfacing of palmar surface of the hand. Japan Journal of Plastic and Reconstructive Surgery 20: 584

Niessen F B, Spauwen P H, Schalkwijk J, Kon M 1999 On the nature of hypertrophic scars and keloids: a review. Plastic and Reconstructive Surgery 104(5): 1435–1458

Ninkovic M, Mooney E K, Ninkovic M, Kleistil T, Anderl H 1999 A new classification for the standardization of nomenclature in free flap wound closure. Plastic and Reconstructive Surgery 103(3): 903–917

Parsons R W 1977 Scar prognosis. Clinics in Plastic Surgery 4: 181

Peacock E E, Madden J W, Trier W C 1970 Biologic basis for the treatment of keloids and hypertrophic scars. Southern Medical Journal 63: 775

Ponten B 1981 The fasciocutaneous flap: its use in soft tissue defects in the lower leg. British Journal of Plastic Surgery 34: 215

Purdue G F, Hunt J L, Layton T R 1985 Burns in motor vehicle accidents. Journal of Trauma 25: 216–219

Purdue G F, Hunt J L, Lang E D 1990 Obesity: a risk factor in the burn patient. Journal of Burn Care and Rehabilitation 11: 32–34

Quinn K J 1987 Silicone gel in scar treatment. Burns 13: 33–37

Rautio J 1991 Resurfacing and sensory recovery of the sole. Clinics in Plastic Surgery 18: 615–626

Rohrich R J, Spicer T E 1986 Wound healing/hypertrophic and keloid scars: an overview. Selected Readings in Plastic Surgery 4: 11–24

Russell W L, Sailors D M, Whittle T B, Fisher D F Jr, Burns R P 1991 Limb salvage versus traumatic amputation: a decision based on a seven part predictive index. Annals of Surgery 213: 473–480

Saltz R, Hochberg J, Given K S 1991 Muscle and musculocutaneous flaps of the foot. Clinics in Plastic Surgery 18: 627–638

Schenk R R, Cheema T A 1984 Hypothenar skin grafts for fingertip reconstruction. Journal of Hand Surgery 8: 49

Sommerlad B C, Creasey J M 1978 The stretched scar: a clinical and histological study. British Journal of Plastic Surgery 31: 34

Spann K, Mileski W J, Atiles L, Purdue G, Hunt J 1996 The 1996 Clinical Research award. Use of a pneumatonometer in burn scar assessment. Journal of Burn Care Rehabilitation 17: 515–517

Tang Y W 1992 Intra- and post-operative steroid injections for keloid and hypertrophic scars. British Journal of Plastic Surgery 45: 371–373

Walton R L, Rothkopf D M 1991 Judgement and approach for management of severe lower extremity injuries. Clinics in Plastic Surgery 18: 525–540

Warden G D 1987 Outpatient care of thermal injuries. Surgical Clinics of North America 67: 147

Xavier T S, Lamb D W 1974 The forearm as donor site for split skin grafts. Hand 6: 243

Yaremchuk M J, Brumback R J, Manson P N 1987 Acute and definitive management of traumatic osteocutaneous defects of the lower extremity. Plastic and Reconstructive Surgery 80: 1–12

Zawacki B E, Azen S P, Imbus S H, Chang Y C 1979 Annals of Surgery 189: 1–5

Zook E G 1981 The perionychium: anatomy, physiology and care of injuries. Clinics in Plastic Surgery 8: 21–31

Peripheral nerve injuries

Grey E. B. Giddins and Rolfe Birch

■ Introduction

This chapter addresses the outcomes of peripheral nerve injuries and in particular the factors affecting their outcome. It highlights the areas of uncertainty such as over timing of surgery. It also addresses some of the medical negligence issues surrounding nerve injuries.

Classification

Two systems are in common use. The first, which describes physiological abnormality in nerve function, was introduced by Seddon in 1942 and is as follows:

■ *Neurapraxia*   There is a block to conduction of nerve impulses without disruption of the axon or its supporting cells. Wallerian degeneration does not occur. Fibrillation potentials are not seen in muscles, and the nerve trunk continues to conduct distal to the lesion. A common example is seen in operations using a tourniquet. If a nerve trunk, exposed in the course of an operation with a suprasystolic cuff in place, is stimulated, a failure of muscular response is seen at about 30 minutes. Release of the tourniquet is rapidly followed by normal muscular response. Other examples include compression or displacement of nerve trunks in fractures or dislocations. The prognosis is good *if the cause is removed*. In neurapraxia some preservation of nerve modalities is found. The largest fibres, A alpha to the skeletal muscle and A beta to the cutaneous sensory receptors, are more vulnerable than the A delta and C fibres responsible for light touch, pain and sudo- and vasomotor function, which are narrower and either lightly or non-myelinated. Pressure sense, light touch and sympathetic function are characteristically preserved in neurapraxia. Electrical conduction is preserved. The distal nerve trunk does not degenerate.

■ *Axonotmesis*   The axon is damaged but the connective tissue sheaths of the endoneurial tube, perineurium and epineurium are intact. The axon undergoes Wallerian degeneration. Distal conduction is lost. From about 3 weeks spontaneous muscular activity is noted by detecting fibrillation potentials. The prognosis is, on the whole, good *if the cause is removed*. A common

example is the radial nerve palsy following fracture of the humerus which recovers at the appropriate rate (1 mm per day) to a normal or near normal level. Nonetheless incomplete recovery frequently occurs not least due to end organ failure (q.v.).

■ *Neurotmesis*   The nerve trunk is divided. There will be no recovery until the nerve is repaired. The clinical features are identical to axonotmesis. All function is lost. The most significant clinical sign in both neurotmesis and axonotmesis is *complete loss of sympathetic function, of sweating and of vasomotor control. The skin becomes red and dry.* Neurotmesis is the most likely diagnosis in open wounds and in high-energy fractures. It is also the most likely diagnosis when a nerve stops working after an operation in which the surgeon's knife has been in the field of that nerve. Differentiation between the two is possible only by awaiting events or by exploring the nerve.

Seddon's classification is useful but his terms are anachronistic. Sunderland (1978) has developed a classification based upon an anatomical idea of progressive disruption of the connective tissue sheath of a nerve. It is graded from 1 to 5: grade 1 is equivalent to neurapraxia, grade 2 to axonotmesis, and grades 3–5 represent differing degrees of neurotmesis. The classification does help in the difficult traction lesion, but the author has not found it particularly helpful in determining clinical action.

The failure of both these systems is their attempt to devise a classification linking clinical with underlying pathological changes, Seddon with conduction and Sunderland with disturbance of internal architecture. A simple distinction between degenerative and non-degenerative lesions seems better, and can be made by clinical examination:

■ *Non-degenerative*.   Conduction block (i.e. neurapraxia): it may be short-lasting or prolonged. Some modalities of sensation persist; nerve action potentials are detectable in the distal trunk; there is no spontaneous muscular activity (fibrillation potentials). This subject has been classified by Gilliatt (1980).

■ *Degenerative*.   Of favourable (axonotmesis) or unfavourable (neurotmesis) prognosis. All modalities are lost; there is no distal conduction; fibrillation potentials appear at about 3 weeks.

The lesion may be mixed, notably in partial transection of nerve. It is safest to assume that all of the lesion is of the worst type present.

Grading of results

The Nerve Injuries Committee of the Medical Research Council introduced the system of grading in 1954 (modified in 1975) as shown in Table 25.1.

This system is inadequate to measure the return of muscle *endurance*. Recovery of muscles such as the dorsi flexors of the ankle to less than M4 is of little functional worth. The system is particularly deficient in the assessment of hand function, this weakness being only partially diminished by the use of Moberg's pick-up test (1958) or scrupulous measurement of the return of two-point discrimination. The hand function assessment charts developed by Wynn Parry & Salter (1976) are particularly good, for they record accuracy of localisation and ability to recognise, and discriminate between different objects and textures; they also give an indication of the overall agility, co-ordination and stamina of the hand. Some examples are shown in Figs 25.1. and 25.2. These are primarily of use in research rather than daily clinical practice.

The MRC system is of least use in describing the outcome of obstetric and adult brachial plexus injuries.

Most of the papers reviewed for this chapter used the MRC system. There seems to be general agreement to group results into three categories of good, fair and poor, as shown in Table 25.2.

Table 25.2 Grading of results used for this chapter

Motor		Sensory
M0		S0
M1	Poor	S1
M2		S2
M3	Fair	S3
M4		S3+
M5	Good	S4

General factors governing prognosis

The factors governing outcome are mainly without the control of the surgeon. The first three are of the greatest importance and in the following order.

Age

There seems to be little doubt that prospects of recovery after repair of a nerve trunk are very much better in children than in adults. This was clearly demonstrated by McEwan (1962) in reviewing the work from Melbourne. Her conclusion was confirmed by Seddon's analysis of his own extremely large series (Table 25.3). We should now introduce a warning note. It is quite wrong to assume that the natural prognosis for nerve injuries in children is always good. Upper limb length discrepancy in the child born with severe obstetric lesion of the brachial plexus is

Table 25.1 The MRC system as widely used

	Motor		Sensory
M0	Paralysis	S0	None
M1	Flicker	S1	Deep pain sensation
M2	Movement with gravity eliminated	S2	Skin touch, pain and thermal sensation ('protective')
M3	Movement against gravity	S3	Skin touch, pain, temperature sensation with accurate localisation: stereognosis deficient. Cold sensitivity and hypersensitivity are usual
M4	Movement against resistance	S3+	Object and texture recognition. Trivial cold sensitivity and hypersensitivity trivial, 2 P.D. <8 mm in hand
M5	Normal	S4	Indistinguishable from normal: 2 P.D. equal to uninjured part

ROYAL NATIONAL ORTHOPAEDIC HOSPITAL TRUST – OCC. THERAPY DEPT.

STERIOGNOSIS ASSESSMENT

NAME: RECORD NO.

<u>MAIN FUNCTIONAL DIFFICULTIES</u>   DOMINANT HAND

<u>WORK</u>

<u>DAILY ACTIVITIES</u>

<u>HOBBIES</u>

<u>STERIOGNOSIS</u>

DATE						
SHAPES (Test one section only)	Interpretation	Time	Interpretation	Time	Interpretation	Time
1. Square						
Oblong						
Triangle						
Diamond						
2. Circle						
Oval						
Semi-circle						
Moon						
AVERAGE TIME						
TEXTURE (Test 6 items)						
Sandpaper						
Formica						
Wood						
Rubber						
Carpet						
Leather						
Velvet						
Fur						
Cotton wool						
Sheepskin						
Plastic						
Metal						
AVERAGE TIME						

Fig. 25.1 An occupational therapy sensory assessment form (continued on page 454)

DATE						
COINS (Test 3 items)	Interpretation	Time	Interpretation	Time	Interpretation	Time
2p						
5p						
10p						
20p						
50p						
£1						
AVERAGE TIME						
OBJECTS – LARGE						
1. Sink plug)						
Cotton reel)						
Plug)						
Bottle) Test 3						
Saucer) items						
Soap)						
Egg cup)						
Tea strainer)						
2. Pencil)						
Fork)						
Metal comb)						
Ball point pen)						
Screwdriver) Test 3						
Teaspoon) items						
Toothbrush)						
Paint brush)						
Peg)						
AVERAGE TIME						
OBJECTS – SMALL						
1. Safety pin						
Paper clip						
Nail						
Screw						
2. Nut						
Rubber						
Thimble						
Screw hook						
Button hook						
Yale key						
Ball of wool						
Ball of string						
AVERAGE TIME						
LOCALISATION SCORE						
PROTECTIVE SENSATION						
COMMENTS						

Fig. 25.1 continued

ROYAL NATIONAL ORTHOPAEDIC HOSPITAL TRUST – OCC. THERAPY DEPT.

LOCALISATION CHART – RIGHT HAND

NAME: RECORD NO:

NAME:		
SCORE		

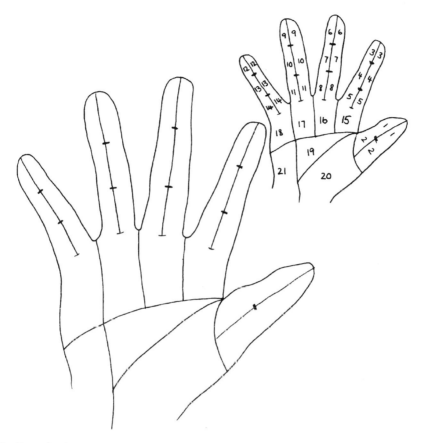

Fig. 25.2 A localisation chart.

Table 25.3 Age and results for median and ulnar: 584 cases at all levels (from Seddon 1975)				
Age	Number of cases	Good	Fair	Poor
		%	%	%
0–10	35	71	29	–
11–15	47	57.6	32	10.4
16–20	106	33	46	21
Over 21	396	~25	~55	~20

as much as 20% and the growth of the hand is even more impaired. A high injury of the sciatic nerve in infancy or in childhood will lead, if repair is unsuccessful, to profound disturbance of development, with shortening and progressive skeletal deformity.

As a rule, the results of nerve repair deteriorate progressively with age. Results are significantly worse for repair of median and ulnar nerves in patients who are over the age of 50 years, decisively so after injuries of the brachial plexus or proximal injuries of the sciatic nerve.

The nature of injury

The amount of destruction of the nerve is least after a clean cut with a knife; it is greater after a closed traction injury and may be so extensive as to be irreparable, as in irradiation neuritis, after injection injury or in burns. This is shown by comparing the outcome of median and ulnar nerve repairs at the wrist in war wounds with those from civilian practice (Table 25.4). Omer (1974) followed a large number of gunshot wounds to nerves. The results were generally poor: they were substantially worse in high-velocity missile injuries or when the wound was above the elbow. He noted some return of function in only 40% of the 67 of his patients with adequate follow-up.

The level of injury

In general, the more proximal the lesion, the worse the prognosis. The MRC Special Report (1954) described the outcome in 290 repairs of the median nerve wounded in war. Useful recovery occurred in 40% of nerves injured from the level of the mid-forearm distally. This fell to about 35% when the nerve was injured from the mid-arm to the mid-forearm, and to 20% in those injured more proximally. This is confirmed in Cooney's 1991 review of five series setting out results of repair of the proximal median nerve. The outlook is even worse after injuries of the brachial plexus. Useful hand function is rarely regained after even the most extensive repair performed within days of injury. Birch et al (1988) reported on 48 cases of reconstruction of the brachial plexus using the free vascularised ulnar nerve graft. The lateral cord or the median nerve was re-innervated in all cases. Recovery into the long flexor muscles to M3 and sensation within the median territory of the hand to S2 was found in 13 cases. Gilbert (1993) analysed the results of 31 of his cases

of obstetric brachial plexus palsy in which the lower trunk had been re-innervated by nerve graft or by nerve transfer. Some recovery into the intrinsic muscles was noted in 16 (51%). These are admirable results, but in no case was normal hand function regained.

The importance of the level of lesion is emphasised by study of the results of repair of the sciatic nerve at the hip. Seddon found no case of recovery into the intrinsic muscles of the foot in his large series.

The nerves

It is often said that mixed nerve trunks do worse, but in fact the consequences of injury to a nerve of cutaneous sensation may be particularly severe. Pain (Chronic regional pain syndrome type II—CRPS II) after injury to the medial cutaneous nerve of the forearm, the superficial radial, ulnar or sural nerves, may be wholly disproportionate and may greatly disturb function. The outlook for certain nerves, in particular the predominantly motor nerves, is potentially good if they are repaired promptly and skilfully. The accessory, musculo-cutaneous, posterior interosseous, deep palmar division of the ulnar and the motor recurrent branch of the median nerves are examples. Of course, these are mixed nerves, containing a high proportion of afferent fibres, and one of the possible reasons for the quality of results is the short distance to the receptor organs.

The length of injured nerve

If a large segment of nerve has been injured or there has been a delay leading to nerve retraction preventing primary repair then the results of surgery will be less good as the results of nerve grafting are less good (Merle et al 1986).

Table 25.4 Age, cause and results in repairs of median and ulnar nerves at wrist (modified from Seddon 1975)

Series		Motor		Sensory	
Zachary (1954), 300 cases, war		Median M3+ or better	40%	Median S3 or better	11%
		Ulnar M4	16%	Ulnar S3 or better	38%
Nicholson & Seddon (1957),110 cases, civil – includes children		Median M3+ or better	65%	Median S3 or better	24.6%
		Ulnar M4	35%	Ulnar S3 or better	68.5%
McEwan (1962), 48 children, 37 adults, civil	Children	Median M3+ or better	60%	Median S3 or better	93%
		Ulnar M4	71%	Ulnar S3 or better	100%
	Adults	Median M3+ or better	60%	Median S3 or better	67%
		Ulnar M4	23%	Ulnar S3 or better	84%

Associated injury: vascular lesion

The long-term function of the limb depends on its innervation, but if blood supply is not restored there will be no limb at all or it will be so impaired by postischaemic fibrosis that nerve regeneration will be valueless.

Seddon strongly favoured primary repair of digital nerves, because the injury to the adjoining digital artery led to extensive scarring within the distal stump prejudicing delayed repair. LeClercq et al (1985) reported on 64 cases of injury to the ulnar nerve and artery. They gained worthwhile results in 73% of cases when the artery was repaired: this fell to only 22% when the ulnar artery was ligated or the repair had thrombosed. Barros d'Sa (1992) sets out the modern approach to vascular injury.

Factors governing prognosis within the control of the surgeon

Technical

Although most experienced surgeons believe that the skill of the surgeon influences the outcome this is as yet unproven. Nonetheless surgeons should be guided by the widely accepted principles of careful surgery, performed by an experienced surgeon, using adequate magnification (loupes/microscope) and ensuring skeletal stability, adequate vascularity and a healthy bed for nerve revascularisation and gliding. It is also assumed that careful and appropriate after-care has been ensured by the surgeon. Common causes of failure following repair of a nerve include neglecting to deal with an injury to the vessels, failure to restore gliding planes, so that the repaired nerve becomes adherent to an adjacent scar or tendon, failure to decompress the distal compartments, including the carpal tunnel, and failure closely to supervise the splinting, physiotherapy and rehabilitation.

If in doubt a surgeon should provide primary wound care and skeletal support (assuming a viable limb) and refer immediately to a centre experienced in nerve repair.

Delay

In general terms the longer the delay before repair is undertaken, the worse the prognosis. This lesson was unequivocally demonstrated by the MRC series and also by the very large American experience of Woodhall & Beebe (1956). Zachary (1954) introduced the term 'critical delay', an interval of time after which nerve repair is a waste of time. Woodhall & Beebe (1956) went further, demonstrating that the decline in results was progressive with increased delay from injury to repair. O'Brien (1975), a pioneer of microsurgical and replantation surgery, demonstrated the superiority of results when nerves were repaired at the time of replantation of the limb against those where a later repair was effected. Merle and his colleagues in Nancy have acquired very extensive experience of the injured hand. In their analysis of 150 repairs of median and ulnar nerves, results following primary repair were decisively better than in later cases (Merle et al 1986). LeClercq et al (1985), from Liège, reported similar findings. Birch & Raji (1991) described results of 108 median and ulnar nerve repairs. There were no failures among the 48 primary sutures; five of the 25 delayed sutures failed, while seven of the 35 delayed grafts failed.

There are three reasons for the poorer results with delay:

- There is progressive deterioration within the distal nerve trunk, the target organs and the skin, changes which become irreversible and ultimately present a wholly unfavourable field for regenerating axons.
- There are progressive and ultimately irreversible changes within the central nervous system, with loss of parent motor neurones and changes within the receptor fields of sensory neurons.
- The secondary changes of wasting, atrophy and deformity lead to such common fixed contractures as equinus at the ankle, extension deformity of metacarpophalangeal joints and internal rotation contracture at the shoulder.

Modern teaching holds that nerve repair should be undertaken promptly and ideally within 5–7 days and certainly a maximum of 10 days. Nonetheless a review of the literature does not completely support this. Experimental studies in animals have compared immediate with delayed repair. The results are not clearcut: in a rat model immediate sciatic nerve repair resulted in a greater myelin content than repair at 3 weeks (Bora et al 1976). An electrophysiological assessment of a primate model showed better results in immediate versus delayed repair at 3 weeks (Grabb 1968).

Other studies have supported delayed nerve repair. The synthetic machinery of the neurons does not function for the first week following injury. Over the next 2 weeks there is reactivation with a doubling of protein content and activity. Thus some authors have recommended nerve repair at 2–3 weeks to take advantage of the up-regulated neurons (Seddon 1975). Experiments 'conditioning' nerves 2 days to 2 weeks prior to a second lesion have shown increased rates of axon growth from the proximal nerve stumps (Brisby & Keen 1985, Lundborg et al 1990). In summary, although it is believed that nerve repair ought to be undertaken within 7–10 days of injury assuming a clean wound and fit patient, this is not necessarily supported by the literature and a repair up to 3 weeks post injury could be considered as acceptable, not least in terms of medical negligence.

Another important question is: what is the maximum delay after which nerve surgery is likely to be futile? Again the literature is not clearcut: axons in the proximal stump can regenerate for at least 1 year following injury (Holmes & Young 1942). Nonetheless, the quality and quantity of the regeneration deteriorates substantially with time. Furthermore, denervated human muscle shows changes as early as 6 weeks, with markedly abnormal motor end plates by 1 year. These changes do not appear to be irreversible until 3 years, and denervated human muscle has been found to be functional even after 1 year (Sunderland 1978). Again the literature is unclear but it appears that repair after 1 year is unlikely to give worthwhile motor or sensory function. Moreover, if there is a long distance from the repair site to the end-organ then repair beyond 6 months may be of little value. These trends are even more marked in patients aged over 50.

Summary

The importance of these different factors is emphasised by Frykman & Gramyk (1991), who collected 553 grafts of upper limb nerves from 18 published series. Ninety percent of digital nerve grafts achieved S3 (fair), 80% of median grafts reached M3, while 78% achieved S3. In the ulnar nerve grafts, 65% reached M3 and 78% achieved S3. They found that age was important, particularly for recovery of sensation after repair of digital and of median nerves and in the return of power for grafts of radial nerves. The length of the grafts and increase in delay were deleterious for recovery of sensation; the level of the lesion was particularly important for motor recovery.

Some specific nerve injuries
The spinal accessory nerve

The spinal accessory nerve is at risk from operations of biopsy of lymph nodes in the posterior triangle of the neck. Paralysis of the trapezius muscle is very troubling, not least as most patients experience severe pain. There is severe impairment of function at the shoulder, as well as impairment of the use of the upper limb as a whole. The characteristic features have been described by Williams et al (1996): pain, drooping of the shoulder, loss of abduction luging of the scapular and facial/ear numbness if there is associated transverse cervical, or greater auricular nerve injury. The natural history is extremely poor, and spontaneous recovery is rare. Of Valtonen & Lilius's patients (1974), 11 were unable to return to any form of work. The result of repair performed within 3 months of injury is good. Useful recovery followed repair of the nerve in seven of eight cases performed at the peripheral nerve injury unit at Stanmore, within 3 months from injury (Birch et al 1991). All repairs carried out after an interval of 1 year failed (see Table 25.5).

Gabel & Nunley (1991) reviewed the subject, pointing out that the incidence of spinal accessory nerves injured in biopsy and excision of cervical lymph nodes was between 3 and 10% in series from the first part of last century, and they go on to suggest that the incidence of such iatrogenic disasters is decreasing. Unfortunately, accidental section of the accessory nerve continues to occur. Delay in diagnosis is the rule.

Severe pain after injury to the accessory nerve is striking, and there are two possible explanations. The first is that the upper limb is no longer supported; the second, that there is a secondary traction upon the brachial plexus. If the scapula is supported by a fascial sling or by transfer of levator scapulae and rhomboids, there may be some improvement in overall function but the pain persists,

Table 25.5 Spinal accessory nerve injuries

Author(s)	Number of cases	Cause	Number of repairs
Valtonen & Lilius (1974)	14	All iatrogenic	None
Norden (1946)	16	15 iatrogenic	3
Gordon et al (1977)	21	All iatrogenic	4
Osgaard et al (1987)	5	All iatrogenic	5
Seddon (1975)	14	8 iatrogenic	1
Birch (1992)	22	17 iatrogenic	15

suggesting that the injury to the nerve itself is a potent cause of pain.

The preferred treatment is prompt repair of the nerve. Grafting appears always to be necessary: a good result is expected if the operation is performed within 3 months of injury.

The long thoracic nerve

Paralysis of serratus anterior leads to loss of control of the scapula, and disturbance of thoraco-scapula movement. There is secondary interference with glenohumeral movement. Deep, dull aching pain is common.

The nerve is most commonly injured in severe traction lesions of the brachial plexus. The next most common cause is iatrogenic, notably following the transaxillary approach to the first rib or the sympathetic chain, and in operations for axillary clearance. Ellis (1985) emphasised the importance of displaying the nerve and protecting it during operations by the transaxillary route. The long thoracic nerve is rarely injured in stab wounds to the neck.

The results of surgery are not reported but anecdotal evidence suggests some motor recovery and good pain relief following repair. Reconstruction options include intercoastal nerve transfer if primary repair is impossible, or transfer of pectoralis major or minor to the lower pole of the scapula. This may give some improved control of the scapula and some pain relief.

The axillary (circumflex) nerve

Complete paralysis of the deltoid muscle leads to substantial loss of power at the shoulder, estimated at about 50% in abduction and 30% in extension and flexion. Petrucci et al (1982) reported on 21 cases treated by neurolysis or nerve grafting and they noted a severe loss of function in the upper limb as a whole. Nonetheless, some patients with an isolated injury to the axillary nerve retain a near normal range of movement at the shoulder. Associated injury to the suprascapular nerve or to the rotator cuff is not uncommon, and must be excluded in patients presenting with axillary nerve palsy who are unable to initiate abduction and external rotation.

The most common causes include the following:

- traction lesions of the brachial plexus
- fracture dislocation at the shoulder
- open wounds, including iatrogenic injuries

The prognosis for spontaneous recovery after traction lesions and open wounds is unfavourable. Recovery after closed fracture or dislocation at the shoulder is more difficult. The best review of the natural history of axillary nerve palsy is that of Watson Jones (1936), who followed 15 cases. Thirteen went on to full recovery and in all but one this was noted at 7 months from the original injury. The deltoid remained paralysed in two cases. Leffert & Seddon (1965), in their study of infraclavicular lesions of the brachial plexus, found spontaneous recovery in only one of six of their cases of circumflex palsy. Blom & Dahlback (1970) studied 73 patients who had suffered shoulder fractures or dislocations. The clinical study was supplemented with electromyography and they found nine cases of complete paralysis and 15 of partial denervation of the deltoid. All of these patients made a full spontaneous recovery. There are a few reports of results of grafts to the axillary nerve; these are set out in Table 25.6.

The wise surgeon examines the deltoid function and the sensory distribution of the nerve in the 'Regimental badge' distribution before attempting reduction, and makes a written note of his observations. It is too commonly assumed that axillary nerve dysfunction following a shoulder injury is a 'neurapraxia'; that is, a non-degenerative lesion with anticipated full recovery. If substantial recovery has not occurred by 6 weeks urgent investigation with EMG studies or referral should be undertaken with a view to rapid exploration of the nerve at the latest by 3 months post injury. This is confirmed by Barnard et al (1997) in their report on 146 cases. It is important, however, to exclude a rotator cuff lesion as the cause of the shoulder dysfunction. Following a high-energy dislocation or fracture dislocation the chances of a severe nerve injury are substantially higher and urgent nerve exploration should be considered. The nerve is invariably

Table 25.6 Results of grafts to the axillary nerve

	Number of repairs	Recovery to M4 or better
Millesi (1980)	5	4
Petrucci et al (1982)	8	7
Friedman et al (1990)	3	3
Birch (1992)	22	13

injured at the entrance to the quadrilateral space. A 'neuroma in continuity' may be found but, as Friedman et al (1990) showed, this indicates such internal disruption of the architecture of the nerve that spontaneous recovery will not occur. Grafting is always necessary and a good result should be expected in over 80% of cases

The radial nerve

The radial nerve palsy is probably the most common of nerve injuries encountered by the orthopaedic surgeon. The literature on the subject is extensive and confusing. There arc three main types of injury:

1. Open wounds including missile injuries or open fractures and iatrogenic injuries. The nerve is severed in over 80% of these and should be repaired if possible. Strachan & Ellis (1971) described an exposure to minimise injury to the posterior interosseous nerve.
2. Extensive injuries to the infraclavicular brachial plexus. These are high-energy injuries, multiple nerve ruptures are found, and the axillary artery is ruptured in 46% of cases (Cavanagh et al 1986). Repair of the radial nerve is of secondary importance to salvaging the limb.
3. Closed fractures of the humerus. Seddon reported 210 cases of radial nerve injury, 74 of these following simple closed fractures of the shaft of the humerus. Just over 70% of these went on to spontaneous recovery. In his monograph of 1975, Seddon referred to the experience of Bohler in Austria. Radial nerve palsy was found in 57 of Bohler's patients after 765 fractures of the humerus, an incidence of 7.4%; 47 (82.5%) of these palsies went on to full spontaneous recovery.

An expectant approach is justified in simple low-energy fractures of the shaft of the humerus *with reasonable apposition of the bone fragments after reduction*. The argument for exploration is stronger where the fracture cannot be reduced, in high-energy injuries, in oblique fractures of the lower part of the humerus or when there is associated dislocation of the shoulder or elbow. If the surgeon deems that the fracture, on its own merits, demands internal fixation, then the nerve should be exposed.

Results of the larger series of radial nerve repair are set out in Table 25.7.

Most of these cases were casulties of the Second World War. It is reasonable to suggest that a properly executed early repair of a clean laceration of the radial nerve will be followed by a good outcome (M4 or better) in about 80% of cases. Results are better for more distal injuries, particularly for posterior interosseous nerves.

The outcome of injury of the superficial sensory branches of the radial nerve is not known. Spontaneous recovery following lacerations does not seem to occur as would be expected. The loss of sensation does not appear to be important but significant pain may occur from the neuroma. It is felt that primary repair may reduce the incidence of symptomatic neuromata but this is not proven. The outcome of repair of the superficial sensory branches of the radial nerve is not known.

Musculo-cutaneous nerve

Common causes of injury to this nerve include:

- rupture in traction lesion of the infraclavicular brachial plexus
- lacerations, including iatrogenic

Results of repair are excellent. Seddon found recovery to at least M4 in eight of nine of his repairs. Osborne et al reported 57 good results in 85 repairs: 12 of 13 clean open wounds gave good results as against 30 of 48 closed traction lesions. Results were better for repair in under 14 days and with grafts under 12 cm.

Median and ulnar nerves

The important work of the Special Committee of the Medical Research Council in this country (1954) and its equivalent in the USA (Woodhall & Beebe 1956) has already been referred to. This established the importance of the type of injury, the level of injury, the age of the

Table 25.7 Results of radial nerve repair		
Author(s)	**Number of cases**	**Recovery to M4 or better (%)**
Seddon (1975), civilian	67	54
Seddon (1954), military (in Medical Research Council 1954)	114	36.9
Woodhall & Beebe (1956), military	197	21.3
Mayer & Mayfield (1947), civilian	39	72

patient and the delay from injury to repair. The results were not good. In a study of 300 military cases of median nerve injury, Zachary (1954) found useful recovery in approximately one-third of cases. In their series of 110 cases of median and ulnar nerve injuries, Nicholson & Seddon (1957) achieved useful recovery in about 50%, and rather less than this for median sensation. Two important contributions were made about this time. Brooks (1955) reported on 33 cases of repair by graft of the median nerve in adults. The gap was at least 7 cm in all of these cases and he achieved at least M3, S3 (at least fair) in two-thirds of his cases. McEwan (1962) reported on the work of the Melbourne School of Plastic Surgery headed by Rank and Wakefield. She described the results after primary repair from the median and ulnar nerves in 37 adults and 48 children. Results for the children were extremely good. Fair or good results were obtained in 60% of the nerve repairs in adults, with the exception of motor recovery for the ulnar nerve, which was surprisingly poor at about one-third.

The fundamental contributions of these pioneers established in particular:

■ There has been a greater appreciation of the importance of the handling of soft tissues, of good skin cover, and of repair of adjacent arteries.

■ There has been a greater understanding of the harm of tension or of disturbance of local circulation on a nerve repair, as a result also of the work associated with Millesi.

The case for primary repair, advanced by Rank et al (1973), was strengthened by experience with replantation when O'Brien (1975) showed, decisively, that the nerve trunks should be repaired at the time of replantation. Merle et al (1986) reported on 150 cases of repair of median and ulnar nerves, obtaining very good results for primary sutures. They recommended that the radial or ulnar arteries always be repaired, and this was emphasised by LeClercq et al (1985), who demonstrated that results after primary repair of the ulnar nerve were very much better when the adjacent artery was successfully repaired. Birch & Raji (1991) reviewed the results of 108 median and ulnar nerve repairs in adults injured between the elbow and the wrist. These were clean wounds: they excluded such injuries as burns, open fractures and iatrogenic lesions. The wounds in the primary repair group were more severe than in the delayed groups, with a much higher incidence of injury to the radial or ulnar arteries and to muscles or tendons. Assessment was detailed, and included review by an occupational therapist and neurophysiological investigations. Results from primary repair were plainly better than those in the delayed group (see Table 25.8).

Millesi has refined techniques of nerve grafting and his own results are particularly impressive, achieving 80% of fair or good for median motor function and 100% fair or good for median sensory function (see Millesi et al 1972, 1976). Frykman & Gramyk (1991) have collected over 200 cases of grafts of median and ulnar nerves from 10 series published after 1972. They selected papers which gave descriptions of individual patients and separate analysis of the outcome for motor and sensory function with adequate records for age, the length of graft and the interval from injury to repair (see Table 25.9).

To sum up, a skilful graft of the median nerve can be expected to achieve a fair or good result in nearly 80% of cases, and slightly less for the ulnar nerve. Frykman & Gramyk stated that 'as with direct nerve repairs the results of nerve grafting deteriorate with increasing age, gap, delay and high levels of injury. The most important effect on nerve recovery after grafting is age, closely followed in importance by gap length, level of injury, and delay. However, the effect of gap and delay were much greater in the sensory than motor recovery, and level of

Table 25.8 Results of 108 nerve repairs in 95 patients (from Birch & Raji 1991)

Grade	Nerve	Primary	Delayed	Graft
Good	Median	19	5	4
	Ulnar	20	2	7
Fair	Median	7	8	8
	Ulnar	2	5	9
Poor	Median	0	2	2
	Ulnar	0	5	

Table 25.9 Results of grafts of median and ulnar nerve (from Frykman & Gramyk 1991)

Median	M5	M4	M3	Ulnar	M5	M4	M3
Motor, 100 cases	30	38	12	Motor, 93 cases	12	26	23
Median	S4	S3+	S3	Ulnar	S4	S3+	S3
Sensory, 104 cases	13	31	37	Sensory, 98 cases	13	20	43
Median Motor: 80% fair or good				Ulnar Motor: 65% fair or good			
Sensory: 78% fair or good				Sensory: 78% fair or good			

injury had a greater effect on motor than sensory recovery'. It should be emphasised that of all of these factors, only one—delay—is within the control of the surgeon, always assuming adequate skill and facilities.

The digital nerves

It is widely assumed that results for repair of digital sensory nerves are good, but closer scrutiny of more detailed series rather dampens this optimism. Seddon strongly favoured primary repair of digital nerves, recognising the importance of injury to the adjacent artery. Tupper et al (1988) closely reviewed 109 cases, and found that 35% of their adults achieved S4, and 48% S3+; no less than 83% of these could be classed as good. However, they found that *no* patient regained normal sensation. Goldie et al (1992) reviewed the results of 30 digital nerve repairs. Normal two-point discrimination was regained in 37% of fingers, but only 27% of patients graded their overall result as excellent and none felt that the finger had regained normal sensation, while 40% complained of persistent hyperaesthesia for up to 2 years.

Steinberg & Koman (1991) collected results from 366 adults and 35 children drawn from seven reported series. Twenty-five percent of adults regained S4, compared with 58% in the children; 48% of adults achieved S3+, compared with 40% of children.

Nerve injuries in the lower limb

Wood (1991) commented on the surprisingly little interest in these common injuries caused by open wounds, open fractures, dislocations and iatrogenic errors, and reflected on the absence of firm principles of management. An example of what is possible is the striking success following repair of an open wound of the lumbo-sacral plexus by Meyer (1987). In fact, the very large series reported by Clawson & Seddon (1960a,b) of results of repair of the sciatic nerve and of the long-term consequences of injury to that trunk do set out some very clear guidelines.

Sciatic nerve

Seddon discussed the sciatic nerve in terms of its two component divisions, the common peroneal and the tibial nerves; he encountered 345 injuries of the former and 229 injuries of the latter. There were 145 nerve repairs, most of these by secondary suture. The two major papers of 1960 were based on analysis of 119 nerve sutures and 13 grafts. All of the patients were adults, and the most common level of lesion was in the thigh.

Of 72 sutures of the common peroneal nerve, 34.7% achieved functional dorsi flexion of the ankle. Of 47 cases of suture of the tibial nerve, 79% regained functional plantar flexion of the foot. The tibialis posterior regained functional strength in one-third. There was no functional recovery in the long flexors of the toes, nor in the intrinsic muscles of the foot. Recovery of sensation ranging from S2–S4 was recorded in just under two-thirds of cases. Two types of fixed deformity were a problem, equinus of the heel and clawing of the toes (30%). Trophic ulcers occurred in 14% of patients. Pain or hypersensitivity of the sole of the foot was a significant problem in 50%. Seddon observed that the discrepancy between function and the neurological deficit was wider for the sciatic nerve than for almost any other. Some of his patients with complete sciatic palsy returned to a vigorous active normal life. Others with seemingly very minor deficits 'felt very sorry for themselves'.

Injuries to the sciatic nerve have particularly severe consequences in children. Failure of recovery for the sciatic nerve at the hip following, say, injection injury, leads to progressive shortening of the limb and, if there is partial recovery, to progressively severe deformity of the foot. Failure of recovery of the common peroneal nerve leads inexorably to an equino varus deformity, which may be prevented by timely transfer of part of the tibialis posterior tendon into the peroneus longus tendon. Failure of recovery of the tibial division leads to atrophy of the foot and the calcaneo valgus deformity, which may be mitigated by timely transfer of peroneus brevis to tibialis posterior.

Nerve injury in fractures and dislocations in the lower limb

Seddon found that less than one-half of his 57 cases of nerve injury after skeletal injury of the lower limb recovered to normal or near normal levels. He pointed out that nerves are at risk from rupture or entrapment after dislocation and that they were more at risk from transection in open fractures. He made one particularly important recommendation: *'Palsy of the sciatic nerve from closed fracture of the shaft of the femur is an indication for urgent exploration of the nerve.'*

The pelvis and hip

The lumbo-sacral plexus is at risk in more severe fracture dislocations of the pelvis. The diagnosis is evident from clinical examination, for sensory loss extends well beyond the territory of the sciatic nerve: the flexors of the hip and extensors of the knee are weak or paralysed and there may be sphincter dysfunction. The injury is a traction lesion and rupture within the spinal canal or avulsion of the spinal nerves from the cord is frequent. The sciatic nerve is at risk in fracture dislocations of the hip and is highest in posterior column fractures. In his review of 830 personal cases, Epstein (1980) identified 68 nerve injuries, an incidence of 8%. Good recovery occurred in 43% and a bad result in 32%. LeTournel & Judet (1981) noted 57 nerve injuries in 469 patients treated by operation, a pre-operative incidence of 12%, which rose to 17.4% in the posterior column group. Their work suggests that early reduction and fixation of the pelvis is helpful for the nerve; in 36 cases of nerve injury treated by early operation recovery was good in 21, but poor in 13. However, they noted the real risk to the sciatic nerve during operation: 30 of their cases developed sciatic nerve palsy after operation and recovery was bad in 13 of these. Meticulous care for the nerve, using femoral traction with flexion of the knee, reduced the incidence of intra-operative injuries from 18 to 9% in their series.

To conclude, it is important to distinguish on clinical examination between injury to the lumbar sacral plexus and the sciatic nerve. Displaced fracture–dislocations of the hip causing injury to the sciatic nerve demand urgent reduction. The nerve should be displayed, removing loose bony fragments which may compress or impale it. It must be acknowledged that there is a significant risk to the sciatic nerve in operations for open reductions and internal fixation, and the prognosis for the recovery of such lesions is not good.

The knee

There are two common patterns of injury to nerves at the knee. The popliteal artery is ruptured in about 3% of supracondylar fractures of the femur and in at least 30% of dislocations of the knee. The artery or its major branches are ruptured in about 10% of displaced fractures of the proximal tibia. Treatment of the vascular injury determines the outcome for the leg as well as for the nerve: the nerve lesion is usually secondary to compression and ischaemia. DeBakey and Simeone (1955) reported 364 amputations in 502 legs after ligation of the popliteal artery. When a policy of repair of the vessel was introduced in the Korean and Vietnam wars, the amputation rate dropped from 73% to 32% (Rich et al 1969). The reader is referred to the important work of Barros d'Sa & Moorehead (1989), who have shown that intra-luminal shunts have simplified treatment of these difficult injuries.

The common peroneal nerve

Platt (1928) described lesions of the common peroneal nerve from adduction injuries of the extended knee. These are severe injuries, and in cases in which the tibial nerve and the popliteal nerves are involved the outlook for the leg is poor. Sedel & Nizzard (1993) and Wilkinson & Birch (1992) found useful results in over half of 44 cases of closed traction rupture.

Nerve injuries during arthroplasty of the hip

Until recently, information on incidence and causations of nerve injuries associated with hip arthroplasties has been relatively sparse. Ratcliffe (1984) collected 50 cases from a survey among orthopaedic surgeons in the UK. Traction was thought to be the most important feature in the 16 femoral nerve palsies which usually followed an antero-lateral approach to the hip. He found no clear relation between the approach and the sciatic nerve palsies. On occasion, direct injury to the nerve by the knife, wire or suture was found; haematoma causing compression or bleeding within the nerve did occur in patients on anticoagulant therapy. He recommended that steps be taken to exclude a lesion within the spinal canal and commented on the rarity of a true common peroneal nerve injury at the knee. In several of his patients urgent re-exploration improved the situation by relieving the nerve from compression or strangulation from wire or suture.

Schmalzried & Amstutz (1991) reviewed over 3000 consecutive hip arthroplasties from the UCLA. They found an incidence of 1% of nerve palsies after primary hip replacement, 2–3% after revision arthroplasty, and an incidence of 5.8% in patients with a primary diagnosis of congenital dislocation of the hip. Femoral and obturator nerve palsies were most often associated with extrusion of cement. In a cadaveric study they demonstrated that the sciatic nerve was at risk from being compressed between the posterior edge of the osteotomised trochanter and the ischium after dislocation, flexion and internal rotation of the hip during a lateral trans-trochanteric approach. Those patients who did well recovered within 6 months, while those with severe pain did badly and 20% were left with severe disability.

They made several recommendations:

- The patient should be warned of the risk of this complication.
- Particular care should be taken to support the limb during operation.
- The sciatic nerve should be regularly exposed during revision arthroplasty.
- In high-risk cases neurophysiological monitoring of the sciatic nerve should be performed, recording from the nerve just distal to the sciatic notch.

Since adopting this protocol, their incidence of nerve palsy in primary cases has been reduced to 0.6% and to 1.8% in revision arthroplasty.

Birch reports having seen 37 cases of injury to the femoral or sciatic nerves. There was no clear relation between the approach and the nerve injury, and no case of isolated injury to the common peroneal nerve was found. All these nerves were injured at the hip. Direct injury was found in 12 cases; in four more cases the nerve was compressed by haematoma or there had been an intra-neural bleed (Bonney 1998). In one case (Birch et al 1992) the sciatic nerve was burnt by cement, and this segment was resected and repaired by graft. The thermal injury to the nerve from curing acrylic cement extended to no more than 1 cm beyond the cement. In two cases nerves were injured indirectly from ischaemia following accidental injury to the iliac or femoral arteries. A combination of traction and compression is the most common cause. In these cases exploration showed the nerve to be entrapped and tethered within the scar tissue, with thickened epineurium and obliteration of longitudinal blood vessels. In some, a degree of conduction block was demonstrable. External neurolysis of the nerve was sometimes followed by improvement of pain and sensation in this group. In four patients colleagues had performed urgent re-exploration before referral, finding one case of transection of the sciatic nerve, one of strangulation by suture and two cases of compression by haematoma. Relief of pain and recovery of a nerve was good in three of these four, and certainly better than equivalent cases in which no such prompt action had been taken.

It is appropriate to suggest some guidelines for this difficult complication. It seems that patients should now be warned of risks of damage to the nerve during operations for hip arthroplasty. Particular care should be taken in high-risk cases: the recommendation from the UCLA that the sciatic nerve be seen and protected throughout the operation appears reasonable. The value of intra-operative monitoring of the nerve remains unclear: its use reflects a particularly high standard of care, but it does not give immunity to the nerve. If monitoring is to be performed it is better done along the exposed sciatic nerve. Most patients now have one form or other of prophylactic anti-coagulation which excludes neurophysiological monitoring by epidural electrodes. If a patient awakens with severe pain or with a complete lesion of either the femoral or sciatic nerve, then the surgeon is best advised to re-explore the nerve urgently. It is much less clear what to do when the injury is partial and there is little pain. The risk of leaving a potentially treatable condition alone must be balanced against the risk of subjecting patients who may be elderly or otherwise infirm to a second anaesthetic, and to an operation which carries with it a risk of introducing sepsis into the field.

Iatrogenic injuries

All persons involved in the treatment of patients are potentially responsible for accidental injury to nerves. Nurses may inject incorrect drugs or choose unsuitable sites. Physiotherapists may cause damage by improper handling of crutches and appliances. Physicians may cause damage by faulty injection of radio-opaque media, anaesthetists by want of careful positioning and padding may allow compression neuropathies, and the opportunities for surgeons to damage nerves are, of course, considerable. For a severe warning of the dangers of poorly organised day surgery, the article by Bonney in the Journal of the Medical Defence Union (1992) and the correspondence from him and Birch in a later issue (1992) are recommended reading.

Injection injuries

The sciatic nerve, the brachial plexus, the nerves to the shoulder and the nerves in front of the elbow are particularly at risk from injection for therapeutic purposes, for cannulation of adjacent vessel, for contrast studies or parenteral feeding and from regional anaesthesia. Seddon (1975) described 24 cases, finding that pain was often severe and recovery frequently limited. He described intense intra-neutral fibrosis often extending far within a nerve. Hudson (1993) confirmed that damage to the nerve was related not only to the chemical nature of the agent but also to whether it was injected within the nerve or adjacent to it. He showed that lignocaine, procaine, hydrocortisone and triamcinalone produced extensive degeneration and fibrosis when injected into the rat sciatic nerve. When a conscious patient complains immediately of very severe pain in the distribution of a nerve during the course of an injection, one must assume that the needle is in the nerve. There is still controversy about the role of operation, but these authors believe that it is wisest to expose the nerve, to incise the epineurium but not the perineurium, and to irrigate the nerve trunk with physiological Ringer's solution.

Irradiation

Vautrin (1954) reported on irradiation neuritis in five patients with different primary cancers. There was progressive and irreversible progression of the lesion. Speiss (1972) studied the pathological changes within the axon and in the myelin sheath from irradiation and considered that it was those with vasculitis which led to progressive endo-neurial fibrosis. It is now clearly established that malignant peripheral nerve sheath tumours may develop within the field of irradiation many years after completion of treatment (Sordillo et al 1981, Ducatman & Scheithauer 1983).

Irradiation neuritis may cause the most intense pain and it may affect all or any part of the plexus; there are no distinct clinical features which allow distinction from recurrent malignant disease. Narakas et al (1989) described the natural history of the condition in 126 patients. Symptoms commenced between 6 and 8 months after treatment. A typical presentation is with a patient complaining of pins and needles in the thumb and index finger between 18 months and 3 years after treatment. A diagnosis of carpal tunnel syndrome may be made, but close examination shows impairment of lateral cord function.

Severe and intractable pain is a dominant feature in 50% of patients. In the majority there is a relentless progression of loss of feeling and of power. Operations upon the brachial plexus rarely improve function, although they may ease pain. The reader is referred to the excellent review of Thomas & Holdorff (1993).

Surgical injuries

These may follow a failure to detect risk factors. Diabetes and thyroid disease predispose to neuropathy. The risks from anaemia, hypertension, ischaemic heart disease and malignant disease are well known, but not all orthopaedic surgeons are aware of a very real hazard of using a tourniquet in the lower limb after arterial reconstruction. The tourniquet should *never* be used after femoro-popliteal bypass grafting: to do so carries a very real risk of losing the leg (Mansfield 1992). Hereditary sensory motor neuropathy and hereditary compression neuropathy are uncommon conditions which should be considered in the differential diagnosis of nerve entrapment syndromes.

The number of nerves divided or otherwise irreparably damaged during the course of operations seen at the Peripheral Nerve Injury Unit of the Royal National Orthopaedic Hospital, and at St Mary's Hospital, is set out in Table 25.10. Orthopaedic surgeons were responsible for one-half of these cases. In one-third, the accident occurred during emergency operations for treatment of a fracture or vascular injury. Delay in diagnosis was a striking feature, exceeding 6 months in nearly one-half of patients. Birch et al (1991) reviewed 68 cases of transection of

Table 25.10 Iatrogenic nerve injuries, excluding nerves of cutaneous sensation; nerves injured at operation at the hip

Operation	ACC	BP	MC	ME	UL	RA	PI	FE	SC	CP	TIB
Wound exploration for fracture, n = 30	–	–	2	3	6	11	4	–	1	2	1
Removal of implant, n = 12	–	–	–	1	2	4	1	–	1	2	1
Lymph node biopsy, n = 22	15	6	–	–	–	–	–	1	–	–	–
Removal of cyst, ganglion or other benign tumour, n = 25	–	11	1	1	1	2	–	2	3	2	2
Cervical sympathectomy, n = 3	–	3	–	–	–	–	–	–	–	–	–
Excision of cervical or first thoracic rib, n = 3	–	3	–	–	–	–	–	–	–	–	–
Varicose vein or arterial surgery, n = 23	–	–	1	–	–	–	–	3	–	18	1

ACC, accessory; BP, brachial plexus; MC, musculocutaneous; ME, median; UL, ulnar; RA, radial; PI, poster interosseous; FE, femoral; SC, sciatic; CP, common peroneal; TIB, tibial.

peripheral nerve trunks. They emphasised that prevention was the best course, using adequate incisions particularly where the normal anatomy had been distorted by scar. They recommended intra-operative nerve stimulation. The best general advice is modified from that of Bonney (1986): if there is an incision (surgical or traumatic) over the line of a nerve and there is dysfunction in the distribution of that nerve, the nerve has been cut until proven otherwise, i.e. there must be documentation that the nerve was seen to be intact at the end of the operation otherwise the nerve should be explored.

Compression neuropathies

Cooper (1991) reviewed compression neuropathies from faulty positioning of patients on the operating table and in the recovery ward. The sciatic and common peroneal nerves are particularly at risk in lithotomy, the brachial plexus in the Trendelenburg position, and the ulnar and lateral femoral cutaneous nerves in the prone position. Hypovolaemia, hypotension and cold, particularly in patients with anaemia or coagulopathy, are significant factors in causation. A permanent deficit occurred in between 5 and 22% of cases of brachial plexus lesion, and in between 10 and 27% of patients with common peroneal palsy. Wadsworth & Williams (1973) emphasised the danger of permanent dysfunction from pressure of the ulnar nerve in the anaesthetised patient. These are not benign lesions: prevention is essential. The head should be positioned in the mid-line, avoiding undue extension or lateral flexion. The shoulder should not be abducted beyond 90° and accidental extension of the shoulder must be prevented. Padding of the elbows and of the knee should be standard practice in all operating theatres.

As already indicated, the tourniquet is potentially dangerous. The surgeon must be cautious in its use, avoiding it wherever possible, ensuring that adequate checks are made of pressure recording equipment, that the cuff is not too narrow and that it is inflated for as short a time as possible. Cuff pressure should be monitored and should not exceed 300 mmHg. In the upper limb typically 250 mmHg suffices for a bloodless field but in fat arms 300 mmHg may be necessary. Tourniquet times should be recorded in the operation notes. It has been stated that the tourniquet should be released after 2 hours and then not reinflated for a good 30 mins. There is no science to back up this assertion nor is it borne out in clinical practice. Although it represents good guidance, upper limb surgeons often apply the tourniquet for up to 3 hours with no obvious harmful effects (Giddins—personal communication). In the lower limb there appears to be less experience of the use of tourniquets for over 2 hours. Nerve lesions caused by tourniquets have historically been estimated to occur in between one in 5000 and one in 8000 cases (Love 1978, Yates et al 1981). Electromyography reveals abnormality as little as 20 minutes after application of a tourniquet; nonetheless, nerves appear to tolerate prolonged compression provided the pressure is not too high. The radial nerve is the most commonly afflicted nerve in the upper limb, followed by the ulnar and median nerves. Almost all go on to recover in between 3 and 6 months (Sunderland 1978), but there are one or two cases reported with permanent deficit (Speigel & Lewin 1945), often associated with persistent disturbance of sweating and pain (Bolton & McFarlane 1978). The basis for prolonged conduction block was established by Ochoa et al (1972), who showed the characteristic deformity of the node of Ranvier, which is displaced away from the compressed segment of the nerve.

In summary, it appears that excess pressure is more harmful than excess time. Nonetheless, efforts should be made to minimise tourniquet time and an active decision made if the time exceeds 2 hours; 3 hours probably represents a maximal safe time in the upper limb.

The brachial plexus

Serious injuries of the brachial plexus are the most complex and difficult of the peripheral nerve lesion. One of the reasons for this is that the central nervous system is so frequently involved by avulsion of spinal nerves directly from the spinal cord. Only a brief outline of prognosis can be given here; the subject is more extensively treated elsewhere (Birch 1992). Bonney (1959) studied 25 patients, finding that 12 remained in severe pain several years after their injury, and Wynn Parry et al (1987) showed that 112 patients out of 122 with pre-ganglionic injury continued to be in severe pain for between 3 and 30 years after their accident. There are estimated to be about 350 cases of complete or partial supraclavicular traction injuries every years in the UK (Goldie & Coates 1992) and about 150 of severe infraclavicular lesions. The incidence of open wounds from knife or gunshot is increasing although traction injuries are not. Rosson (1988) reviewed over 200 patients injured in motorcycle accidents, finding that 90% were aged less than 25 years, nearly one-half held only a provisional licence and that in over one-third the motorcycle had an engine capacity of 125 cc or less. The dominant limb was injured in over 60%, and there were severe injuries to the head, the chest and the viscera or to other limbs in 50%. More than one-third of these patients remained unemployed more than 1 year after the accident. Arterial injury is common, occurring in over 10% of cases in supraclavicular injury and in over 30% of the infraclavicular lesions. The incidence of pre-ganglionic injury is high and injury to the spinal cord is not uncommon in complete lesions. A Brown Sequard's Syndrome is detected in about 10% of such cases.

It is now possible to give a reasonable indication of the results of the different operations of nerve repair and nerve transfers:

- Repair of ruptures in the posterior triangle achieves worthwhile function at shoulder level and in the elbow in about two-thirds of cases.
- Nerve transfer has improved the outlook for shoulder and elbow function in patients with pre-ganglionic injuries to C5, C6 and C7.
- In complete lesions a combination of conventional grafting with nerve transfer gives a chance of some modest return of hand function in children and young adults.
- Re-innervation of the limb secures significant pain relief in many patients.
- Delay in repair is harmful—the earlier the repair is performed the better. After 6 months failure is the rule.
- Results after primary grafting of nerves at the same time as urgent repair of ruptured axillary or subclavian vessels are better than in cases of delayed nerve repair.
- A closely monitored programme of rehabilitation is extremely important (Wynn Parry et al 1987).

The obstetric brachial plexus palsy (OBPP)

Platt (1973), writing at a time when incidence was diminishing, described OBPP as a vanishing condition, but this no longer seems to be the case. The incidence in the literature is between 0.6 and two cases per 1000 live births. Two groups of infants are particularly at risk; the larger group includes the heavy baby (> 4 kg) with shoulder dystocia. A much smaller proportion of babies born by breech delivery and with very low birthweight have the most severe injuries. An analysis of 200 consecutive babies seen in the Peripheral Nerve Injury unit shows a substantially higher mean birthweight than the national average. Nonetheless, the national average birthweight is increasing, suggesting that the incidence will increase.

The clinical course

In many cases recovery occurs within a few days when the injury is a conduction block, but if paralysis persists for 3 weeks then nerve injury is degenerative and prognosis is less certain. A widely used classification for these children is useful as a guide to prognosis:

- *Group 1: C5 and C6.* The shoulder and elbow flexors are paralysed, and the arm lies in the classical posture described by Erb and Duchenne. About 90% of children make complete spontaneous recovery at the shoulder and elbow, and hand function is always normal.
- *Group 2: C5, C6 and C7.* Paralysis of the shoulder, of the elbow and of the extensors of the wrist. There will be spontaneous recovery to normal levels to the hand in 75%, for elbow flexion in 75%, and for the shoulder in a little over 50%.
- *Group 3: C5 to T1.* Paralysis is complete, but there is no Claude Bernard Horner syndrome. Full spontaneous recovery occurs for the limb as a whole in no more than one-third of children. The chief defect is usually at the shoulder.
- *Group 4: C5 to T1, with Claude Bernard syndrome.* This is the worst of all, with ruptures or pre-ganglionic injury of all spinal nerves. Spontaneous recovery never occurs.

For further discussion about indications for operation and results and for treatment of the complex deformities in this condition, the reader is referred to the reviews of Narakas (1987) and Gilbert (1993).

Acknowledgements

The authors gratefully acknowledges the many colleagues who have been kind enough to refer patients: this work would be impossible without such professional generosity. Thanks also to George Bonney, for constant stimulation in this field; Christopher Wynn Parry, for introducing the authors to the concept of rehabilitation; and Mrs Margaret Taggart, for the collation of many records and results.

■ References

Barros d'Sa A 1992 Arterial injury. In: Eastcott H A G (ed.) Arterial surgery, 3rd edn. Churchill Livingstone, Edinburgh, pp 355–414

Barros d'Sa A, Moorhead R J 1989 Combined arterial and venous intra luminal shunting in major trauma of the lower limb. European Journal of Vascular Surgery 3: 577–581

Birch R 1992 Advances in diagnosis and treatment of closed traction lesions of the supraclavicular brachial plexus. In: Catterall A (ed.) Recent advances in orthopaedics. Churchill Livingstone, Edinburgh, pp 65–76

Birch R, Raji A R M 1991 Repair of median and ulnar nerves. Journal of Bone and Joint Surgery 73B: 154–157

Birch R, Bonney G, Dowell J, Hollingdale J 1991 Iatrogenic injuries of peripheral nerves. Journal of Bone and Joint Surgery 73B: 280–282

Birch R, Dunkerton M, Bonney G, Jamieson A M 1988 Experience with the free vascularised ulnar nerve graft in repair of supraclavicular lesions of the brachial plexus. Clinical Orthopaedics No. 237: 96–104

Birch R, Wilkinson M C P, Vijayan K P, Gschmeissner S 1992 Cement burn of the sciatic nerve. Journal of Bone and Joint Surgery 74B: 731–733

Blom S, Dahlback L O 1970 Nerve injuries in dislocations of the shoulder joint after fracture of the neck of the humerus. Acta Chirurgica Scandinavica 136: 461–466

Bolton C F, McFarlane R M 1978 Human pneumatic tourniquet paralysis. Neurology 28: 787–793

Bonney G 1959 Prognosis in traction lesions of the brachial plexus. Journal of Bone and Joint Surgery 41B: 4–35

Bonney G 1986 Iatrogenic injuries of nerves. Journal of Bone and Joint Surgery 68B: 9–13

Bonney G 1998 *Iatropathic Injury in Surgical Disorders of the Peripheral Nerves*. Birch R, Bonney G, Wynn Parry CB (eds) Churchill Livingstone, Edinburgh

Brooks D 1955 The place of nerve grafting in orthopaedic surgery. Journal of Bone and Joint Surgery (American) 37: 299–326

Cavanagh S P, Bonney G, Birch R 1986 The infraclavicular brachial plexus: the case for primary repair. Journal of Bone and Joint Surgery 69B: 489 (abstract)

Clawson D K, Seddon H J 1960a The results of repair of the sciatic nerve. Journal of Bone and Joint Surgery 42B: 205–212

Clawson D K, Seddon H J 1960b The later consequences of sciatic nerve injury. Journal of Bone and Joint Surgery 42B: 213–225

Cooney W P 1991 Median nerve repairs: the results of treatment. In: Gelberman R H (ed.) Operative nerve repair and reconstruction. J B Lippincott, Philadelphia, ch 26, pp 379–391

Cooper E 1991 Nerve injury associated with patient positioning in the operating room. In: Gelberman R H (ed.) Operative nerve repair and reconstruction. J B Lippincott, Philadelphia, pp 1231–1242

DeBakey M E, Simeone F A 1955 Acute battle incurred arterial injury. In: Surgery and World War Two: Vascular surgery. Medical Department, US Army. US Government Printing Office, Washington DC, pp 60–148

Ducatman B S, Scheithauer B W 1983 Post irradiation neurofibrosarcoma. Cancer 51: 1028–1033

Ellis H 1985 Transthoracic sympathectomy. In: Greenhalgh R M (ed.) Vascular surgical techniques. Butterworth, London, pp 147–151

Epstein H 1980 Traumatic dislocation of the hip. Williams and Wilkins, Baltimore

Friedman A H, Nunley J A, Goldman R D, Urbaniak R J 1990 Repair of isolated axillary nerve lesions following infra-clavicular brachial plexus injuries. Neurosurgery 27(3): 403–407

Frykman G K, Gramyk K 1991 Results of nerve grafting. In: Gelberman R H (ed.) Operative nerve repair and reconstruction. J B Lippincott, Philadelphia, ch 39, pp 553–567

Gabel G, Nunley J A 1991 The spinal accessory nerve. In: Gelberman R H (ed.) Operative nerve repair and reconstruction. J B Lippincott, Philadelphia, ch 32, pp 445–452

Gilbert A 1993 Obstetrical brachial plexus palsy. In: Tubiana R (ed.) The hand, vol 4. W B Saunders, Philadelphia, English translation, ch 38, pp 575–601

Gilliat R W 1980 Acute compression block. In: Summer A J (ed.) The physiology of peripheral nerve disease. W B Saunders, Philadelphia, pp 287–315

Goldie B S, Coates C J 1992 Brachial plexus injuries – a survey of incidence and referral pattern. Journal of Hand Surgery (British) 17B: 86–88

Goldie B S, Coates C J, Birch R 1992 The long term results of digital nerve repair in no man's land. Journal of Hand Surgery 17B: 75–77

Gordon S L, Graham W P, Black J T, Miller S H 1977 Accessory nerve function after surgical procedures in the posterior triangle. Archives of Surgery 112: 264–268

Hudson A R 1993 Peripheral nerve surgery. In: Dyck P J, Thomas P K (eds.) Peripheral neuropathy, 3rd edn. W B Saunders, Philadelphia, pp 1674–1690

LeClercq D C, Carlier A J, Khuc T, Depierreux L, Lejeune G N 1985 Improvement in the results in 64 ulnar nerve sections associated with arterial repair. Journal of Hand Surgery, Suppl 10A: 997–999

Leffert R D, Seddon H J 1965 Infra-clavicular brachial plexus injuries. Journal of Bone and Joint Surgery (British) 47: 9–22

LeTournel E, Judet R 1981 Fractures of the acetabulum. Springer-Verlag, Berlin

Love B R T 1978 The tourniquet. Australian and New Zealand Journal of Surgery 48: 66–70

Mallet J 1972 Paralysie obstetricale. Revue Chirurgie Orthopédique 58(suppl 1): 115

Mansfield A O 1992 Personal communication. London Vascular Society Meeting, St. Mary's Hospital, London

Mayer J H, Mayfield F H 1947 Surgery of the posterior interosseous branch of the radial nerve. Surgery, Gynecology and Obstetrics 84: 979–982

McEwan L E 1962 Median and ulnar nerve injuries. Australian and New Zealand Journal of Surgery 32: 89–104

Medical Research Council 1954 Peripheral nerve injuries – Special Report No. 282. HMSO, London

Merle M, Amend P, Cour C, Foucher G, Michon J 1986 Microsurgical repair of peripheral nerve lesions: a study of 150 injuries of the median and ulnar nerves. Peripheral Nerve Repair and Regeneration 2: 17–26

Meyer V E 1987 Specific problems of skeletal management in upper limb replantation. In: Urbaniak J R (ed.) Microsurgery for major limb reconstruction. C V Mosby, St Louis, Missouri, pp 56–61

Millesi H 1980 Nerve grafts: indications, techniques and prognosis. In: Omer G E, Spinner M (eds.) Management of peripheral nerve problems. W B Saunders, Philadelphia, pp 425–426

Millesi H, Meissl G, Berger A 1972 The interfascicular nerve grafting of the median and ulnar nerves. Journal of Bone and Joint Surgery (American) 54: 727–750

Millesi H, Meissl G, Berger A 1976 Further experience with interfascicular grafting of median, ulnar and radial nerves. Journal of Bone and Joint Surgery (American) 58: 209–218

Moberg E 1958 Objective methods for determining the functional value of sensibility in the hand. Journal of Bone and Joint Surgery 40B: 454–476

Narakas A O 1987 Obstetrical brachial plexus injuries. In: Lamb D W (ed.) The paralysed hand. Churchill Livingstone, Edinburgh, pp 116–135

Narakas A O 1989 Lesions due nerf axillaire et lésions associé du nerf suprascapulaire. Review Medicale de la Suisse Romande 109: 545–556

Narakas A O, Brunelli G, Clodius L, Merle M 1989 Traitement chirurgical des plexopathies postactinique. In: Alnot J Y, Narakas A O (eds.) Les paralysies du plaxus brachial. Monographie due Groupe d'Etudes de la Main, no. 15. Expansion Scientifique Française, Paris, pp 240–249

Nicholson O R, Seddon H J 1957 Nerve repair in civil practice: results of treatment of median and ulnar nerve lesions. British Medical Journal 2: 1065–1071

Norden A 1946 Peripheral injuries to the spinal accessory nerve. Acta Chirurgica Scandinavica 94: 515–532

O'Brien B McC 1975 Microsurgery in the treatment of injuries. In: McKibben B (ed.) Recent advances in orthopaedics. Churchill Livingstone, Edinburgh

Ochoa J, Fowler T J, Gilliat R W 1972 Anatomical changes in peripheral nerves compressed by pneumatic tourniquet. Journal of Anatomy 113: 433–455

Omer G E 1974 Injuries to nerves of the upper extremity. Journal of Bone and Joint Surgery (American) 56: 1615–1624

Osgaard O, Eskesen V, Rosenjorn A 1987 Microsurgical repair of iatrogenic accessory nerve lesions in the posterior triangle of the neck. Acta Chirurgica Scandinavica 153: 171–173

Petrucci F S, Morelli A, Raimondi P L 1982 Axillary nerve injuries: 21 cases treated by nerve graft and neurolysis. Journal of Hand Surgery 7: 271–278

Platt H 1928 On the peripheral nerve complications of certain fractures. Journal of Bone and Joint Surgery 10: 403–414

Platt H 1973 Obstetrical paralysis: a vanishing chapter in orthopaedic surgery. The Bulletin of the Hospital of Joint Diseases 34: 4–21

Rank B K, Wakefield A R, Hueston J T 1973 Surgery of repair as applied to hand injuries, 4th edn. Churchill Livingstone, Edinburgh

Ratcliffe A H C 1984 Vascular and neurological complications. In: Ling R S M (ed.) Complications of total hip replacement (current problems in orthopaedics). Churchill Livingstone, Edinburgh, pp 18–29

Rich N M, Bouch J H, Hughes C W 1969 Popliteal artery injuries in Vietnam. American Journal of Surgery 118: 531–534

Rosson J W 1988 Closed traction lesions of the brachial plexus: an epidemic among young motor cyclists. Injury 19: 4–6

Schmalzried T P, Amstutz H C 1991 Nerve injury in total hip arthroplasty. In: Gelberman R H (ed.) Operative nerve repair and reconstruction. J B Lippincott, Philadelphia, pp 1245–1254

Seddon H J 1942 A classification of nerve injuries. British Medical Journal 2: 237–239

Seddon H J 1975 Surgical disorders of the peripheral nerves, 2nd edn. Churchill Livingstone, Edinburgh

Sedel L, Nizzard RR 1993 Nerve Grafting for traction injuries of the common peroneal nerve. A report of 17 cases. Journal of Bone and Joint Surgery 75B: 772–774

Sordillo P P, Helson L, Hajdu S L Malignant schwannoma. Cancer 47: 2503–2509

Speigel I J, Lewin P 1945 Tourniquet paralysis. Journal of the American Medical Association 129: 432–435

Speiss H 1972 Schadigungen am Peripheren Nervensystem durch Ionisierende Strahlen. In: Schriften reihe Neurologie, Neurology Series, Bd 10. Springer-Verlag, New York

Steinberg D R, Koman L A 1991 Factors affecting the results of peripheral nerve repair. In: Gelberman R H (ed.) Operative nerve repair and reconstruction. J B Lippincott, Philadelphia, ch 24, pp 349–364

Strachan J, Ellis V 1971 Vulnerability of the posterior interosseous nerve during radial head resection. Journal of Bone and Joint Surgery (British) 53B: 320–323

Sunderland S 1978 Nerves and nerve injuries, 2nd edn. Churchill Livingstone, Edinburgh

Sunderland S, McArthur R A, Nan D A 1993 Repair of a transected sciatic nerve. Journal of Bone and Joint Surgery (American) 75: 911–914

Thomas P K, Holdorff V 1993 Neuropathy due to physical agents. In: Dyck, P J, Thomas P K (eds.) Peripheral neuropathy, 3rd edn. W B Saunders, Philadelphia, pp 990–1014

Tupper J W, Crick J C, Matteck L R 1988 Fascicular nerve repair: a comparative study of epineurial and fascicular (perineurial) techniques. Orthopedic Clinics of North America 19(1): 57–69

Valtonen E J, Lilius H J 1974 Late sequelae of iatrogenic spinal accessory nerve injury. Acta Chirurgica Scandinavica 140: 453–455

Vautrin C 1954 Deficit moteur du membre supérieur après radiotherapie cervico-axallaire à dose élevée. Memoire d'Electro-Radiologie 40, Institute du Radium, Université de Paris

Wadsworth T J, Williams J R 1973 Cubital tunnel external compression syndrome. British Medical Journal 1: 662–666

Watson Jones R 1936 Fractures in the region of the shoulder joint. Proceedings of the Royal Society of Medicine 29: 1058–1072

Wood M B 1991 Peripheral nerve injuries to the lower extremity. In: Gelberman R H (ed.) Operative nerve repair and reconstruction. J B Lippincott, Philadelphia, ch 35, pp 489–504

Woodhall B, Beebe G W 1956 Peripheral nerve regeneration. Veterans Administration Monograph. Washington, DC, US Government Printing Office

Wynn Parry C B, Salter M 1976 Sensory re education after median nerve lesions. Hand 8: 250–257

Wynn Parry C B, Frampton V, Monteith A 1987 Rehabilitation of patients following traction lesions of the brachial plexus. In: Tertzis J K (ed.) Microreconstruction of nerve injuries. W B Saunders, Philadelphia, pp 483–495

Yates S K, Hurst R N, Brown W F 1981 The pathogenesis of pneumatic tourniquet paralysis in man. Journal of Neurology, Neurosurgery and Psychiatry 44: 759–767

Zachary R B 1954 Results of nerve sutures. In: Seddon H J (ed.) Peripheral nerve injuries. Medical Research Council Special Report Series, no. 282. London, HMSO, pp 354–388

Introduction

As we enter the 21st century it seems important to reflect that we have now entered an era when credible psychiatric classification systems have begun to allow us to begin to use well-defined operational criteria to make more accurate diagnoses. The use of well-defined clinical criteria and targeted drug and behavioural therapies has led to better detection and treatment of some disorders. No longer do we have to tolerate the notion that psychiatry is a medical backwater. The biological basis of psychopathology has become the focus of intensive research so that the impact of life events now appears to have a psychophysiological resonance. It is important to realise that the group of psychological disorders that we call 'functional' are not, in reality, under conscious control, as the biological basis of central nervous system disorders becomes increasingly apparent.

Carpenter (1996), the Cambridge neurophysiologist, has described the modern relationship between the concepts of 'mind' and 'brain' by stating:

In a nutshell, 'brain versus mind' is no longer a matter for much argument. Functions such as speech and memory, which not so long ago were generally held to be inexplicable in physical terms, have now been irrefutably demonstrated as being carried out by particular parts of the brain, and to a large extent imicable by suitably programmed computers. So far has brain encroached on mind that it is now simply superfluous to invoke anything other than neural circuits to explain every aspect of Man's overt behaviour.

The accurate assessment of the psychological impact of traumatic experiences has been viewed historically as being difficult, subjective and unreliable. This is in stark contrast to universal recognition that traumatic events generate both physical and psychological consequences. The trauma literature is full of evidence that traumatic experiences inevitably impact on cognitive and emotional processing in victims, irrespective of whether or not an individual or a group of individuals has been involved. Only successful mental processing of the traumatic memory imprint converts victims into true survivors.

Of course, trauma victims make their own, individual interpretations of their experiences and this leads to a variety of psychological and behavioural responses, but it is very important to see that there is also a spectrum of well-defined psychological syndromes with key characteristics common to all. An example of such a well-defined psychological reaction to trauma is post-traumatic stress disorder. Another would be depression. Modern editions of the major psychiatric classification manuals, such as the 10th edition of the International Classification of Diseases (ICD-10, 1992) and, more so, the 4th edition of the Diagnostic and Statistical Manual of the American Psychiatric Association (DSM-IV, 1994), attempt to identify core features of these reactions in order to 'operationalise' the diagnostic criteria. Fortunately, reliable measures of these features are now available. This facilitates accurate assessment of the effects of trauma on individuals and on populations.

Reliable instruments which can measure changes in mood, emotions and behaviour mean that they can be used as powerful adjuncts to clinical opinion in the assessment of trauma victims in both clinical and medico-legal work. With their help diagnosis, treatment and prognosis can be approached and monitored more confidently and less speculatively. The much vaunted 'on the balance of probabilities, doctor...?' is a soul-searching question that can be avoided more often than not if modern, criterion-based classifications are found. This chapter sets out to explore this area in depth.

Nomenclature

In the past, authors have described the psychological effects of trauma as presenting in three distinct ways:

1. as persistent somatic symptoms with no demonstrable organic basis (Tarsh & Royston 1985);
2. as psychological symptoms such as depression or anxiety (Parker 1977); and
3. as a mixture of organic and psychological symptoms (Woodyard 1982).

The complexity of potential reactions has been reflected in the wide range of diagnostic labels attached to symptom clusters, such as post-concussional syndrome (Taylor 1967) and accident neurosis (Miller 1961). More recently, the concept of post-traumatic stress disorder (PTSD) was introduced in the 3rd edition of the Diagnostic and Statistical Manual of the American

Psychiatric Association (DSM-III 1980), prompted by the psychological problems noticed in US combat veterans in the aftermath of the Vietnam war. Woodyard (1982) described a model for three types of 'compensation syndrome', which he named:

1. Exaggeration
2. Compensation neurosis
3. Malingering

Parker (1977) preferred the term 'accident neurosis', since this was not complicated by subjective implications concerning aetiology. Trimble (1984) used 'post-traumatic neurosis' as a general term for the symptom complex. However, the use of 'neurosis' as an integral part of the terminology is best avoided when referring to the cluster of symptoms which appear following psychological trauma because the range of psychological reactions includes psychotic disturbance (White et al 1987) with abnormal cognitions (delusions) and abnormal perceptions (hallucinations). White (1981) described a large population of patients who develop symptoms when no legal action is involved, and so the use of 'compensation' and 'litigation' in such circumstances seems fundamentally flawed. The use of a general term such as 'post-traumatic state' permits the inclusion of the whole range of psycho-behavioural responses to trauma without specifying discrete psychopathologies. This is too loose a framework for use in either clinical or medico-legal work. For example, the issue of attributability cannot be settled as easily for depression as it can be for PTSD. Depression may be the result of secondary stresses whereas the re-experiencing of a specific event in the form of flashbacks and nightmares effectively 'pins that event down' as responsible for the symptoms. Hoffman (1986) discussed possible models for such formulations.

PTSD represents an extensively researched, reliable and valid symptom cluster within the spectrum of traumatic stress reactions. It has been recognised since 1980, when it was first identified in DSM-III.

History

The word 'trauma' is from the ancient Greek and means 'puncture' or 'pierce'. This conveys powerfully the sense of penetrating impact which is a very useful image to keep in mind when considering whether or not an event has had a traumatising effect. PTSD acts as a suitable paradigm for the impact of stress on individuals. Although the term was introduced as recently as 1980, the syndrome was known. It was appropriate for the DSM-III to herald in the new classification because the

return of a large number of combat veterans from Vietnam who exhibited war-related psychological stress reactions precipitated an urgent research programme to elucidate the nature of these disabling conditions (Kentsmith 1986). The research programme revealed a remarkably consistent pattern of behavioural disturbance which was given the then new PTSD classification, and emphasised its value as a diagnostic construction. A rapidly growing library of literature confirmed the relevance of PTSD as a valid reaction applicable to a large variety of traumatised populations, such as rape victims, abused children, refugees, and victims of disasters, domestic violence and accidents. Of particular interest in this chapter is the recent work undertaken to investigate the psychiatric consequences of road traffic accidents (Mayou et al 1993). This will be discussed in detail in the following section on PTSD.

History makes it clear that PTSD was recognised in ancient Greece and Rome. Homer described the core features of PTSD in Achilles in the Iliad (c. 850 BC). Shakespeare did likewise in his character Hotspur in Henry IV, Part I (the exact reference is Henry IV, Part I, Scene II, lines 44–69). Samuel Pepys wrote graphic descriptions of PTSD in his diaries documenting the effects of the Great Fire of London in 1666. Charles Dickens was involved in a railway disaster in Kent in 1865 and subsequently described the effects on himself, drawing attention to his very own development of the cardinal features of PTSD. Such descriptions clearly demonstrate an awareness throughout history of the psychological effects of trauma. Wars and large-scale disasters have provided a rich source of such information. In the main, normal, previously fit people were involved.

The 20th century witnessed great advances in the understanding of the physiology and psychology of such reactions (Van der Kolk et al 1987; Friedman 1991). The Vietnam war threw up some surprises with regard to the post-traumatic state, and can be seen to be a landmark in changing attitudes towards the reaction to overwhelming stress. For example, there was the recognition that it was not uncommon for veterans to display *delayed* reactions, which had all the features of the reaction manifested in the immediate aftermath of exposure to trauma. Sometimes the delay amounted to several years, the subject showing no evidence of being affected in the interim. This puzzling phenomenon has, understandably, often created doubt in the minds of clinicians, lawyers and lay public alike about the validity of the relationship between the traumatic event and the psychological reaction. DSM-IV (1994) gave out the strong message that the development of a post-traumatic stress reaction does not imply vulnerability in the survivor, but rather that the reactions are attributable to the traumatic event and that identical reactions can be delayed in onset. Another major psychiatric classification system, the ICD-10 (10th edition of the International Classification of Diseases, 1992), contains the following statement on the question of personality vulnerability:

Predisposing factors such as personality traits or previous history of neurotic (anxiety-related) illness may lower the threshold for the development of the syndrome (PTSD) or aggravate its course, **but they are neither necessary nor sufficient to explain its occurrence**.

It is extremely important to emphasise that psychological reactions to trauma are everyday phenomena, definitely not reserved solely for human involvement in wars and major peacetime disasters. Records from wars and disasters, and reports following assault, rape and road traffic accidents, reveal a common core of symptoms. To make this point, the 1980s saw an unprecedented number of disasters in the UK. Most of these incidents involved large numbers of physically injured victims who required orthopaedic, surgical and medical attention. This has had the effect of bringing into the civilian arena the lessons learnt from military medical experience. The same types of psychological stress reactions were identified and the need for accurate medico-legal assessment of the psychological effects of the trauma has reached a new and higher level of awareness.

Psychological, social and biological dimensions

It is important to consider what is meant by the term 'psychological' when used in this context. Clearly, the meaning has to include cognition, mood and behaviour and the impact of such disturbance on the victim's social and occupational functioning, family and general quality of life. This is considerable and represents an important health problem. The biological dimension also exists in new links being forged between chronic traumatic stress and physical complications such as coronary artery disease, infections, hypertension and immunopathologies, as well as the constellation of psychosomatic illnesses (Friedman 1991). In PTSD a unique disturbance of neurotransmitters, adrenalin overproduction and endorphin underproduction has been described (Van der Kolk et al 1987, Friedman 1991). Turnbull (1997) drew attention to the association between these neuro-modulatory influences and chronic whiplash injury.

The elucidation of the underlying biological dimension of the impact of traumatic stress has led to exciting therapeutic developments (Van der Kolk et al 1987). What have been termed the 'psychological' effects of trauma should now be more aptly termed the 'psychosociobiological' effects, and such conditions might require treatments which take into account the multidimensional quality of the syndrome.

Incidence

The incidence of psychological problems following trauma is very difficult to assess (Weighill 1981). This is because of the poor standard of classification in the literature and the highly selective populations that have been studied. Many studies describe patients selected because they are claiming compensation. This represents only a small proportion of total accident cases: Harris (1981) estimated that only 12% of all accident victims become involved in compensation claims.

In general terms, the incidence of significant post-traumatic psychopathology which translates into disability increases as the degree of traumatic interface with perpetrators increases. Studies of natural disasters anticipate an incidence of PTSD and other chronic post-traumatic reactions at 1 year of about 5%. For road traffic accidents this rises to between 10 to 20%; for combat-related trauma it is about 25%; while for assault 50%, rape 75% and torture victims, it is about 90% at 1 year.

In some studies the incidence has been found to be even higher. Studies of groups not selected because of litigation indicate that there is a high incidence of psychological problems following trauma. White (1981) reviewed 163 unselected accident victims; psychological sequelae were seen 1 year after the accident in 75% of the group and some 25% were classified as suffering from moderately severe to severe problems. Braverman (1976), in a study of skiing-related trauma where no litigation or compensation was involved, interviewed 21 patients: 11 demonstrated a definite psychiatric reaction, and of these, three had developed a post-traumatic stress reaction. Fowlie & Aveline (1985) studied air crews following ejection from aircraft. No compensation was involved. Self-report measures in the form of psychological questionnaires revealed that 71% of the group suffered psychological problems after ejection; 40% reported that these problems remained unresolved at the time of enquiry.

Studies of litigant groups are poorly standardised in terms of classification of symptoms. They are also, by definition, pre-selected and therefore comparison between studies is difficult. Woodyard (1980) undertook a survey of 600 unselected compensation cases and identified 16% of the subjects as suffering from a 'compensation syndrome'. This excluded 8% whom he defined as exaggerating their symptoms. Parker (1977), in a study of 750 unselected accident litigants, identified 13% as exaggerating or deceiving. Parker also demonstrated an incidence of 39% of anxiety-related problems in the groups after excluding patients with head injury, bereavement reactions or other obvious aetiological factors. When patients have sustained a head injury then, in one study (Kelly 1972), the incidence of anxiety-related symptoms was 67 to 75%. The subject of malingering is considered in more detail later in this chapter.

There exists a closer agreement on the frequency of occurrence of more clearly defined patterns of stress reaction. PTSD was seen in 10% of subjects studied by Hoffman (1986). Post-traumatic psychosis is rare, occurring in only 2% of subjects reported by Parker (1977). The aetiology of 'compensation psychosis' is undecided (White et al 1987), but was thought likely to be the result of extremely high levels of anxiety triggering off a stress-induced psychotic reaction.

Symptoms

Neurosis

The term 'neurosis' is used to describe psychological disturbances which do not bear the hallmark of psychotic illnesses (delusions and hallucinations and disturbance of 'ego boundaries' such as passivity—the 'made to do' or 'made to think' phenomena) but which imply intense levels of anxiety at their core. Studies of patients with 'post-traumatic neurosis' report a wide range of symptoms. In his study of 750 consecutive accident victims, Parker (1977) listed the most common complaints in a subgroup of 296 neurotic patients. Topping the list was tension headache, which was described as differing from headache of proven organic origin by the typical use of colourful language in its description, hand gestures to indicate pressure features such as 'bearing down' or 'band-like' sensations, and the observation that analgesics gave little or no relief—and yet were used in considerable dosages and over prolonged periods. In the same patient group, the second most common symptom was increased irritability. Parker described the combination of headache and irritability as commonplace in the neurotic group whereas headache without irritability was seen more often in the patients who grossly exaggerated their symptoms.

Trimble (1984) described the neurotic symptoms following trauma as primarily anxiety and depression, with secondary manifestations such as palpitations, insomnia,

panic attacks, breathlessness and phobias. He claimed that the presence of these symptoms, whether or not they were associated with apparent physical illness, favoured a diagnosis of neurosis and made the diagnosis of malingering unlikely. Kelly (1981) described the primary symptoms of post-traumatic syndrome as headache, vertigo, poor concentration, unreliable memory, insomnia, and depression manifested by fatigue, impotence, loss of libido, and unreasonable resentment and anger. Hodge (1971) described symptoms of anxiety, insomnia, recurrent dreams of the accident, emotional instability, fear of driving, a preoccupation with symptoms, and hostility combined with feelings of 'righteous indignation'.

In a study of 500 cases which were the subject of litigation, Thompson (1965) reported that the most frequently encountered constellation of symptoms were anxiety and its somatic expression, with particular emphasis on the cardiovascular, gastrointestinal and respiratory systems. Panic attacks, emotional tension, depression, hyperventilation, phobias and repetitive dreams were also observed.

With hindsight, perhaps the most significant point that emerged from these studies was the observation that the psychological and behavioural reactions to traumatic experiences in those exposed took a standardised form. The relatively stereotyped reaction included elements of re-experiencing the trauma, increased physiological and psychological arousal, and phobic avoidance. This observation leads directly on to the next classification—post-traumatic stress disorder.

Post-traumatic stress disorder

Davidson (1992) described how:

each doctor needs to maintain a high level of awareness that patients may have experienced trauma, that PTSD can often account for a variety of common symptoms, and that it may also be at the root of a persisting, treatment-resistant depressive or anxiety state. . .while the hallmark symptoms of PTSD are pathognomonic, especially the intrusive recollections, flashbacks, and re-experiencing of trauma through nightmares etc., PTSD is still a diagnosis which is frequently missed, even by psychiatric professionals. The reasons why a doctor might perhaps overlook the diagnosis include:

a) not asking the patient about the experience of trauma;
b) patient reluctance to disclose painful material;
c) physician discomfort in discussing events which might be gruesome, horrifying or unimaginable;
d) the fact that chronic PTSD often presents with non-specific symptoms such as headache, insomnia, irritability, depression, tension, substance abuse, interpersonal or professional dysfunction.

Psychological defence mechanisms which involve *denial* are frequently found in certain sections of the community. Denial is a very useful psychological defence often found in emergency service workers, police officers, military personnel, medical and nursing staff etc., because exposure to trauma through its victims is an inevitable part of their everyday occupations. Dealing with trauma victims successfully requires the ability to deny the uncomfortable reality of their own vulnerability. Trauma victims themselves are plunged into the new reality that human life is fragile and can be extinguished rapidly and unexpectedly. This may have a profound, enduring impact and it will often affect those in contact with them in both the short-and the long-term. Denial reactions can be very adaptive when used appropriately (for example, when an urgent but risky or noxious task needs to be completed), but they can also be responsible for distortions of thinking when over-used. Such awkwardness can lead to the following distortions:

- viewing victims as responsible for their own misfortune
- viewing suffering as an expression of underlying weakness
- viewing suffering as having a 'hidden agenda' such as financial compensation (Alexander 1990)

Those who are familiar with medico-legal reporting and Court appearances will be very familiar with the above distortions and will, no doubt, have been frustrated by them.

Since PTSD was first identified in DSM-III (DSM-III, APA, 1980) it has undergone two slight revisions in DSM-III-Revised (1987) and DSM-IV (1994), but the initial concept has been upheld.

PTSD occurs in individuals who have been exposed to a catastrophic event. This means a traumatically stressful event. It is not enough to have been exposed to war-zone stress, rape, childhood abuse, natural or technological disasters. In the latest revision of the concept (DSM-IV, 1994), it is also necessary that individuals exposed to the stressful situation experienced a powerful emotional reaction such as fear, terror, horror, helplessness or the feeling that they were going to die. This represents the 'piercing' impact of traumatic events and also a very important change in the concept of what constitutes a legitimate traumatising event. A traumatic event cannot simply be judged to have been traumatic by objective description, it has to have been experienced as traumatic subjectively by the victim. Certain factors such as stressor intensity, suddenness, duration of exposure, amount of warning, significance of physical injuries and the time over which the trauma evolved can be assessed more objectively. However, the medico-legal significance of this is that it is not possible for another person to judge whether or not an event has been traumatic or not. A thorough examination of the impact that the event had on a victim is required in all cases to uncover the subjective element in the history. This is why criterion A in the definition of PTSD in DSM-IV has such a special significance and has been called the 'gatekeeper criterion'. If criterion A is not satisfied and some of the symptom clusters normally associated with PTSD develop following exposure to a serious life-stressor (such as a bereavement, divorce, major disappointment—events which are unpleasant but are not life-threatening), then by definition an adjustment disorder is diagnosed.

Sometimes there are special difficulties in elucidating exactly what happened and that brings us back to the psychological defence, denial. For example, unconscious denial may blur memory for extremely traumatic events or even obliterate available memory altogether. Sometimes, depersonalisation (out-of-body) experiences, which represent the extreme version of dissociation, will be consciously denied by victims because of the potential reaction of others and basic fears for their own sanity. In fact, depersonalisation is a relatively common experience for those victims involved in life-threatening situations, especially where entrapment is a factor (fractured limbs, jammed car doors etc.) and should be actively pursued when taking the history of the immediate reaction to a trauma (Turnbull 1999, 2000).

Dalenberg (1999) clearly saw dissociative experiences as being the most emotionally disturbing to the patient of the spectrum of PTSD symptoms. Dissociation typically is described as disruption in the integration of consciousness, identity, memory or perception. As a major PTSD symptom it deserves special clinical (and therefore medico-legal) attention. It is important to recognise dissociative symptoms for the following reasons:

1. Depersonalisation or derealisation is distressing for virtually anyone who must live through it. The feeling of estrangement from the self or one's environment is terrifying for the dissociative patient as is the experience of not being in control.
2. Dissociation can result in practical problems for the patient, interfering with the performance of social and occupational activities. Memory problems also interfere with long-term relationships.
3. Dissociative patients are poor predictors of danger. Both the under- and overprediction of danger can precipitate crises.
4. Dissociation is an impediment to self-understanding. This can provide obstructions to progress in therapies which are cognitively-oriented.

5. Dissociative symptoms may make the patient appear to be an unreliable reporter of his own cognitive and emotional life. This can make it difficult to make an accurate diagnosis and also lead to the taking of different histories depending upon the attitude of the history-taker. In litigation run on adversarial grounds the doctors reporting on behalf of the Claimant may be perceived by the patient/client as being 'friendly' and non-threatening. The quality of such an assessment may reflect the intrusive symptoms of PTSD. By stark contrast, doctors reporting for the Defendants may be perceived as threatening and the resulting history, accurately recorded by the Defendant's medical experts, may reflect the more avoidant aspects of the clinical condition. In some cases this can lead to unnecessary prolongation of litigation simply because the two sides of medical experts have based their opinions on the opposite poles of the intrusion versus avoidance spectrum of symptoms which exists in PTSD (Turnbull 1997a).

When it is established that a person has been traumatised, three major symptom clusters develop as the acute stress disorder (in DSM-IV, 1994) or the exactly equivalent acute stress reaction (ICD-10, 1992) and, should these persist beyond 1 month then, by definition, a PTSD has developed.

The first symptom cluster of *re-experiencing symptoms* means that the trauma essentially continues to have a life of its own in the form of untriggered recurrent thoughts, flashbacks and nightmares. Alternatively, the traumatic memories might be stimulated by cues that remind the victim of the trauma.

The second cluster is characterised by *avoidance and numbing*. This is because individuals suffering from PTSD find the re-experiencing of symptoms so intolerable and so difficult to deal with that a number of behavioural and cognitive strategies are brought into play to minimise intrusive recollections. There are *avoidance symptoms*, such as avoiding situations that will predictably remind the victim of the traumatic event, and *numbing symptoms*, shutting down the emotions, dissociation, psychogenic amnesia, inability to have feelings, and social withdrawal.

The third cluster of *hyperarousal symptoms* closely resemble the symptoms characteristic of anxiety states—increased irritability, insomnia etc.—but what is most strongly characteristic of PTSD is *hypervigilance*, because those who have been traumatised never want to repeat the experience and are 'on guard'. Hypervigilance can be so extreme that it can mimic a paranoid state and this is not a hypothetical possibility because it can lead to making the wrong diagnosis, mistaking a severe PTSD for a psychosis.

Because of the internal psychological conflict between intrusiveness and avoidance, PTSD symptoms can come to the surface several months or even many years after the traumatising event once the suppressive avoidance dimension weakens or fails. This is called *delayed-onset PTSD*. Diagnostic criteria for PTSD (DSM-IV) are:

A. The person has been exposed to a traumatic event in which both of the following were present:
   (1) the person experienced, witnessed, or was confronted with an event or events that involved actual or threatened death or serious injury, or a threat to the physical integrity of self or others; and
   (2) the person's response involved intense fear, helplessness, or horror (note: in children, this may be expressed instead by disorganised or agitated behaviour).

B. The traumatic event is persistently re-experienced in one (or more) of the following ways:
   (1) recurrent and intrusive distressing recollections of the event, including images, thoughts or perceptions (note: in young children, repetitive play may occur in which themes or aspects of the trauma are expressed);
   (2) recurrent distressing dreams of the event (note: in children, there may be frightening dreams without recognisable content);
   (3) acting or feeling as if the traumatic event were recurring (includes a sense of reliving the experience, illusions, hallucinations and dissociative flashback episodes, including those that occur on waking or when intoxicated);
   (4) intense psychological distress at exposure to internal or external cues that symbolise or resemble an aspect of the traumatic event; and
   (5) physiological reactivity on exposure to internal or external cues that symbolise or resemble an aspect of the traumatic event.

C. Persistent avoidance of stimuli associated with the trauma and numbing of general responsiveness (not present before the trauma), as indicated by three (or more) of the following:
   (1) efforts to avoid thoughts, feelings or conversations associated with the trauma;
   (2) efforts to avoid activities, places or people that arouse recollections of the trauma;
   (3) inability to recall an important aspect of the trauma;

(4) markedly diminished interest or participation in significant activities;

(5) feeling of detachment or estrangement from others;

(6) restricted range of affect (e.g. unable to have loving feelings); and

(7) sense of a foreshortened future (e.g. does not expect to have a career, marriage, children or normal life span).

D. Persistent symptoms of increased arousal (not present before the trauma), as indicated by two (or more) of the following:

(1) difficulty falling or staying asleep;

(2) irritability or outbursts of anger;

(3) difficulty concentrating;

(4) hypervigilance;

(5) exaggerated startle response.

E. Duration of the disturbance (symptoms in criteria B, C and D) is more than 1 month.

F. The disturbance causes clinically significant distress or impairment in social, occupational or other important areas of functioning.

The issue of vulnerability

The acute PTSD phenomenon is best regarded as representing an attempt to adapt positively to a life-threatening event with positive survival potential (Van der Kolk et al 1987). The flashback memories afford ongoing opportunities to absorb the meaning of what was, in fact, a survival experience.

There is considerable evidence in favour of the concept that normal individuals develop acute PTSD in response to abnormal, and usually life-threatening, stress exposure (Turnbull & Busuttil 1992). There is no convincing evidence to support the concept of a specific vulnerability to the development of acute PTSD because it develops as a direct consequence of exposure to a traumatising experience as described above. The development of chronic PTSD probably represents an obstruction to mental processing of the traumatic memories once they have been imprinted, leading to persistent symptom clusters, and this is where vulnerabilities have their effect (ICD-10 (1992); Turnbull 1994). These factors have practical significance in medico-legal assessments of trauma victims, for example they help to assess prognosis.

Assessment of pre-vulnerability to the development of chronic PTSD must look carefully at:

(1) previous life-experiences and, especially, previous exposure to trauma (which may not have been resolved);

(2) habitual coping skills;

(3) general arousability;

(4) history of psychiatric illness; and

(5) neuroticism as a personality trait.

Secondary stressors, i.e. those which develop after the traumatic impact, also have to be searched for because of their maintaining or exacerbating potential. These include:

(1) the extent of loss or destruction of property;

(2) the number of deaths during the trauma;

(3) the ultimate meaning and significance of the trauma;

(4) preoccupation with physical injuries; and

(5) the development of co-morbid conditions such as depression, anxiety states, substance abuse.

PTSD has a persistent, underpinning biological dimension which accompanies this development (Friedman 1991). The persisting biological changes energise 'satellite' psychopathologies, and it has been estimated that over 50% of cases of PTSD develop a co-morbid psychiatric illness (Davidson & Baum 1986) where panic disorder and major depressive disorder are the most commonly encountered co-morbid disorders.

Mayou et al (1993) determined the psychiatric consequences of being a road traffic accident victim by following up 188 consecutive patients seen in the A&E department of the John Radcliffe Hospital, Oxford, for a period of 1 year. They found that acute, moderately severe emotional distress was common. Almost one-fifth of subjects suffered an acute stress syndrome characterised by mood disturbance and horrific memories of the accident. Anxiety and depression usually improved over the 12 months, although 10% of patients had significant mood disorders at 1 year. PTSD occurred in 10% of patients. Phobic travel anxiety as a driver or passenger is more common than PTSD and frequently disabling. Emotional disorder was associated with having pre-accident psychological or social problems and, in patients with multiple injuries, continuing medical complications. PTSD was not associated with a neurotic predisposition but was strongly associated with horrific memories of the accident. They concluded that psychiatric symptoms and disorder are frequent after major and less severe road accident injury. Post-traumatic symptoms are common and disabling. They advised that early information and advice might reduce psychological distress and travel anxiety and contribute not only to road safety but also to the assessment of 'nervous shock'.

The measurement of PTSD

The measurement of PTSD has been the focus of considerable research. Specific psychological instruments have been devised which have received international approval (Keane et al 1984). The syndrome of PTSD was first accorded legal recognition in British courts following the Piper Alpha disaster of 1987 (Alexander 1990).

Psychophysiological assessment methods for PTSD, which will hopefully improve the accuracy of its diagnosis (Pitman et al 1987), are still in the process of development. There are new and exciting developments in brain scanning methods including PET (positron-emission-tomography) and dynamic MRI, which have elucidated the function of various parts of the brain. For example, it has been possible to 'see' the generation of 'flashback' memories following exposure to a triggering stimulus on PET (Van der Kolk 1994). Probably, psychophysiological assessments will help to measure severity of post-traumatic syndromes and provide an objective means of making the diagnosis. They will be in addition to taking a clinical history, matching the results with DSM-IV criteria and using psychological tests.

Psychological tests

In the case of PTSD, psychological (psychometric) testing falls into two distinct categories: the tests which measure PTSD symptomatology and those which have a more general application or measure secondary syndromes such as depression.

The Clinician-Administered PTSD Scale for DSM-IV (CAPS 1998) measures PTSD symptom frequency and intensity. The test also assesses presence or absence of the disorder (Blake et al 1990, revised 1998). A maximum score of 68 for symptom intensity is possible. It should be used in the specialist trauma clinic setting.

The Revised Impact of Event Scale (Revised-IES, Horowitz et al 1979) is a 15-item, self-rating scale designed to assess the extent to which a traumatic event has affected an individual's life over the most recent 14 days. It measures intrusive and avoidance phenomena of PTSD; that is, thoughts and images related to the trauma which intrude into the mind involuntarily and efforts made by the individual to avoid being reminded of the trauma. The scale is commonly used as a screening tool for PTSD; however, studies have shown that it is also useful for making the diagnosis of the disorder. A cut-off score of 35 or above for making the diagnosis has been demonstrated in a British population (Neal et al 1994). A maximum score of 75 is possible. Because this is a self-report scale and has a high degree of validity it is recommended for use not only by psychiatrists and psychologists but also by surgeons and personal injury lawyers.

The General Health Questionnaire-28 (GHQ-28, Goldberg & Hillier 1979) is a 28-item, self-rating scale which screens for psychological disorder in the general population. The threshold score for identifying 'caseness', i.e. above which there is an increasing likelihood that the person would be suffering from significant psychiatric symptoms, is 5, and the maximum possible score is 28. It focuses on breaks in normal function rather than life-long traits and, therefore, detects the appearance of new phenomena of a distressing nature. The GHQ-28 has subscales which measure:

- somatic symptoms
- anxiety/insomnia
- social dysfunction
- severe depression

The Beck Depression Inventory (BDI, Beck et al 1979) measures depressive symptoms over the past 7 days. It is a 21-item, self-rating scale and is one of the most widely used, validated and reliable tests used in the assessment of depression. The Cognitive–Affective subscale measures the severity of depressive thoughts and feelings, the Somatic–Performance subscale the severity of the physical and social aspects of depression. A score of 0–9 is within the normal range; 10–18 indicates mild–moderate depression, 19–29 moderate–severe depression and 30–63 extremely severe depression.

The Revised-IES should be used much more frequently by non-mental health professionals. This would lead to the identification of PTSD much earlier as a complication of some difficult orthopaedic problems such as chronic whiplash and chronic pain syndromes (Turnbull 1997). The underlying biological dimension of PTSD can exacerbate chronic musculoskeletal and pain syndromes, especially the over-production of adrenaline and underproduction of endorphins.

Phobic symptoms

Phobia following trauma may represent 'stretching' of the phobic elements of PTSD into a syndrome in its own right. Thompson (1965) found 21% in his series of 500 accident victims. The phobias were not of a classical form and were in the main related to the injury, such as fear of driving following a car crash or fear of heights following a fall. In the two cases in which there was evidence of a classical claustrophobia (fear of enclosed places), there was a history of pre-existing neurosis. The phobia pattern following trauma may be directly derived from the circumstances of the injury (Hodge 1971). Patients will demonstrate avoidance or reduction of the activity related to the trauma (Kuch et al 1985).

Hysterical symptoms

Woodyard (1982) believed compensation neurosis to be characterised by symptoms including tension headache, depression, irritability, aggression and loss of libido. Pain out of proportion to the severity or site of the injury was present, and showed only a transient response to conventional methods of treatment. Dissociation or conversion symptoms were described as frequent. In the former the patient maintains for a considerable length of time some line or course of action in which he appears not to be actuated by the normal self—or, alternatively, the usual self seems not to have access to recent memories that one would normally expect the patient to have (examples would be trances, fugues and amnesia). In the latter, symptomatic changes of physical function occur, which unconsciously—and in a distorted form—give expression to latent and covert anxieties that have previously been repressed or over-controlled. In each case the fundamental anxiety is dispelled, and this is termed the 'primary gain'. However, there is always the question of 'secondary gain', where the advantage is the result of conscious manipulation (the primary gain is, by definition, beyond the conscious control of the individual), and this is of importance in compensation cases following accidental injury. The classical hysteric is nothing if not suggestible; and susceptibility to suggestion, especially in those of a relatively unsophisticated nature, could be an important determinant of the development of a hysterical symptom of dissociative or conversion type. This has to be borne in mind by the assessor of the degree of physical injury. Woodyard concluded that dissociation or conversion symptoms were frequent occurrences following accidental injury. He also described patchy, variable hyperaesthesia unrelated to dermatomes or peripheral nerves.

Tarsh & Royston (1985) studied a group of 35 accident victims selected for gross somatisation and symptoms with no adequate organic aetiology. They classified 10 of the patients as suffering from illness of an hysterical or hypochondriacal type which would have legitimately led to referral to a psychiatrist. Of these patients, five had hysterical disuse of the upper limb; two involved the fingers only, while three involved either hand or hand plus arm. Two of the 10 had severe hysterical gait disorder and the remaining three had profound, totally disabling hypochondriasis.

Thompson (1965) classified 73 of his 500 patients as suffering from hysterical neurosis. In 96% the symptom was located at the site of the injury; 92% displayed passive indifference ('la belle indifference') and 21% had a mixed anxiety/hysterical neurosis. Hysterical symptoms were most common in the industrial injury cases, a finding also reported by Parker (1977).

It remains to be said that in the investigation of a large series of patients who had suffered as a result of accidental injuries, Tarsh & Royston (1985) found that the great majority did not recover from their disabilities following legal settlement of their compensation claims, although the attitudes of primary relatives did change as they accepted the validity of the compensation claims. Hohl (1974) and Pennie & Agambar (1990) concentrated their interest on soft tissue injuries of the neck, and both studies concluded that there is no evidence to suggest that symptoms resolve on the settlement of litigation.

It is possible that the reduction of anxiety levels in litigants which would inevitably follow the acceptance of the concept that psychological effects of trauma are as valid as physical sequelae would inevitably lead to a reduction of the development of anxiety-linked conditions such as hysterical reactions, which have been regarded as 'maladaptive'. Characteristic reactions to trauma often lead to the development of phenomena—intrusive recollections being a good example—which lead to high levels of anxiety and doubts about self-vulnerability. Intrusive recollections which take the form of flashbacks are often very frightening and can be confused by the sufferer as hallucinations and evidence of the development of psychotic breakdown. The extremely high levels of anxiety so engendered might act as a breeding-ground for various neurotic phenomena, including hysterical dissociation and conversion reactions. Such reactions are commonly encountered in studies of hostages who characteristically experience extreme anxiety (Turnbull & Busuttil 1992). A word of caution about the assumption that an observed phenomenon has a hysterical basis: memories of the trauma are imprinted on the amygdala from which flashbacks emanate, as demonstrated on PET scans. Sensations which imprint on the amygdala include not only the images from the obvious visual, auditory, olfactory, taste and physical pressure 'channels', but also from emotional and pain sources. Therefore, flashbacks may, legitimately, re-create the re-experiencing of the widest possible range of afferent inputs. This can lead to manifestations which appear to be strange and non-anatomical which are, in reality, flashbacks to the original traumatic experience rather than anxiety-based. A colourful example was the intermittent, strange gait accompanied by falling over which could not be explained in terms of anatomy or straightforward orthopaedic disability but which became meaningful once it had been discovered that the intermittency was connected with stimuli which resembled the original trauma—being struck from behind in a stationary car by a lorry with failed brakes when there was no visual pre-warning. Another, less esoteric and much more frequently encountered example was the episodic exacerbation of whiplash pain which was, in reality, the re-experiencing of the original pain in flashback form.

Psychosis

Psychosis may develop as an acute reaction following head injury. As the acute phase resolves the patient may recover completely or may be left with continuing problems (Lishman 1978). Achte et al (1967) described psychosis developing as a delayed feature of head injury, observing schizophrenia, paranoid psychosis, depressive psychosis and hypomanic psychosis in a series of 3552 soldiers with head injury. Bracken (1987) reported that a search of the literature revealed 20 cases of manic psychosis following head injury. Lishman (1978) concluded that the generally accepted view was that psychosis following head injury should be seen as indicating a constitutional predisposition in the majority of cases, with the injury serving as a trigger for the appearance of the symptoms. It should be reiterated that flashbacks to real events are often still misinterpreted as hallucinations and can convey real memories in any or all of the special senses.

Malingering

Although hysterical mechanisms are, by definition, unconscious, a major problem confronting psychiatrists and orthopaedic surgeons in medico-legal work is where to draw the dividing line between hysteria and conscious simulation or malingering. ('Malingering' is a term derived from the French 'malingre', meaning 'sickly'.) Fortunately, hysterical symptoms are becoming less common due to improved education and awareness of psychological mechanisms, permitting the expression of emotional conflicts for what they actually are, and making the communication of suffering via hysterical symbolism redundant. Hysterical phenomena appear to lie on a spectrum from the genuinely unconscious to the conscious. This parallels the development from 'primary' gain through to 'secondary' gain described above. Malingering appears to lie at the extreme, conscious end of the spectrum.

Malingering is defined as the conscious simulation of symptoms or of disability (Enelow 1971), or the deliberate imitation of disease or disability for gain (Woodyard 1982). The diagnosis of malingering may only be made with any degree of certainty when the patient is observed, outwith the clinical setting, performing an act that he claimed to be impossible. Woodyard (1982) suggested that symptoms which were clearly absurd were an indicator of malingering; he cited as an example the loss of memory following a back injury. Trimble (1984) pointed out that malingering must be diagnosed on positive criteria, but noted that there was a lack of experimental evidence which would allow such criteria to be defined. Hurst (1940) set two diagnostic criteria which give a positive diagnosis of malingering:

(1) The patient is observed to perform an act that he claims he is not able to do.
(2) The patient admits to malingering.

Miller & Cartilige (1972), reviewing earlier studies, stated that when symptoms were entirely subjective, the distinction between malingering and neurosis (including hysteria) rested in the last resort on the credibility of a witness. Again, the point is made that the likelihood of such maladaptive responses to accidental injury is minimised by recognition that psychological reactions to trauma are legitimate at the time of the initial assessment.

Looking at PTSD in particular, the syndrome implies a definite causal link to what is often a compensatable event. Therefore, when evaluating possible PTSD with external incentives at stake it becomes necessary carefully to assess causality, intentionality and motivation as well as traumatic events and symptoms. Also, when incentives are at issue, clinicians must report their opinions to a third party. This difficult situation demands an objective, thorough and sensitive clinical assessment in which clinicians must struggle with the implications of believing or disbelieving their patients. Distinguishing malingering from PTSD is often not a simple matter (Armstrong & High 1999). Simple listing of symptoms, even if obtained in a well-validated structured interview, is not enough. Verbal descriptions are also not enough. Observation of emotions connected with the history is essential to the determination of the reliability of information. Other sources of information such as medical and occupational records and family members must also be considered.

Malingering is the intentional production of false symptoms motivated by external incentives. An alternative is 'factitious disorder'. This also involves the intentional production of false symptoms, but is motivated by the compulsion to assume a sick role.

Resnick (1997), Pitman (1996) and Rogers (1997) have all offered guidelines for the detection of malingering:

(1) when the claimant does not co-operate with the assessment,
(2) calls attention to distress but is evasive about symptom details (the opposite is true in genuine PTSD),
(3) describes behaviour inconsistent with reported symptoms, e.g. inability to work with ongoing involvement in recreational activities, and
(4) blames all life problems on the trauma and PTSD—genuine PTSD patients tend to avoid treatment, feel guilty and try to appear normal;
(5) the majority of malingerers are not men—there is no evidence for gender differences in frequency;

(6) malingerers are not sociopathic—no studies have proven a link between these two behaviours;

(7) there is no connection between the vividness and emotional impact of a trauma story and its truthfulness;

(8) true PTSD sufferers are able to describe criterion A peritraumatic horror, helplessness and/or dissociation. Absence of, or vagueness about, these 'state of mind' aspects of PTSD when recounting relatively recent traumatic experiences is suspicious;

(9) direct questions should be avoided—standardised structured interviews are highly suggestive to malingerers and are mainly useful where malingering is not an issue—symptoms should be carefully explored;

(10) wishing to be believable, malingerers often assert their closeness towards family, not realising that this is inconsistent with emotional numbing—true PTSD avoidance serves the purpose of controlling painful or distressing symptoms—malingered avoidance tends to have an external incentive such as enhancing monetary compensation;

(11) with unsophisticated malingerers, inserting an unlikely symptom such as decreased need for sleep into a series of questions about PTSD symptoms often reveals inconsistencies;

(12) careful observation of behavioural responses such as staring, startling and somatic reactions when traumatic material is discussed can help to distinguish between a true PTSD sufferer and a malingerer, and

(13) a safeguard when using self-report scales is to ask for detailed examples of any symptoms reported.

Assessment

The accident

Hoffman (1986) discussed the importance of a detailed investigation of the history of the accident when assessing a patient who has suffered a personal injury. Pilowsky (1985) pointed out that the patient may suppress the more horrific aspects of the accident unless closely questioned. He also emphasised the importance of obtaining the patient's perception of the danger involved in the trauma; even trivial accidents may be perceived as life-threatening by the patient, and this perception often dictates the psychological response to the trauma. These cases of crypto-trauma are often missed without careful history-taking. DSM-IV reflects this realisation by re-working the first criterion in the definition of PTSD to include 'high-magnitude stressful incidents in the perception of the exposed individual'. This alteration more easily absorbs everyday incidents such as road traffic accidents and assault as triggers for a full-blown post-traumatic stress reaction which is no longer regarded as being capable of development only after exposure to mass disasters.

Injury type

Whiplash injury

Whiplash, or hyperextension injury of the neck, carries a high risk of post-traumatic neurotic symptoms; 50% may develop psychoneurotic illness (Gay & Abott 1968). Hodge (1971) stated that the type of accident which produces a whiplash injury is also the type which produces the traumatic stress reactions. In a study of 100 cases of whiplash injury after settlement of compensation, Gotten (1956) reported that 54 patients showed no appreciable symptoms, 34 had minor discomfort and 12 had severe symptoms. This would support McNab (1973), who stated that, out of a group of 266 whiplash injury patients, after settlement 45% still had symptoms despite satisfactory resolution in their favour in the Courts.

Alexander (1982) coined the term 'accident neurosis' to describe patients who complain of a similar constellation of symptoms after an accident involving head trauma or injury to some other part of the body, especially the back, neck or limbs. Regardless of the nature and site of the principal injury, the following features are common to all patients: a higher incidence in men, unskilled workers and following industrial accidents and a high frequency of compensation litigation, which correlates poorly with the severity of the injury. The symptomatology is mixed and variable, anxiety, depression and hysterical conversion being common, with a tendency for histrionic exaggeration in addition to a range of more classical post-concussional symptoms. Despite the well-publicised work of Miller (1961), return to work and complete recovery from disability are uncommon even after settlement of any compensation claim (Weighill 1983, Tarsh & Royston 1985). Traumatic incidents which cause whiplash injuries will frequently have involved sufficient bodily impact also to cause minor head injury. See Hohl (1974), Pennie & Agambar (1990) and Gargan & Bannister (1990) for the results of their studies of the prognosis for whiplash injuries. There have been two major international conferences on the subject of whiplash injury organised in the UK recently which have brought together all of the disciplines which are involved in this difficult and multi-dimensional condition (Lyons Davidson, 1997, 2000).

Head injury

Post-concussional syndrome may follow closed or penetrating head injury. A minor head injury is defined as one warranting brief inpatient overnight observation in hospital but with a post-traumatic amnesia of less than 12 hours. Despite the transient nature of the period of unconsciousness caused by minor head injury and the rapid, immediate recovery, a substantial minority of patients develop a cluster of persistent and troublesome complaints termed the post-concussional syndrome which has been reviewed by Montgomery et al (1991). Much of the symptomatology is psychological in nature: irritability, poor concentration, loss of confidence, anxiety, depression, and intolerance of noise and bright lights. Fatigue, headache, dizziness, vertigo and intolerance of alcohol are somatic components of the syndrome (McMillan 1991). The post-concussional syndrome is suggested to take three principal forms in the work of Montgomery et al (1991). The first is the classical form described above. The second is accident neurosis, with a more mixed, variable cluster of symptoms. The third important complication of minor head injury is a depressive syndrome. The depressive symptoms may emerge from or blend imperceptibly with those of the post-concussional syndrome. Unlike accident neurosis, there is no tendency for histrionic over-elaboration of symptoms or signs, and recovery is not complicated by the question of compensation.

The degree to which the post-concussional syndrome, accident neurosis and post-traumatic depression overlap remains unclear. It may be that they are all part of a wide spectrum of response to head injury. Post-concussional symptoms provide the central core of all three states, appearing in pure culture in the post-concussional syndrome. Post-concussional symptoms represent the common sequelae of blunt head injury. In the other syndromes additional features are superimposed: a compensation claim and histrionic exaggeration of symptoms and signs in accident neurosis; and affective symptoms and depressed mood in post-head-injury depression. Such a hypothesis can account for the reported heterogenous nature of symptoms following minor head injury.

PTSD following head injury presents a special difficulty. Since the vast majority of minor head injuries do not occur during an event 'that is outside the range of usual human experience', as required by the DSM-III-R and DSM-IV diagnostic criteria for PTSD, it might be argued that it is unlikely that PTSD contributes significantly to the usual spectrum of post-head-injury symptomatology, although it might have relevance in a few special cases. The new thinking about the first criterion in PTSD, which is crystallised in DSM-IV, suggests that the attitude of the individual victim and his perspective of disaster and life-threat must be taken into account. The focus of the incident-related memories of

the accident which caused the head injury might also lie outside the accident itself and, for example, lead to flashbacks and other intrusive recollections of intensive care at a time when registrable memory is restored to normal. Current practice is that if the other features of PTSD are fulfilled and the recollections of available memory fulfil the criteria for genuine intrusive recollections of the traumatic event, then the diagnosis of PTSD can be made. Therefore, PTSD may represent a more significant post-head-injury complication than has previously been the case.

McMillan (1991) described stress reactions following severe head injury as being indistinguishable from PTSD with intrusive re-experiencing of available memories associated with the events of the trauma, hyperarousal and avoidance features. These cases made it clear that PTSD can occur even when there is loss of consciousness and organic amnesia for the event and its immediate sequelae. Classification of symptoms described below in such cases are consistent with DSM-III, DSM-III-R and DSM-IV criteria for diagnosis of PTSD:

1. Experience of sequelae of car accident.
2. (a) Recurrent and intrusive thoughts.
   (b) Psychological distress at anniversary of trauma.
3. (a) Avoidance of thoughts associated with accident.
   (b) Avoidance of situations associated with sequelae.
   (c) Diminished interest in friends/socialising and career.
   (d) Feelings that career would not progress further and ambitions foreshortened.
4. (a) Early wakening.
   (b) Irritability/temper outbursts.
   (c) Poor concentration.
   (d) Physiological reactivity on exposure to symbolic stimulus (e.g. palpitations).
5. Duration longer than 1 month.

The relative role of organic and psychogenic factors in the genesis of post-concussional symptoms has been a matter of heated debate over the years. In a review of the literature, Trimble (1984) suggested that this is related to organic injury. In a study of 670 patients, Lishman (1968) showed that the degree of psychiatric disability correlated with the length of post-traumatic amnesia; this was confirmed by Guthkelch (1980) in a prospective study of 398 head injury patients. Kelly (1972) noted an incidence of 65 to 75% neurotic symptoms in a prospective study of 152 head injuries. Trimble (1984) reported that many studies showed considerable psychiatric morbidity following head injury, and that no studies have shown neurotic symptoms to be influenced by compensation in head injury cases. The prognosis of neurosis following head injury is poor if the patient has not returned to work by the time the settlement has occurred (Kelly & Smith 1981).

Erichsen (1866) used the term 'spinal concussion' to account for the occurrence of post-concussional symptoms as described after railway accidents. The pathological evidence for organic cerebral change is sparse, since few cases came to autopsy. Montgomery et al (1991) examined 26 consecutive admissions to an A&E department with minor head injuries. Their findings suggested both cortical and brain stem damage following minor head injury. This psychobiological monitoring over the subsequent 6 month period revealed three patterns of recovery. Half recovered within 6 weeks, a minority demonstrated continuing dysfunction over 6 months with persisting brain stem dysfunction, and less than a third showed an exacerbation of symptoms with no evidence of brain stem dysfunction, the exacerbation being a consequence of psychological and social factors.

Loss of consciousness

Adler (1943) followed up patients who had been involved in the Coconut Grove Disaster and observed that unconsciousness improved outcome, especially if prolonged for more than 1 hour. McMillan (1991) recorded the single case study of a road traffic accident victim who developed PTSD despite loss of consciousness and organic amnesia for the event and its immediate sequelae. Mayou et al (1993) showed that PTSD was strongly associated with horrific memories of the accident and did not occur in victims who were rendered unconscious and had no available memory of the accident. There is no memory basis for the subsequent development of flashbacks, nightmares or any other re-experiencing phenomena. Also, amnesia for the event leads to less avoidance reaction because triggering cues are not recognised.

There is evidence that brain trauma together with impairment of consciousness can improve recovery from trauma. Changes in key neurotransmitters may alter the process of traumatic memory consolidation (Glue et al 1993) and this offers hope of new therapeutic approaches to the prevention of PTSD.

Back injury

In a study of 509 patients with low back injury, Krusen & Ford (1958) showed that only 56% of compensation cases improved compared with 89% of non-compensation cases. However, the compensation cases were referred for treatment much later than the non-compensation group. In his study of 52 cases of neurosis/malingering Woodyard (1982) found that spinal injury carried a greater risk of residual symptoms than other injuries. Fifteen of the 19 patients with residual symptoms had suffered lumbar or cervical injury. This was supported by Balla & Moraitis (1970), in a study of 82 Greek patients with back or neck injuries.

Other factors

Studies of patients with post-traumatic disorders have commented on two main sets of factors which may influence the presentation and course of the reaction: namely, pre-existing illness, and ethnic and cultural factors.

Pre-existing illness

Parker (1977) found that 20% of his patients had obvious neurotic symptoms prior to the accident, and that 24% had clear obsessional personality traits. In a study of psychosocial aspects of post-accident anxiety, Modlin (1967) noted the presence of rigid personality characteristics in a group within his study. Studies of patients with low back pain (Leavitt 1985) have shown that those without any organic findings have scores on the Minnesota Multiphasic Personality Inventory (MMPI) which indicate significant elevation of hypochondriasis and hysteria scales. Pheasant et al (1979) showed that these elevated scores were good prognostic indicators of poor response to surgery in low back problems. Assessment of pre-trauma personality, based as it is on retrospective data, is often not reliable. This may account in part for the great variations in proportions of patients who were reported to have pre-existing problems. Thompson (1965) reported that 87% of his group of post-traumatic neurosis patients had pre-existing neurotic traits. However, Culpan & Taylor (1973) found that previous personality seemed to be of no particular significance in the majority of post-traumatic neurotics.

Here again, PTSD might provide a valuable clinical clue in the observation that obsessional personality traits tend to be found in a high proportion of chronic post-traumatic states (Van der Kolk et al 1987). The degree of control over emotional expression which is characteristic of obsessional personalities tends to prevent healthy processing of the recollections of the traumatic event. This in turn tends to lead to delay in the resolution of the traumatic material in PTSD and the development of a prolonged chronic PTSD out of an initially adaptive post-traumatic stress reaction. Since the chronic version of PTSD represents a high-anxiety state the syndrome then goes on to be shaped by the personality characteristics of the individual who has been exposed to a high-magnitude and, often, life-threatening stressor. Mayou et al (1993) provided the most up-to-date evidence to support the general trend in thinking that pre-existing psychiatric illness tends to be exacerbated by traumatic exposure but that PTSD behaves differently, developing de novo without pre-existing vulnerability.

Ethnic and cultural factors

Tarsh & Royston (1985) confirmed the findings of Balla & Moraitis (1970) that immigrant status may be important in the prognosis of post-traumatic disorders with back and other injuries. They discussed the role of the family in the maintenance of illness after trauma and pointed out the importance of identifying family over-protectiveness. There may be role changes resulting from the illness, which are difficult to reverse. These factors require consideration when assessing the patient's reaction to trauma. However, the extensive world literature on PTSD contains no convincing evidence that particular ethnic or cultural factors confer any advantage or disadvantage in relation to the development of the syndrome.

Trauma and physical health

In recent years the relationship between mental and physical health has become increasingly fascinating. Holistic approaches have become more popular among doctors and patients alike. Mainly in the US, studies of military populations examining the relationship between combat or other military exposure (e.g. prisoner-of-war experiences) and health outcomes have increasingly found that PTSD and other post-trauma conditions provide important links between trauma exposure and physical health (Green & Schnurr 2000). Likewise, exposure to traumatic events has been linked with health complaints in the general population. Ullman & Siegel (1996) found that a history of trauma predicted poorer health perceptions, more chronic physical limitations and increased prevalence of chronic medical conditions, controlling for age, gender, social class and psychiatric disorder in a community setting. Felliti et al (1998) looked at a population of nearly 10 000 people and found that there was a significantly increased risk of developing serious psychiatric and physical health problems in those who were exposed to childhood trauma or childhood abuse. Many psychological, physiological and behavioural components of PTSD are themselves associated with poor physical health and could mediate the relationships among trauma, PTSD and adverse health outcomes (Friedman & Schnurr 1995, Schnurr & Jankowski 2000). For example, cardiovascular reactivity, disturbed sleep physiology and dysregulation of certain hormones such as adrenaline might promote physical illness. Depression is also associated with a range of poor health outcomes (Schulberg et al 1987) and recent findings implicate biological aspects of depression as causal factors in cardiovascular disease (Musselman et al 1998).

The evidence for an association between previous exposure to trauma and the subsequent development of physical illness is sufficiently strong to recommend that a trauma history is taken as a routine in all medical settings, especially in patients who somatise, exhibit high levels of distress and who are frequent attenders. This is another situation in which the use of self-rating scales might be of value in screening.

Sutherland, Hutchison & Alexander (2000) have described fascinating preliminary results of their study of persistent metabolic distortions in post-traumatic psychopathology and their contribution to a catabolic state which is associated with delay in healing and physical recovery in orthopaedic patients. They have identified basic markers of metabolic disturbance (C-Reactive Protein and Soluble Interleukin-6-Receptor) which correlate with indices of post-traumatic psychopathology which might be of value in monitoring the recovery process, and they emphasise that holistic treatment which addresses both physical and psychiatric issues is the most effective formula.

Busuttil (1997) described the development of a Coping Scale derived from evaluation of stressor variables in the context of psychological morbidity after road traffic accidents. Three hundred and seventy one survivors were contacted 1–4 months post accident. Most had not suffered serious physical injuries. The aim was to evaluate predictive variables for PTSD other than serious physical trauma, by using a questionnaire which looked for identified features of post-traumatic psychopathology. The following observations were made:

1. Even when there was no serious injury, 30% of road traffic accident survivors had PTSD symptoms. Overall, 51% had significant scores for anxiety, depression and PTSD. There was a high incidence of co-morbidity.
2. The presence of serious injury increased the likelihood of developing PTSD by almost 100% (24% in the non-serious injury group compared with 43% in the serious injury group).
3. Litigation was not a predictive factor variable for PTSD (when the diagnosis of PTSD was made using the Impact of Event Scale [IES] with a cut-off score of 30).
4. In this group of road traffic accident survivors accident and injury variables were least predictive of PTSD using regressive models. Coping style accounted for 47% of the variance and social support for a further 20%.

Robertson et al (2000) have demonstrated that high quality information in the form of a leaflet about post-traumatic reactions distributed to patients attending A&E departments and a traumatic stress clinic is very well-received. This opens up opportunities to reduce resistance to identification of post-traumatic psychopathology in patients who have been exposed to everyday traumatic events (such as road traffic accidents) after which we already known that the prevalence of post-traumatic syndromes is considerable and often undiscovered. Klein et al (2000) have developed the Aberdeen Trauma Screening Index to identify those of heightened risk of developing post-traumatic psychopathology following orthopaedic trauma. Again, the challenge is one of correct identification of psychopathology at an early stage to facilitate holistic recovery.

Of course, the identification of post-traumatic psychopathology needs to be accompanied by the development of effective treatments. This theme is addressed in the following section on prognosis.

Prognosis

The prognosis in cases of psychological reactions to trauma has been the subject of much discussion. Miller (1961), in a study which has had undue influence on contemporary views, argued that virtually all post-accident neurosis patients recover after the settlement of litigation. However, this study of 50 highly selected cases from a series of 500 litigants was of an unrepresentative neurotic group, and the conclusions have not been supported by other workers.

Kelly & Smith (1981), in a study of 43 cases of post-traumatic syndrome, showed that 17 of the patients had returned to work prior to settlement. Failure to return to work by settlement day indicated a poor prognosis. Such patients rarely returned to work at all.

Mendelson (1982) confirmed that, in an unselected series of 101 patients involved in litigation following trauma, only 35 resumed work prior to settlement. Of the rest, 53 were followed up, nine had returned to work following settlement and 44 were not working at an average of 15 months after settlement. This study agreed with Kelly & Smith (1981) that the older the patient, the less likely is the possibility of return to work. Woodyard (1982) studied 52 cases where return to work could be assessed; only 27% were at work in less than 6 months and 61% were out of work for at least a year. Of these 41 patients, only six returned to their previous employment and 18 never returned to work.

In a study of 35 litigants with gross somatic symptoms with no demonstrable organic pathology, Tarsh & Royston (1985) found that return to work was unusual and full recovery rare. The authors concluded that in this selected group the prognosis for recovery was as bad as if the illness had a physical basis. Balla & Moraitis (1970) studied 82 patients of Greek origin after industrial or traffic injuries. They acknowledged that legal proceedings were a complicating factor which might adversely affect the prognosis. They showed that a settlement of legal matters had little or no influence on most patients—their symptom pattern remained unaltered.

In a study of 509 patients with low back injury, Krusen & Ford (1958) discussed the role of compensation in dictating outcome. The group studied included 54% who were eligible for compensation while the remainder were not seeking compensation. Of the compensation group, 56% improved compared with 89% of the non-compensation group. There was a correlation between duration of symptoms before treatment and lack of improvement. This finding has been confirmed by Kelly (1981) in cases of post-traumatic syndrome. Mendelson (1982), in a review of the effect of legal settlement on compensation claims, concluded that compensation and financial gain are only part of a complex of factors, such as the psychological impact of the accident, cultural and ethnic variables and family relationship changes, which all determine prognosis and outcome.

There is cause to be more optimistic about treatment outcomes for post-traumatic syndromes. Certainly, the fundamental understanding that PTSD is associated with 'blocked' memory processing (Siegel 1997) has strongly reinforced the concept that methods which specifically aim to facilitate memory-processing have a definite part to play in the treatment of PTSD and other post-traumatic psychopathologies, especially if these conditions are identified early. Cognitive therapy (Foa & Rothbaum 1998), exposure therapy (Keane 1995), eye-movement desensitisation and re-processing (EMDR; Shapiro 1989), and group therapy (Busuttil et al 1995) all work well. In general terms, trauma-focused treatments appear to be more effective than anxiety management treatments. Addressing the traumatic impact at an appropriate time seems to be a central connecting theme for early identification and screening, psychological first aid, critical incident stress debriefing and treatments.

Modern developments in the identification and treatment of PTSD and other post-traumatic psychopathologies briefly described above mean that it is no longer acceptable to give a final prognosis in cases where Claimants have not received treatment. Treatment of post-traumatic psychopathology also has a significant bearing on the outcome of physical injuries and the ultimate level of disability.

Medico-legal reports

Guidance for compiling a psychiatric report for litigation following personal injury is available. Hoffman (1986) suggested the following outline:

- source of information
- history of the accident
- post-accident course
- history
- family history and psychiatric history
- personal history and life events (paying particular attention to previous trauma)
- mental state examination
- independent information
- summary
- prognosis
- attributability to the accident

More general guidance on involvement with the Courts is given by Grounds (1985) and Gibbens (1974). These articles deal solely with the psychiatrist in Court.

Summary

- Psychological reaction to trauma arises in a variety of clinical forms. The differential diagnosis of the response involves careful psychiatric investigation, and may require detailed psychological testing.
- PTSD represents a highly standardised reaction to life-threat.
- PTSD commonly occurs following everyday traumatic experiences such as road traffic accidents and other physical trauma which are initially assessed by orthopaedic surgeons.
- Biological disturbances associated with post-traumatic psychopathologies are associated with delayed healing of physical injuries.
- More holistic treatments improve the speed of recovery, the eventual quality of recovery and clarify the prognosis.
- Compensation and financial gain have not been shown to be major motivating factors in the development of post-traumatic psychological states, or in their perpetuation. There is no evidence to suggest that symptoms disappear with settlement of litigation.
- Guidelines for identifying malingering are given.
- Treatment of post-traumatic psychopathology is frequently very successful. This is best done in the early stages if treatment is to have maximum benefit.
- The prognosis of post-traumatic psychological reactions will be affected by stressors which will tend to increase anxiety, such as prolonged litigation, limiting physical injury and general factors such as unemployment and financial problems. These other factors do not have the same significance in PTSD, in which the impact of the stressor itself has primary importance.

- The role of the orthopaedic surgeon in the management of post-traumatic psychological reactions is to be aware of the problem, to identify cases in which a reaction is present, to normalise the attitude towards the reaction, and to initiate early referral for further assessment and treatment.
- The use of self-report psychometric tests by orthopaedic surgeons and lawyers should be encouraged.
- The British legal system now recognises the validity of the concept of primary psychological injury, or psychological injury in conjunction with physical injury.

References

Achte K A, Hillbom E, Aalberg V 1967 Post-traumatic psychoses following war brain injuries. Reports from the Rehabilitation Institute for Brain-injured Veterans in Finland, vol I, Helsinki

Adler A (1943) Neuropsychiatric complications in victims of Boston's Coconut Grove Disaster. Journal of the American Medical Association, 123, 1098–1101

Alexander D A 1990 Psychological intervention for victims and helpers after disasters. British Journal of General Practice 40: 345–348

Alexander D A 1996 Trauma research: A new era. Journal of Psychosomatic Research 41 1: 1–5

Alexander M P 1982 Traumatic brain injury. In: Benson D F, Blumer D (eds) Psychiatric aspects of neurologic disease, 2. Grune and Stratton; New York, pp 219–249

American Psychiatric Association 1980 Diagnostic and statistical manual of mental disorders III. APA, Washington, DC

American Psychiatric Association 1987 Diagnostic and statistical manual of mental disorders III – revised. APA, Washington, DC

American Psychiatric Association 1994 Diagnostic and statistical manual of mental disorders IV. APA, Washington, DC.

Armstrong J G, High J R 1999 Guidelines for differentiating malingering from PTSD National Center for PTSD Clinical Quarterly 8(3) 46–48

Balla J I, Moraitis S 1970 Knights in armour; a follow-up study of injuries after legal settlement. Medical Journal of Australia 2: 355–361

Beck A, Ward C, Mendelson M, Mock J, Erbaugh J 1961 An inventory for measuring depression. Archives of General Psychiatry 4: 561–571

Beck A, Rush A, Shaw B F, Emery G 1979 Cognitive therapy for depression. New York Guildford Press

Blake D, Weathers F, Nagy L, Kaloupek D, Charney D, Keane T 1990 Clinician-administered PTSD scale (CAPS-I). Revised clinician administered PTSD scale for DSM-IV (CAPS-II) Boston Mass Behavioral Science Division Boston National Center for Post-Traumatic Stress Disorder.

Bracken P 1987 Mania following head injury. British Journal of Psychiatry 150: 681–682

Braverman M 1976 Validity of psychosomatic reactions. Journal of Forensic Sciences 22: 654–662

Busuttil W, Turnbull G J, Neal L A, Rollins J, West A G, Blanch N, Herepath R 1995 Incorporating psychological debriefing techniques within a brief group psychotherapy programme for the treatment of post-traumatic stress disorder. British Journal of Psychiatry 167: 495–502.

Busuttil A M C 1997 Coping and Psychological Morbidity after Road Traffic Accidents: The Development of a Coping Scale and an Evaluation of Stressor Variables, Coping and Social Support in relation to Post-Traumatic Stress Disorder. (unpublished) Doctoral Thesis, University of Surrey.

Carpenter R H S 1996 A last look at the brain: Motivation and behaviour. In Neurophysiology, Third Edition. Arnold: London 286–289

Culpan R, Taylor C 1973 Psychiatric disorders following road traffic and industrial injuries. Australia and New Zealand Journal of Psychiatry 7: 32–39

Dalenberg C J 1999 The management of dissociative symptoms in patients. National Center for PTSD Clinical Quarterly, 8,(2)

Davidson L M, Baum A 1986 Chronic stress and post-traumatic stress disorders. Journal of Consulting and Clinical Psychology 54(3): 303–308

Davidson J 1992 Drug therapy of post-traumatic stress disorder. British Journal of Psychiatry 160: 309–314

Dyregov A 1989 Caring for helpers in disaster situations: psychological debriefing. Disaster Management 2: 25–30

Enelow A J 1971 Compensation in psychiatric disability and rehabilitation. CC Thomas, Springfield, Illinois

Erichsen J E 1866 On railway and other injuries of the nervous system. Walton & Maberly, London

Felliti V J, Anda R E, Nordenberg D, Williamson D E, Spitz A M, Edwards V, Koss M P, Marks J S 1998 Relationship of childhood abuse and household dysfunction to many of the leading causes of death in adults. American Journal of Preventive Medicine 14: 245–258.

Foa E B, Rothbaum B O 1998 Treating the trauma of rape: Cognitive-behavioral therapy for PTSD. New York: Guildford Press

Fowlie D G, Aveline M O 1985 The emotional consequences of ejection, rescue and rehabilitation in RAF aircrew. British Journal of Psychiatry 146: 609–613

Friedman M J 1991 Biological approaches to the diagnosis and treatment of post-traumatic stress disorder. Journal of Traumatic Stress 4(1): 67–92

Gargan M F, Bannister G C 1990 Long term prognosis of soft tissue injuries of the neck. Journal of Bone and Joint Surgery 72B: 901–903

Gay J R, Abbott K H 1968 Common whiplash injuries of the neck. Journal of the American Medical Association 152: 220–225

Gibbens T C N 1974 Preparing psychiatric court reports. British Journal of Hospital Medicine 12: 278–284

Glue P, Nutt D J, Coupland N J 1993 Stress and psychiatric disorder: reconciling social and biological approaches. In Stress: An Integrated Approach (eds) S C Stanford & P Salmon p53–73 London: Academic Press.

Goldberg D P, Hillier V F 1979 A scaled version of the general health questionnaire. Psychological Medicine 9: 139–145

Gotten N 1956 Survey of 100 cases of whiplash injury after settlement litigation. Journal of the American Medical Association 162: 865

Green B L, Schnurr P P 2000 9 1 National Center for PTSD Clinical Quarterly 1–5.

Grounds A 1985 The psychiatrist in court, British Journal of Hospital Medicine 34(1): 55–58

Guthkelch A N 1980 Post-traumatic amnesia, post concussional symptoms and accident neurosis. European Neurology 19: 91–102

Harris D 1981 Financial needs: an academic viewpoint. Naidex 1981 conference, Warwickshire, October, pp 231–233

Hodge J R 1971 The whiplash neurosis. Psychosomatics 12: 245–250

Hoffman B F 1986 How to write a psychiatric report for litigation following personal injury. American Journal of Psychiatry 143: 164–169

Hohl M 1974 Soft tissue injuries of the neck in automobile accidents: factors influencing prognosis. Journal of Bone and Joint Surgery 56A: 1675–1681

Homer 1974 The iliad (Fitzgerald R trans) Anchor/Doubleday, New York (original c. 800 B.C.)

Horowitz M J, Wilner N, Alvarez W 1979 Impact of event scale: A measure of subjective stress Psychological Medicine 41: 209–218

Hurst A F 1940 Medical diseases of war. Edward Arnold, London

Keane T M, Malley P F, Fairbank J A 1984 Empirical development of an MMPI subscale for the assessment of combat-related post-traumatic stress disorder. Journal of Consultational Clinical Psychology 53: 888–891

Keane T 1995 The role of exposure therapy in the psychological treatment of PTSD National Center for PTSD Clinical Quarterly 5(1): 3–6

Kelly R E 1972 The post-traumatic syndrome. Pahlevi Medical Journal 3: 530

Kelly R 1981 The post-traumatic syndrome. Journal of the Royal Society of Medicine 74: 242–245

Kelly R, Smith B N 1981 Post-traumatic syndrome: another myth discredited. Journal of the Royal Society of Medicine 74: 275–277

Kentsmith D K 1986 Principles of battlefield psychiatry. Military Medicine 151(2): 89–96

Klein S 2000 The Aberdeen trauma screening index Paper presented at Third World Conference for the International Society for Traumatic Stress Studies Melbourne, March 2000 Book of Abstracts No. 204.

Krusen E M, Ford D E 1958 Compensation factor in low back injuries. Journal of the American Medical Association 166: 1128–1133

Kuch K, Swinson R P, Kirby M 1985 Post-traumatic stress disorder after car accidents. Canadian Journal of Psychiatry 30: 426–427

Leavitt F 1985 The value of the MMPI conversion V in the assessment of psychogenic pain. Journal of Psychosomatic Research 29. 125–131

Lishman W A 1968 Brain damage in relation to psychiatric disability after head injury. British Journal of Psychiatry 114: 373

Lishman W A 1978 Organic psychiatry. Blackwell, Oxford

Mayou R, Bryant B, Duthie R 1993 Psychiatric consequences of road traffic accidents. British Medical Journal 307: 647–651

McMillan T M 1991 Post-traumatic stress disorder and severe head injury. British Journal of Psychiatry 159: 431–433

McNab I 1973 The whiplash syndrome. Clinical Neurosurgery 20: 232–241

Mendelson G 1982 Not cured by verdict: effect of legal settlement on compensation claimants. Medical Journal of Australia 2: 132–134

Miller H 1961 Accident neurosis. British Medical Journal 1: 919–925, 992–1228.

Miller H, Cartilige H 1972 Simulation and malingering after injuries to the brain and spinal cord. Lancet i: 580–585

Modlin H C 1967 The post accident anxiety syndrome: psychosocial aspects. American Journal of Psychiatry 123: 1008

Montgomery E A, Fenton G W, McLelland R J, MacFlynn G, Rutherford W H 1991 The psychobiology of minor head injury. Psychological Medicine 21: 375–384

Musselman D L, Evan D L, Nemeroff C B 1998 The relationship of depression to cardiovascular disease. Archives of General Psychiatry 55: 580–592.

Neal L A, Busuttil W, Rollins J, Herepath R, Strike P, Turnbull G J 1994 Convergent validity of measures of post-traumatic stress disorder in a mixed military and civilian population. Journal of Traumatic Stress 7: 447–455

Parker N 1977 Accident litigants with neurotic symptoms. Medical Journal of Australia 2: 318–322

Parkes C M 1997 A typology of disasters, chapter 7 in Psychological Trauma – A Developmental Approach (eds) D Black M. Newman J. Harris-Hendriks G. Mezey Gaskell: Royal College of Psychiatrists also, Newman, M. Psychological consequences of road traffic accidents, chapter 8(I): Summerfield, D. The impact of war and atrocity on civilian populations, chapter 10(A): Turner S. & McIvor R. Torture, chapter 13.

Pennie B H, Agambar L J 1990 Whiplash injuries: A trial of early management. Journal of Bone and Joint Surgery 72B: 277–279

Pheasant H C, Gilbert D, Goldfarb J, Herron L 1979 The MMPI as a predictor of outcome in low back surgery. Spine 4: 78–84

Pilowsky I 1985 Cryptotrauma and accident neurosis. British Journal of Psychiatry 147: 310–311

Pitman R K, Orr S P, Forgue D F 1987 Psychophysiologic assessment of post-traumatic stress disorder imagery in Vietnam combat veterans. Archives of General Psychiatry 44: 970–975

Pitman R K, Sparr L F, Saunders L S, McFarlane A C 1996 Legal Issues in Posttraumatic Stress Disorder in B A van der Kolk A C McFarlane L Weisaeth (eds) Traumatic Stress. New York: Guildford Press 378–397.

Resnick P J 1997 Malingering of Posttraumatic Disorders in R Rogers (ed) Clinical assessment of malingering and deception New York: Guildford Press

Robertson C 2000 What do patients want to know about trauma? Paper presented at Third World Conference for the International Society for Traumatic Stress Studies Melbourne March 2000 Book of Abstracts No 202

Rogers R 1997 Clinical assessment of malingering and deception. New York: Guildford Press

Schulberg H C, McClelland M, Burns B J 1987 Depression and physical illness: The prevalence causation and diagnosis of co-morbidity. Clinical Psychology Review 7: 145–167.

Shapiro F 1989 Efficacy of the eye-movement desensitisation procedure in the treatment of traumatic memories. Journal of Traumatic Stress 2: 199–223.

Siegel D 1997 Memory and trauma in Psychological Trauma – A Developmental Approach. Gaskell: The Royal College of Psychiatrists 44–54

Sutherland A G, Hutchison J D, Alexander D A 2000 It's not enough just to fix the fracture – The metabolic effects of post-traumatic psychopathology. Third World Conference for the International Society for Traumatic Stress Studies Melbourne March 2000 Book of Abstracts No.200

Tarsh M J, Royston C 1985 A follow-up study of accident neurosis. British Journal of Psychiatry 146: 18–25

Taylor A R 1967 Post-concussional sequelae. British Medical Journal 2: 67

Thompson G N 1965 Post-traumatic psychoneurosis – a statistical survey. American Journal of Psychiatry 121: 1043–1048

Trimble M R 1984 Post-traumatic neurosis. Wiley, Chichester

Turnbull G J, Busuttil W 1992 Debriefing of British prisoners of war and released Lebanon hostages during 1991. Paper presented at the World Congress of the International Society of Traumatic Stress Studies, Amsterdam, Proceedings

Turnbull G J 1994 Classification of PTSD. In: Black D, Newman M, Mezey G, Hendricks J H (eds) Psychological trauma: a developmental approach. Gaskell, London (in press), ch 4

Turnbull G J 1997a PTSD and chronic whiplash injury. Paper presented at Lyons Davidson International Conference on Whiplash Injury, Bristol, Proceedings

Turnbull G J 1997b Post-traumatic stress disorder: A psychiatrist's guide. Journal of Personal Injury Litigation, 4/97: 234–243

Turnbull G J 2000 Trauma to the mind Paper presented at Lyons Davidson International Conference on Whiplash Injury, Bath, Proceedings.

Ullman S E, Siegel J M 1996 Traumatic events and physical health in a community sample. Journal of Traumatic Stress 9: 703–720.

Van der Kolk B A, Greenberg M, Boyd H, Krystal J 1987 Inescapable shock, neurotransmitters, and addition to trauma: toward a psychobiology of post-traumatic stress. Biological Psychiatry 20: 314–325

Van der Kolk B A 1996 Trauma and memory in Traumatic Stress: The Effects of Overwhelming Experience on Mind, Body, and Society, chapter 12 (eds) B Van der Kolk A C McFarlane L Weisaeth The Guildford Press: New York London

Walker J L 1981 The psychological problem of the Vietnam veteran. Journal of the American Medical Association 246(7): 781–782

Weighill V E 1981 Compensation neurosis: a review of the literature. Journal of Psychosomatic Research 27: 97–104

White A C 1981 Psychiatric study of patients with severe burn injuries. British Medical Journal 284: 465–467

White A C, Armstrong D, Rowan D 1987 Compensation psychosis. British Journal of Psychiatry 150: 692–694

Woodyard J E 1980 Compensation claims and prognosis. Journal of Social and Occupational Medicine 30: 2–5

Woodyard J E 1982 Diagnosis and prognosis in compensation claims. Annals of the Royal College of Surgeons of England 64: 191–194

World Health Organisation 1992 The ICD-10 Classification of Mental and Behavioural Disorders: Clinical Descriptions and Diagnostic Guidelines. Geneva. WHO.

Chapter 27

Post-traumatic reflex sympathetic dystrophy

Roger M. Atkins

■ Introduction

Reflex sympathetic dystrophy (RSD) is a syndrome characterised by pain, autonomic dysfunction, oedema, joint stiffness and contracture. Because its features vary with aetiology and site affected, the condition has a number of synonyms. The International Association for the Study of Pain (1986) listed 67 different terms in the English, French and German literature. Mitchell et al (1864) noted the burning nature of the pain following nerve trauma and used the term *causalgia* (from Greek 'burning pain'). Südeck (1900, 1901) investigated conditions characterised by severe osteoporosis, including some cases of RSD, and the condition was named *Südeck's atrophy* by Nonne (1901). Leriche (1923, 1926) implicated the sympathetic nervous system in *post-traumatic osteoporosis* and De Takats introduced the term *reflex sympathetic dystrophy* in 1937. Homans (1940) proposed *minor causalgia* to imply a relationship between Mitchell's causalgia renamed *major causalgia*, and similar conditions arising without direct nerve injury. *Causalgic state* (De Takats 1945) and *mimo causalgia* (Patman et al 1973) followed to add to the confusion. Today the term *causalgia* is reserved for the original Mitchell use in which a nerve injury produces severe RSD associated with burning pain (Stanton-Hicks et al 1995).

Steinbrocker (1947) introduced the term *shoulder hand syndrome* for a condition which may be separate from true RSD and *algoneurodystrophy* was suggested by Glik & Helal (1976). *Algodystrophy*, from the Greek 'painful disuse', was introduced by French rheumatologists in the late 1960s.

Sympathetically maintained pain consists of pain, hyperpathia and allodynia which are relieved by selective sympathetic blockade. The relationship between RSD and sympathetically maintained pain is disputed (Stanton-Hicks et al 1995). In RSD a proportion of the pain is usually sympathetically maintained and is therefore relieved by sympathetic blockade. However, in RSD a process is also taking place which leads to initial tissue oedema followed by severe contracture. This is not an inevitable part of sympathetically maintained pain (Janig 1990). The term is now falling out of favour.

In an attempt to clarify the taxonomy of the bewildering array of different diagnoses, nomenclatures and syndromes, the International Association for the Study of Pain (1986) suggested that the generic term 'Complex Regional Pain Syndrome' (often referred to as CRPS) should be adopted. Complex Regional Pain Syndrome type 1 refers to straightforward RSD in all its manifestations while Complex Regional Pain Syndrome type 2 is reserved for all cases of RSD where there was definite damage to a peripheral nerve which is the cause of the syndrome.

Incidence

The classic teaching is that RSD is a very rare complication of trauma, occurring in only 1 in 2000 injuries involving an extremity (Plewes 1956). The full blown condition is certainly uncommon (Louyot et al 1967) and consequently the incidence is considered to be low in retrospective series (Bacorn & Kurtz 1953; Green & Gay 1956; Plewes 1956; Lidström 1959; Frykman 1967; Stewart et al 1985). However, prospective studies show that RSD occurs more commonly following fracture in a mild, sub-clinical form. Following tibial fracture and osteoporotic distal radial fracture, the incidence is 30% (Aubert 1980; Atkins et al 1989; Atkins et al 1990; Bickerstaff 1990; Sarangi et al 1993). The majority of these cases will resolve without specific treatment; however, some minor long-term sequelae which are usually sub-clinical are common (Field et al 1992; Field & Atkins 1997).

RSD may occur at any age but it is most common in middle-aged adults. It affects both sexes and all races but is more common in women (Wilder et al 1992). In children, the presentation and clinical course differ from that in adults (Wilder et al 1992). The condition may be more prevalent in the winter months (Aubert 1980).

Causation

The most common precipitating cause for RSD is trauma, which accounts for 30 to 77% of cases (Plewes 1956; Serre et al 1973; Schiano et al 1976; Doury et al 1981). The severity of the precipitating trauma varies from the very severe injuries described by Mitchell et al (1864), who studied sequelae of gunshot wounds in the American Civil War, to simple contusions (Serre et al 1973). The condition may be caused by the trauma of a surgical operation. Doury et al (1981), reviewing 132 post-traumatic cases, found that one-third were caused by bruising and sprains, while one-quarter followed fracture. Minor trauma therefore accounts for the majority of cases, although the condition is more prevalent after crushes and injuries which involve nerve damage (CRPS 2 in the new taxonomy). It has been suggested that the immobilisation which is a consequence of the trauma, rather than the trauma itself, may be the precipitating factor (Watson Jones 1952; Bernstein et al 1978; Serre et al 1973; Muller et al 1979; Fam & Stein 1981) and overvigorous rehabilitation has also been postulated (Savin 1974). The true situation is probably that the condition is a common but unpredictable result of trauma rather than of its treatment (Aubert 1980; Atkins et al 1989; Atkins et al 1990; Bickerstaff 1990; Sarangi et al 1993). Overvigorous mobilisation may prolong the disease and immobilisation will allow contractures to develop. However, it is not necessarily evidence of an unacceptable standard of surgical treatment for a patient to develop RSD.

Apart from trauma, reported causes of RSD include spinal cord disease (De Takats 1945; Evans 1947), nerve root irritation (Oppenheimer 1938; Rosen & Graham 1957; Drucker et al 1959; Serre et al 1973; Karlson et al 1977; Bernini & Simeone 1981), spinal anaesthesia (Drucker et al 1959), myelography (Moretton & Wilson 1971), cerebrovascular accidents (Moskowitz et al 1958; Eto et al 1980), subarachnoid haemorrhage (Rosen & Graham 1957), brain tumours (Walker et al 1983) and herpes zoster infection (Südeck 1901; Richardson 1954; Baer 1966). Upper limb RSD is classically associated with cardiac problems (Steinbrocker 1947; Froment et al 1956) and thrombosis (De Takats 1945).

Pathogenesis

RSD may be considered to be either an exaggerated response to a painful event affecting an extremity or an abnormality of the usual healing processes following injury. However, if trauma is the usual precipitating cause of RSD, it is not clear why one fracture should give rise to RSD while an identical injury in another patient or even in a different limb in the same patient does not. Following tibial fracture, the incidence is not significantly altered by the method of treatment and open anatomic reduction and rigid internal fixation do not abolish the condition (Sarangi et al 1993). Following distal radial fracture, quality of reduction does not seem to influence the incidence (Atkins et al 1990) and this series found no relation between the severity of the fracture and the incidence,

while others report that RSD is more common after more serious fractures (Bickerstaff 1990). There is an association between the application of an excessively tight plaster of Paris cast for a Colles' fracture and the subsequent development of RSD but it is not clear whether this is the cause of the RSD or merely a reflection of the swelling which is a feature of the condition (Field & Atkins 1994).

The pathogenesis of RSD probably contains two linked elements, one involving local tissues and the other, a central reflex. Local tissue effects of RSD have been difficult to investigate because of a lack of a large homogeneous population of patients with early RSD. It seems likely that after the initial tissue damage directly resulting from the injury, an imbalance in capillary homeostasis continues and is associated with increased pressure and exudation causing prolonged oedema. Local tissue anoxia follows, which stimulates afferent pain fibres and causes release of local mediators, maintaining the abnormal state (Ficat et al 1971; Ficat et al 1973; Renier et al 1973; Cooke & Ward 1990).

The abnormalities in sensory perception, such as allodynia and hyperpathia, are probably related to an abnormal difference in cutaneous sensory threshold between the affected and contralateral limbs and this sensitisation may be reversed by sympathetic blockade (Francini et al 1979; Procacci et al 1979). In addition, sympathetic activity can activate mechanoreceptors and peripheral nociceptors directly (Campbell et al 1988). It has been suggested that alpha-adrenergic receptors may become expressed on nociceptors following soft tissue or nerve injury and that these receptors can be directly activated by sympathetic discharge through the release of adrenaline.

Chronic irritation of a peripheral sensory nerve as a result of the initial trauma and subsequent soft tissue damage (Livingston 1943) could lead to a self-sustaining cycle producing increased afferent input and an abnormal level of activity in the internuncial neuronal pool of the spinal cord. This would lead to the continuous stimulation of sympathetic and motor efferent nerve fibres. Doupe et al (1944) suggested the development of an artificial synapse between sensory afferents and sympathetic efferents (an ephase), allowing a direct cross-stimulation and formation of the pain cycle.

Roberts (1986) has suggested that an initial painful stimulus activates unmyelinated nociceptors which leads to sensitisation of wide dynamic range (WDR) neurones in the dorsal horn. The sensitised neurones are further activated by low threshold mechanoreceptors, which explains allodynia. Low threshold mechanoreceptors can also be activated by sympathetic efferent activity and so a vicious cycle incorporating the central nervous system is set up. This concept is controversial (Schwartzman 1992). The gate control theory of pain transmission further developed the concept of a fine-tuning mechanism activated by cells in the substantia gelatinosa of the dorsal horn of the spinal cord (Melzak & Wall 1965). These cells can modulate the afferent impulses which are carried by small C-fibres and large A-fibres so that selective activation of the C-fibres inhibits the cells of the substantia gelatinosa and 'opens the gate' to pain transmission. A-fibre activity can stimulate the substantia gelatinosa to increase its inhibitory effect on pain transmission and 'close the gate'.

Some patients with RSD are undoubtedly emotionally labile and have a low threshold for pain (De Takats 1943). Pelissier et al (1981) and Subbarao & Stillwell (1981) noted a tendency towards hysterical or depressive neuroticism in RSD patients, although Vincent et al (1982) found no such abnormality. A number of authors have suggested that there is a psychogenic component to the pain of RSD (Bergan & Conn 1968; Wirth & Rutherford 1971; Hill 1980; Pack et al 1970; Lankford & Thompson 1977) and adult patients may require psychiatric help (Omer & Thomas 1971; Bernstein et al 1978). In contrast, such problems are rare in children (Wilder et al 1992). It must be remembered that these studies are investigating a chronic, painful and debilitating condition which may itself affect the patient's psychological balance.

Clinical features

The dominant feature of RSD is pain but the condition is very variable in presentation and clinical course and a description of a classical severe case will be given. The disease is most easily divided into two phases, the early phase which is dominated by vasomotor instability and swelling, and the late phase when joint contracture and atrophy of the affected part is the leading feature (Steinbrocker & Argyros 1958; Bonica 1979; Doury et al 1981; Wilson 1990). Some authors further subdivide the early phase according to whether the limb is predominantly vasodilated (Stage 1) or vasoconstricted (Stage 2).

The condition normally affects the periphery, usually hand or foot. The knee is being increasingly recognised (Katz & Hungerford 1987; Cooper et al 1989) but the elbow is normally spared even when the entire arm is affected. Involvement of the shoulder is common and it seems probable that at least some examples of frozen shoulder are true RSD, while the hip is rarely affected except in pregnancy.

The condition usually begins between a week to a month after the precipitating trauma. As the swelling and pain from the original injury begin to subside, a new pain begins which is more diffuse, particularly unpleasant and which does not follow a dermatomal distribution. Abnormalities of pain perception are extremely common and there is controversy as to whether these are an essential feature for the diagnosis (Merskey 1979). The most commonly described alterations are allodynia (pain provoked by stimuli which are not usually considered painful, such as gentle touch) and hyperpathia (a temporal and spatial summation of an allodynic response). Hyperalgesia (increased sensitivity to a noxious stimulus) and triggering (where a minor sensory stimulus to one small area causes unbearable pain) are common. The pain is often burning (causalgic), it is out of all proportion to the precipitating stimulus and the sufferers often state that it is simply the worst pain which they have ever experienced. In a severe case the phenomenon of sensory overflow occurs, where a cold draft, a loud noise or even an emotional stress will cause unbearable pain. The pain is unremitting (although sleep is often unaffected) and it becomes worse with proximal radiation as the condition progresses. Tenderness is universal and this is the basis of dolorimetry (Steinbrocker 1949; Hollander & Young 1963; McCarty et al 1965, McCarty et al 1968; Kozin et al 1976a; Atkins & Kanis 1989; Sarangi et al 1991), which may be used to quantify the severity of the condition.

Vasomotor instability and oedema are usually present from an early stage, although these features are less marked when the RSD affects more proximal parts of the limb. In classic descriptions, the vasomotor instability is initially of a vasodilated type, the limb being dry, hot and pink. Within a few days or weeks, however, the limb becomes vasoconstricted and appears blue and cold. At this stage there tends to be excessive sweating. During this early part of the condition, oedema is marked and loss of joint mobility is due to a combination of swelling and the fact that pain is exacerbated by movement of joints. As the condition progresses, the vasomotor instability tends to remit and the oedema resolves as the condition enters the late phase.

In the late phase of RSD, the entire limb is atrophic. The skin is thin with loss of the normal joint creases and the subcutaneous fat has disappeared. Hair growth is abnormal, with the hairs usually becoming fragile and of uneven width and curling. Occasionally, there is excessive growth of hair. The nails are also affected, becoming brittle and brown. Pits and ridges are common and the nail may occasionally become curved in any direction. Involvement of the palmar and plantar fascia causes thickening and contracture, giving rise to a condition similar to Dupuytren's disease.

Tendon sheaths become constricted leading to triggering and increased resistance to movement. Although the tendons themselves probably do not shorten significantly, muscle contracture combined with tendon adherence leads to a reduction of tendon excursion and fixed length phenomena are common. The joint capsules and collateral ligaments become shortened, thickened and adherent, leading to fixed joint contracture. These late physical changes are irreversible (Drucker et al 1959; Lankford & Thompson 1977).

RSD in children

Bernstein et al (1978) provided the first large, systematic report of RSD in children, describing the syndrome in 23 patients between the ages of 9 and 16 years, with a mean age of 12.4 years. Prior to 1978, few individual cases of RSD in children had been reported.

There are a number of differences between the condition in children and in adults. Children do not develop the severe disabling pain experienced by adults and trophic changes are rare. The characteristic radiographic changes seen in adults do not occur, and a much milder diffuse osteopenia is usually seen. Bone scan abnormalities may be minimal or absent. These differences probably relate to the differences in bone metabolism between children and adults rather than to a fundamental alteration of the process of RSD.

A high proportion of the children in Bernstein et al's 1978 series had a history of overt parental conflict (10 out of 12); a tendency to accept responsibility beyond their years was recognised in 11 of 13 children, and all showed a marked indifference to the implications of their illness for future functioning. Children seemed to be easier to treat than adults and responded to simple physical therapy methods. Similar findings were reported by Ruggeri et al (1982).

Investigations and differential diagnosis
Scintigraphic changes

Bone involvement is universal in RSD. In the early stage there is bone oedema, usually accompanied by an increase in blood flow although occasionally it is reduced. This is reflected by an increase in uptake on the early phase of the scan (Kozin et al 1981). Most characteristic is the increased uptake seen in the delayed scan. It used to be thought that the increased uptake was confined to the peri-articular regions (Kozin et al 1976b; Mackinnon & Holder 1984), suggesting that RSD was primarily a joint disease. However, quantitative examination of digitised scans shows that there is increased uptake throughout the affected region (Demangeat et al 1988; Atkins et al 1993). This increased uptake is not always seen in children.

Later in the condition, the bone scan returns to normal.

Radiographic changes

Patients with RSD develop a localised high-turnover osteoporosis due to increased osteoclastic resorption. This is partly stimulated by immobilisation and is dependent on the presence of an intact thyroid and parathyroid (McKay et al 1977). The osteoporosis may be generalised, but an X-ray appearance of small rounded areas of translucency up to 10 mm in diameter superimposed on the generalised reduction in bone density is more distinctive. Patchy osteoporosis, subchondral or subperiosteal enhancement of osteoporosis, metaphyseal banding and profound osteoporosis are all common (Genant et al 1975; Kozin et al 1976b). However, none of these appearances is diagnostic of RSD, they are simply features of rapid bone loss. Curiously, despite the severe bone loss, fracture through regions affected by RSD is very uncommon, presumably because the patient so effectively protects the limb because of the pain. The extent of osteoporosis may be quantitated using densitometry (Bickerstaff et al 1993).

RSD does not cause arthritis and joint space preservation is an important differentiation from early arthritis. Südeck's technique of radiographing the two hands or feet on one plate for comparison of bone density remains useful.

Other investigations

Reports of the appearances of RSD on MRI scanning are few and tend to be anecdotal. The changes seen early in the condition are those of bone and soft tissue oedema.

Thermography may help in the diagnosis of RSD (Uematsu et al 1981; Perelman et al 1987). Patients with RSD affecting the knee (Katz & Hungerford 1987) showed more than 1°C decrease in cutaneous temperature around the affected knee. Similar findings were described by Cooke et al (1993) in cases of upper limb RSD, while their studies also showed changes in microcirculatory velocity and volume, total limb blood flow and total digit flow. The same authors described paradoxical responses in symptomatic hands when the asymptomatic hand was subjected to a cold challenge by immersion in water at 20°C for 1 minute. Opinions are divided as to whether these investigations are of diagnostic use.

Synovial biopsy shows proliferation with non-specific subsynovial fibrosis which increases in the later stages (Ogilvie-Harris & Roscoe 1987). Bone biopsy (Basle et al 1983) shows alteration of medullary vascularity with reduced arteriolar flow, interstitial oedema and stasis. Osteocyte degeneration is seen with demineralisation of lamellar bone trabeculae. Massive and irregular osteoclastic bone resorption occurs with reactionary osteoblastic formation of new, irregular bone trabeculae.

The full blood count, erythrocyte sedmentation rate, viscosity and C reactive protein levels are normal as is the remainder of the serum biochemistry. The patient will be systemically well, usually without weight loss and general clinical examination is normal.

Sympathetic blockade has been regarded in the past as an essential diagnostic investigation by a number of authors (Toumey 1948; Patman et al 1973; Katz & Hungerford 1987). Regional sympathetic blockade of the stellate ganglion (upper limb) and lumbar sympathetic chain (lower limb) should produce relief of pain, albeit temporary, in patients with RSD. The results of such sympathetic blockade using local anaesthetic also have direct prognostic implications in respect of certain treatment methods which may be offered in cases which have been resistant to physiotherapeutic methods of treatment.

Clinical assessment

RSD is essentially a clinical diagnosis and there is no single diagnostic test. In a classic case there is all too little doubt as to the diagnosis. However, in a marginal case, the most common differential diagnosis is that of a swollen, tender limb. Direct effects of the original trauma, fracture, cellulitis, arthritis and malignancy are the most common alternative diagnoses and investigations will be directed towards the exclusion of these. By the use of clinical examination and the simple investigations of plain radiographs and bone scanning, it is usually possible to come to an objective opinion as to whether the patient is truly suffering from RSD and whether he is exaggerating his symptoms. However, there are pitfalls. A patient with RSD may very genuinely fear an episode of severe pain if he moves a joint. To some degree the pain is subconsciously reinforced, though, so that when a patient is distracted, he is able to move the limb more normally.

Many of the physical findings are relatively subjective, and in a medico-legal context it may be necessary to establish a patient's veracity. While it is easy for a patient to complain of unendurable pain, it is less common for an uninformed person accurately to mimic allodynia and hyperpathia. From a practical point of view, a patient who is experiencing severe allodynia and hyperpathia will usually be unable to bear clothes touching the affected part. It is simple for a patient to present with a limb which he refuses to move because of pain; however, RSD is an inevitably contracting condition and if the patient with the condition cannot move the limb, soft tissue and atrophy will occur. Their absence makes the diagnosis very

unlikely. Furthermore, in those patients with the condition who do not develop fixed contracture, the prognosis seems to be good for recovery. Although vasomotor instability and sweating may be variable, soft tissue atrophy and abnormalities of nail and hair growth are objective physical signs. In a clinically doubtful case, the finding of a normal bone scan, combined with complete absence of osteoporosis radiographically, all but rules out RSD in an adult.

Management

Severe, full blown RSD is rare and extremely difficult to treat; however, in the orthopaedic setting mild RSD is common, and although it may be self limiting it is painful and distressing. The majority of patients who develop RSD are sensible people who are extremely worried at the development of pain that they cannot understand; but the occasional patient who exhibits the 'Südecky' personality type will tend to have a poor prognosis and should be treated particularly vigorously. Injudicious surgery may make RSD far worse. Finally, the best results are obtained when the condition is treated early.

The key to successful management is to make the diagnosis early, treat the patient sympathetically and avoid surgery where possible, so it is necessary to keep a very high index of clinical suspicion concerning the diagnosis. It is not reprehensible to have caused a case of RSD through surgery. It is, however, unfortunate if diagnosis and subsequent treatment are delayed and such a delay may contribute to a poor outcome.

The first line treatment of RSD is reassurance, sympathetic physiotherapy and simple analgesia. Non-steroidal anti-inflammatory drugs appear to give better pain relief than opiates. The aim of these treatments is to maintain the range of joint movement so that when the condition has passed off there are no residual contractures. This will be sufficient in the large majority of cases. Immobilisation and splintage are generally best avoided. If used, joints must be placed in a safe position and splintage must be seen as a temporary pain-relieving adjunct to mobilisation.

Second line treatment is complex, controversial and often unsuccessful and many patients are left with pain and significant disability. At this stage a pain specialist should be involved and treatment should be continued on a shared basis. Treatment of RSD is bedevilled by anecdote and unsupported opinion and the situation is made worse by differing diagnostic criteria. The tendency for the condition to self-resolve in the early stages, a large placebo effect of treatment and the lack of universally accepted methods for quantification of the condition make it very difficult to assess the true efficacy of treatment. Indeed the very statement that early treatment gives optimal results may merely illustrate the tendency of early cases to resolve. The condition requires well-constructed prospective, randomised and blinded trials of treatment but unfortunately there are very few in the literature. Corticosteroids (Kozin et al 1981; Christensen et al 1982), regional local anaesthetic block with methylprednisolone (Poplawski et al 1983), calcitonin (Gobelet et al 1986; Bickerstaff & Kanis 1991), alpha-adrenergic blockade (Abram & Lightfoot 1981; Ghostine et al 1984), vasodilator therapy (Prough et al 1985; Moesker et al 1985), transcutaneous nerve stimulation (Kesler et al 1988) and acupuncture (Chan & Chow 1981; Fielka et al 1993) have all been reported to work in some cases.

Until recently, sympathetic blockade has been the mainstay of treatment for the intractable case although its efficacy is uncertain (Jadad et al 1995). The exact form of sympathetic interruption varies. Lumbar paravertebral blockade was effective compared to conservative management in a retrospective study (Wang et al 1985), and in the upper limb, intravenous guanethidine blockade has been compared successfully to stellate ganglion blockade (Bonelli et al 1983). The advantage of guanethidine blockade is that, although it requires careful supervision, it is easier to administer than paravertebral sympathetic blockade. Recently, however, it has been suggested that a significant part of the effect of guanethidine blockade is due to placebo and that it is ineffective and, indeed, that its use may prolong some features of the condition (Glynn et al 1981; Jadad et al 1995; Livingstone & Atkins 2001).

Epidural blockade has also been used, particularly in RSD of the knee (Cooper et al 1989). The combination of sympathetic blockade and analgesia allows mobilisation using continuous passive motion. However, Pountain et al (1993) found these treatments to be of little use in the chronic condition.

Recent therapeutic strategies have emphasised the use of centrally acting analgesic drugs, such as amitryptiline, carbamazepine and gabapentine, but once again there is a paucity of well-controlled studies.

The use of surgery to correct fixed contractures is controversial and uncommon, for it represents a painful stimulus and may exacerbate the condition or precipitate a new attack. This risk must be balanced against the proposed benefit very carefully. Contractures usually involve all of the soft tissues and surgical releases will need to be radical. Surgery should be delayed until the active phase of RSD has completely passed and ideally there should

be a gap of at least a year since the patient last experienced pain and swelling. The operation must be performed carefully with minimal trauma. Expectations must be limited and it is essential to provide adequate analgesia in the postoperative period, for which indwelling epidural catheters have been advocated. It has been suggested that any tendency of surgery to precipitate RSD can be minimised by a prophylactic lumbar sympathetic block or guanethidine.

■ References

Abram S E, Lightfoot R W 1981 Treatment of long-standing causalgia with prazosin. Regional Anaesthesia 6: 79–81

Atkins R M 1989 Algodystrophy. DM Thesis Oxford

Atkins R M, Kanis J A 1989 The use of dolorimetry in the assessment of post traumatic algodystrophy of the hand. British Journal of Rheumatology 28: 404–409

Atkins R M, Duckworth T, Kanis J A 1989 Algodystrophy following Colles' fracture. Journal of Hand Surgery 14B: 161–164

Atkins R M, Duckworth T, Kanis J A 1990 Features of algodystrophy following Colles' fracture. Journal of Bone and Joint Surgery 72B: 105–110

Atkins R M, Tindale W, Bickerstaff D, Kanis J A 1993 Quantitative bone scintigraphy in reflex sympathetic dystrophy. British Journal of Rheumatology 32: 41–45

Aubert P G 1980 Etude sur le risque algodystrophique. Thèse pour le doctorat en médecin diplome d' ètat. University of Paris, Val de Marne

Bacorn R W, Kurtz J F 1953 Colles' fracture: a study of 2000 cases from the New York State Workmen's Compensation Board. Journal of Bone and Joint Surgery (Am) 35A: 643–658

Baer R D 1966 Shoulder hand syndrome. Its recognition and management. South Medical Journal 59: 790–794

Basle M F, Rebel A, Renier J C 1983 Bone tissue in reflex sympathetic dystrophy syndrome. Sudeck's atrophy. Structural and ultrastructural studies. Metabolic Bone Disease and Related Research 4: 305–311

Bergan J J, Conn J 1968 Sympathectomy for pain relief. Medical Clinics of North America 52: 147–159

Bernini P M, Simeone F A 1981 Reflex sympathetic dystrophy associated with low lumbar disc herniation. Spine 6: 180–184

Bernstein B H, Singsen B H, Kent J J, Kornreich H, King K, Klix R, Hanson U 1978 Reflex neurovascular dystrophy in children. Journal of Paediatrics 93: 211–215

Bickerstaff D R 1990 The natural history of post traumatic algodystrophy. MD Thesis University of Sheffield

Bickerstaff D R, Kanis J A 1991 The use of nasal calcitonin in the treatment of post traumatic algodystrophy. British Journal of Rheumatology 30: 291–294

Bickerstaff D R, Charlesworth D, Kanis J A 1993 Changes in cortical and trabecular bone in algodystrophy. British Journal of Rheumatology 32: 46–51

Bonelli S, Conoscente F, Movilia P G, Restelli L, Francucci B, Grossi E 1983 Regional intravenous guanethidine vs. stellate ganglion block in reflex sympathetic dystrophies: a randomised trial. Pain 16: 297–307

Bonica J J 1979 Causalgia and other reflex sympathetic dystrophies. Advances in Pain Research and Therapy 3: 141–166

Campbell J N, Raga S N, Meyer R A 1988 Painful sequelae of nerve injury. In: Dubner R, Gebhart G F, Bond M R (eds) Proceedings of the 5th World Congress on Pain. Elsevier Science Publishers, Amsterdam, pp 135–143

Chan C S, Chow S P 1981 Electroacupuncture in the treatment of post-traumatic sympathetic dystrophy (Südeck's atrophy). British Journal of Anaesthesia 53: 899–901

Christensen K, Jensen E M, Noer I 1982 The reflex sympathetic dystrophy syndrome. Response to treatment with systemic corticosteroids. Acta Chirurgica Scandinavica 148: 653–655

Cooke E D, Ward C 1990 Vicious circles in reflex sympathetic dystrophy—a hypothesis: discussion paper. Journal of the Royal Society of Medicine 83: 96–99

Cooke E D, Steinberg M D, Pearson R M, Flemming C E, Toms S L, Elinsade J A 1993 Reflex sympathetic dystrophy and repetitive strain injury: Temperature and microcirculatory changes following mild cold stress. Journal of the Royal Society of Medicine 86: 690–693

Cooper D E, DeLe J C, Ramamurphy S 1989 Reflex sympathetic dystrophy of the knee. Treatment using epidural anaesthesia. Journal of Bone and Joint Surgery (Am) 71: 365–369

De Takats G 1937 Reflex dystrophy of the extremities. Archives of Surgery 34: 939–956

De Takats G 1943 The nature of painful vasodilatation in causalgic states. Archives of Neurology 53: 318–326

De Takats G 1945 Causalgic states in peace and war. JAMA 128: 699–704

Demangeat J, Constantinesco A, Brunot B, Foucher G, Farcot J 1988 Three-phase bone scanning in reflex sympathetic dystrophy of the hand. Journal of Nuclear Medicine 29: 26–32

Doupe J, Cullen C H, Chance G Q 1944 Post-traumatic pain and the causalgic syndrome. Journal of Neurology, Neurosurgery and Psychiatry 7: 33–48

Doury P, Dirheimer Y, Pattin S 1981 Algodystrophy: diagnosis and therapy of a frequent disease of the locomotor apparatus. Springer–Verlag, Berlin

Drucker W R, Hubay C A, Holden W D, Bucknovic J A 1959 Pathogenesis of post traumatic sympathetic dystrophy. American Journal of Surgery 97: 454–465

Eto F, Yoshikawa M, Ueda S, Hirai S 1980 Post hemiplegic shoulder hand syndrome with special reference to related cerebral localisation. Journal of American Geriatric Society 28: 13–17

Evans J A 1947 Reflex sympathetic dystrophy: report on 57 cases Annals of Internal Medicine 26. 417–426

Fam A G, Stein J 1981 Disappearance of chondrocalcinosis following reflex sympathetic dystrophy. Arthritis Rheumatology 24: 747–749

Ficat P, Allet J, Pujol M, Vidal R 1971 Traumatisme dystrophie reflexe et osteonecrose de la tête femorale. Annals Chirurgica 25: 911–917

Ficat P, Allet J, Lartigue G, Pujol M, Tramm A 1973 Algodystrophie reflexe post traumatique. Etude hemodynamique et anatomopathologique. Revue Chirurgie 59: 401–414

Field J, Atkins R M 1994 Algodystrophy following Colles' fracture is associated with secondary tightness of casts. Journal of Bone and Joint Surgery 76B: 901–905

Field J, Atkins R M 1997 Algodystrophy is an early complication of Colles' fracture. What are the implications? Journal of Hand Surgery 22B: 178–182

Field J, Warwick D, Bannister G C 1992 The features of algodystrophy 10 years after Colles' fracture. Journal of Hand Surgery 17B: 318–320

Fielka V, Resch K L, Ritter-Diuetrich D et al 1993 Acupuncture for reflex sympathetic dystrophy. Archives of International Medicine 82: 728–732

Francini F, Zoppi M, Maresca M, Procacci P 1979 Skin potential and EMG changes induced by electrical stimulation. 1. Normal man in arousing a non-enrousing environment. Applied Neurophysiology 42: 113–124

Froment D, Perrin A, Goni N A, Jandet R 1956 Periarthrites scapulo-humerales et autres manifestations neurotrophiques d' origine coronarienne. Troisieme Conference du Rhumatisme, Aix les Bains

Frykman G 1967 Fracture of the distal radius and its complications including the shoulder hand syndrome. Acta Orthopaedica Scandinavica (suppl) 108

Genant H, Kozin F, Bekerman C, McCarty D, Sims J 1975 The reflex sympathetic dystrophy syndrome. Radiology 117: 21–32

Ghostine S Y, Comair Y G, Turner D M, Kassell N F, Azar C G 1984 Phenoxybenzamine in the treatment of causalgia. Report of 40 cases. Journal of Neurosurgery 60: 1263–1268

Glik E N, Helal B 1976 Post traumatic neurodystrophy. Treatment by corticosteroids. Hand 8: 45–47

Glynn C J, Baselow R W, Walsh J A 1981 Pain relief following post ganglionic sympathetic blockade with intravenous guanethidine. British Journal of Anaesthesia 53: 1297–1301

Gobelet C, Meier J, Schaffner W, Bischol-Delaloye A, Gerster J, Burckhardt P 1986 Calcitonin and reflex sympathetic dystrophy syndrome. Clinical Rheumatology 5: 382–388

Green J T, Gay F H 1956 Colles' fracture residual disability. American Journal of Surgery 91: 636–642

Hill G J 1980 Outpatient surgery. W B Saunders and Co, Philadelphia, p 684

Hollander J L, Young D G 1963 The palpameter: an instrument for quantitation of joint tenderness. Arthritis Rheumatology 6: 277

Homans J 1940 Minor causalgia. A hyper aesthetic neurovascular syndrome. New England Journal of Medicine 222: 870–874

International Association for the Study of Pain 1986 Subcommittee on Taxonomy. Classification of chronic pain. Pain (suppl 3): 529

Jadad A R, Carroll D, Glynn C J, McQuay H J 1995 Intravenous regional sympathetic blockade for pain relief in reflex sympathetic dystrophy: A systematic review and a randomised, double-blind crossover study. Journal of Pain and Symptom Management 10: 13–20

Janig W 1990 The sympathetic nervous system in pain: Physiology and pathophysiology. In: Stanton-Hicks M (ed.) Pain in the sympathetic nervous system. Kluwer Academic Publishers, Massachussetts, pp 17–89

Karlson D H, Simon H, Wegner W 1977 Bone scanning in diagnosis of reflex sympathetic dystrophy secondary to herniated lumbar discs. Neurology 27: 791–793

Katz M M, Hungerford D S 1987 Reflex sympathetic dystrophy affecting the knee. Journal of Bone and Joint Surgery 69: 797–803

Kesler R W, Saulsbury F T, Miller L T, Rowlingson J C 1988 Reflex sympathetic dystrophy in children: treatment with transcutaneous electric nerve stimulation. Pediatrics 82: 728–732

Kleinert H E, Cole N M, Wayne L, Harvey R, Kutz J E 1972 Post-traumatic sympathetic dystrophy. Journal of Bone and Joint Surgery (AM) 54: 899–903

Kozin F, McCarty D J, Sims J, Genant H 1976a The reflex sympathetic dystrophy syndrome. I. Clinical and histological studies: evidence for bilaterality, response to corticisteroids, and articular involvement. American Journal of Medicine 60: 321–331

Kozin F, Genant H K, Bekerman C, McCarty D J 1976b The reflex sympathetic dystrophy syndrome. II. Roentgenographic and scintigraphic evidence of bilaterality and of periarticular accentuation. American Journal of Medicine 60: 332–338

Kozin F, Ryan L M, Carerra G F, Soin J S, Wortmann R L 1981 The reflex sympathetic dystrophy syndrome (RSDS); III. Scintigraphic studies, further evidence for the therapeutic efficacy of systemic corticosteroids and proposed diagnostic criteria. American Journal of Medicine 70: 23–30

Lankford L L, Thompson J E 1977 Reflex sympathetic dystrophy, upper and lower extremity. Diagnosis and management. C V Mosby, St Louis, pp 163–178

Leriche R 1923 Oedeme dur aigu post-traumatique de la main avec impotence fonctionelle complete. Transformation soudaine cinq heures après sympathectomie humerale. Lyon Chirurgica 20: 814–818

Leriche R 1926 Traitement par la sympathectomie periarterielle des osteoporoses traumatiques. Bulletin of Members of Society Chirurgica, 52: 247–251

Lidström A 1959 Fractures of the distal end of radius. A clinical and statistical study of end results. Acta Orthopaedica Scandinavica (suppl) 41

Livingston W K 1943 Pain mechanisms: a physiologic interpretation of causalgia and its related states. Macmillan, New York, p 212

Livingstone J, Atkins R M 2001 (in press). The treatment of algodystrophy of the hand with intravenous guanethidine blockade. A prospectively randomised double blind study. Journal of Bone and Joint Surgery

Louyot P, Gaucher A, Montet Y, Combebias J F 1967 Algodystrophie du membre inferior. Revue Rheumotologia Maladie Osteoarthritic 34: 733–737

Mackinnon S E, Holder L E 1984 The use of three phase radio nucleatide bone scanning in the diagnosis of reflex sympathetic dystrophy. Journal of Hand Surgery 9A; 556–563

McCarty D J, Gatter R A, Phelps P 1965 A dolorimeter for the quantification of articular tenderness. Arthritis Rheumatology 8: 551–559

McCarty D J, Gatter R A, Steele A O 1968 A 20 lb dolorimeter for quantitation of articular tenderness. Arthritis Rheumatology 11: 696–698

McKay N N S, Woodhouse N J Y, Clarke A K 1977 Post-traumatic reflex sympathetic dystrophy syndrome (Südeck's atrophy): effects of regional guanethidine infusion and salmon calcitonin. British Medical Journal 1: 1575–1576

Melzak R, Wall P D 1965 Pain mechanisms: a new theory. Science 150: 971–979

Merskey H 1979 Pain terms: A list with definitions and notes on usage. Pain 6: 249–252

Mitchell S W, Morehouse C R, Keen W W 1864 Gunshot wounds and other injuries of nerves. J B Lippincott, Philadelphia

Moesker A, Boersma F T, Scheijgrond H W, Cortvriendt W 1985 Treatment of post traumatic sympathetic dystrophy (Südeck's atrophy) with guanethidine and ketanserin. Pain Clinic 1: 171–176

Moretton L B, Wilson M 1971 Severe reflex algodystrophy (Südeck's atrophy) as a complication of mylography. Report of two cases. American Journal of Roentgenology 10: 156–158

Moskowitz E, Bishop H F, Pe H, Shibutlni K 1958 Post hemiplegic reflex sympathetic dystrophy. JAMA 167: 836–838

Muller M E, Allgower M, Schneider R, Willenegger H 1979 Manual of internal fixation. Techniques recommended by the AO group, 2nd edition

Nonne N 1901–1902 Über die Radiolographische nachweisbare akute und kronische 'Knochenatrophie' (Südeck bie Nerven-Erkrankungen). Fortschritte auf dem Gebiete der Rontgenstrahlen 5: 293–297

Ogilvie-Harris D J, Roscoe M 1987 Reflex Sympathetic dystrophy of the knee. Journal of Bone and Joint Surgery (Br) 69: 5, 804–806

Omer G, Thomas S 1971 Treatment of causalgia: review of cases at Brook General Hospital. Texas Medicine 67: 93–96

Oppenheimer A 1938 The swollen atrophic hand. Surgery Gynaecology and Obstetrics 67: 446–454

Pack T J, Martin G M, Magnus J L, Kavanaugh G J 1970 Reflex sympathetic dystrophy: Review of 140 cases. Minnesota Medicine 53: 507–512

Patman R D, Thompson J E, Persson A V 1973 Management of post traumatic pain syndromes. Report of 113 cases. American Journal of Surgery 177: 780–787

Pelissier J, Touchon J, Besset A, Chartier J, Blotman F, Baldy Molinier M, Simon L 1981. La personnalite du sujet souvrant d'algodystrophie sympathique reflexe. Etudes psychometrques par le test MMPI. Rheumatologie 23: 351–354

Perelman R B, Adler D, Hympreys M 1987 Reflex sympathetic dystrophy: electronic thermography as an aid to diagnosis. Orthopaedics Review 16: 53–58

Plewes L W 1956 Südek's atrophy of the hand. Journal of Bone and Joint Surgery 38B: 195–203

Poole C 1973 Colles' fracture. A prospective study of treatment. Journal of Bone and Joint Surgery 55B: 540–544

Poplawski Z J, Wiley A M, Murray J F 1983 Post-traumatic dystrophy of the extremities. A clinical review and trial of treatment. Journal of Bone and Joint Surgery 65A: 642–655

Pountain G D, Chard M D, Smith E M, Hazleman B L, Jenner J R, Hughes D L 1993 Comparison of guanethidine blocks and epidural analgesia in longstanding algodystrophy of the lower limb. British Journal of Rheumatology 32 S2: 53

Procacci P, Francini F, Maresca M, Zoppi M 1979 Skin potential and EMG changes induced by cutaneous electrical stimulation. 2. Subjects with reflex sympathetic dystrophies. Applied Neurophysiology 42: 125–134

Prough D S, McLeskey C H, Poehling C G et al 1985 Efficacy of oral nifedipine in the treatment of reflex sympathetic dystrophy. Anesthesiology 62: 796–799

Renier J C, Brugeon C A, Boasson M, Dillaber T C 1973 Algodystrophie du membres inferieur. Archives Medicin Oeust 3: 107–118

Richardson A T 1954 Shoulder hand syndrome following herpes zoster. American Journal of Physiologic Medicine 2: 132–134

Roberts W J 1986 A hypothesis on the physiological basis for causalgia and related pains. Pain 24: 297–311

Rosen P S, Graham W 1957 The shoulder hand syndrome: historical review with observations on 73 patients. Canadian Medical Association Journal 77: 86–91

Ruggeri S B, Athreya B H, Doughty R, Gregg J R, Das M M 1982 Reflex sympathetic dystrophy in children. Clinical Orthopaedics and Related Research 163: 225–230

Sarangi P, Ward A, Smith E J, Atkins R M 1991 The use of dolorimetry in the assessment of post traumatic algodystrophy of the foot. The Foot 1: 157–163

Sarangi P, Smith E J, Ward A, Atkins R M 1993 Algodystrophy and osteoporosis following Colles' fracture. Journal of Bone and Joint Surgery 75B: 833–834

Savin R 1974 La responsabilite de la re-education fonctionnelle dans le declenchenent des algodystrophie reflexes post-traumatiques des membres. Memoirs CES Rheumatologies, University of Paris

Schiano A, Eisinger J, Aquaviva P C 1976 Les algodystrophies. Laboratoire Armour-Montagu, Paris

Schwartzman R J 1992 Reflex sympathetic dystrophy and causalgia. Neurologic Clinic 10: 953–973

Serre H, Simon L, Claustre J, Sany J 1973 Formes cliniques des algodystrophies sympathetiques des membres inferieurs. Rheumatoligie (Aix les Bains) 23: 43–54

Stanton-Hicks M, Janig W, Hassenbusch S, Haddox J D, Boas R, Wilson P 1995 Reflex sympathetic dystrophy: changing and taxonomy. Pain 63: 127–133

Steinbrocker O 1947 Painful homolateral disability of the shoulder and hand with swelling and atrophy of the hand. American Journal of Medicine 6: 80–84

Steinbrocker O 1949 A simple pressure gauge for measured palpation in physical diagnosis and therapy. Archives of Physiologic Medicine 30: 289

Steinbrocker O, Argyros T G 1958 The shoulder hand syndrome: present status as a diagnostic and therapeutic entity. Medical Clinics of North America 42: 1533–1553

Stewart H D, Innes A R, Burke F D 1985 The hand complications of Colles' fractures. Journal of Hand Surgery 10B: 103–106

Subbarao J, Stillwell G K 1981 Reflex sympathetic dystrophy syndrome of the upper extremity: analysis of total outcome of management in 125 cases. Archives of Physiologic Medicine and Rehabilitation 62: 549–554

Südeck P 1901–1902 Reflektorische knochenatrophie. Fortschritte auf dem Gebiete der Rontgenstrahlen 5: 277–293

Südeck P, Über D 1900 Akute (reflektorische) knochenatrophie. Archive Klinische Chirurgie 762: 147–156

Toumey J W 1948 Occurrence and management of reflex sympathetic dystrophy (causalgia of the extremities). Journal of Bone and Joint Surgery 30: 883–894

Uematsu S, Hendler N, Hungerford D S, Long D, Ono N 1981 Thermography and electromyography in the differential diagnosis of chronic pain syndromes and reflex sympathetic dystrophy. Electromyography and Clinical Neurophysiology 21: 165–182

Vincent G, Ernst J, Henniaux M, Beaubigny M 1982 Essais d'aproche psychologique dans les algoneurodystrophies. Revue de Rhumatisme 49: 767–769

Walker J, Belsole R, Jermain B 1983 Shoulder hand syndrome in patients with intracranial neoplasms. Hand 15: 347–351

Wang J K, Johnson K A, Ilstrup D M 1985 Sympathetic blocks for reflex sympathetic dystrophy. Pain 23: 13–17

Watson Jones, Sir R 1952 Fractures and joint injuries. E S Livingstone, Edinburgh and London, 4th edition

Wilder R T, Berde C B, Wolohan M, Vieyra M A, Masek B J, Micheli L J 1992 Reflex sympathetic dystrophy in children. Journal of Bone and Joint Surgery (Am) 74A: 910–919

Wilson P R 1990 Sympathetically mediated pain: diagnosis, measurement, and efficacy of treatment. In: Stanton-Hicks M (ed.) Pain and the sympathetic nervous system. Kluwer Academic Publishers, Massachusetts, pp 90–123

Wirth F P, Rutherford R B 1971 A civilian experience with causalgia. Archives of Surgery 100: 633–638

Chapter 28

Recognised arm conditions and work

Tim R. C. Davis

To many workers with arm pain and men on the Clapham omnibus it seems obvious. If the pain came on at work, then the work caused the painful condition. Unfortunately, this logic is incorrect as most musculoskeletal pain due to chronic conditions usually first presents during a period of maximum activity, and for many people this occurs at work. If one first developed pain due to an osteoarthritic hip during a marathon, few would argue that the osteoarthritis was caused by the marathon. Although the term 'work-related upper limb disorders' (WRULD) is commonly used in legal circles, it is not found in standard medical and hand surgery textbooks and the conditions gathered under this label do not share a common pathology. Their only common feature is that they may all temporarily become more painful during or after use, whether at work or at home. For most it is not known whether use causes or worsens the underlying pathology, or simply aggravates the pain of the condition. Furthermore, it is not known whether their long-term prognoses are affected by continuing to work in the presence of pain. There is little benefit in grouping recognised arm conditions under the WRULD banner, which implies causation, but if a banner is required then 'use-related upper limb disorder' is surely more appropriate.

Standard medical textbooks frequently simply state the author's opinion on causation without any supporting references, and thus the medical expert must read the relevant published research in order to provide a considered opinion. This must be done with caution as the perfect study has not yet been written (Vender et al 1995), papers can be found to support almost any opinion and abstracts of papers often overstate their conclusions and can easily be misinterpreted. In order to interpret the results of epidemiological and other published studies correctly, it is vital to recognise their limitations, which include:

1. Most epidemiological studies of arm pain have a cross-sectional design and thus demonstrate only associations between work and disease. Such studies cannot tell whether a disease is caused by or aggravated by work, or whether an association is due to a predisposing factor which was not assessed (for example, age, sex or social class).

2. Cross-sectional epidemiological studies investigate survivor populations consisting of those who are sufficiently fit to remain in the workforce. If previous workers resigned because they suffered from the disease under investigation, then the study may fail to detect a work–disease association.

3. No study, however large, is capable of concluding that a particular condition is always, or is never, caused by work. An epidemiological study would have to be exceedingly large to demonstrate that a condition which commonly occurs in the general population, and is thought to develop spontaneously in most cases, may be caused by work practices in a few instances. Furthermore, if the disorder is caused by the combination of a number of factors (multifactorial), then only very large studies will be able to distinguish the relative importance of each factor.

4. Studies which fail to show an association between work and a particular arm pathology are useful only if they are sufficiently large to have a reasonable chance of demonstrating a positive result. For example, if a condition occurs in 5% of the general population and 10% of a workforce, all studies which recruit less than 440 workers and 440 controls will have less than 80% power. Such studies have an unacceptably high (greater than 20%) chance of failing to show a significant difference when in fact one does exist.

Epidemiological surveys of arm pain among the workforce are exceedingly difficult to perform. When assessing their results one must consider the following potential problems:

1. Did the study investigate symptoms or diseases? Although an arm condition of a particular pathological severity may produce only niggling pain at work in an office worker, it may be sufficiently painful to prevent a heavy manual labourer from working. Thus epidemiological surveys which study 'reported arm pain' or 'arm pain causing sick leave' (symptoms) usually demonstrate higher prevalences in heavy manual labourers than in office workers. If all of the study population is interviewed and examined, including those who have not complained of arm pain, this difference may disappear.

2. Are the diagnostic criteria used in the study acceptable (Davis 1998, Harrington et al 1998)? Frequently, the cause of arm pain is diagnosed from questionnaire responses. Although this may appear satisfactory for some diagnoses, Dimberg (1987) found that less than 50% of lateral elbow pain reported in a questionnaire was due to epicondylitis. If a study reports a disease prevalence rate which one considers surprisingly high then one should check that the diagnostic criteria were sufficiently rigorous.

3. How was a case of a disease defined? Frequently, the definition of a case of arm pain in epidemiological studies is that the pain was present for 1 week, or occurred once a month, during the past year. Thus many of the cases included in these studies may have been transient and relatively mild which is in complete contrast to the cases usually seen for medical reports. Can one extrapolate the findings for mild cases to severe cases?

4. Were individual conditions analysed separately or were they all lumped together (Silverstein et al 1987, English et al 1995)? Frequently, arm diagnoses are lumped together, often with a large group of 'tenosynovitis and peritendinitis', which in most studies is a misdiagnosis indicating the presence of forearm pain and tenderness. This lumping approach assumes that the effect of work, if any, on all the conditions is the same.

5. Was there a control group and was it of sufficient size and properly matched to the study group? The prevalences of most painful arm conditions is dependent on age and sex. Furthermore, pain is a subjective sensation and social and psychological factors undoubtedly alter its perceived intensity. For example, the term 'repetitive strain injury' ('RSI') may cause concern in a group of workers and the resultant anxiety may amplify the intensity of any arm pain which they experience. Thus the control and study groups should be matched for social and psychological, as well as demographic, parameters.

6. How was the work content assessed? Work content in many epidemiological surveys is deduced from the worker's job title, possibly with the addition of a few questions which enquire into the main work activities. Other studies use complex work content questionnaires but only infrequently are the work activities assessed first hand by the researchers (a costly process). Work is usually categorised according to its repetitiveness and forcefulness and other factors, such as vibration, are frequently not considered. Although the work practices of meat cutters in one pork processing plant may be associated with trigger digit (Moore & Garg 1994), this does not mean that all meat cutters are at risk of developing this condition—in other factories their work practices may be significantly different.

7. Were recreational and sporting activities and other possible causes or exacerbants of disease, such as smoking, assessed?

8. Is it certain that the symptoms first started after the onset of the work? As most epidemiological studies are of a cross-sectional design, this is not always easy to ascertain.

9. Do the results of one's favoured study concur with those of other studies? If not, are the other studies of a lesser quality?

The diagnosis

When one assesses someone for a medical report who has previously sustained a fracture or dislocation, there is usually little argument as to the diagnosis which is there for all to see on the X-rays which are routinely stored for several years. The situation is often very different with cases of arm pain alleged to have been caused by work. In such cases one has to rely on a careful history which is usually taken several years after the onset of the condition, and the contemporary GP notes which frequently simply state 'epicondylitis', 'tenosynovitis' or 'RSI', with no record of the clinical findings on which the 'diagnosis' was made. It is thus vital to obtain as good a history as possible of the presenting symptoms and the responses to standard treatments which are known to have high success rates. For example, if someone was diagnosed as suffering with De Quervain's disease or carpal tunnel syndrome but his condition did not even temporarily improve with steroid injections and was not helped by surgery, then one should question the original diagnosis. Furthermore, it is important not to develop tunnel vision and assume that the presumed diagnosis, which may have been made by a GP, hospital consultant, physiotherapist, trade union representative or the 'Claimant', is correct and simply ask questions about symptoms which one expects to be present and look for clinical signs which one expects to be present. If one does this with a person with diffuse arm pain of unknown origin in whom a diagnosis of epicondylitis has been made, one may obtain a good history and demonstrate all the relevant clinical signs of epicondylitis, but totally miss the fact that the patient is also troubled with other symptoms, such as shoulder/neck pain and hand tingling, and that other signs are present such as tenderness around other epicondyles and bony prominences and pain on resisted wrist and finger flexion, as well as on resisted wrist and finger extension. It is thus vital to enquire about symptoms which one does not expect to be present, as well as those which one does expect, and to examine the whole of both arms and record both the negative and positive findings.

One should always check the Claimant's history against the contemporary GP and hospital records to ensure that the arm condition did not develop before the work exposure which was thought to have caused the condition, and that the present condition is not just a recurrence of a pre-existing problem. One should also note the clinical findings at the time of onset of the problem (if any were recorded), which may be completely different to the present condition.

Diagnostic criteria

Not infrequently, the Plaintiff's and Defendant's medical experts fail to agree on the diagnosis, and this is often due to the interpretation of the clinical findings. If one presses hard enough one can always elicit tenderness over bony prominences such as the lateral epicondyle and radial styloid process, and pulling discomfort (rather than sharp pain) on the back of the thumb during resisted thumb extension or Finkelstein's test is often erroneously interpreted as demonstrating the presence of de Quervain's disease. Further problems arise as no test is entirely specific for a particular condition and false positives can occur with tests such as Phalen's and Tinel's. A recent meeting sponsored by the Health and Safety Executive suggested minimum diagnostic criteria (Table 28.1) for diagnosing disease in epidemiological studies (Davis 1998, Harrington et al 1998), and their use in medico-legal practice as minimal diagnostic criteria for ongoing disease would also be advantageous.

After review of the relevant notes and assessment of the patient one may either diagnose (on the 'balance of probability') a recognised arm condition which everyone agrees exists or feel unable to make a diagnosis. In addition, and in this author's biased opinion unwisely, one can make a controversial diagnosis such as 'RSI' or 'adverse mechanical tension', or inappropriately diagnose a condition such as 'tenosynovitis' even though the history and clinical findings are completely wrong for the condition.

Arm pain of unknown origin

In practice this can be localised pain with localised clinical signs, suggesting some underlying localised pathology which one is unable to diagnose, or more diffuse arm pain which is accompanied by diffuse 'soft' subjective clinical findings such as tenderness, though no hard clinical signs such as muscle-wasting or definite swelling. The cause of the diffuse arm pains remains uncertain, with some considering that the sufferers are malingerers and others considering that their pain has a strong psychological component and that the minor aches and pains of everyday life have been amplified by the fear that there is something seriously wrong, the possibility of compensation and/or misinformation provided by doctors, physiotherapists, ergonomists, newspapers or trade unions. Others still consider diffuse arm pains are due to physical disease which has been caused by work, and is due to a pathology which not everyone agrees exists. 'RSI' is one such 'condition/phenomenon' which was made popular in Australia during the 1980s, at a time when the country was suffering an epidemic of arm pain. This 'condition' was presumed to be caused by work and was compensatable, but was diagnosed by the presence of obscure arm pain without any hard clinical findings. Controversy still exists as to the nature of these diffuse arm pains, as well as their pathogenesis (do they develop spontaneously or as a result of work practices?), and all manner of underlying pathologies have been suggested. It has recently been proposed that they may be due to abnormal nerve function, possibly secondary to restricted nerve mobility ('adverse mechanical tension'), and there is no doubt that some non-specific diffuse arm pains can be reproduced by the upper limb equivalents of the sciatic stress test (Quintner 1989). One recent study has reported remarkably significant differences between the sensory vibration thresholds in the hands of 'RSI' sufferers, office workers and students, and concluded that these differences were attributable to office work which thus causes 'RSI' (Greening & Lynn 1998). Another study by the same workers has suggested that the median nerve is more constrained in the carpal tunnel in 'RSI' sufferers (labelled non-specific diffuse forearm pain in their study) than in controls (Greening et al 1999). However, these findings have not yet been confirmed by other workers, and the relevance and proposed pathomechanics of the observed differences are as yet unproven. Furthermore, any proposed causative link with any particular work practices remains hypothetical while the underlying pathological process causing the pain remains unknown. The fact that the pain develops or becomes worse at work, or with other use, does not demonstrate causation: if someone develops chest pain (angina) due to coronary artery disease when playing a round of golf, no one would suggest that the golf had

Table 28.1 Suggested minimum diagnostic criteria for upper limb disorders in epidemiological studies (Harrington et al 1998)

Carpal tunnel syndrome

Pain, paraesthesia or sensory loss in the median nerve distribution *and one of*
  Tinel's test positive
  Phalen's test positive
  Nocturnal exacerbation of symptoms
  Motor loss with wasting of abductor pollicis brevis
  Abnormal nerve conduction time

Tenosynovitis of the wrist

Pain on movement localised to the affected tendon sheaths at the wrist *and*
Reproduction of the pain by resisted active movement of the affected tendons with the forearm stabilised.

De Quervain's disease

Pain which is centred over the radial styloid *and*
Tender swelling of the first extensor compartment *and either*
  Pain reproduced by resisted thumb extension *or*
  Positive Finkelstein's test.

Lateral epicondylitis

Lateral epicondylar pain *and*
Epicondylar tenderness *and*
Pain on resisted extension of the wrist.

Shoulder capsulitis (frozen shoulder)

History of unilateral pain in the deltoid area *and*
Equal restriction of active and passive glenohumeral movement in a capsular pattern (external rotation > abduction > internal rotation)

Shoulder tendonitis

History of pain in the deltoid region *and*
Pain on one or more active movements:
  abduction for supraspinatus tendonitis
  external rotation for infraspinatus and teres minor tendonitis
  internal rotation for subscapularis tendonitis

Bicipital tendonitis should be considered with a history of anterior shoulder pain and pain on resisted active flexion of the elbow or supination of the forearm.

caused the coronary artery disease. It simply temporarily increased the demands on the heart and thus temporarily caused cardiac muscle ischemia due to the coronary artery disease which had been developing for years due to hereditary and environmental factors such as smoking. Furthermore, no doctor would then advise that all exercise be avoided, for fear that this might make the coronary artery disease worse.

Factitious injuries

A factitious injury is one in which the persistent clinical symptoms and signs (which can be most impressive) are self-induced as a result of psychological disease or malingering (Kasdan 1995). The 'sufferers', who may even request amputation of the 'diseased' arm, usually present with severe disability following a trivial injury, but occasionally with a possible work-induced condition. In the author's opinion, however, few, if any, 'RSI' sufferers are malingerers. Factitious injury must be considered when bizarre clinical signs are present, and are out of all proportion to the initiating injury/insult. Severe hand and forearm swelling can be produced by the application of a tourniquet to the upper arm, and swelling on the back of the hand (Secretan's disease) can be caused by repeatedly banging the involved area against a hard surface. Abnormal hand postures, such as the clenched fist position, are also a manifestation of factitious disease.

Proposing work causation

When writing a report, if one considers that a particular case of disease has been caused by work, it is wise to offer a proposed pathogenesis. Thus, if one considers that a case of De Quervain's disease has been caused by 'repetitive pinching at work', one should provide a reasonable explanation as to how this activity could have caused the first extensor compartment to become too small for the extensor pollicis brevis and abductor pollicis longus tendons, or how these tendons and the surrounding tenosynovium became too large for the first extensor compartment. To do this one must be aware of the pathological features of the condition.

Tenosynovitis and peritendinitis

These two conditions are frequently misdiagnosed and in many studies there is considerable doubt as to whether the investigators were actually studying tenosynovitis or forearm pain of uncertain origin (Viikari-Juntura 1983). Tenosynovitis is an inflammation of the synovial sheath surrounding tendons and thus can affect only tendons in regions where they are covered with tenosynovium. Thus tenosynovitis can affect:

1. The finger, thumb and wrist flexor tendons as they pass under or through the flexor retinaculum.
2. The finger, thumb and wrist extensor tendons as they pass under the extensor retinaculum.
3. The finger and thumb flexor tendons within the digital flexor sheaths.

Tenosynovitis presents as a localised painful swelling directly over the involved tendon. When the tendon is moved, crepitus may be detected and resisted contraction and passive stretching of the involved musculotendinous unit are painful.

The vast majority of cases of tenosynovitis seen in hand clinics are due to inflammatory arthropathies, but there are also occasional cases of localised hand tenosynovitis following an episode of unaccustomed activity. If there is no previous history of tenosynovitis or joint synovitis and no other evidence of musculoskeletal inflammation, it is reasonable to attribute such tenosynovitis to the unaccustomed use of the hand. Such 'work-related' tenosynovitis resolves quickly and only infrequently recurs on resumption of the initiating hand activity. It does not cause chronic pain or disability.

Peritendinitis crepitans (intersection syndrome) is a rare though well-defined condition which presents as a painful swelling on the dorsoradial aspect of the distal forearm, at the point where the abductor pollicis longus and extensor pollicis brevis tendons cross over the extensor carpi radialis brevis and longus tendons. There is a relatively well-accepted association between this condition and strenuous hand activity and it is not uncommon in oarsmen and canoeists. The condition has been well described in the car manufacturing industry (Thompson et al 1951) and was attributed to unaccustomed hand usage, return to work following a period of absence and direct blunt trauma to the distal forearm. The condition is said to be readily treatable and should not cause chronic disability.

De Quervain's disease

Although orthopaedic and hand surgery textbooks frequently state that this condition is obviously caused by unaccustomed repetitive use of the thumb, such statements are rarely supported with references and the situation is not so clear cut. However, it is generally agreed that De Quervain's disease sometimes develops following a direct blow to the radial border of the wrist, or as a complication of a wrist fracture.

De Quervain's disease is not a type of acute tenosynovitis and its pathology is identical to that of trigger finger, with glycose-aminoglycan infiltration and fibrocartilage transformation of the first extensor compartment (Clarke et al 1998). It is the author's opinion that De Quervain's disease is frequently incorrectly diagnosed. There should be a well-localised tender swelling over the radial styloid process, and resisted thumb extension and forced passive thumb flexion with wrist ulnar deviation (modified Finkelstein's test) should cause *sharp* pain and not just dorsal thumb discomfort. De Quervain's disease is much less common than basal thumb osteoarthritis epicondylitis and carpal tunnel syndrome, and one study detected no cases in 667 workers during a 30 month observation period (Kurppa et al 1991).

Two studies primarily concerned with the treatment of De Quervain's disease (Anderson et al 1991, Witt et al 1991) suggest that the condition is twice as common in females as males and that about two-thirds of cases occur in the dominant hand. It most commonly occurs between the ages of 40 and 50 years, although it can present throughout adulthood and a significant number of cases develop during and after pregnancy. Although neither of these two studies included a control population, occupational analysis of the 154 patients in both studies did not show any obvious associations with any particular employments and a third of cases occurred in housewives. In contrast another study (English et al 1995) has suggested that De Quervain's disease and other thumb conditions (trigger thumb, ganglia and basal thumb osteoarthritis) are more common in nurses, secretaries and assembly line workers and are associated with pinching, wrist flexion and extension and maintaining a bent thumb position at work. Unfortunately, the results of this study are difficult to interpret as the control group was poorly matched, and all the thumb conditions were analysed collectively (only 27 of the 69 thumb cases were De Quervain's disease).

Trigger finger

The pathology of trigger digit is identical to that of De Quervain's disease and it is at least twice as common in females as males. It can present throughout adulthood but most commonly occurs between the ages of 40 and 70 years, usually affecting either the thumb or the middle and ring fingers (Fauna et al 1989, Marks & Gunther 1989, Newport et al 1990). One study concerning the treatment of this condition found that most cases occurred in housewives, retired people and sedentary workers (Anderson & Kaye 1991), and a survey of patients with trigger digits in Nottingham has shown that their employment spectrum is similar to that of the general population (Trezies et al 1998). However, Moore & Garg (1994) demonstrated an association between trigger digit and meat-cutting. Although the results of this single study by no means prove that constant use of a knife at work can cause trigger finger, these data should not be immediately dismissed.

Dupuytren's disease

Dupuytren's disease is endemic within those of northern (and to a lesser extent eastern) European extraction. It is less common in those with Mediterranean, Japanese or American-Indian ancestry and rare in those of Chinese and Afro-Caribbean descent. The disease has a strong hereditary propensity and close relations of patients presenting with the condition frequently also have the disease (Ling 1963). Epilepsy, diabetes, high alcohol intake and smoking (Burge et al 1997) are predisposing factors for this disease, which can also affect the hands, feet and penis (Peyronie's disease). Dupuytren's disease is more common in men than women and occurs more frequently with increasing age.

Early (1962) collected data which suggest that Dupuytren's disease is equally common in office and manual workers and that the severity of the disease is not influenced by work (Table 28.2). Bennett (1982) subsequently challenged the validity of Early's work on the basis that his control group of office workers was predominantly female, but careful review of Early's paper suggests that this criticism is unfounded. Furthermore, Hueston (1963), a plastic surgeon with a particular interest in Dupuytren's disease, personally examined the hands of over 6000 people and found no association between occupation and Dupuytren's disease. In contrast, Mikkelsen (1978) considered that Dupuytren's disease was nearly three times as common in heavy manual workers who also developed more severe disease. Although Mikkelsen's study is large, the majority of his cases of Dupuytren's disease were mild and without contracture. It is not clear who examined the 17 000 pairs of hands included in this study and it is possible that manual workers' skin callosities were incorrectly diagnosed as early Dupuytren's disease.

There is no doubt that Dupuytren's disease can develop following a specific injury to the hand (penetrating wound, fracture, burn), or a fracture or dislocation of the ipsilateral wrist or arm. Two related studies (Kelly et al 1992, Stewart et al 1991) demonstrated that 8.5% of patients with Colles' fractures developed Duputyren's disease in the ipsilateral hand within 6 months of their

Table 28.2 Prevalence of Dupuytren's disease (percent) according to age and sex (Early 1962)

Age	15–24	25–34	35–44	45–54	55–64	65 –74	75+
Men	0.1	0.2	1.2	4.1	10.1	14.1	18.1
Women	0	0	0	0.5	1.4	6.2	9.0

injury. However, many of these patients subsequently developed Dupuytren's disease in the contralateral hand, which suggests that they would have developed Dupuytren's disease regardless of their injuries, although their injuries probably brought forward the clinical onset of this condition.

Carpal tunnel syndrome (CTS)

CTS is a common condition, with as many as 18% of the general population experiencing symptoms suggestive of this condition, and neurophysiological studies demonstrating a 7 to 16% prevalence rate for delayed median nerve conduction in the carpal tunnel (Ferry et al 1999). Prevalence rates of 9.2% and 0.6% for adult females and males respectively have been calculated in Belgium (De Krom et al 1992); however, most cases are probably very mild, and never sufficiently severe to warrant surgery, as the carpal tunnel decompression rates in Maine, USA, and the Trent region, UK, are only 144 per 100 000 per year and 55 per 100 000 per year respectively (Burke 2000). The age distribution of 508 consecutive patients undergoing carpal tunnel in CTS surgery at the Queens Medical Centre, Nottingham, is shown in Fig. 28.1.

Although CTS can be secondary to inflammation of the tenosynovium (tenosynovitis) in patients with rheumatoid arthritis or other inflammatory arthropathies, histological studies have demonstrated that the tenosynovium in CTS is only rarely inflamed (Neal et al 1987). Also, although some doctors consider that cases of CTS in workers may be secondary to work-induced tenosynovitis, the histopathology of the tenosynovium of the carpal tunnel in CTS is identical in workers and non-workers (houseminders and the unemployed) with myxoid degenerative changes and synovial oedema and fibrosis, and no

inflammation (Chell et al 1999). Interestingly, this small study also suggested that myxoid degeneration within the flexor retinaculum was more common in women performing 'high force' work.

The sensitivity and specificity of the clinical diagnostic criteria for CTS, including Phalen's and Tinel's tests, are disputed, and some workers consider that the diagnosis cannot be made without confirmatory nerve conduction studies (Nathan et al 1993). This opinion contrasts with the practice of many surgeons in the UK who usually diagnose CTS using only a careful history and examination. However, the exclusive use of clinical assessments in epidemiological field surveys is probably subject to errors, especially if clinical histories are obtained by questionnaire, and neurophysiological tests are probably beneficial although the definitions of 'normal' and 'abnormal' median nerve conduction in the carpal tunnel are disputed and the relationship between clinical CTS and median nerve slowing is not clear-cut.

Repetitive forceful use of the hand has been implicated as a potential cause of CTS. The definitions and methods of assessment of repetitiveness and forcefulness vary from study to study but Silverstein et al (1987) defined high-force tasks as those with an estimated average hand force of more than 4 kg. Highly repetitive tasks were defined as those with a cycle time of less than 30 seconds or 'with more than 50% of the cycle time involved in performing the same kind of fundamental cycles'. These authors (Silverstein et al 1987) performed a detailed ergonomic assessment of 652 workers and categorised their work into one of four groups, according to whether it required high or low hand force and had a high or low repetition rate. Of these workers, 2.1% had symptoms and signs consistent with CTS and the prevalence of this presumed syndrome was significantly associated with high-force/repetition work. However, no correlation was demonstrated between the prevalence of CTS and the position of the hand, wrist and thumb during work. Vibration was not specifically assessed in this study and many of the workers in the high-force/repetition group were also exposed to this factor which is thought to cause or aggravate CTS and cause other peripheral neuropathies. Furthermore, one cannot say whether the excess of presumed CTS was caused by the work, or whether the work simply exacerbated the condition in 'at risk' people. Silverstein et al's 1987 study is frequently criticised because CTS was diagnosed by clinical assessment and not nerve conduction studies. This is a reasonable criticism, as Nathan et al (1993) found that about 50% of the workers with numbness and tingling in the hand do not have nerve conduction evidence of CTS, but most would agree that it is

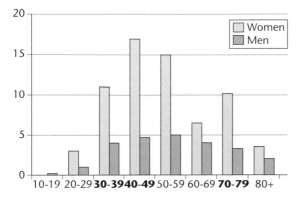

Fig. 28.1 Age/sex prevalence of carpal tunnel surgery patients.

possible to have intermittent symptoms of the syndrome with normal nerve conduction studies.

Nathan et al (1988) reported median nerve slowing within the carpal tunnel in 39% of 471 workers. Although the prevalence of this nerve conduction abnormality in workers (not hands) appeared to differ according to the forcefulness and repetitiveness of the work, the authors considered that their findings did not demonstrate any association between type of work and median nerve conduction abnormalities. This was because:

- There was no significant association between the prevalence of hands (not workers) with abnormal nerve conduction studies and type of work.
- Work requiring use of both hands was not associated with an increased prevalence of bilateral nerve conduction abnormalities.
- Duration of employment was not a predictor of abnormal nerve conduction studies.

Vibration was not assessed in Nathan's study and some workers with abnormal nerve conduction studies may have had no symptoms (Nathan et al 1993). Furthermore, as 39% of the study population demonstrated abnormal sensory median nerve conduction, one might wonder whether the reference normal range was correct. In a subsequent study (Nathan et al 1992), nerve conduction studies were repeated 5 years later in 316 of the original 471 workers, and the prevalence of sensory median nerve conduction abnormalities was found to be unchanged, and was positively associated with basal metabolic index (weight/height^2) and the wrist depth/width ratio. The authors concluded that the prevalence of CTS among these workers was predominantly determined by personal factors (age, obesity, smoking, basal metabolic rate) and not by type of work. Another study of median nerve conduction (Schottland et al 1991) also demonstrated that nerve conduction abnormalities correlate with age, and in addition found that they occurred equally often in new recruits as in established workers in the poultry-processing industry. Unfortunately, this study was statistically not particularly powerful, and another neurophysiological study has concluded that nerve conduction abnormalities are associated with repetitive work (Barnhart et al 1997), although their data analysis may have demonstrated improved ulnar nerve, rather than diminished median nerve, function. A further study has also concluded that nerve conduction abnormalities are associated with work factors (force and repetitiveness), and that personal factors (age, weight) accounted for only 8% of the abnormalities (Werner et al 1994). This contrasts with Nathan & Keniston's conclusion that 80% of nerve conduction variability could be explained by personal factors, and only 13% was attributable to work factors (Nathan & Keniston 1993).

The studies mentioned above all investigated manual workers and only a few papers have studied the prevalence of CTS in office workers. However, Hales et al (1994) found only clinical evidence of CTS in four of 517 (0.2%) predominantly female VDU workers.

Thus, the relationship between work and CTS remains controversial. Furthermore, if CTS is associated with particular work practices, it is impossible to state whether the work caused the CTS or exacerbated an asymptomatic CTS and brought forward the onset of symptoms in a person whose personal factors put him at risk of developing this condition. The Industrial Injuries Advisory Council (1992) reviewed the evidence regarding work causation of CTS in 1992 and concluded that there was insufficient evidence to classify it as a prescribed disease, unless there was a significant exposure to vibration. However, they felt that the possibility of work-causation could not be ruled out in all cases, and that each individual case should be considered on its merits. A unilateral case of CTS in a young slim male worker whose involved hand is regularly exposed to vibration is far more likely to be work-induced/exacerbated than a case of bilateral CTS in an overweight 40-year-old woman who works on a production line.

Hand/arm vibration syndrome (vibration white finger)

Lumberjacks, grinders, car mechanics, platers, road workers, welders and others who regularly use hand-held power tools are at risk of developing the hand-arm vibration syndrome (HAVS). Vibration can cause a vasospastic hand condition (20%), a peripheral neuropathy (48%) or a combination of both (32%). The delay (referred to as the latency period) between the start of the vibration exposure and the development of symptoms can be as short as six months or as long as 17 years, but the symptoms must develop during, or a few months after, the period when the sufferer was using vibrating tools (Ekenvall, 1987). Symptoms which develop more than a year after the cessation of the vibration exposure are probably due to other factors. Although it is widely accepted that vibration causes vascular and neurological damage to the hand, some wonder if the vascular component is as common and disabling as generally perceived, and whether the sensorineural component does indeed occur (Hadler, 1999).

The vasospastic condition presents as intermittent cold-induced skin blanching of the fingers which extends proximally from the finger-tips and has a well localised proximal border. The fingers involved should be those exposed to the most vibration. The attacks usually last for 20–60 minutes and are followed by a period of hyper-aemia which is characterised by finger redness and tingling which may be very painful. In contrast, the more common spontaneous Raynaud's phenomenon usually occurs in females, does not have a well-defined proximal border and is usually symmetrical and involves all the fingers. The vasospastic changes of HAVS were originally graded according to the Taylor and Pelmear Scale (Table 28.3).

However, they are now usually graded according to severity by the Stockholm classification (Gemne et al 1987) which is shown in Table 28.4.

Vibration can also damage peripheral nerves in the hand and cause finger paraesthesia and numbness and hand weakness and pain. The sensory symptoms are due to CTS in 25% of cases (Pelmear & Taylor 1994), but whether vibration causes the pathology of CTS to develop or aggravates a CTS which is developing for other reasons is uncertain. In the remaining 75% of cases the sensory symptoms are caused by vibration-induced digital nerve or skin sensory receptor damage (Rosen et al 1993); in severe cases this may cause permanent, disabling numbness and tingling. This vibration-induced neuropathy, which is often diffuse and frequently not localised to the median or ulnar nerve sensory territories, is graded as shown in Table 28.5 (Brammer et al 1987).

Fortunately, the results of carpal tunnel decompression in CTS associated with vibration exposure are good (Bostrom et al 1994), and the vasospastic symptoms are thought to subside gradually after prolonged (years) avoidance of vibration. The prognosis for the vibration-induced digital nerve/receptor damage is less certain, but cessation of vibration exposure should prevent deterioration.

Epicondylitis

Lateral and medial epicondylitis and rotator cuff tears have similar degenerative microscopic features (Chard et al 1994) and are not types of tenosynovitis. The characteristic features are of a non-inflammatory, myxoid degenerative process in which disorganised and immature collagen forms and immature fibroblastic and vascular elements are found. Acute inflammatory cells are almost always absent and chronic inflammatory cells are only occasionally scattered within the connective tissue. Thus the term epicondylitis is inappropriate and degenerative tendinosis of the common extensor/flexor origin might be more apt (Kraushaar & Nirschl 1999). The cause of the pain in this condition is unknown, although it is not due to inflammation and may be mediated by chemical factors.

Although it has been proposed that epicondylitis is caused by multiple 'microtraumatic' events, the link between 'repetitive trauma' and the histopathological changes of this condition has never been demonstrated

Table 28.3 Taylor and Pelmear scale of the stages of Raynaud's phenomenon in hand/arm vibration syndrome

Stage	Condition of digits	Work and social interference
0	No blanching of the digits	No complaints
0_T	Intermittent tingling	No interference with activities
0_N	Intermittent numbness	No interference with activities
1	Blanching of one or more fingertips with or without tingling and numbness	No interference with activities
2	Blanching of one or more fingertips with tingling and numbness. Usually confined to winter	Slight interference with home and social activities. No interference at work
3	Extensive blanching. Frequent episodes in summer as well as winter	Definite interference at work, at home and with social activities. Restriction of hobbies
4	Extensive blanching. Frequent episodes during the summer and winter	Occupation changed to avoid further vibration exposure because of severity of symptoms and signs

Table 28.4 The Stockholm classification of the vascular component of hand/arm vibration syndrome

Grade 1	Skin blanching distal to the distal interphalangeal joint
Grade 2	Skin blanching distal to the proximal interphalangeal joint
Grade 3	Skin blanching distal to the metacarpophalangeal joint
Grade 4	Skin blanching distal to the metacarpophalangeal joint and trophic skin changes

Table 28.5 The staging of vibration neuropathy of hand/arm vibration syndrome

Stage 1 (1SN)	Intermittent numbness, with or without tingling
Stage 2 (2SN)	Intermittent or persistent numbness, reduced sensory perception
Stage 3 (3SN)	Intermittent or persistent numbness, reduced tactile discrimination and/or manipulative dexterity

and remains hypothetical. Furthermore, although the presence of microscopic or macroscopic tears in the degenerate common extensor origin is considered by some to demonstrate that the condition arises as a result of overuse, such tears are by no means invariably present and are probably not the initiating factor in the pathological process. This is because such tears are most unlikely to cause myxoid degeneration in the surrounding tendon, and it is more likely that the tears (which may involve only collagen bundles and may only be seen with electron microscopy) occur as a secondary feature due to weakening of the common extensor origin as a result of pre-existing degenerative 'disease'. In other words, the presence of tears may simply reflect the fact that the 'diseased' common extensor origin is very weak and readily tears during daily life. Certainly, the evidence from population and work-force studies suggests that factors other than arm usage at work are important in the initiation of this widespread condition.

Epicondylitis is most common in the 40–50 age group where it has estimated prevalences of 10% in women and 3% in men (Allander et al 1974, Verhaar 1994), and its incidence in the UK has been estimated at 4.23/1000/year (Hamilton 1986). Questionnaire studies which do not include an additional clinical examination overestimate the prevalence of this epicondylitis (Dimberg 1987), while the use in other studies of localised epicondylar tenderness alone as the diagnostic criterion of the condition also produces errors, as this sign is open to considerable subjective and objective interpretation: if one presses hard enough one can always elicit tenderness. Better criteria are localised epicondylar pain and tenderness which is exacerbated by resisted wrist extension (lateral epicondylitis) or flexion (medial epicondylitis) (Harrington et al 1998). Furthermore, one should palpate both epicondyles and the decianon processes of both arms to confirm that the epicondylar tenderness is not diffuse as in 'fibromyalgia'.

Although epicondylitis is undoubtedly most troublesome to manual workers, this does not infer that their work has caused or worsened the prognosis of the epicondylitis, and studies of workers in the fish-processing (Chiang et al 1993, Ohlsson et al 1994), meat-processing (Viikari-Juntura et al 1991) and engineering (Dimberg 1987) industries have failed to show that the prevalence of this condition is determined by the type of work performed. In these studies the prevalence rates of epicondylitis among the workforce were 14.5% (Chiang et al 1993), 4% (Ohlsson et al 1994), 5.3% (Dimberg 1987) and 0.8% (Viikari-Juntura et al 1991). The Industrial Injuries Advisory Council (1992) reviewed the evidence regarding work causation of lateral and medial epicondylitis in 1992 and concluded that there was insufficient evidence for prescription of these disorders in relation to occupation.

Radial tunnel syndrome

Radial tunnel syndrome occurs as a result of compression of either the radial or the posterior interosseous nerve in the proximal forearm, and several structures have been implicated here (Roles & Maudsley 1972). There are no epidemiological data on this rare condition and its diagnostic criteria are not well established. Although it may cause proximal forearm pain during or after exertion, there is no scientific evidence to suggest that the pathology is caused by any particular work activity.

Ganglia

Ganglia are common and arise either from a joint (typically the wrist or distal interphalangeal joints) or the synovial lining of a tendon. They commonly become more pronounced and uncomfortable with activity but there is little to suggest that they develop as a result of particular work practices. Prevalence rates of 3% and 3.5% have been reported among office (Hales et al 1994) and slaughterhouse (Viikari-Juntura 1983) workers respectively. Though the majority of ganglia develop spontaneously, this author believes that some form following definite and significant wrist injuries.

Neck/shoulder problems

Neck and shoulder pain are very common among the general population and their prevalences increase with age (Allander et al 1974, Bovim et al 1994). The journals contain a large number of papers assessing ergonomic factors responsible for neck and shoulder pain at work but the vast majority study symptoms and not diseases. Many consider only transient neck/shoulder discomfort and thus their relevance to disease causation and aggravation is doubtful. Furthermore, analysis of those studies which do describe the nature of the pain suggests that the diagnosis in many instances is imprecise ('shoulder/neck pain of uncertain origin' or 'soft-tissue neck condition'). Recent work has focused on the effects of psychological and social, rather than ergonomic, factors on the prevalence of shoulder/neck pain and these appear important for both clerical and manual workers (Linton & Kamwendo 1989, Hales et al 1994, Pietri-Taleb et al 1994). Working with one's arms above head-height has been associated with an increased prevalence of shoulder pain but not with a specific disease.

Stenlund et al (1992) observed worryingly high rates of radiological acromioclavicular joint osteoarthritis among rockblasters (62%), bricklayers (59%) and foremen (36%). However, the severity of this osteoarthritis was the same in all three groups and advanced degenerative changes were never observed.

Rotator cuff disease is usually degenerate in nature and is found in 17% of cadaver shoulders under the age of 40, and in 40 to 50% of older specimens (Chard et al 1994). Herberts et al (1984) reported prevalences of 18% for welders and 2% for male clerks, while Stenlund et al

(1993) found evidence of this condition in 40% of rock-blasters and 8 to 17% of bricklayers and foremen. Ohlsson et al (1994) found prevalence rates of 27% and 8% among female fish-processors and female sedentary workers respectively. Hales et al (1994) recorded a 6% prevalence rate for rotator cuff disease amongst VDU workers and found no association with age, gender, recreational activities or keystroke rate. The unanswered question is, as always, does manual labour cause disease or aggravate pre-existing disease?

Summary

- The relationship between the causation, as opposed to aggravation of symptoms, of upper limb disorders and work is often uncertain. Much published literature on this subject is methodologically unsound.
- It is not always possible to diagnose the cause of arm pain, which is common in the general population.
- The report should provide a reasonable explanation of the pathogenesis of the condition if a positive association is claimed.
- True tenosynovitis can occasionally follow an episode of unaccustomed activity and invariably resolves quickly. Peritendinitis crepitans is often associated with strenuous hand activity but should not cause chronic disability.
- De Quervain's disease may follow a direct blow, but its association with particular employment or activities is uncertain.
- Trigger finger is commonly found in housewives and retired people.
- Dupuytren's disease may follow a specific injury to the hand, although the injury probably only brings forward the presentation of the condition.
- The relationship between work and CTS is controversial. Personal factors, such as age, sex and weight, must be considered.
- Workers who regularly use strongly vibrating power hand-tools are at risk of developing the hand-arm vibration syndrome.
- Studies have failed to show that the prevalence of epicondylitis is determined by the type of work performed.
- There is no scientific evidence to suggest that radial tunnel syndrome is caused by any particular work activity.
- There is an increased prevalence of shoulder pain associated with working with the arms above head-height, but it is not associated with a specific disease. Rotator cuff disease is usually degenerate in nature.

References

Allander E, Chard M D, Cawston T E 1974 Prevalence, incidence and remission rates of some common rheumatic diseases or syndromes. Rotator cuff degeneration and lateral epicondylitis: a comparative histological study. Scandinavian Journal of Rheumatology 53: 30–34

Anderson B C, Kaye S 1991 Treatment of flexor tenosynovitis of the hand ('trigger finger') with corticosteroids. Archives of Internal Medicine 151: 153–156

Anderson B C, Manthey R, Brouns M C 1991 Treatment of De Quervain's tenosynovitis with corticosteroids. Arthritis and Rheumatism 34: 793–798

Barnhart S, Demers P A, Miller M, Longstreth W T, Rosenstock L 1997 Carpal tunnel syndrome among ski manufacturing workers. Scandinavian Journal of Work and Environmental Health 17: 46–52

Bennett B 1982 Dupuytren's contracture in manual workers. British Journal of Industrial Medicine 39: 98–100

Bostrom L, Gothe C J, Hansson S, Lugnegard H, Nilsson B Y 1994 Surgical treatment of carpal tunnel syndrome in patients exposed to vibration from handheld tools. Scandinavian Journal of Plastic and Reconstructive Hand Surgery 28: 147–149

Bovim G, Schrader H, Sand T 1994 Neck pain in the general population. Spine 19: 1307–1309

Brammer A J, Taylor W, Lundborg G 1987 Sensorineural stages of the hand-arm vibration syndrome. Scandinavian Journal of Work and Environmental Health 13: 279–283

Burge P, Hoy G, Regan P, Milne R 1997 Smoking, alcohol and the risk of Dupuytren's contracture. Journal of Bone and Joint Surgery 79: 206–210

Burke F 2000 Carpal tunnel syndrome: reconciling 'demand management' with clinical need. Journal of Hand Surgery 25B

Chard M, Cawston T, Riley G, Gresham G, Hazleman B 1994 Rotator cuff degeneration and lateral epicondylitis: a comparative histological study. Annals of Rheumatic Diseases 53: 30–34

Chell J, Stevens A, Davis T R C 1999 Does work affect the histology of the tenosynovium in patients with carpal tunnel syndrome? Journal of Bone and Joint Surgery (in print)

Chiang H C, Ko Y C, Chen S S 1993 Prevalence of shoulder and upper-limb disorders among workers in the fish-processing industry. Scandinavian Journal of Work and Environmental Health 19: 125–131

Clarke M, Lyall H, Grant J, Matthewson M 1998 The histopathology of De Quervain's disease. Journal of Hand Surgery 23B: 732–734

Davis T 1998 Diagnostic criteria for upper limb disorders in epidemiological studies. Journal of Hand Surgery 23B: 567–569

De Krom M, Knipschild P G, Kester A D M et al 1992 Carpal tunnel syndrome: prevalence in the general population. Journal of Clinical Epidemiology 45: 373–376

Dimberg L 1987 The prevalence and causation of tennis elbow (lateral humeral epicondylitis) in a population of workers in an engineering industry. Ergonomics 30: 573–580

Early P F 1962 Population studies in Dupuytren's contracture. Journal of Bone and Joint Surgery 44B: 602–613

Ekenvall L 1987 Clinical assessment of suspected damage from hand-held vibrating tools. Scandinavian Journal of Work and Environmental Health 13: 271–274

English C J, MacLaren W M, Court-Brown C et al 1995 Relations between upper limb soft tissue disorders and repetitive movements at work. American Journal of Industrial Medicine 27: 75–90

Fauna P, Andersen H J, Siminsen O 1989 A long-term follow-up of the effect of repeated corticosteroid injections for stenosing tenovaginitis. Journal of Hand Surgery 14B: 242–243

Ferry S, Pritchard T, Keenan J, Croft P, Silman A 1999 Estimating the prevalence of delayed median nerve conduction in the general population. British Journal of Rheumatology 37: 630–635

Gemne G, Pyykko I, Taylor W, Pelmear P L 1987 The Stockholm Workshop scale for the classification of cold-induced Raynaud's phenomenon in the hand-arm vibration syndrome (revision of the Taylor–Pelmear scale). Scandinavian Journal of Work and Environmental Health 13: 275–278

Greening J, Lynn B 1998 Vibration sense in the upper limb in patients with repetitive strain injury and a group of at-risk office workers. International Archives of Occupational and Environmental Health 71: 29–34

Greening J, Smart S, Leary R 1999 Reduced movement of median nerve in carpal tunnel during wrist flexion in patients with non-specific arm pain. Lancet 354: 217–218

Hadler N 1999 Occupational musculoskeletal disorders: Lippincott Williams & Wilkins, Philadelphia

Hales T R, Sauter S L, Peterson M R 1994 Musculoskeletal disorders among visual display terminals in a telecommunications company. Ergonomics 37: 1603–1621

Hamilton P G 1986 The prevalence of humeral epicondylitis: a survey in general practice. Journal of the Royal College of General Practitioners 36: 464–465

Harrington J, Carter J, Birrell L, Gompertz D 1998 Surveillance case definitions for work related upper limb syndromes. Occupational and Environmental Medicine 55: 264–271

Herberts P, Kadefors R, Hogfors C, Sigholm G 1984 Shoulder pain and heavy manual work. Clinical Orthopaedics and Related Research 191: 166–178

Hueston J T 1963 Dupuytren's Contracture E. & S. Livingstone, Edinburgh and London

Industrial Injuries Advisory Council 1992 Work related upper limb disorders. Department of Social Security, London

Kasdan M 1995 Factitious injuries of the upper extremity. Journal of Hand Surgery 20A: S57–S60

Kelly S A, Burke F D, Elliot D 1992 Injury to the distal radius as a trigger to the onset of Dupuytren's disease. Journal of Hand Surgery 17B: 225–229

Kraushaar B, Nirschl R 1999 Tendinosis of the elbow (Tennis Elbow). Journal of Bone and Joint Surgery 81A: 259–278

Kurppa K, Viikari-Juntura E, Kuosma E, Huuskonen M P K 1991 Incidence of tenosynovitis or peritendinitis and epicondylitis in a meat-processing factory. Scandinavian Journal of Work and Environmental Health 17: 32–37

Ling R S M 1963 The genetic factor in Dupuytren's disease. Journal of Bone and Joint Surgery 45B: 709–718

Linton S J, Kamwendo K 1989 Risk factors in the psychosocial work environment for neck and shoulder pain in secretaries. Journal of Occupational Medicine 31: 609–613

Marks M R, Gunther S F 1989 Efficacy of cortisone injection in the treatment of trigger fingers and thumbs. Journal of Hand Surgery 14A: 722–727

Mikkelsen O A 1978 Dupuytren's disease—the influence of occupation and previous hand injuries. Hand 10: 1–8

Moore J S, Garg A 1994 Upper extremity disorders in a pork processing plant: relationship between job risk factors and morbidity. American Industrial Hygiene Association Journal 55: 703–715

Nathan P A, Keniston R C 1993 Carpal tunnel syndrome and its relation to general physical condition. Hand Clinics 9: 253–261

Nathan P A, Keniston R C, Meadows K D, Lockwood R S 1993 Predictive values of nerve conduction measurements at the carpal tunnel. Muscle and Nerve 16: 1377–1382

Nathan P A, Keniston R C, Myers L D, Meadows K D 1992 Obesity as a risk factor for slowing of sensory conduction of the median nerve in injury. Journal of Occupational Medicine 34: 379–383

Nathan P A, Meadows K D, Doyle L S 1988 Occupation as a risk factor for impaired sensory conduction of the median nerve at the carpal tunnel. Journal of Hand Surgery 13B: 167–170

Neal N C, McManners J, Stirling G A 1987 Pathology of the flexor sheath in the spontaneous carpal tunnel syndrome. Journal of Hand Surgery 12B: 229–232

Newport M L, Lane L B, Stuchin S A 1990 Treatment of trigger finger by steroid injection. Journal of Hand Surgery 15A: 748–750

Ohlsson K, Hansson G-A, Balogh I 1994 Disorders of the neck and upper limbs in women in the fish processing industry. Occupational and Environmental Medicine 51: 826–832.

Pelmear P L, Taylor W 1994 Carpal tunnel syndrome and hand-arm vibration syndrome. Archives of Neurology 51: 416–420

Pietri-Taleb F, Riihimaki H, Viikari-Juntura E, Linstrom K 1994 Longitudinal study on the role of personality characteristics and psychological distress in neck trouble among working men. Pain 58: 261–267

Quintner J L 1989 A study of upper limb pain and paraesthesiae following neck injury in motor vehicle accidents: assessment of the brachial plexus tension test of Elvey. British Journal of Rheumatology 28: 528–533

Roles N, Maudsley R 1972 Radial tunnel syndrome: resistant tennis elbow as a nerve entrapment. Journal of Bone and Joint Surgery 54B: 499–506

Rosen I, Stromberg T, Lundborg G 1993 Neurophysiological investigation of hands damaged by vibration: comparison with idiopathic carpal tunnel syndrome. Scandinavian Journal of Plastic and Reconstructive Hand Surgery 27: 209–216

Schottland J R, Kirschberg G J, Fillingim R, Davis V P, Hogg F 1991 Median nerve latencies in poultry processing workers: an approach to resolving the role of industrial cumulative 'trauma' in the development of carpal tunnel syndrome. Journal of Occupational Medicine 33: 627–631

Silverstein B, Fine L, Stetson D 1987 Hand-wrist disorders among investment casting plant workers. Journal of Hand Surgery 12A: 838–844

Silverstein B A, Fine L J, Armstrong T J 1987 Occupational factors and carpal tunnel syndrome. American Journal of Industrial Medicine 11: 343–358

Stenlund B, Goldie I, Hagberg M, Hogstedt C 1993 Shoulder tendinitis and its relation to heavy manual work and exposure to vibration. Scandinavian Journal of Work and Environmental Health 19: 43–49

Stenlund B, Goldie I, Hagberg M, Hogstedt C O M 1992 Radiographic osteoarthrosis in the acromioclavicular joint resulting from manual work or exposure to vibration. British Journal of Industrial Medicine 49: 588–593

Stewart H D, Innes A R, Burke F D 1991 The hand complications of Colles' fractures. Journal of Hand Surgery 10B: 103–107

Thompson A R, Plewes L W, Shaw E G 1951 Peritendinitis crepitans and simple tenosynovitis: a clinical study of 544 cases in industry. British Journal of Industrial Medicine 8: 150–160

Trezies A, Lyons A, Fielding K, Davies T R C 1998 Is occupation an aetiological factor in the development of trigger finger? Journal of Hand Surgery 23B: 539–540

Vender M I, Kasdan M L, Truppa K L 1995 Upper extremity disorders: a literature review to determine work-relatedness. Journal of Hand Surgery 20A: 534–541

Verhaar J A N 1994 Tennis elbow. Anatomical, epidemiological and therapeutic aspects. International Orthopaedics 18: 263–267

Viikari-Juntura E 1983 Neck and upper limb disorders among slaughterhouse workers. An epidemiological and clinical study. Scandinavian Journal of Work and Environmental Health 9: 283–290

Viikari-Juntura E, Kurppa K, Kuosma E 1991 Prevalence of epicondylitis and elbow pain in the meat-processing industry. Scandinavian Journal of Work and Environmental Health 17: 38–45

Werner R A, Albers J W, Franzblau A, Armstrong T J 1994 The relationship between body mass index and the diagnosis of carpal tunnel syndrome. Muscle and Nerve 17: 632–636

Witt J, Pess G, Gelberman R H 1991 Treatment of De Quervain tenosynovitis: a prospective study of the results of steroids and immobilisation in a splint. Journal of Bone and Joint Surgery 73A: 219–222

Radiology in medico-legal practice

David Wilson

Introduction

This chapter aims to help the reader to understand the significance of a radiology report as a crucial legal document in the absence of the images themselves. It also describes the layout of a radiology medico-legal report and details the background information that is required. Lastly, it covers technical issues relating to the value and reliability of each imaging technique.

In medico-legal cases radiographs (plain films) have an immediate attraction to clinicians and the legal profession in that they are a hard copy and permanent record of the state of the patient at the time of the examination. This can be a double-edged sword. Sometimes the images show a pre-existing disease, which may wrongly be attributed to the injury. Alternatively, an apparently normal examination may be wrongly considered to exclude significant disease should the practitioners overlook the deficiencies and blind areas of each imaging technique.

Ionising radiation

The National Radiation Protection Board and the Royal College of Radiologists strongly advise and require that radiation is used only when the potential benefits to the patient outweigh the disadvantages (RCR Working Party 1995). There are direct effects of radiation which are unlikely to be seen in routine practice. These are the results of direct cellular damage and include burning, cell death and necrosis. Much more significant is the risk of inducing malignancy, which is a matter of chance. Even a small quantity of radiation may induce a tumour. Strictly, there is no safe radiation dose. The dose limits imposed for radiation workers are intended to keep the statistical chance of induced neoplasm to a level equivalent to other risks in everyday life. There is no legal limitation to the amount of radiation that can be used for medical diagnostic purposes, hence the need to balance risk against potential clinical benefit. In general, it is unlikely that an examination using ionising radiation and prescribed for the sole purpose of medico-legal assessment would be regarded of sufficient benefit to the patient to outweigh these risks. If it is appropriate to perform an examination as part of the follow-up or ongoing care of the patient,

then it is entirely reasonable to use it for medico-legal purposes as well. These considerations apply even more strongly to nuclear medicine studies and CT where the radiation load is higher. The use of helical CT, although quicker, may increase the radiation dose to the patient and so should be used with utmost care. Arguably, ultrasound and MRI can be used with relative safety, as there are no known long-term toxic effects from either investigation. However, as these are relatively new procedures it is possible that as yet unknown long-term effects may result, so it is recommended that their use be kept to a minimum.

Contraindications to MRI

There are important and specific contraindications to MRI. Metallic bodies in the central nervous system (typically surgical clips), metal foreign bodies within the orbit, implanted pacemakers, implanted stimulation devices, certain types of prosthetic heart valve and certain older types of intrauterine contraceptive devices are all contraindications to MR scanning. The magnetic field could exert force on ferromagnetic objects which might cause damage if they are in delicate locations. Implanted joint replacements and fracture fixation devices are not usually a contraindication to MR, although they may degrade the quality of the study in areas close to the prosthesis or implant. Otherwise, as far as is known, MR examinations are unlikely to cause any permanent deleterious effects.

Film archives

The original radiological report is a 'legal document'. It is regarded as the essential permanent record of the examination; however, films and digitally stored images are usually kept for a number of years. It is expensive to file and retain images and by the time cases reach the stage of litigation it is common for the original image to have gone missing. Often the only evidence is the original written report. UK general hospitals generally retain films for 8 years, but some have a policy of recycling the films after 4 years. Exceptionally a permanent record is held, although this tends to occur only in smaller specialised units. Some hospitals store radiographs as a microfilm or 100 mm film archive. This is usually a permanent store, but the images are inevitably degraded. Optical disc archives are better but the digitising process still leads to some loss of detail. An image matrix of 4000 × 4000 pixels (dots on the image) is necessary to give reproduction indistinguishable from the original and many systems fall far short of this standard. Computer-generated images are stored without loss of detail and are usually a reliable record. Some practices ask patients to retain their own films. Unfortunately, the author's own experience has shown that the loss rate is worse than the most dilatory of records departments.

Films are routinely copied for the purpose of medico-legal reporting. However, this process may degrade the image quality and obliterate patient information such as the name or date of examination. Other patients' films may be included in the packet. For these reasons care should be taken in identifying the images and if there is doubt the original should be obtained. This is particularly important when an important decision is based on difficult or subtle changes on the images.

Format of the medico-legal report

Review reports of radiographic material should indicate by whom the report was prepared, at whose request it was written and the date that the films were performed and reviewed. There should be an initial statement that the author understands his duty to the Court ('As an expert witness I understand my duties to the Court and have complied with that duty.'). At the end of the report the author should state, 'I believe that the facts I have stated in this report are true and that the opinions I have expressed are correct', before signing and dating the document. It is wise to number each page and give an abbreviated title to the document on each page. In longer reports numbering of paragraphs may be useful. Material available at the time of reporting should be listed, including written medical reports, referral letters and previous radiographs. Note should be made of the annotation on the radiographs, particularly the location of the examination, the date and the patient's name. Care should be taken not to report images that have insufficient demographic information or where the detail is obscured by the copying process. Each film should be assessed for its technical adequacy. Under-penetrated films should not be relied upon as they may mask pathology. It is unwise to try and report ultrasound films performed by another examiner. Ultrasound is a hands-on technique and depends on the observer's overview of the moving images. Pictures are taken of representative sections but they do not reproduce the whole examination. The information on printed copies of MR and CT examinations may be incomplete, as the reporting radiologist will have had access to images on a workstation, providing a much wider range of data with the advantage of all potential window levels and 3D reconstruction. It may be necessary to go back to archived digital data if there are specific problems. Digitally stored images are often kept longer than plain films. They are normally held at the institution where the examination was performed. Different machines store the images in their own format and if the equipment has been replaced or upgraded it may be difficult to recall images. Older machines used tape storage that is not as reliable as an optical disc archive and may be difficult to read if the old machine has been removed. Sometimes the manufacturer may be able to convert old data to a readable media. No storage medium is entirely secure and most rely on the hard copy of the images as the permanent archive.

The abnormalities observed on the images should be recorded and their significance analysed in separate section.

In general, the report should be dispassionate and should address the questions posed in the letter of instruction. When there are alternative explanations these should be enumerated and compared. An opinion should be formed by the expert as to the likeliest conclusion based on a 'balance of probabilities'. Note that this test is not necessarily as precise as might be expected in clinical practice and merely represents an informed view.

The latest reforms in Civil Procedures require a strict and tight timetable for preparation and delivery of reports. The expert should undertake the work only if it can reasonably be presented within the deadlines that will be indicated in the letter of instruction.

Relationship to previous clinical material

Radiographs and other images should also be reported in the context of the clinical circumstances. Investigations should be designed to respond to particular clinical questions. Screening studies 'fishing' for any abnormalities are more likely to throw up confusing normal variants and signs of the ageing process that are difficult to judge out of the clinical context. Therefore, if a consultant radiologist is asked to comment on old or new examinations as part of a medico-legal presentation, it should be in the context of the history and clinical examinations. It is useful for the radiologist to have access to the preliminary medical report and it will improve the quality of the evidence if specific questions are placed at the time of examination or review. Reporting radiologists should declare what material has been available at the time of examination and should list current and previous images that are reviewed.

The absence of previous examinations that have been undertaken should be noted.

When the patient is examined, it may become apparent that other investigations have been performed which may be pertinent to your report. It is quite in order to ask to see these studies. Refusal by the patient or his solicitors of such a request may be important information itself.

Strengths and weaknesses of imaging
Plain radiographs

There is extensive experience in the use of plain radiographs in the diagnosis of trauma, degenerative disease and a wide variety of other conditions. The diagnosis of fractures, malalignment and osteoarthritis is well documented in standard texts and needs little further comment in this article. It should be noted there are significant weaknesses in plain radiographs as a diagnostic tool and the reporting clinician and radiologist should be aware of this.

Occult fractures

Plain radiographs cannot diagnose all fractures. The example of occult scaphoid injuries is typical, but there is also evidence that trabecular micro-fractures may lead to significant symptoms and disability, although they are often invisible on the initial examination. Plain films taken weeks or months later may show areas of sclerosis, but sometimes these signs are absent. The advent of modern imaging, in particular nuclear medicine and MRI, has confirmed that many bone injuries are not recognised on plain films. Despite this, significant malalignment should be apparent on a plain radiograph, provided the images cover the area affected and provide at least two projections taken at about 90° to each other. A single view may easily overlook important pathology including displaced fractures.

Plain films may also be used for signs of soft tissue injury. The presence of an effusion seen by displacement of fat planes, for example in the lateral radiographs of the elbow, is highly specific. However, care must be taken if in the painful elbow fat pad displacement is not seen because a true lateral could not be obtained. Soft tissue swelling and calcification may also be apparent. The examiner should be aware that despite these positive signs, normal radiographs do not in themselves exclude soft tissue injuries. For example, the majority of patients with internal derangement of the knee have normal plain radiographs and many patients with sciatica have a normal spine X-ray! All too often legal advisers assume that a normal radiograph excludes significant disease. Clinicians will be well aware that serious and sometimes life-threatening pathology may be hidden under a normal radiographic image.

Injuries to muscle, ligament, tendon insertion, articular cartilage, the brain, and thoracic and abdominal viscera cannot be excluded by plain radiography.

Ageing

Degenerative joint disease is a form of pathology but of course increases in frequency as each individual ages. Asymptomatic degenerative disease is common. All findings must be related to their clinical context. For example, 30% of normal asymptomatic adults aged 30 years have intervertebral disc prolapse that might be taken as an indication for surgery if they were also complaining of sciatica. An experienced radiologist should be able to advise whether the changes seen on imaging are merely in keeping with the patient's age. However, this will be a judgement based on examination of many cases and there are no firm measures of how much spondylosis or osteoarthritis is expected for a specified age. Injury to a joint may accelerate osteoarthritis, either locally or in adjacent joints that are loaded by an abnormal movement. If the changes are more severe in a limb or part of the body that has been affected by a previous injury than would be expected in a patient of that age, then it may be supposed that this is as a result of trauma. Plain radiographs and other imaging may also show osteoarthritis in early films taken at or near the time of injury. The signs would normally take many months to develop and therefore if they are present within a few days or weeks of an injury, it is unlikely that they are as a result of the incident in question.

Plain film signs of osteoarthritis are joint space narrowing, subchondral sclerosis, subchondral lucencies, marginal osteophytes, fragmentation of bony articular surface, loose bodies in the joint, and, eventually, malalignment of the joint surfaces. Note that joint space narrowing is the earliest sign. Subchondral sclerosis and lucencies follow. Osteophytes are a late sign of degenerative joint disease but the presence of marginal spurs alone does not confirm a diagnosis of osteoarthritis. Some individuals, particularly those with manual occupations, or those involved in regular sporting activity, may show traction spurs and prominent ligamentous insertions which do not represent osteoarthritis. On the other hand the absence of joint space narrowing, although useful in excluding a diagnosis of severe osteoarthritis, does not in itself exclude early fragmentation of the cartilage surface. The most powerful technique available is to study a series of plain radiographs taken over a period of months or years. Sometimes comparison with the opposite limb helps but this should not be regarded as routine.

Fragments of ossified material apparently in a joint may actually be in the soft tissues. Radiographs taken in isolation cannot confirm a loose body in the joint. Clinical signs, cross-sectional imaging and arthroscopy should be considered if the diagnosis of a loose fragment needs confirmation.

Healing

The age of a fracture can be judged by the extent and maturity of the healing process. The more complex the fracture the more slowly it is likely to heal and other delaying factors must be taken into account. The specific age of an injury can usually only be estimated at the best in weeks, months or years. It is rarely possible to place specific figures on this, although accuracy improves when a series of films are studied. Well-aligned fractures may heal without any residual scar. Several years down the line the radiographs can be surprisingly normal. A normal-looking bone may have been fractured in the past. The older the patient at the time of injury, the less likely it is that full repair and remodelling will occur. On the other hand, irregularity of trabecular pattern, cortical thickening and contour changes can be used as evidence of previous injury, but cannot necessarily date it in relation to the incident in question. In the child, assessment of fracture healing can give some idea of the age of injury and specific fractures can be highly suggestive of non-accidental injury (Rao & Carty 1999)

Variants

There are numerous normal variants, which are well recorded, in two major textbooks, Keats' Normal Variation and Kohler & Zimmer's Borderlines of Normal and Early Pathological Findings in Skeletal Radiography (Keats 1991, Kohler & Zimmer 1993). These textbooks cover the majority of variants; however, they are not comprehensive. Accessory ossicles will be well corticated and have smooth margins. They are easily confused with old avulsed fragments. Benign bone tumours, including fibrous cortical defects and enchondromas, are common and are usually of no clinical significance. If when these have been consulted and matters are still unresolved then and only then is it justified to consider further radiation exposure. This additional radiation burden could not be justified if the only indication were for medico-legal assessment without any potential clinical benefit.

Nuclear medicine

Scintigraphy provides valuable functional images but poor anatomic definition and weak specificity. Areas of increased activity imply disease of traumatic degenerative, inflammatory, infective or neoplastic nature. Nuclear medicine is rarely specific for one of these pathologies but correlation with clinical features and plain radiographs may lead to a firm diagnosis. Scintigraphy is more sensitive than plain radiographs to early arthropathy and is useful in the diagnosis of osteonecrosis and stress fractures. Nuclear medicine examination requires an intravenous injection with the introduction of a radiopharmaceutical and it is therefore an invasive test with a significant radiation burden. The same principles apply as to other tests involving a radiation dose.

Ultrasound

Ultrasound is used for the examination of soft tissues, particularly the abdominal viscera and muscle. In injury it may detect haematomas and partial muscle ruptures. Unfortunately, the technique is very observer dependent and the images are unlikely to be interpretable by another radiologist. For medico-legal purposes it is best to rely only on previously written reports. Comparison with the images taken at the time of the examination is unlikely to be contributory either to include or exclude additional features. There are no known contraindications to ultrasound examination and therefore it could appropriately be used as an additional examination to assist in the preparation of a report on causation or prognosis.

Magnetic resonance imaging

Like ultrasound, MRI is fortunate in having no known deleterious effects and therefore it is a technique that arguably can be employed in patients who require diagnosis for non-clinical purposes. It is particularly sensitive to intra-osseous and soft tissue disease and in many circumstances a normal MRI study will exclude significant pathology. As far as is known, MRI is the most sensitive technique for detecting stress fractures, micro-fractures and intra-articular disease. In joint injury, its one major weakness is that current standard imaging does not exclude early articular surface damage. In the diagnosis of chondral disease, arthroscopy is more sensitive. However, thinning, fragmentation and separation of fragments of articular cartilage may be detected with MR and it is certainly the most sensitive imaging technique for these diagnoses. Scars from previous fractures are visible within the trabecular bone as an area of reduced signal on all sequences. It is sometimes difficult to differentiate calcified areas from fibrotic tissue. A comparison with plain radiographs and CT will be necessary if it is important to make this distinction. MR is useful in the assessment of the growing epiphysis and may show bridging and tethering not seen on plain radiographs. It is highly sensitive to osteonecrosis and would be positive within 12 or 24 hours. The insult leaves residual changes, probably in perpetuity. Each MR examination is designed for a particular purpose and as much information as possible should be given to the examining radiologist prior to the procedure. An undirected examination could overlook significant disease. On the other hand, if the problem posed is the exclusion of a variety of conditions, then MR can be a very powerful test. Therefore, details of method and technique are important in judging whether the MR examination is adequate to answer the question posed.

The age of injuries may be judged by the presence or absence of oedema and haematoma. Swelling and oedema normally settle within weeks, or sometimes months, of an injury. It is rarely possible to be more specific than broad generalisations as to the date of the lesion. In particular, it is not possible to judge the age of a disc prolapse. An old prolapse may lead to persisting irritation with oedema, while a new injury may have associated congestion swelling or may show little in the way of associated abnormality, depending on the location and nature of the lesion.

Computed tomography

CT uses a substantial quantity of ionising radiation, limiting its application and restricting the size of the region that can safely be examined. It is useful in confirming or refuting diagnoses suspected on plain radiographs and in judging the extent and nature of a bony injury. It can image soft tissue, but compared to MRI it is less sensitive to ligament and muscle damage. CT is very useful in the diagnosis of intra-abdominal and intra-thoracic injury, especially to the soft tissue structures not imaged well by other techniques. A normal CT of the chest comes close to excluding any significant trauma.

Imaging advances

In the context of assessing a patient's imaging, it is important to consider the hospital where the images were obtained and the expertise available. It is all too easy for a specialist centre to conclude that the imaging that was performed in a less specialised department was inadequate. Realistically, the radiologist performing the imaging may be a generalist without the extensive knowledge of a particular diagnosis or may not have access to the latest technology.

One should also keep in mind the immense advances in technology over the last decade in all types of imaging. A patient may have had images that by today's standards appear archaic but which were state of the art several years ago. Always ask yourself the question; 'Were the images and reports previously obtained of acceptable standard for the institution and year that they were performed?'

Attending Court

It is wise to determine in advance how to address the members of the Court and to ensure timely presence. Many cases are settled in advance and often immediately prior to the hearing. The expert should be prepared to give advice to council during these negotiations. It is prudent to define fees based on attendance rather than the giving of evidence. Solicitors will be aware of the considerable demands on an expert's time but may not be able to give much notice of cancellation of booked attendance in Court. The fee structure should take this into account and it may be varied according to the notice given for cancellation.

The radiologist may be faced with particular difficulties in Court. It is essential that any expert witness should decline to make comment on areas outside his/her own area of expertise. A radiologist should defer all clinical issues to the appropriate expert. In general, he/she should comment on the indications for an imaging test, the performance and interpretation of the investigation, the quality of the study and the particular findings of those studies. It is also anticipated that the radiologist will be able to give advice on which other imaging investigations are appropriate, their potential for solving the problem and how urgently they should be arranged. The radiologist should resist being lured into opinions on prognosis, or the appropriateness or competence of treatment. To express a view on areas outside one's own expertise invites criticism of the opinions presented on areas where one is an expert.

In Court, the radiologist may be asked to demonstrate the findings on the original images. This presents particular difficulties as neither light boxes nor background lighting are likely to be suitable for optimum viewing. If a lesion is likely to be difficult to see in these circumstances then the expert's duty is to inform the Court of this problem.

Conclusion

Diagnostic imaging is a powerful tool that may be used in both the detection and the exclusion of trauma and injury. The particular pitfall which radiologists know but which Barristers frequently choose not to remember is that an apparently normal examination does not exclude the presence of pathology.

Ionising radiation should be used carefully and the examiner will be required to justify its use, given that the potential advantage to the patient should outweigh the risks.

Table 29.1   **Checklist for a radiological medical report**
Page numbers and headings
Statement
'I understand that my duty in writing this report is to help the Court on matters within my expertise. I understand that this duty overrides any obligation to the person from whom I receive instructions or by whom I am paid.'
Author's name, status and qualifications
Date of report
Subject of report
Report to whom (with his/her reference numbers)
Material available
List of documents
List of films with date, location taken, quality and findings
List of original reports that are available
Your interpretation of the images
What you cannot see on the images
Analysis of findings (list alternative hypotheses)
Opinion (answer the questions in your letter of instruction)
Statement
'I believe that the facts I have stated in this report are true and that the opinions I have expressed are correct.'
Signature

Summary

- In general, it is unlikely that an examination using ionising radiation and prescribed for the sole purpose of medico-legal assessment would be regarded as of sufficient benefit to the patient to outweigh the risks of the radiation.
- Screening studies 'fishing' for abnormality are more likely to throw up normal variants and signs of ageing that may confuse, rather than clarify, the issues in a medico-legal case.
- The major weakness of MRI in joint surgery is that current standard imaging sequences do not exclude early articular cartilage damage.
- It is not possible to judge the age of an intervertebral disc prolapse on MRI.
- An apparently normal imaging investigation does not exclude the presence of pathology.

▇ Acknowledgements

The author thanks Dr Gina Allen MRCGP MRCP FRCR and Mr Christopher Bulstrode MA FRCS for the advice that they gave during the preparation of this manuscript.

▇ References

Keats T E 1977 An atlas of normal developmental roentgen anatomy, 2nd ed. Year Book Medical Publishers

Keats T E 1991 Normal roentgen variants that may simulate disease, 5th ed. Year Book Medical Publishers

Rao P, Carty H 1999 Non-accidental injury: review of the radiology. Clinical Radiology Jan 54(1): 11–24

RCR Working Party 1995 Making the best use of a department of radiology, 3rd ed. Royal College of Radiologists, London

Schmidt X, Holthusen X (eds) 1993 Kohler & Zimmer's Borderlands of normal and early pathologic findings in skeletal radiography, 4th ed. Georg Thiem Verlag

Chapter

30

Vibration white finger

Jack Collin

Introduction

The hand-arm vibration syndrome comprises a collection of vascular and neurological symptoms, signs and pathological changes in the upper limb caused by exposure to injurious vibration. The vascular manifestations of the syndrome constitute the disease of vibration white finger.

- Vibration white finger has been a prescribed industrial disease in the UK since 1985.
- The local symptoms and signs of vibration white finger in an affected hand are in practice indistinguishable from those of other causes of Raynaud's syndrome. The condition can be classified as Raynaud's syndrome of occupational or environmental origin.
- The severity of symptoms and signs is related to individual susceptibility and the magnitude, wave frequency, impulsiveness and duration of vibration exposure.
- The key to diagnosis is a detailed occupational history of vibration exposure and its relationship to onset, severity and progression of symptoms. Other causes of Raynaud's syndrome and neurological symptoms should be excluded.
- The neurological symptoms and signs of hand arm vibration syndrome are contentious. They are commonly associated with vibration white finger but may occur independently and may progress at a different rate to the vascular disturbances.
- Diagnostic tests may be useful to provide objective confirmation of the existence of disease but do not establish its causation.
- The absence of objective physical signs on examination or failure to provide positive confirmation of disease by diagnostic testing does not overturn a diagnosis based on the clinical history of symptoms and their relationship to vibration exposure.

Raynaud's syndrome

The term Raynaud's syndrome is used to group together those conditions both known and unknown which have in common the occurrence of digital changes in colour and sensation known as Raynaud's phenomenon. Raynaud's disease is currently reserved as the name for Raynaud's syndrome of idiopathic origin and since the unknown causes of the syndrome are almost certainly numerous its use should be discarded.

The common causes of Raynaud's syndrome are shown in Table 30.1. The connective tissue disorders account for the majority of cases in which a definite diagnosis is established. Raynaud's syndrome is present in 95% of patients with scleroderma (Medsger 1985), and the syndrome may precede the onset of other manifestations of scleroderma by many years.

In patients with idiopathic Raynaud's syndrome and those with an underlying systemic disease, the symptoms are bilateral and symmetrical. Symptoms confined to one hand suggest a local cause such as thoracic outlet syndrome or atherosclerotic arterial occlusion. In patients with vibration white finger, only limbs exposed to vibration are affected and so in most patients one hand is predominantly or exclusively affected.

Symptoms and signs of vibration white finger

The majority of patients present for clinical examination many years after the onset of the first symptoms and at an advanced stage of the disease. They describe the episodic vascular symptoms and signs of Raynaud's phenomenon in one or both hands but not the feet. Episodes may be triggered by exposure to a vibration stimulus, cold temperature, a reduction in temperature or even normal ambient temperatures.

Raynaud's phenomenon is episodic blanching of the fingers and hands due to intense vasospasm of the digital and palmar arteries. If the vasospasm persists the hands may become cyanosed (purple in colour) as most of the oxygen is removed by the tissues of the hands from the little blood which is supplied to them. The episode terminates by the occurrence of intense reddening of the hands (reactive hyperaemia), often accompanied by pain and tingling. The severity of the reactive hyperaemia is greater when the vasospasm has been severe and prolonged since it is caused by marked dilatation of the capillary bed in response to tissue anoxia.

Table 30.1	Common causes of Raynaud's syndrome
Idiopathic	
Primary Raynaud's syndrome or Raynaud's 'disease'	
Connective tissue disorders	
Systemic sclerosis	
Systemic lupus erythematosus	
Rheumatoid disease	
The vasculitides	
Dermatomyositis	
Haematological disorders	
Polycythaemia	
Cryoglobulinaemia	
Cold agglutinins	
Arterial disease	
Atherosclerosis	
Thoracic outlet syndrome	
Buerger's disease	
Drugs	
Ergot and derivatives	
β-adrenergic blockers	
Occupational or environmental	
Vibration white finger	
Heavy metal poisoning	
Polyvinyl chloride	

In severe cases of vibration white finger there may be permanent changes in the tips of the fingers with reduction of the bulk of the finger pulp and spindling of the fingers. Eventually, in approximately 1% of cases there may be progression to digital gangrene, requiring amputation of one or more fingers (Yodaiken et al 1985).

The clinical condition of each hand can be classified according to the Stockholm workshop scale for cold-induced Raynaud's phenomenon in the hand-arm vibration syndrome (Gemne et al 1987).

Stage 1—Occasional attacks affecting only the tips of one or more fingers

Stage 2—Occasional attacks affecting distal and middle (rarely also proximal) phalanges of one or more fingers

Stage 3—Frequent attacks affecting all phalanges of most fingers

Stage 4—As for Stage 3 with trophic changes in the finger tips

Sensorineural symptoms

Original scales to classify the severity of symptoms in the hand-arm vibration syndrome were a hybrid of vascular and neurological components. It is now clear that the vascular component (vibration white finger) can develop independently of the neurological changes of the hand-arm vibration syndrome (Brammer et al 1987a). In addition, patients with no vasospastic symptoms but severe sensorineural impairment have been described (Brammer et al 1987b).

It is thought that the small unmyelinated nerve fibres that transmit pain and temperature sensations are most susceptible to damage by vibration. Reduced pain and temperature discrimination are likely to be the first neurological signs of the disease. In more severe cases tactile discrimination is impaired and there may be loss of manipulative dexterity. The sensorineural changes of the hand-arm vibration syndrome can be staged as follows (Brammer et al 1987):

Stage 1 (SN)—Intermittent numbness with or without tingling

Stage 2 (SN)—Intermittent or persistent numbness, reduced sensory perception

Stage 3 (SN)—Intermittent or persistent numbness, reduced tactile discrimination and/or manipulative dexterity

Occupational history

Careful recording of all occupational exposure to vibrating tools is essential. Many of the tools used in industry will be unknown to most doctors and lawyers and an explanation of their use and vibration characteristics should be elicited from the patient. For each tool the time of first use and the subsequent daily, weekly and annual duration of use should be recorded together with any protective measures taken or introduced.

The first occurrence of symptoms associated with vibration exposure should be noted. The progression and nature of the symptoms over time and with variations in vibration exposure should be established. The first occurrence and progression of symptoms precipitated by cold or not induced directly by vibration must be recorded. The occurrence of symptoms before occupational exposure to vibration suggests pre-existing Raynaud's syndrome and a non-occupational cause is likely.

The time from the start of the vibration exposure to the onset of symptoms varies depending on individual susceptibility and the nature and intensity of vibration exposure. Low frequency vibration produces most subjective discomfort, is generally thought to be more damaging and its importance is 'weighted' relative to high frequency vibration (Wasserman 1989). The resonance frequency of the hand and fingers is between 100 and 200 Hz, and at this frequency the amplitude of the induced oscillation is greatest and may exceed that of the source. Other characteristics of vibration relevant to the causation of vibration injury are its velocity, acceleration and displacement. The most that can be expected of the patient is for him to be able to say how 'strong' or 'severe' was the vibration transmitted by the tools of his trade.

Diagnostic tests

The main function of diagnostic investigations is to exclude other known causes of Raynaud's syndrome. The most useful clinical observation is whether the symptoms and signs are unilateral or bilateral.

If symptoms are exclusively or predominantly unilateral, primary Raynaud's syndrom and most causes of sec-

ondary Raynaud's syndrome can be confidently excluded. In such patients normal arterial pulses at the wrist, equal blood pressures measured in each arm and the absence of a cervical rib on radiography of the thoracic outlet largely exclude local atherosclerosis or thoracic outlet syndrome.

In patients with bilateral symptoms a history of bilateral vibration exposure is important to establish and if the symptoms are symmetrical the vibration exposure of each arm should be comparable. There is no infallible test for any of the connective tissue diseases but measurement of erythrocyte sedimentation rate (ESR) and serological tests for antinuclear antibodies, anticentromere antibodies, antineutrophil cytoplasmic antibodies (ANCA) and anticardiolipin antibodies are essential requirements for the diagnosis in the absence of clear-cut clinical manifestations of a specific connective tissue disease. Haemoglobin estimation and tests for cold agglutinins and cryoglobulin will exclude a haematological cause of Raynaud's syndrome.

Positive diagnostic tests
Cold provocation tests

Many variations of the cold provocation test have been described, including the skin temperature restitution test (Hack et al 1986) and the finger systolic pressure test (Olsen 1982). In its simplest form the hands are immersed in cold water at 10°C for 5 minutes and the colour of the fingers assessed by visual inspection on withdrawal (Pyykko et al 1986).

Ambient finger skin temperature test

The skin temperature of the fingers in patients with vibration white finger may be lower than normal. Smoking is prohibited for at least an hour before the test. The patient then stays in a room at 20–22°C for 30 minutes before the skin temperature on the back of the middle phalanx of the fingers is measured. A skin temperature below 26°C is abnormal (Matoba & Sakurai 1987).

Other tests described for objective demonstration of vascular manifestations of the hand-arm vibration syndrome include the nail compression test (Matoba & Sakurai 1987), capillaroscopy, (Vayssaorat et al 1987), laser Doppler velocimetry (Wollersheim et al 1989) and angiography. All the tests fall well short of 100% sensitivity and specificity and do not differentiate between the many causes of Raynaud's syndrome.

Pathogenesis and pathology

The pathogenesis of vibration-induced vascular and neurological changes is poorly understood. Most theories attribute the conditions to either central sympathetic hyperreactivity or local vascular changes. Vibration-exposed workers show differences in cardiac function (Bovenzi 1986) and other manifestations of central autonomic dysfunction (Miyashita et al 1982). Some pharmacological studies suggest that in patients with vibration white finger there may be a functional dominance of alpha 2 over alpha 1 adrenoceptors.

Some patients with vibration white finger have a reduced number of finger nailfold capillaries (Vayssaorat et al 1987) and hypertrophy of vascular smooth muscle may occur in the digital arteries and arterioles (Takeuchi et al 1986). The smooth muscle hypertrophy may be a response to prolonged vasoconstriction and eventually may progress to arterial occlusion with the development of digital gangrene.

The neuropathy of hand-arm vibration syndrome appears to occur in two phases. First there is the occurrence of reversible neural oedema after which secondary irreversible destruction of the myelin sheaths and axons occurs (Brammer & Pyykko 1987).

Treatment and prognosis

Vibration exposure should stop or if this is not possible should be reduced to a minimum. Tobacco smoking should stop since it exacerbates digital vasospasm and is the most important cause of peripheral arterial occlusive disease, the co-existence of which will worsen the prognosis for ischaemic fingers. Avoidance of cold and wet conditions will decrease the number and severity of episodes of digital vasospasm. The patient's core temperature should be maintained by wearing warm clothing outdoors and by ambient temperature control indoors. The hands should be protected from exposure to cold and dampness by wearing sheepskin mittens which provide more effective finger insulation than gloves. In severe cases battery-heated mittens may be required.

There is no specific pharmacological treatment that is generally effective but some patients obtain relief from calcium channel blockers such as nifedipine. It is essential to use a long-acting formulation of the drug such as Adalat Retard® and side effects can be minimised by commencing the drug in low dosage with the first few administrations being taken before retiring to bed at night. Alternative drugs worth trying if nifedipine proves to be ineffective are the 5-hydroxytryptamine antagonist katanserin or the angiotensin-converting enzyme inhibitor captopril. It may be worthwhile trying one or more of these preparations consecutively in individual patients but none should be persisted with unless benefits convincingly outweigh side effects of the drug.

In most patients with vibration white finger of mild to moderate severity progression of the disease will be prevented by cessation of exposure to further vibration injury. In patients with severe disease the condition may continue to worsen despite the removal of the initiating cause and they may progress to digital gangrene and amputation.

Prevention

Employers owe their employees working with vibrating tools a duty of care which extends to education in the risks of vibration exposure and instruction in methods of prevention of vibration injury.

Tool provision and maintenance

The design of many vibrating tools has been progressively improved to reduce their weight and the amount of vibration transmitted to the operator. Old and particularly poorly maintained tools are generally a greater hazard than new tools. Heavier tools require a greater grip strength to operate and consequently transmit more vibration to the operator.

Gloves and grip force

Instructing workers to hold the vibrating tool loosely and providing antivibration gloves can reduce the amount of vibration injury. Neither of these measures is popular since they reduce both the manipulability and control of the tool. Low grip force maintains joint elasticity and reduces vibration transmission up the arm. Protective gloves act both as shock absorbers and to reduce co-existent cold-induced vasospasm.

Duration of vibration exposure

The most important preventive measure is to restrict the duration and concentration of exposure to the vibrating tool. Table 31.2 shows the restrictions imposed on chain saw use in the State forests of Japan (Saito 1987). No such restrictions have been imposed in British industry but the existence of such restrictions in another major industrial nation sets a standard for care of which a responsible employer should be cognisant.

United Kingdom disablement benefit

It was first proposed that vibration white finger should be prescribed as an Industrial Disease in 1950 but government reports in 1954, 1970, 1975 and 1981 recommended against such action: 'A condition which will give rise to a large number of claims of which the great majority will have to be disallowed either because the disablement was so trivial or because of the difficulty of distinguishing

Table 30.2 Restrictions on the operating time of chain saws in the State forests of Japan

	Maximum	Minimum
One operating cycle	10 mins	
Operating time per day	2 hours	
Consecutive operating days	2 days	
Operating days per week	4 days	
Operating hours per month	32 hours	
Operating days per year	120 days	
Non-operating period each year		2 months

Table 30.3 Prescribed Industrial Disease A11, vibration white finger (DSS 1989)

Episodic blanching occurs throughout the year, affecting the middle or proximal phalanges, or in the case of the thumb the proximal phalanx of:

- In the case of a person with five fingers (including thumb) on one hand, any three of those fingers
- In the case of a person with only four such fingers, any 2nd of those fingers
- In the case of a person with less than four such fingers, any one of those fingers or, as the case may be, the one remaining finger

between occupational and non-occupational cases'. In 1985 vibration white finger became prescribed Industrial Disease number A11 (Taylor 1985; Table 31.3).

Contributory negligence and causation

Two issues can reasonably be raised by the defence in an action alleging negligence by an employer: namely, the use of vibrating tools outside the Defendant's employment, and cigarette smoking by the Plaintiff.

Many workmen who use vibrating tools frequently change employers during their career and often are self-employed for varying periods. In addition, power tools in regular use at home for DIY work may contribute substantially to total exposure to injurious vibration. A careful work and recreational activity history is essential if fair apportionment of exposure times is to be achieved.

Cigarette smoking, although not directly involved in the production of vibration vascular or sensorineural injuries, is likely to be a significant contributory factor. Tobacco smoking is the most important cause of peripheral arterial occlusive disease, and for patients in whom other causes such as diabetes mellitus or hypercholesterolaemia predominate smoking substantially worsens the prognosis. Buerger's disease, a rare form of early onset occlusion of small arteries resulting in digital gangrene, is believed to be caused by an idiosyncratic susceptibility to

smoking induced vascular injury. Buerger's disease may be clinically indistinguishable from severe vibration white finger.

In addition to causing accelerated onset atherosclerosis, tobacco smoking causes acute digital vasospasm which may compound vasospasm induced by vibration. Chronic smoking by binding around 10% of available haemoglobin with high-affinity carbon monoxide is liable to induce secondary polycythaemia. Both polycythaemia and the hyperfibrinogenaemia usually present in smokers increase blood viscosity and reduce blood flow and oxygen delivery to the tissues.

■ References

Bovenzi M 1986 Some pathophysiological aspects of vibration induced white finger. European Journal of Applied Physiology 55: 381–389

Brammer A J, Piercy J E, Auger P L 1987a Sensorineural stages of the hand-arm vibration syndrome. Scandinavian Journal of Work and Environmental Health 13: 279–283

Brammer A J, Piercy J E, Auger P L 1987b Assessment of impaired tactile sensation: A pilot study. Scandinavian Journal of Work and Environmental Health 13: 380–384

Brammer A J, Pyykko I 1987 Vibration induced neuropathy detection by nerve conduction measurements. Scandinavian Journal of Work and Environmental Health 13: 317–322

Department of Social Security If you have an industrial disease. Aug 1989 N12,

Gemne G, Pyykko I, Taylor W, Pelmear P L 1987 The Stockholm Workshop Scale for the classification of cold induced Raynaud's phenomenon in the hand-arm vibration syndrome (revision of the Taylor–Pelmear scale). Scandinavian Journal of Work and Environmental Health 13: 275–278

Hack M, Boilat M A, Schweizer C, Lob M 1986 Assessment of vibration-induced white finger: Reliability and validity of two tests. British Journal of Independent Medicine 43: 284–287

Matoba T, Sakurai T 1987 Physiological methods used in Japan for the diagnosis of suspected hand-arm vibration syndrome. Scandinavian Journal of Work and Environmental Health 13: 334–336

Medsger T A 1985 Systemic sclerosis (scleroderma), eosinophilic fasciitis and calcinosis. In: McCarty D J (ed.) Arthritis and allied conditions, 10th ed. Lea and Febiger

Miyashita K, Shiomi S, Itoh N, Kasamatsu T, Iwata H 1982 Development of the vibration syndrome among chain sawers in relation to their total operating time. In: Brammer A J, Taylor W (eds) Vibration effects on the hand and arm in industry. John Wiley, New York, pp 269–276

Olsen N 1988 Diagnostic tests in Raynaud's phenomenon in workers exposed to vibration: A comparative study. British Journal of Independent Medicine 45: 426–430

Pyykko I, Farkkila M, Korhonen O, Starck J, Jantte V 1986 Cold provocation tests in the evaluation of vibration induced white finger. Scandinavian Journal of Work and Environmental Health 12: 254–259

Saito K 1987 Prevention of the hand-arm vibration syndrome. Scandinavian Journal of Work and Environmental Health 13: 301–304

Takeuchi T, Futatsuka M, Imanishi H, Yomada S 1986 Pathological changes observed in the finger biopsy of patients with vibration induced white finger. Scandinavian Journal of Work and Environmental Health 12: 280–283

Taylor W 1985 Vibration white finger: A newly prescribed disease. British Medical Journal 291: 921–922

Vayssaorat M, Patri B, Mathieu J F 1987 Raynaud's phenomenon in chain saw users. Hot and cold finger systolic pressures and nailfold capillary findings. European Heart Journal 8: 417–422

Wasserman D E 1989 To weight or not to weight...that is the question. Journal of Occupational Medicine 31: 909

Wollersheim H, Reyenga J, Thein T H 1989 Post occlusive reactive hyperaemia of fingertips monitored by laser Doppler velocimetry in the diagnosis of Raynaud's phenomenon. Microvascular Research 38: 286–295

Yodaiken R E, Jones E, Kunicki R 1985 The Raynaud phenomenon of occupational origin. In: Davis E (ed.) Advances in microcirculation, vol 12. Karger, Basel, pp 6–33

Medicolegal aspects of cauda equina syndrome

John Hutchinson and Jeff Livingstone

Introduction

The cauda equina (literally 'horse's tail') refers to motor and sensory nerves below the termination of the spinal cord and within the spinal canal. Damage to any part of this structure results in the cauda equina syndrome (CES). The most consistent presenting features are urological or rectal dysfunction in association with saddle anaesthesia due to compression of the sacral nerve roots. Other clinical features may include low back pain, sciatica and motor or sensory deficit in the lower limbs (Jennet 1956; Tanden & Sankaren 1967; Kennedy et al 1999; Shapiro 2000). The early recognition and emergency treatment of CES may be related to the degree of functional recovery.

Pathophysiology

The differential growth of the spinal cord and vertebral column is responsible for the formation of the cauda equina which consists of lumbar and sacral nerve roots. The spinal cord reaches to the level of the second lumbar vertebral body in most adults and is attached to the coccyx via a fibrous remnant, the filum terminale.

Injury to the cauda equina nerves results in:

- Urological dysfunction which presents as a spectrum of disorders including altered urethral sensation, loss of desire to void, poor stream, retention, micturition by straining and incontinence (Neilsen et al 1980; O'Flynn et al 1992).
- Autonomic bowel dysfunction with perirectal numbness and loss of rectal and anal sphincter control.
- Motor weakness in the lower limbs.
- Sensory loss in the lower limbs classically with saddle (S4) and perineal (S5) sensory loss.
- Sexual dysfunction due to sensory loss. Erection is generated by a reflex arc via pudendal nerves (afferent) and the pelvic splanchnic nerves (efferent). Ejaculation is mediated via L1 and is often spared.

The majority of authors believe that CES is defined by the onset of rectal or bladder dysfunction (Ahn et al 2000).

Aetiology

Cauda equina syndrome accounts for 1 to 5% of spinal pathology (Kennedy et al 1999). Lumbar intervertebral disc prolapse is the most common cause, representing between 1 and 2.5% of surgeries for disc protrusion in some centres (Jennet 1956; Kostuik et al 1986; Kennedy et al 1999; Ahn 2000; Shapiro 2000). The disc spaces most often involved differ; however, the L4-5 and L5-S1 were involved in 90% of series—although a higher incidence of herniation in proximal levels was noted in a recent meta-analysis (Ahn et al). Most cases involve massive or central disc prolapse but posterolateral and smaller herniations with associated spondylosis are also described on MR imaging (Tandon et al 1967; Kennedy et al 1999). Myelograms reveal complete block in over 60% (Kostuik et al 1986).

Acute trauma as a cause of CES is rare and is described following spinal fractures and ballistic injuries (Benzel et al 1987; Gertzbein et al 1988). However, the role of trauma in CES due to lumbar disc herniation is less well defined. A precipitating trauma was associated with 62% of cases in a meta-analysis of 322 cases (Ahn et al 2000). Kostuik identified traumatic events in four of 10 patients with acute onset CES. The role of trauma was less well defined in 21 patients with a more insidious onset. Two patients had undergone chiropractic manipulation. Haldeman & Rubinstein (1992) reviewed the medical literature from 1911 to 1989 and found ten reported cases of CES in patients undergoing manipulation without anaesthesia and 16 cases with manipulation under anaesthesia. They described a further three cases of their own. Their conclusions were that CES following manipulation is extremely rare and that a cause/effect relationship was assumed when there was a temporal relationship between manipulation and symptoms. The cases they described emphasised a lack of appreciation of CES by both the chiropractor and at initial medical contact, leading to a delay in diagnosis.

Metastatic invasion, primary tumours, discitis, iatrogenic injury, epidural haematoma and epidural abscess may also cause cauda equina compression (Fearnside & Adams 1978; Chow et al 1996; Faraj et al 1996; Rittmeister et al 1999).

CES secondary to lumbar disc herniation

Mode of presentation

Men in the fourth to fifth decade of life tend to be the most prone to disc herniation and subsequent CES (Shapiro

2000). The syndrome presents with a sudden onset of symptoms in 69% of patients with a history of associated back pain of greater than 3 years in up to 80% (Ahn et al 2000). Kostuik (1986), in a series of 31 patients, reported 10 patients with acute onset and 21 with a more gradual onset over a few days to several weeks.

Tandon & Sankaren (1997) divided patients into three presenting groups:

1. sudden onset of CES with no history of backache
2. acute onset of bladder dysfunction following a long history of backache
3. gradual onset of CES from a background of chronic low backache and sciatica

Shapiro (2000) analysed the presentation of 44 cases in which 32% were type 1 with no history of back pain, 20% type 2 and 48% type 3. Kennedy et al (1999) found the incidence of type 1 presentation much rarer (only one in 19 cases).

Clinical features

Urological dysfunction was present in all patients but symptoms range from post-micturition residual volume to painful retention of urine. Loss of bladder control necessitating catheterisation was more frequent with acute onset of CES and was required in 63% (Kennedy et al 1999). Patients with a gradual onset may use manual compression on the abdomen or breath holding to assist bladder emptying. Reduced anal tone and absent perianal wink was recorded in 78% of the Kennedy et al series.

Saddle hypoaesthesia was present in 100% patients in two series and considered pathognomonic for CES by these authors (Kennedy et al and Shapiro). Complete perineal sensory loss is less frequent (seven of 19 patients) but is associated with a poor outcome following decompression Kennedy et al 1999).

Sciatica was present in over 95% of cases and is bilateral in between 45 to 90%, often with one leg affected more severely than the other. Long-standing unilateral sciatica frequently progresses to bilateral symptoms just prior to development of CES. Kostuik (1986) reported that all patients had decreased straight leg raise (mean 30° and all had a positive Lasègue sign).

Peripheral motor weakness is described in most patients (over 95%) involving the foot (EHL in 11 of 19 patients described by Kennedy et al), with up to 80% unable to stand or ambulate because of pain or weakness. Lesions at the lumbosacral junction may not cause motor or reflex changes and a diagnosis of CES may be missed unless sensation in the saddle area is examined. Ankle jerks were reduced or absent in 60% and knee jerks in only 40%.

Timing of surgery

As the incidence of CES in lumbar disc disease is small there are few series of adequate size that are powerful enough to investigate the relationship between delay to surgical decompression and prognosis for recovery.

Three retrospective studies published have documented that early decompression is associated with a better outcome. Kennedy et al (1999) reviewed 19 patients and found the mean time to decompression in 14 patients who did well was 14 hours (6–24 hours) compared to 30 hours (20–72) in those who fared poorly. Shapiro (2000) reviewed 44 patients of whom 20 were decompressed within 48 hours (17 underwent surgery within 12 hours). The remaining 24 patients had a mean delay of 9 days. There was a significant chance of persistent bladder/sphincter problems, motor deficit, persistent pain and sexual dysfunction in those treated after 48 hours. The meta-analysis of 322 cases by Ahn (2000) confirmed that there are significant advantages in treating patients within 48 hours of the onset of symptoms in terms of motor, sensory and urinary/rectal function.

Kostuik advocated surgery within 48 hours but stated that the timing of surgery was less important than the severity of the initial problem (Kostuik et al 1986). Those with gradual deterioration and early urological dysfunction without retention or incontinence may fare better if treated before they develop complete CES.

Prognosis for recovery

The most important prognostic factor for recovery in CES is believed to be decompression within 48 hours of the onset of symptoms. Complete perianal hypoaesthesia, and significant bladder and/or rectal sphincter dysfunction preoperatively, also correlate with a poor recovery.

Patients' satisfaction with bladder function does not equate with recovery as there may be a significant residual volume (Scott 1965).

In patients treated early bladder control may return within days with 95% recovering continence and normal bladder function at 6 months. Normal anal tone recovers within 2 months. Motor function recovers to 4/5 power in the early postoperative period with near full recovery by 6 months to 1 year. Recovery of saddle and perineal sensation recovers within a few weeks. Most males and females are able to return to sexual activity but may notice reduced strength of erection and difficulty in achieving orgasm due to residual sensory impairment. In Kostuik et al's 1986 series 23% of men undergoing surgery within 48 hours remained impotent.

In those decompressed after 48 hours 63% were still using intermittent catheterisation at 1 year. Persistent motor deficits can be expected in over 50% at 1 year. Both sexes have significant impairment of sexual function with males unable to achieve erection, and in females the fear of urinary incontinence during intercourse causes additional emotional distress.

Ahn (2000) compared pre-operative variables and postoperative outcomes using logistic regression analysis and odds ratios; however, the variables assessed were not recorded in all the series reviewed. Patients who underwent surgery after 48 hours were at 2.5 times the risk of continuing urinary deficit, 9.1 times at risk of a continuing motor deficit and rectal dysfunction and 3.5 times the risk of continuing to have a sensory deficit.

Summary

Cauda equina syndrome results from compression of peripheral nerve roots distal to the conus medullaris within the spinal canal.

CES is rare and occurs in 2% of patients undergoing lumbar disc surgery and a high index of suspicion is required for its diagnosis.

In 70% patients there is a history of chronic back pain with or without sciatica and the syndrome develops acutely within 24 hours in over 50%.

Most authors agree that CES is heralded by the development of urinary or rectal dysfunction but not necessarily acute retention.

Decompression within 48 hours probably results in a significantly better recovery than surgery after 48 hours.

References

Ahn M U, Ahn N U, Buchowski J M, Garret E S, Sieber A N, Kostuik J P 2000 Cauda equina syndrome secondary to lumbar disc herniation. A meta-analysis of surgical outcomes. Spine 12: 1515–1522

Benzel E C, Hadden T A, Coleman J C 1987 Civilian gunshot wound to the spinal cord and cauda equina. Neurosurgery 20: 281–285

Chow G H, Gebhard J S, Brown C W 1996 Multifocal metachronous epidural abscess of the spine. A case report. Spine 21:9; 1094–1097

Faraj A, Krishna M, Mehdian S M 1996 Cauda equina syndrome secondary to lumbar spondylodiscitis caused by streptococcus milleri. European Spine Journal 5:2: 134–136

Fearnside M R, Adams C B 1978 Tumours of the cauda equina. Journal of Neurology, Neurosurgery and Psychiatry 41: 24–31

Gertzbein S D, Court Brown C M, Marks P 1988 The neurological outcome following surgery for spinal fractures. Spine 13: 641–644

Haldeman S, Rubinstain S M 1992 Cauda equina syndrome in patients undergoing manipulation of the lumbar spine. Spine 17: 1469–1473

Jennet W 1956 A study of 25 cases of compression of the cauda equina by prolapsed intervertebral discs. Journal of Neurology, Neurosurgery and Psychiatry 19: 109–116

Kennedy J G, Soffe K E, McGrath A, Stephens M M, Walsh M G, McManus F 1999 Predictors of outcome in cauda equina syndrome. European Spine Journal 8: 317–322

Kostuik J P, Harrington I, Alexander D, Rand W, Evans D 1986 Cauda equina syndrome and lumbar disc herniation. Journal of Bone and Joint Surgery 68A: 386–391

Nielsen B, McNully M, Schmidt K et al 1980 A urodynamic study of cauda equina syndrome due to lumbar disc herniation. Urology International 35: 167–170

O'Flynn K J, Murphy R, Thomas D G 1992 Neurogenic bladder dysfunction in lumbar intervertebral disc prolapse. British Journal of Urology 69: 38–40

Rittmeister M, Leyendecker K, Kurth A, Schmitt E 1999 Cauda equina compression due to a laminar hook. European Spine Journal 8:5: 417–420

Scott P J 1965 Bladder paralysis in cauda equina lesions from disc prolapse. Journal of Bone and Joint Surgery 47B: 224–235

Shapiro S 2000 Medical realities of cauda equina syndrome secondary to lumbar disc herniation. Spine 25: 348–352

Tandon P N, Sankaren B 1967 Cauda equina syndrome due to lumbar disc prolapse. Indian Journal of Orthopaedics 1: 112–116

Index

Page references in **bold type** refer to figures or tables